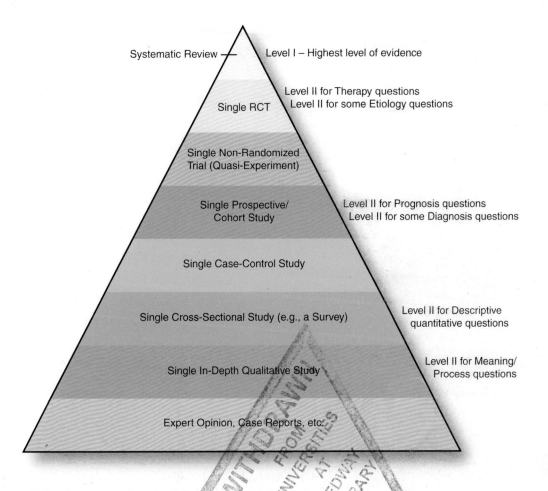

**FIGURE 2.1** ● Evidence hierarchy: levels of evidence.

# Essentials of Nursing Research
## Appraising Evidence for Nursing Practice

● Denise F. Polit, PhD, FAAN
President, Humanalysis, Inc.
Saratoga Springs, New York
Professor, Griffith University School of Nursing
Brisbane, Australia
www.denisepolit.com

● Cheryl Tatano Beck, DNSc, CNM, FAAN
Distinguished Professor, School of Nursing, University of Connecticut
Storrs, Connecticut

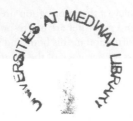

edition 8

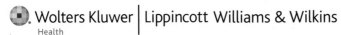

Wolters Kluwer | Lippincott Williams & Wilkins
Health

Philadelphia · Baltimore · New York · London
Buenos Aires · Hong Kong · Sydney · Tokyo

*Acquisitions Editor:* Christina C. Burns
*Product Manager:* Helen Kogut
*Editorial Assistant:* Dan Reilly
*Design Coordinator:* Joan Wendt
*Illustration Coordinator:* Brett MacNaughton
*Manufacturing Coordinator:* Karin Duffield
*Prepress Vendor:* SPi Global

4th edition

Printed in China

**Not authorised for sale in the United States, Canada, Australia, New Zealand, Puerto Rico, or the U.S. Virgin Islands.**

**Library of Congress Cataloging-in-Publication Data**
Polit, Denise F.
Essentials of nursing research : appraising evidence for nursing practice / Denise Polit, Cheryl Tatano Beck. — 8th ed.
   p. ; cm.
  Includes bibliographical references and index.
  ISBN 978-1-4511-7679-7
 I. Beck, Cheryl Tatano. II. Title.
  [DNLM: 1. Nursing Research. 2. Evidence-Based Nursing. WY 20.5]
  610.73072—dc23

2012023962

*To*

**Our Families—Husbands, Children, Grandchildren**

*Husbands:* Alan and Chuck
*Children:* Alex, Alaine, Lauren, Norah and Curt, Lisa
*Grandchildren:* Julia and Maren

# REVIEWERS

Susan E. Bernheiel, EdD, MSN, CNE
Professor of Nursing
Mercy College of Northwest Ohio
Toledo, Ohio

Elizabeth W. Black, MSN, RN
Assistant Professor, Nursing
Gwynedd-Mercy College
Gwynedd Valley, Pennsylvania

Diane M. Breckenridge, PhD, MSN, RN
Associate Professor
School of Nursing
La Salle University
Philadelphia, Pennsylvania

Colleen Carmody-Payne, EdD, MS, RN
Assistant Professor
Center for Professional and International Studies
Keuka College
Penn Yan, New York

Barbara Cheyney, MS, BSN, RN-BC
Adjunct Faculty
Seattle Pacific University
Seattle, Washington

Christine Coughlin, EdD, RN
Associate Professor
School of Nursing
Adelphi University
Garden City, New York

Darlene Del Prato, PhD, RN
Assistant Professor
State University of New York Institute
    of Technology
Utica, New York

Cheryl Hettman, PhD, RN
Chairperson and Associate Professor
California University of Pennsylvania
California, Pennsylvania

Patrick E. Kenny, EdD, RN-BC, ACRN, APRN-
    PMH, NE-BC
Assistant Professor of Nursing
DeSales University
Center Valley, Pennsylvania

Kereen Forster Mullenbach, PhD, MBA,
    MSN, RN
Assistant Professor
Radford University
Radford, Virginia

Judee E. Onyskiw, PhD, MN, BScN, RN
Faculty, and Research and Scholarship Advisor
Grant MacEwan University
Edmonton, Alberta

Sabita Persaud, PhD, RN
Assistant Professor
Bowie State University
Bowie, Maryland

Rosemarie DiMauro Satyshur, PhD, RN
Assistant Professor
School of Nursing
University of Maryland
Baltimore, Maryland

Linda J. Scheetz, EdD, RN, FAEN
Associate Professor
Department of Nursing
SUNY New Paltz
New Paltz, New York

Denise Schilling, PT, PhD
Associate Professor/Chair
Department of Physical Therapy Education
Western University of Health Sciences
Pomona, California

# USER'S GUIDE

Learning Objectives focus student's attention on critical content

## LEARNING OBJECTIVES

**On completing this chapter, you will be able to:**

- Discuss the rationale for an emergent design in qualitative research, and describe qualitative design features
- Identify the major research traditions for qualitative research and describe the domain of inquiry of each
- Describe the main features of ethnographic, phenomenologic, and grounded theory studies
- Discuss the goals and methods of various types of research with an ideological perspective
- Define new terms in the chapter

Key New Terms alert students to important terminology

## KEY TERMS

| | | |
|---|---|---|
| Basic social process (BSP) | Critical theory | Hermeneutics |
| Bracketing | Descriptive phenomenology | Interpretive phenomenology |
| Case study | Descriptive qualitative study | Narrative analysis |
| Constant comparison | Emergent design | Participant observation |
| Core variable | Ethnonursing research | Participatory action research |
| Critical ethnography | Feminist research | (PAR) |

**Example of qualitative comparisons:**

Baum and colleagues (2012) explored the experiences of 30 Israeli mothers of very-low-birth-weight babies when the babies were still in neonatal hospitalization. The researchers discovered that there were three patterns with regard to attribution of blame for not carrying to full term: those who blamed themselves, those who blamed others, and those who believed that premature delivery was fortunate because it saved their baby's life.

Examples help students apply content to real-life research

Tip boxes describe what is found in actual research articles

☞ **TIP:** Experimental designs can be depicted graphically using symbols to represent features of the design. In these diagrams, the convention is that R stands for randomization to treatment groups, X represents receipt of the intervention, and O is the measurement of outcomes. So, for example, a pretest–posttest design would be depicted as follows:

$$R\ O_1\ X\ O_2$$
$$R\ O_1\ O_2$$

☀-Space does not permit us to present these diagrams for all designs, but many are shown in the supplement to this chapter on thePoint₩.

How-to-tell Tip boxes explain confusing issues in actual research articles

☞ **HOW-TO-TELL TIP:** How can you tell if a phenomenological study is descriptive or interpretive? Phenomenologists often use terms that can help you make this determination. In a descriptive phenomenological study such terms may be bracketing, description, essence, and Husserl. The names of Colaizzi, Van Kaam, or Giorgi may appear in the methods section. In an interpretive phenomenological study, key terms can include being-in-the-world, hermeneutics, understanding, and Heidegger. The names van Manen, Benner, or Diekelmann may appear in the method section. These names are discussed in Chapter 16 on qualitative data analysis.

**Critiquing Guidelines** boxes lead students through key issues in a research article

## RESEARCH EXAMPLES WITH CRITICAL THINKING EXERCISES

**Research Examples** highlight critical points made in the chapter and sharpen critical thinking skills

This section presents examples of different types of qualitative studies. Read these summaries and then answer the critical thinking questions, referring to the full research report if necessary.

### EXAMPLE 1 ● A Grounded Theory Study

**Study:** Preserving the self: The process of decision-making about hereditary breast cancer and ovarian cancer risk reduction (Howard et al., 2011).

**Statement of Purpose:** The purpose of the study was to understand how women make decisions about strategies to reduce the risk of hereditary breast and ovarian cancer (HBOC), such as cancer screening and risk-reducing surgeries.

### CRITICAL THINKING EXERCISES

Visit thePoint website for a discussion of all questions. ☀

1. Answer the relevant questions from Box 14.1 on page 00 regarding this study.
2. Also consider the following targeted questions:
   a. Was this study cross-sectional or longitudinal?
   b. Could this study have been undertaken as an ethnography? A phenomenological inquiry?
3. If the results of this study are trustworthy, in what ways do you think the findings could be used in clinical practice?

**Critical Thinking Exercises** provide opportunities to practice critiquing actual research articles

**Summary Points** review chapter content to ensure success

## SUMMARY POINTS

- Qualitative research involves an **emergent design**—a design that emerges in the field as the study unfolds.
- Although qualitative design is elastic and flexible, qualitative researchers plan for broad contingencies that can pose decision opportunities for study design in the field.
- Ethnography focuses on the culture of a group of people and relies on extensive field work that usually includes **participant observation** and in-depth interviews with **key informants**. Ethnographers strive to acquire an **emic** (insider's) perspective of a culture rather than an **etic** (outsider's) perspective.
- Nurses sometimes refer to their ethnographic studies as **ethnonursing research**. Most ethnographers study cultures other than their own; *autoethnographies* are ethnographies of a group or culture to which the researcher belongs.
- Phenomenologists seek to discover the *essence* and *meaning* of a phenomenon as it is experienced by people, mainly through in-depth interviews with people who have had the relevant experience.
- In **descriptive phenomenology**, which seeks to describe lived experiences, researchers strive to **bracket** out preconceived views and to *intuit* the essence of the phenomenon by remaining open to meanings attributed to it by those who have experienced it.
- **Interpretive phenomenology (hermeneutics)** focuses on interpreting the meaning of experiences, rather than just describing them.
- **Grounded theory** researchers try to account for people's actions by focusing on the main concern that their behavior is designed to resolve. The manner in which people resolve this main concern is the **core variable**. The goal of grounded theory is to discover this main concern and the **basic social process (BSP)** that explains how people resolve it.
- Grounded theory uses **constant comparison**: categories elicited from the data are constantly compared with data obtained earlier.
- A controversy in grounded theory concerns whether to follow the original Glaser and Strauss procedures or to use procedures adapted by Strauss and Corbin; Glaser has argued that the latter approach does not result in *grounded theories* but rather in *conceptual descriptions*. More recently, Charmaz's **constructivist grounded theory** has emerged,

**Special icons** alert students to important content found on thePoint ☀ and in the accompanying Study Guide 📖

# NEW! INTERACTIVE CRITICAL THINKING ACTIVITY

This new interactive activity brings the content from the text to an easy-to-use tool that enables students to apply new skills that they learn in each chapter. Students are guided through appraisals of real research examples and then ushered through a series of questions that challenge them to think about the quality of evidence from the study. Responses can be printed or e-mailed directly to instructors for homework or testing.

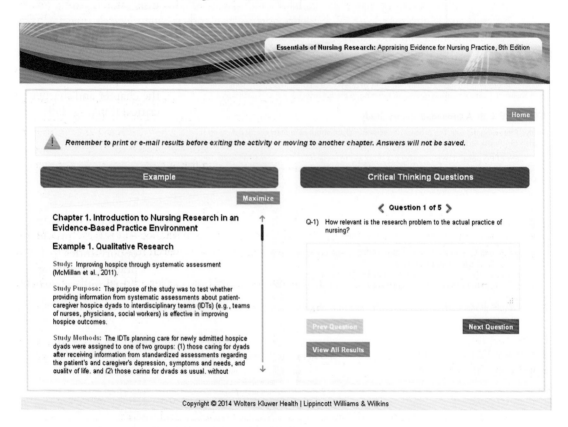

**Essentials of Nursing Research:** Appraising Evidence for Nursing Practice, 8th Edition

Home

⚠ *Remember to print or e-mail results before exiting the activity or moving to another chapter. Answers will not be saved.*

| Example | Critical Thinking Questions |
|---|---|

Maximize

❮ Question 1 of 5 ❯

**Chapter 1. Introduction to Nursing Research in an Evidence-Based Practice Environment**

**Example 1. Qualitative Research**

Study: Improving hospice through systematic assessment (McMillan et al., 2011).

Study Purpose: The purpose of the study was to test whether providing information from systematic assessments about patient-caregiver hospice dyads to interdisciplinary teams (IDTs) (e.g., teams of nurses, physicians, social workers) is effective in improving hospice outcomes.

Study Methods: The IDTs planning care for newly admitted hospice dyads were assigned to one of two groups: (1) those caring for dyads after receiving information from standardized assessments regarding the patient's and caregiver's depression, symptoms and needs, and quality of life, and (2) those caring for dyads as usual, without

Q-1)  How relevant is the research problem to the actual practice of nursing?

Prev Question   Next Question

View All Results

Copyright © 2014 Wolters Kluwer Health | Lippincott Williams & Wilkins

# PREFACE

This publication marks the eighth time we have worked on this textbook, its accompanying *Study Guide for Essentials of Nursing Research*, and student learning ancillaries and instructor teaching materials available on thePoint. This integrated learning–teaching package is designed to teach students how to read and critique research reports and to appreciate the application of research findings to nursing practice.

We continue to enjoy immensely our job of developing a suite of educational tools that convey the important innovations in research methodology while providing updates on nurse researchers' use of new methods.

We are confident that we have introduced numerous improvements to both the content and organization of the text—but at the same time, we have retained many features that have made this book a classic throughout the world. We think that this book and its student resources on thePoint, along with the additional activities provided in its accompanying print Study Guide, will make it easier and more satisfying for nurses to pursue a professional pathway that incorporates thoughtful appraisals of evidence.

## Legacy of *Essentials of Nursing Research*

This edition, like its predecessors, is focused on the art—and science—of research critiques. It offers guidance to students who are learning to appraise research reports and use research findings in practice.

Among the basic principles that helped to shape this and earlier editions of this book are:

1. An assumption that competence in doing and appraising research is critical to the nursing profession
2. A conviction that research inquiry is intellectually and professionally rewarding to nurses
3. An unswerving belief that learning about research methods need be neither intimidating nor dull

Consistent with these principles, we have tried to present research fundamentals in a way that both facilitates understanding and arouses curiosity and interest.

## New to This Edition

### New Organization of Qualitative and Quantitative Materials

In previous editions we made efforts to balance material on qualitative and quantitative research methods, to ensure that each would be given similar emphasis. This balance may have been obscured, however, by intermingling content on both approaches within chapters. In this edition, we blended material on qualitative and quantitative research only in early chapters—for example, in the chapters on evidence-based practice (EBP) and research ethics. Then, we devoted an entire section of the book (Part III) to quantitative research methods and another section (Part IV) to methods for qualitative inquiry. We think this new organization offers greater continuity of ideas and hope it will better meet the needs of students and faculty.

### Streamlining—and New Online Content

We have condensed and revised the content of the book to make it more manageable for use in a one-semester course. For this edition, we are offering online Chapter Supplements (e.g., details about the history of nursing research) on the**Point** website so that instructors can choose which supplementary material to assign to students. A list of all Chapter Supplements available online at the**Point** are included on page xviii.

### New Chapter on Mixed Methods Research

We have added a new chapter on mixed methods research, which involves the blending of qualitative and quantitative data in a single inquiry. This new chapter represents a formal recognition of the surge of interest in mixed methods research among nurse researchers in the past decade.

### Increased Emphasis on Evidence-Based Practice

To an even greater extent than in the past, in this edition we emphasize that research is a crucial enterprise for building an evidence base for nursing practice. In particular, we have devoted more attention in this edition to the issue of asking well-worded questions for EBP and to searching for such evidence.

### New Interactive Critical Thinking Activity

This new interactive activity brings the content from the text to an easy-to-use tool that enables students to apply new skills that they learn in each chapter. Students are guided through appraisals of real research examples and then ushered through a series of questions that challenge them to think about the quality of evidence from the study. Responses can be printed or e-mailed directly to instructors for homework or testing.

### Enhanced Assistance for Instructors

One of the biggest improvements in this edition is the assistance we provide for teaching research methods to students—many of whom may be anxious about the course content and may also question its relevance to their nursing practice. We offer numerous suggestions in the Instructor's Manual on the**Point** website on how to make learning about—and teaching—research methods more rewarding.

## Organization of the Text

The content of this edition is organized into five main parts.

- **Part I—Overview of Nursing Research and Evidence-Based Practice** introduces fundamental concepts in nursing research. Chapter 1 summarizes the background of nursing research, discusses the philosophical underpinnings of qualitative research versus quantitative research, and describes major purposes of nursing research. Chapter 2 offers guidance on using research to build an evidence-based practice. Chapter 3 introduces readers to key research terms, and presents an overview of steps in the research process for both qualitative and quantitative studies. Chapter 4 focuses on research journal articles, explaining what they are and how to read them. Chapter 5 discusses ethics in nursing studies.
- **Part II—Preliminary Research Steps** further sets the stage for learning about the research process by considering aspects of a study's conceptualization. Chapter 6 focuses on the development of research questions and the formulation of research hypotheses. Chapter 7 discusses how to retrieve research evidence and the role of research literature reviews. Chapter 8 presents information about theoretical and conceptual frameworks.
- **Part III—Quantitative Research** presents material on the design and conduct of quantitative nursing studies. Chapter 9 describes fundamental design principles and discusses many specific aspects of quantitative research design. Chapter 10 introduces the topics of sampling and data collection in quantitative studies. Chapter 11 describes the concept of *measurement* and criteria for assessing data quality in quantitative studies. Chapter 12 reviews methods of quantitative analysis. The chapter assumes no prior instruction in statistics and focuses primarily on helping readers to understand why

statistics are needed, what tests might be appropriate in a given situation, and what statistical information in a research article means. Chapter 13 discusses ways of appraising rigor in quantitative studies, and approaches to interpreting statistical results.

- **Part IV—Qualitative Research** presents content relating to the design and conduct of qualitative nursing studies. Chapter 14 addresses the various research traditions that have contributed to the growth of constructivist inquiry and qualitative research. Chapter 15 describes sampling and data collection in qualitative research, and how these differ from approaches used in quantitative studies. Chapter 16 discusses qualitative analysis, with an emphasis on ethnographic, phenomenologic, and grounded theory studies. Chapter 17 elaborates on criteria for appraising trustworthiness and integrity in qualitative studies.

- **Part V—Special Topics in Research** discusses topics that are of increasing importance in research. The emphasis of Chapter 18 is on mixed methods research, but the chapter also discusses other special types of research such as surveys and outcomes research. Finally, Chapter 19 describes systematic reviews, including how to understand and appraise both meta-analyses and metasyntheses.

## Integrated Learning Solution: *Our Text, Study Guide, and Student and Faculty Resources on* thePoint⁎

### Key Features of the Text

We have retained many of the key features that were successfully used in previous editions to assist consumers of nursing research:

- **Clear, "User-Friendly" Style**. Our writing style is designed to be easily digestible and nonintimidating. Concepts are introduced carefully and systematically, difficult ideas are presented clearly, and readers are assumed to have no prior knowledge of technical terms.

- ⁎ **Critiquing Guidelines**. Each chapter includes guidelines for conducting a critique of various aspects of a research article. The guidelines provide a list of questions that walk students through a study, drawing attention to aspects of the study that are amenable to appraisal by research consumers. *Electronic versions of the guidelines are available on* thePoint⁎.

- **Research Examples**. Each chapter concludes with summaries of one or two actual research examples designed to highlight critical points made in the chapter. In addition, these research examples are used to stimulate students' thinking about interesting areas of research inquiry. We have chosen many international examples to communicate to students that nursing research is growing in importance worldwide.

- ⁎ **Critical Thinking Exercises**. Each of the Research Examples is followed by critical thinking exercises designed to help hone the student's skill in critiquing key aspects of research articles. Additional Critical Thinking Exercises in each chapter pertain to the full-length research articles in Appendices A and B of the book.

- **Tips for Consumers**. The textbook is filled with practical guidance and "tips" on how to translate the abstract notions of research methods into more concrete applications. In these tips, we have paid special attention to helping students *read* research reports, which are often daunting to those without specialized research training.

- **Graphics**. Colorful graphics, in the form of supportive tables, figures, and examples, reinforce the text and offer visual stimulation.

- **Chapter Objectives**. Learning objectives are identified in the chapter opener to focus students' attention on critical content.

- **Key Terms**. Each chapter includes a list of new terms, and we have made the list less daunting by including only *key* new terms. New terms are defined in context (and bolded) when used for the first time in the text. A *glossary* at the end of the book provides additional support for those needing to look up the meaning of a methodologic term.

- **Bulleted Summary Points**. A succinct list of summary points that focus on salient chapter content is provided at the end of each chapter.
- **Full-Length Research Articles**. The appendices in the textbook include **four full-length studies**—two quantitative, one qualitative, and one mixed methods—that students can read, analyze, and critique.
- ☀ **Critiquing Supports**.
  - Some of the **Critical Thinking Exercises** at the end of each chapter focus on the full-length articles in Appendix A (a quantitative study) and Appendix B (a qualitative study). *Students can get immediate feedback about their grasp of the material by visiting the* **Point** *to find our "answers" (our expert thoughts about each question in these exercises)*.
  - This edition also includes **full critiques of the two full-length studies** in Appendix C (a quantitative study) and Appendix D (a mixed methods study). Students can use our critiques as models for a comprehensive research critique.

## Key Features of the Study Guide

 *Study Guide for Essentials of Nursing Research, 8e* augments the text and provides students with **application exercises** for each text chapter.

- **Critiquing opportunities** abound in the *Study Guide,* which includes **eight research articles in their entirety**. The studies represent a range of nursing topics and types of study, including:
  - A randomized controlled trial
  - A correlational/mixed methods study
  - An evaluation of an evidence-based practice project
  - A grounded theory study
  - A phenomenologic study
  - An ethnography
  - A meta-analysis
  - A metasynthesis (meta-ethnography)
- The **Application Exercises** in each chapter are based on these eight studies and guide students in reading, understanding, and critiquing them.
- Answers to the set of "Questions of Fact" in each chapter are presented in Appendix I of the *Study Guide,* so that students can receive immediate feedback about their responses.
- **Although critiquing skills are emphasized in the Study Guide**, other activities support students in learning fundamental research terms and principles including:
  - Fill-in-the-blank exercises
  - Matching exercises
  - Study questions
- Answers to questions for which there is an objective answer are provided in Appendix I.

☀ *Student Resources Available on* the**Point**

- **Interactive Critical Thinking Activity** brings the Critical Thinking Exercises from the textbook (except those pertaining to the studies in Appendices A and B) to an interactive tool. The new format makes it easy for students to respond to the series of targeted questions about the Research Examples. Responses can be printed or e-mailed directly to instructors for homework or testing.
- **19 Full Journal Articles** (one corresponding to each chapter) are provided for additional critiquing opportunities. Several of these are the full journal articles for studies used as the end-of-chapter Research Examples. All journal articles that appear on the**Point** website are identified in the text with ☀.

- **Hundreds of Student Review Questions** to assist students in self-testing. This review program provides a rationale for both correct and incorrect answers, helping students to identify areas of strength and areas needing further study.
- **Internet Resources with relevant and useful websites** related to chapter content can be "clicked" on directly without having to retype the URL and risk a typographical error.
- **Chapter Supplements** to further students' exploration of specific topics. A full list of the Supplements appears on page xviii.
- **Critiquing Guidelines** from the text are available in MSWord for your convenience.
- **Answers to the Critical Thinking Exercises** for Appendixes A and B of the textbook offer suggestions for possible responses.
- **An e-book available at no additional cost with the purchase of your text!**

### *The Instructor's Resources Available on* the**Point**

- **Instructor's Manual** includes a chapter corresponding to every chapter in the textbook and contains the following:
  - **Statement of Intent.** Discover the authors' goal for each chapter.
  - **Special Class Projects.** Find numerous ideas for interesting and meaningful class projects. Check out the Icebreakers and activities relating to the Great Cookie Experiment with accompanying SPSS data files.
  - **Test Questions and Answers.** Application questions, short answer questions, and essay questions are specifically designed to test students' ability to comprehend research reports.
  - **Answers to the Interactive Critical Thinking Activity.** Suggested answers to the questions in the new Interactive Critical Thinking Activity are available to instructors. Students can either print or e-mail their responses directly to the instructor for testing or as a homework assignment.
  - **Self-Test PowerPoint Slides.** For each chapter, a series of 5 "test questions" relating to key concepts in the chapter are followed immediately by answers to the questions. The aim of these slides is not to evaluate student performance, but to offer an opportunity for students to obtain quick feedback about whether they have grasped important concepts. All the questions are "application" type questions, to enhance the likelihood that students will see the relevance of the concepts to clinical practice. We hope instructors will use the slides to clarify any misunderstandings and, importantly, to reward students with immediate positive feedback about newly acquired skills.
- **PowerPoint Presentations** offer the traditional summaries of key points in each chapter for use in class presentations. These slides are available in a format that permits easy adaptation and also include audience response questions that can be used on their own or are compatible with i-clicker and other audience response programs and devices.
- **Test Generator Questions** offer hundreds of multiple choice questions to aid instructors in assessing their students' understanding of the chapter content.
- **Image Bank** includes figures from the text and Chapter Supplements that you can include in your own class presentations.
- **Chapter Supplements** include additional information that instructors can use to further their students' understanding and knowledge of a specific topic.

It is our hope and expectation that the content, style, and organization of this eighth edition of *Essentials of Nursing Research* will be helpful to those students desiring to become skillful and thoughtful readers of nursing studies and to those wishing to enhance their clinical performance based on research findings. We also hope that all of the resources that we offer will help to develop an enthusiasm for the kinds of discoveries and knowledge that research can produce.

# ACKNOWLEDGMENTS

Denise F. Polit, PhD, FAAN

Cheryl Tatano Beck, DNSc, CNM, FAAN

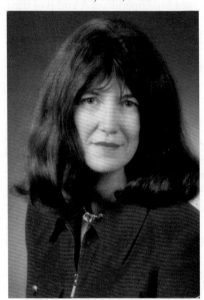

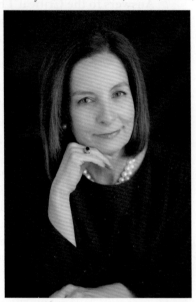

This eighth edition, like the previous seven editions, depended on the contribution of many generous people. Many faculty and students who used the text have made invaluable suggestions for its improvement, and to all of you we are very grateful. Suggestions were made to us both directly in personal interactions (mostly at the University of Connecticut and Griffith University in Australia) and via e-mail correspondence. In addition to all those who assisted us during the past three decades with the earlier editions, there are some who deserve special mention for this new work.

We would like to acknowledge the comments of the reviewers of the seventh edition of *Essentials*, whose anonymous feedback influenced our revisions. Several of the comments triggered several important changes, including the reorganization of the content, and for this we are indebted.

Other individuals made specific contributions. Although it would be impossible to mention all, we note with thanks the nurse researchers who shared their work with us as we developed examples, including work that in some cases was not yet published. We also extend our warm thanks to those who helped to turn the manuscript into a finished product. The staff at Lippincott Williams & Wilkins has been of tremendous assistance in the support they have given us over the years. We are indebted to Christina Burns and Helen Kogut and all the others behind the scenes for their fine contributions.

Finally, we thank our family, our loved ones, and our friends, who provided ongoing support and encouragement throughout this endeavor and who were tolerant when we worked long into the night, over weekends, and during holidays to get this eighth edition finished.

# CONTENTS

**Part 1  Overview of Nursing Research and Its Role in Evidence-Based Practice  1**

    **1**  Introduction to Nursing Research in an Evidence-Based Practice Environment  1

    **2**  Fundamentals of Evidence-Based Nursing Practice  20

    **3**  Key Concepts and Steps in Qualitative and Quantitative Research  40

    **4**  Reading and Critiquing Research Articles  61

    **5**  Ethics in Research  80

**Part 2  Preliminary Steps in Research  99**

    **6**  Research Problems, Research Questions, and Hypotheses  99

    **7**  Finding and Reviewing Research Evidence in the Literature  116

    **8**  Theoretical and Conceptual Frameworks  132

**Part 3  Quantitative Research  149**

    **9**  Quantitative Research Design  149

    **10** Sampling and Data Collection in Quantitative Studies  176

    **11** Measurement and Data Quality  199

    **12** Statistical Analysis of Quantitative Data  214

    **13** Rigor and Interpretation in Quantitative Research  249

**Part 4  Qualitative Research  265**

    **14** Qualitative Designs and Approaches  265

    **15** Sampling and Data Collection in Qualitative Studies  283

    **16** Analysis of Qualitative Data  300

    **17** Trustworthiness and Integrity in Qualitative Research  321

**Part 5  Special Topics in Research  339**

    **18** Mixed Methods and Other Special Types of Research  339

    **19** Systematic Reviews: Meta-Analysis and Metasynthesis  355

**Glossary**  374

**Appendix A**  Howell and Colleagues' (2007) Study: *The Relationship Among Anxiety, Anger, and Blood Pressure in Children*  395

**Appendix B**  Beck and Watson's (2010) Study: *Subsequent Childbirth After a Previous Traumatic Birth*  403

**Appendix C**  McGillion et al.'s (2008) Study: *Randomized Controlled Trial of a Psychoeducation Program for the Self-Management of Chronic Cardiac Pain*  413

**Critique of McGillion and Colleagues' Study**  429

**Appendix D**  Sawyer et al.'s (2010) Study: *Differences in Perceptions of the Diagnosis and Treatment of Obstructive Sleep Apnea and Continuous Positive Airway Pressure Therapy Among Adherers and Nonadherers*  441

**Critique of Sawyer and Colleagues' Study**  467

**Index**  475

## CHAPTER SUPPLEMENTS AVAILABLE ON thePoint

**Supplement for Chapter 1**  The History of Nursing Research
**Supplement for Chapter 2**  Assessing Implementation Potential for EBP Projects
**Supplement for Chapter 3**  Deductive and Inductive Reasoning
**Supplement for Chapter 4**  Guide to an Overall Critique of a Quantitative Research Report and Guide to an Overall Critique of a Qualitative Research Report
**Supplement for Chapter 5**  Elements of Informed Consent
**Supplement for Chapter 6**  Simple and Complex Hypotheses
**Supplement for Chapter 7**  Finding Evidence for an EBP Inquiry in PubMed
**Supplement for Chapter 8**  Prominent Conceptual Models of Nursing Used by Nurse Researchers
**Supplement for Chapter 9**  Selected Experimental and Quasi-Experimental Designs: Diagrams, Uses, and Drawbacks
**Supplement for Chapter 10**  Vignettes and Q Sorts
**Supplement for Chapter 11**  Level II Evidence for Diagnosis Questions
**Supplement for Chapter 12**  Multiple Regression and Analysis of Covariance
**Supplement for Chapter 13**  Research Biases
**Supplement for Chapter 14**  Qualitative Descriptive Studies
**Supplement for Chapter 15**  Transferability and Generalizability
**Supplement for Chapter 16**  A Glaserian Grounded Theory Study: Illustrative Materials
**Supplement for Chapter 17**  Whittemore and Colleagues' Framework of Quality Criteria in Qualitative Research
**Supplement for Chapter 18**  Practical (Pragmatic) Clinical Trials
**Supplement for Chapter 19**  Publication Bias in Meta-Analyses

# part 1

# Overview of Nursing Research and Its Role in Evidence-Based Practice

## chapter 1

## Introduction to Nursing Research in an Evidence-Based Practice Environment

### LEARNING OBJECTIVES

*On completing this chapter, you will be able to:*

- Describe why research is important in nursing and discuss the need for evidence-based practice
- Describe broad historical trends and future directions in nursing research
- Describe alternative sources of knowledge for nursing practice
- Describe major characteristics of the positivist and constructivist paradigms, and discuss similarities and differences between the traditional scientific method (quantitative research) and constructivist methods (qualitative research)
- Identify several purposes of qualitative and quantitative research
- Define new terms in the chapter

### KEY TERMS

| | | |
|---|---|---|
| Assumption | Evidence-based practice | Quantitative research |
| Cause-probing research | Generalizability | Research methods |
| Clinical nursing research | Paradigm | Scientific method |
| Constructivist paradigm | Positivist paradigm | Systematic review |
| Empirical evidence | Qualitative research | |

# NURSING RESEARCH IN PERSPECTIVE

We know that many of you readers are not taking this course because you plan to become nurse researchers. Yet, we are also confident that many of you *will* participate in research-related activities during your careers, and virtually all of you will be expected to be research-savvy at a basic level. Although you may not yet appreciate the relevance of research to a career in nursing, we hope that you will come to see the value of nursing research during this course, and will be inspired by the efforts of the thousands of nurse researchers now working worldwide to develop better methods of patient care. You are embarking on a lifelong journey in which research will play an increasingly important role. We hope to prepare you to enjoy the voyage.

## What Is Nursing Research?

You have already done a lot of research. When you use the Internet to find the "best deal" on a backpack you want, or on an airfare to visit a friend, you start with a question (Where can I get the best deal?), collect the information, and then come to a conclusion. This "everyday research" has much in common with formal research—but, of course, there are important differences, too.

As a formal enterprise, **research** is *systematic* inquiry that uses disciplined methods to answer questions and solve problems. The ultimate goal of formal research is to gain knowledge that would be useful for many people. **Nursing research** is systematic inquiry designed to develop trustworthy evidence about issues of importance to nurses and their clients. In this book, we emphasize **clinical nursing research**, that is, research designed to guide nursing practice. Clinical nursing research typically begins with questions stemming from practice problems—problems you may have already encountered.

**Example of nursing research questions:**
- Does a 6-month program of aerobic exercise result in improvements in executive function, global cognition, and quality of life in community-dwelling elders with mild or moderate Alzheimer's disease (Yu et al., 2012)?
- What are the experiences of people who suffer from facial lipoatrophy with regard to the reconstructive treatments they receive (Gagnon, 2012)?

**☞ TIP:** You may have the impression that research is abstract and irrelevant to practicing nurses. But nursing research is about *real* people with *real* problems, and studying those problems offers opportunities to solve or ameliorate them through improvements to nursing care.

## The Importance of Research to Evidence-Based Nursing

Nursing has experienced profound changes in the past few decades. Nurses are increasingly expected to understand and undertake research, and to base their practice on evidence from research—that is, to adopt an **evidence-based practice (EBP)**. EBP, broadly defined, is the use of the best evidence in making patient care decisions, and such evidence typically comes from research conducted by nurses and other health care professionals. Nurse leaders recognize the need to base specific nursing decisions on evidence indicating that the decisions are clinically appropriate, cost-effective, and result in positive client outcomes.

In the United States and elsewhere, research plays an important role in terms of nursing credentialing and status. The American Nurses Credentialing Center—an arm of the American Nurses Association—has developed a Magnet Recognition Program to recognize health care organizations that provide high-quality nursing care. To achieve Magnet status, practice environments must demonstrate a sustained commitment to EBP and nursing research. Changes to nursing practice are happening every day because of EBP efforts.

> **Example of evidence-based practice:**
> Many clinical practice changes reflect the impact of research. For example, "kangaroo care," the holding of diaper-clad preterm infants skin-to-skin, chest-to-chest by parents, is now widely practiced in neonatal intensive care units (NICUs), but in the early 1990s only a minority of NICUs offered kangaroo care options. The adoption of this practice reflects good evidence that early skin-to-skin contact has clinical benefits, and no negative side effects. Some of this evidence came from rigorous studies by nurse researchers (e.g., Cong et al., 2009, 2011; Ludington-Hoe et al., 2006).

## Roles of Nurses in Research

In the current EBP environment, every nurse is likely to engage in one or more activities along a continuum of research participation. At one end of the continuum are users (*consumers) of nursing research*—nurses who read research reports to keep up-to-date on findings that may affect their practice. EBP depends on well-informed nursing research consumers.

At the other end of the continuum are the *producers of nursing research*: nurses who actively design and undertake studies. At one time, most nurse researchers were academics who taught in schools of nursing, but research is increasingly being conducted by practicing nurses who want to find what works best for their clients.

Between these two end points on the continuum lie a variety of research activities in which nurses engage. Even if you never conduct a study, you may (1) help to develop an idea for a clinical study; (2) assist researchers by collecting research information; (3) offer advice to clients about participating in a study; (4) solve a clinical problem by searching for research evidence; or (5) discuss the implications of a new study in a **journal club** in your practice setting, which involves meetings to discuss research articles. In all the possible research-related activities, nurses who have some research skills are better able than those without them to make a contribution to nursing and to EBP. That means that, at some level, *you* will be contributing to the advancement of nursing.

## Nursing Research: Past and Present

Most people would agree that research in nursing began with Florence Nightingale in the mid-19th century. Based on her skillful analysis of factors affecting soldier mortality and morbidity during the Crimean War, she was successful in bringing about some changes in nursing care and in public health. For many years after Nightingale's work, however, research was absent from the nursing literature. Studies began to appear in the early 1900s, but most concerned nurses' education.

Forces combined in the 1950s to put nursing research on an accelerating upswing in the United States. An increase in the number of nurses with advanced skills and degrees, an increase in the availability of research funding, and the establishment of the journal *Nursing Research* helped to propel nursing research in the mid-20th century. During the 1960s, practice-oriented research began to emerge, and research-oriented journals started publication in several countries. During the 1970s, there was a decided change in emphasis in nursing research from areas such as teaching and nurses themselves to improvements in client care. Nurses also began to pay attention to the utilization of research findings in nursing practice.

The 1980s brought nursing research to a new level of development. Of particular importance in the United States was the establishment in 1986 of the National Center for Nursing Research (NCNR) at the National Institutes of Health (NIH). The purpose of NCNR was to promote and financially support research projects and training relating to patient care. Nursing research was strengthened and given more visibility when NCNR was promoted to full institute status within the NIH: in 1993, the *National Institute of Nursing Research* (NINR) was established. The birth and expansion of NINR helped put nursing research more into the mainstream of research activities enjoyed by other health disciplines. Funding opportunities expanded in other countries as well.

The 1990s witnessed the birth of several more journals for nurse researchers, and specialty journals increasingly came to publish research articles. International cooperation around the issue of EBP in nursing also began to develop in the 1990s. For example, Sigma Theta Tau International sponsored the first international research utilization conference, in cooperation with the faculty of the University of Toronto, in 1998.

> **TIP:** For those interested in learning more about the history of nursing research, we offer an expanded summary in the Chapter Supplements on thePoint website.

## Future Directions for Nursing Research

Nursing research continues to develop at a rapid pace and will undoubtedly flourish in the 21st century. In 1986, NCNR had a budget of $16 million, whereas NINR funding in fiscal year 2011 was about $150 million. Among the trends foreseen for the near future are the following:

- *Continued focus on EBP.* Concerted efforts to use research findings in practice are sure to continue, and nurses at all levels will be encouraged to engage in evidence-based patient care. This means that improvements will be needed in the quality of nursing studies, and in nurses' skills in locating, understanding, critiquing, and using relevant study results.
- *Stronger evidence through confirmatory strategies.* Practicing nurses rarely adopt an innovation on the basis of poorly designed or isolated studies. Strong research designs are essential, and confirmation is usually needed through deliberate *replication* (i.e., repeating) of studies with different clients and in different clinical settings to ensure that the findings are robust.
- *Greater emphasis on systematic reviews.* **Systematic reviews** are a cornerstone of EBP and have assumed increasing importance in all health disciplines. Systematic reviews rigorously integrate research information on a topic so that conclusions about the state of evidence can be reached.
- *Expanded local research in health care settings.* Small studies designed to solve local problems will likely increase. This trend will be reinforced as more hospitals apply for (and are recertified for) Magnet status in the United States and in other countries.
- *Expanded dissemination of research findings.* The Internet has had a big impact on the dissemination of research information, which in turn helps to promote EBP. Through technological advances, information about innovations and research findings can be communicated more widely and more quickly than ever before.

○ *Increased focus on cultural issues and health disparities.* The issue of health disparities has emerged as a central concern in nursing and other health disciplines, and this in turn has raised consciousness about the cultural sensitivity of health interventions. There is growing awareness that research must be sensitive to the health beliefs, behaviors, epidemiology, and values of culturally and linguistically diverse populations.

What are nurse researchers likely to be studying in the future? Although there is tremendous diversity in research interests, research priorities have been articulated by NINR, Sigma Theta Tau International, and other nursing organizations. As but one example, NINR's 2010 budget request identified three broad areas of research emphasis: promoting health and preventing disease; symptom management, self-management, and caregiving; and end-of-life research (NINR website: http://ninr.nih.gov/ninr/).

> **☞ TIP:** All websites cited in this chapter, plus additional websites with useful content relating to the foundations of nursing research, are in the Internet Resources on thePoint website. This will allow you to simply use the "Control/Click" feature to go directly to the website, without having to type in the URL and risk a typographical error. Websites corresponding to the content of most chapters of the book are also in the Internet Resources on thePoint website.

## Sources of Evidence for Nursing Practice

Nurses make clinical decisions based on a large repertoire of knowledge. As a nursing student, you are gaining skills on how to practice nursing from your instructors, textbooks, and clinical placements. When you become a registered nurse (RN), you will continue to learn from other nurses and health care professionals. Because evidence is constantly evolving, learning about best-practice nursing will persist throughout your career.

Some of what you have learned thus far is based on systematic research, but much of it is not. What *are* the sources of evidence for nursing practice? Where does knowledge for practice come from? Until fairly recently, knowledge primarily was handed down from one generation to the next based on clinical experience, trial and error, tradition, and expert opinion. These alternative sources of knowledge are different from research-based information.

### Tradition and Authority

Within nursing, certain beliefs are accepted as truths—and certain practices are accepted as effective—simply based on custom. Tradition may, however, undermine effective problem solving. There is growing concern that many nursing actions are based on tradition, custom, and "unit culture" rather than on sound evidence. Another common source of knowledge is an authority, a person with specialized expertise. Reliance on authorities (such as nursing faculty or textbook authors) is unavoidable. Like tradition, however, authorities as a source of information have limitations. Authorities are not infallible—particularly if their expertise is based primarily on personal experience; yet, their knowledge is often unchallenged.

> **Example of "myths" in nursing textbooks:**
> A recent study suggests that nursing textbooks may contain many "myths." In their analysis of 23 widely used undergraduate psychiatric nursing textbooks, Holman and colleagues (2010) found that all books contained at least one unsupported assumption (myth) about loss and grief—i.e., assumptions not supported by current research evidence. And, many evidence-based findings about grief and loss failed to be included in the textbooks.

> **☞ TIP:** The consequences of not using research-based evidence can be devastating. For example, from 1956 through the 1980s, Dr. Benjamin Spock published several editions of *Baby and Child Care*, a parental guide that sold over 19 million copies worldwide. As an authority figure, he wrote the following advice: "I think it is preferable to accustom a baby to sleeping on his stomach from the beginning if he is willing." (Spock, 1979, p. 164). Research has clearly demonstrated that this sleeping position is associated with heighted risk of sudden infant death syndrome (SIDS). In their systematic review of evidence, Gilbert and colleagues (2005) wrote, "Advice to put infants to sleep on the front for nearly half a century was contrary to evidence from 1970 that this was likely to be harmful" (p. 874). They estimated that if medical advice had been guided by research evidence, more than 60,000 infant deaths might have been prevented.

### Clinical Experience and Trial and Error

Clinical experience is a functional source of knowledge. Yet, personal experience has limitations as a source of evidence for practice because each nurse's experience is too narrow to be generally useful, and personal experiences are often colored by biases. Trial and error, a related source, involves trying alternatives successively until a solution to a problem is found. Trial and error can be practical, but the method tends to be haphazard and solutions may be idiosyncratic.

### Assembled Information

In making clinical decisions, health care professionals also rely on information that has been assembled for various purposes. For example, local, national, and international *benchmarking data* provide information on such issues as the rates of using various procedures (e.g., rates of cesarean deliveries) or rates of clinical problems (e.g., nosocomial infections). *Quality improvement and risk data*, such as medication error reports, can be used to assess practices and determine the need for practice changes. Such sources offer some information that can be used in practice, but provide no mechanism to actually guide improvements.

### Disciplined Research

Disciplined research is considered the best method of acquiring reliable knowledge that humans have developed. Evidence-based health care compels nurses to base their clinical practice to the extent possible on rigorous research-based findings rather than on tradition, authority, intuition, or personal experience—although nursing will always remain a rich blend of art and science.

# PARADIGMS AND METHODS FOR NURSING RESEARCH

The questions that nurse researchers ask, and the methods they use to answer their questions, spring from a researcher's view of how the world "works." In research parlance, a **paradigm** is a world view, a general perspective on the world's complexities. Disciplined inquiry in nursing has been conducted mainly within two broad paradigms. This section describes the two paradigms and outlines the research methods associated with them.

## The Positivist Paradigm

The paradigm that dominated nursing research for decades is called *positivism*. Positivism is rooted in 19th century thought, guided by such philosophers as Newton and Locke.

**TABLE 1.1　Major Assumptions of the Positivist and Constructivist Paradigms**

| Type of Assumption | Positivist Paradigm | Constructivist Paradigm |
|---|---|---|
| The nature of reality | Reality exists; there is a real world driven by real natural causes | Reality is multiple and subjective, mentally constructed by individuals |
| Relationship between researcher and those being researched | The researcher is independent from those being researched | The researcher interacts with those being researched; findings are the creation of the interactive process |
| The role of values in the inquiry | Values and biases are to be held in check; objectivity is sought | Subjectivity and values are inevitable and desirable |
| Best methods for obtaining evidence | • Deductive processes→ hypotheses testing<br>• Emphasis on discrete, specific concepts<br>• Focus on the objective and quantifiable<br>• Corroboration of researchers' predictions<br>• Fixed, prespecified design<br>• Controls over context<br>• Measured, quantitative information<br>• Statistical analysis<br>• Seeks generalizations | • Inductive processes→ hypothesis generation<br>• Emphasis on the whole<br><br>• Focus on the subjective and nonquantifiable<br>• Emerging insight grounded in participants' experiences<br>• Flexible, emergent design<br>• Context-bound, contextualized<br>• Narrative information<br><br>• Qualitative analysis<br>• Seeks in-depth understanding |

Positivism is a reflection of a broader cultural movement (*modernism*) that emphasizes the rational and the scientific.

As shown in Table 1.1, a fundamental assumption of positivists is that there is a reality *out there* that can be studied and known. (An **assumption** is a principle that is believed to be true without verification). Adherents of positivism assume that nature is ordered and regular, and that a reality exists independent of human observation. In other words, the world is assumed not to be merely a creation of the human mind. The related assumption of *determinism* refers to the positivists' belief that phenomena are not haphazard, but rather have antecedent causes. If a person has a stroke, the scientist in a positivist tradition assumes that there must be one or more reasons that can be potentially identified. Within the **positivist paradigm**, much research activity is aimed at understanding the underlying causes of natural phenomena.

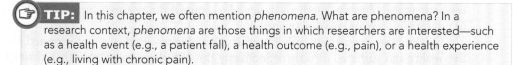

**TIP:** In this chapter, we often mention *phenomena*. What are phenomena? In a research context, *phenomena* are those things in which researchers are interested—such as a health event (e.g., a patient fall), a health outcome (e.g., pain), or a health experience (e.g., living with chronic pain).

Because of their belief in objective reality, positivists prize objectivity. Their approach involves the use of orderly, disciplined procedures with tight controls over the research situation to test hunches about the nature of phenomena being studied and relationships among them.

Strict positivist thinking has been challenged and undermined, and few researchers adhere to the tenets of pure positivism. Postpositivists still believe in reality and seek to understand it, but they recognize the impossibility of total objectivity. Yet, they see objectivity as a goal and strive to be as neutral and unbiased as possible. Postpositivists also appreciate the barriers to knowing reality with certainty, and therefore seek *probabilistic* evidence—i.e., learning what the true state of a phenomenon *probably* is, with a high degree of likelihood. This modified positivist position remains a dominant force in nursing research. For the sake of simplicity, we refer to it as positivism.

## The Constructivist Paradigm

The **constructivist paradigm** (sometimes called the *naturalistic paradigm*) began as a countermovement to positivism with writers such as Weber and Kant. The constructivist paradigm is a major alternative system for conducting research in nursing. Table 1.1 compares four major assumptions of the positivist and constructivist paradigms.

For the naturalistic inquirer, reality is not a fixed entity but rather a construction of the people participating in the research; reality exists within a context, and many constructions are possible. Naturalists take the position of relativism: if there are multiple interpretations of reality that exist in people's minds, then there is no process by which the ultimate truth or falsity of the constructions can be determined.

The constructivist paradigm assumes that knowledge is maximized when the distance between the inquirer and participants in the study is minimized. The voices and interpretations of those under study are crucial to understanding the phenomenon of interest, and subjective interactions are the best way to access them. Findings from a constructivist inquiry are the product of the interaction between the inquirer and the participants.

## Paradigms and Methods: Quantitative and Qualitative Research

**Research methods** are the techniques researchers use to structure a study and to gather and analyze relevant information. The two paradigms correspond to different methods of developing evidence. A key methodologic distinction is between **quantitative research**, which is most closely allied with positivism, and **qualitative research**, which is associated with constructivist inquiry—although positivists sometimes undertake qualitative studies, and constructivist researchers sometimes collect quantitative information. This section gives an overview of the methods linked to the two alternative paradigms.

### The Scientific Method and Quantitative Research

The traditional, positivist **scientific method** involves using a set of orderly procedures to gather information. Quantitative researchers typically move in a systematic fashion from the definition of a problem to the solution of the problem. By *systematic*, we mean that investigators progress through a series of steps, according to a prespecified plan. Quantitative researchers use objective methods designed to control the research situation with the goal of minimizing *bias* and maximizing validity.

Quantitative researchers gather **empirical evidence**—evidence that is rooted in objective reality and gathered directly or indirectly through the senses rather than through personal beliefs or hunches. Evidence for a quantitative study is gathered systematically, using formal instruments to collect needed information. Usually (but not always) the information is **quantitative**—that is, numeric information that results from some type of formal measurement and that is analyzed statistically. Quantitative researchers strive to go beyond the specifics of a research situation; the ability to generalize research findings to individuals other than those who took part in the study (referred to as **generalizability**) is an important goal.

The traditional scientific method has been used productively by nurse researchers studying a wide range of questions. Yet, there are important limitations. For example, quantitative researchers must deal with problems of *measurement*. To study a phenomenon, scientists must measure it, that is, attach numeric values that express quantity. For example, if the phenomenon of interest were patient stress, researchers would want to assess if stress is high or low, or higher under certain conditions or for some people. Physiologic phenomena like blood pressure and temperature can be measured with accuracy and precision, but the same cannot be said of most psychological phenomena, such as stress or resilience.

Another issue is that nursing research focuses on human beings, who are inherently complicated and diverse. The traditional scientific method typically focuses on a relatively small aspect of human experiences (e.g., weight gain, depression) in a single study. Complexities tend to be controlled and, if possible, eliminated rather than studied directly, and this narrowness of focus can sometimes obscure insights. Relatedly, quantitative research within the positivist paradigm has sometimes been accused of a narrowness and inflexibility of vision that does not capture the full breadth of human experience.

> **TIP:** Students often find quantitative studies more intimidating and difficult to read and understand than qualitative ones. Try not to worry too much about the jargon at first— remember that each study has a *story* to tell, and grasping the main point of the story is what is initially important.

## Constructivist Methods and Qualitative Research

Researchers in constructivist traditions emphasize the inherent complexity of humans, their ability to shape and create their own experiences, and the idea that truth is a composite of realities. Consequently, constructivist studies are heavily focused on understanding the human experience as it is lived, through the careful collection and analysis of **qualitative** materials that are narrative and subjective.

Researchers who reject the traditional scientific method believe that a major limitation is that it is *reductionist*—that is, it reduces human experience to only the few concepts under investigation, and those concepts are defined in advance by the researcher rather than emerging from the experiences of those under study. Constructivist researchers tend to emphasize the dynamic, holistic, and individual aspects of human life and try to capture those aspects in their entirety, within the context of those who are experiencing them.

Flexible, evolving procedures are used to capitalize on findings that emerge during the study, which typically take place in naturalistic settings. The collection of information and its analysis typically progress concurrently. As researchers sift through information, insights are gained, new questions emerge, and further evidence is sought to confirm the insights. Through an inductive process (going from specifics to the general), researchers integrate information to develop a theory or description that illuminates the phenomena under observation.

Constructivist studies yield rich, in-depth information that can potentially clarify the varied dimensions of a complicated phenomenon. Findings from qualitative research are typically grounded in the real-life experiences of people with first-hand knowledge of a phenomenon. Nevertheless, the approach has several limitations. Human beings are used directly as the instrument through which information is gathered, and humans are highly intelligent—but fallible—tools. The subjectivity that enriches the analytic insights of skillful researchers can yield trivial "findings" among less competent ones.

Another potential limitation involves the subjectivity of constructivist inquiry, which sometimes raises concerns about the idiosyncratic nature of the conclusions. Would two constructivist researchers studying the same phenomenon in similar settings arrive at similar conclusions? The situation is further complicated by the fact that most constructivist studies involve a small group of participants. Thus, the generalizability of findings from constructivist inquiries is an issue of potential concern.

> 👉 **TIP:** Researchers often do *not* discuss or even mention the underlying paradigm of their studies in their reports. The paradigm provides the context, without being explicitly referenced.

## Multiple Paradigms and Nursing Research

Paradigms are lenses that help to sharpen researchers' focus on phenomena of interest, not blinders that limit intellectual curiosity. We think that the emergence of alternative paradigms for studying nursing problems is a healthy and desirable trend that can maximize the breadth of new evidence for practice. Nursing knowledge would be thin if it were not for the rich array of methods available in the two paradigms—methods that are often complementary in their strengths and limitations.

We have emphasized differences between the two paradigms and associated methods so that distinctions would be easy to understand. It is equally important, however, to note that these two paradigms have many features in common, some of which are mentioned here:

- *Ultimate goals.* The ultimate aim of disciplined research, regardless of paradigm, is to answer questions and solve problems. Both quantitative and qualitative researchers seek to capture the truth with regard to an aspect of the world in which they are interested.
- *External evidence.* Although the word *empiricism* has come to be allied with the classic scientific method, researchers in both traditions gather and analyze evidence empirically, that is, through their senses.
- *Reliance on human cooperation.* Evidence for nursing research comes primarily from humans, and so human cooperation is essential in both qualitative and quantitative research. To understand people's characteristics and experiences, researchers must persuade them to participate in the study *and* to speak candidly.
- *Ethical constraints.* Research with human beings is guided by ethical principles that sometimes interfere with research goals. Ethical dilemmas often confront researchers, regardless of paradigms or methods.
- *Fallibility.* Virtually all studies have limitations. Every research question can be addressed in different ways, and inevitably there are tradeoffs. Financial constraints are often an issue, but limitations exist even in well-funded research. This means that *no single study can ever definitively answer a research question.* The fallibility of any single study makes it important to understand and critique researchers' methods when evaluating evidence quality.

Thus, despite philosophic and methodologic differences, researchers using the traditional scientific method or constructivist methods often share basic goals and face many similar constraints and challenges. The selection of an appropriate method depends on researchers' philosophy and world view, but also on the research question. If a researcher asks, "What are the effects of cryotherapy on nausea and oral mucositis in patients undergoing chemotherapy?" the researcher needs to examine effects through the careful quantitative assessment of patients. On the other hand, if a researcher asks, "What is the process by which parents learn to cope with the death of a child?" the researcher would be hard pressed to quantify such a process. Personal world views of researchers help to shape their questions.

In reading about the alternative paradigms, you likely were more attracted to one of the two paradigms—the one that corresponds most closely to your view of the world. It is important, however, to learn about and respect both approaches to disciplined inquiry, and to recognize their respective strengths and limitations. In this textbook, we describe methods associated with both qualitative and quantitative research in an effort to help you become *methodologically bilingual*.

 **HOW-TO-TELL TIP:** How can you tell if a study is qualitative or quantitative? As you progress through this book, you should be able to identify most studies as qualitative versus quantitative based simply on the study's title, or based on terms in the summary at the beginning of an article. At this point, though, it may be easiest to distinguish the two types of studies based on how many numbers appear in the article, especially in tables. Qualitative studies may have no tables with quantitative information, or only one numeric table describing participants' characteristics (e.g., the percentage who were male or female). Quantitative studies typically have several tables with numbers and statistical information. Qualitative studies often have "word tables" or diagrams and figures illustrating processes inferred from the narrative information gathered.

# THE PURPOSES OF NURSING RESEARCH

Why do nurses do research? The general purpose is to answer questions or solve problems of relevance to nursing. Beyond this broad description, several different systems have been devised to classify different goals. We describe two such classification systems—not because it is important for you to categorize a study as having one purpose or the other, but rather because this will help us to illustrate the broad range of questions that have intrigued nurses, and to further show differences between qualitative and quantitative inquiry.

 **TIP:** Sometimes a distinction is made between basic and applied research. *Basic research* is appropriate for discovering general principles of human behavior and bio-physiologic processes; *applied research* is designed to indicate how these principles can be used to solve problems in nursing practice.

## Research to Achieve Varying Levels of Explanation

One way to classify research purposes concerns the extent to which studies are designed to provide explanations. A fundamental distinction that is especially relevant in quantitative research is between studies whose primary goal is to *describe* phenomena, and those that are **cause probing**—that is, studies designed to illuminate the underlying causes of phenomena.

Using a descriptive/explanatory framework, the specific purposes of nursing research include identification, description, exploration, prediction/control, and explanation. When researchers state their study purpose, they often use these terms (e.g., The purpose of this study was to *explore*....). For each purpose, various types of questions are addressed—some more amenable to qualitative than to quantitative inquiry, and vice versa.

### Identification and Description

Qualitative researchers sometimes study phenomena about which little is known. In some cases, so little is known that the phenomenon has yet to be clearly identified or named or

**TABLE 1.2** **Purposes on the Descriptive–Explanatory Continuum, and Types of Research Questions**

| Purpose | Types of Questions: Quantitative Research | Types of Questions: Qualitative Research |
|---|---|---|
| Identification | | What is this phenomenon? What is its name? |
| Description | How prevalent is the phenomenon? How often does the phenomenon occur? | What are the dimensions or characteristics of the phenomenon? What is important about the phenomenon? |
| Exploration | What factors are related to the phenomenon? What are the antecedents of the phenomenon? | What is the full nature of the phenomenon? What is really going on here? What is the process by which the phenomenon evolves? |
| Prediction and Control | If phenomenon X occurs, will phenomenon Y follow? Can the phenomenon be prevented or controlled? | |
| Explanation | What is the underlying cause of the phenomenon? Does the theory explain the phenomenon? | Why does the phenomenon exist? What does the phenomenon mean? How did the phenomenon occur? |

has been inadequately defined. The in-depth, probing nature of qualitative research is well suited to answering such questions as, "What is this phenomenon?" and "What is its name?" (Table 1.2). In quantitative research, by contrast, researchers begin with a phenomenon that has been previously studied or defined.

**Qualitative example of identification:**
Rosedale (2009) studied the experiences of women after breast cancer treatment. She identified, through in-depth conversations with 13 women, descriptions of intense loneliness that she identified as *survivor loneliness*.

Description of phenomena is an important purpose of research. In descriptive studies, researchers count, delineate, and classify. Nurse researchers have described a wide variety of phenomena, such as patients' stress, health beliefs, and so on. Quantitative description focuses on the prevalence, size, and measurable aspects of phenomena. Qualitative researchers describe the nature, dimensions, and salience of phenomena, as shown in Table 1.2.

**Quantitative example of description:**
Covelli and colleagues (2012) described the prevalence of biologic measures of hypertension risk (e.g., elevated salivary cortisol, cardiovascular reactivity) among African American adolescents.

## Exploration

Exploratory research begins with a phenomenon of interest; but rather than simply describing it, exploratory researchers examine the nature of the phenomenon, the manner in which it is manifested, and other factors to which it is related—including factors that might be *causing* it. For example, a *descriptive* quantitative study of patients' preoperative stress might document the degree of stress that patients experience. An *exploratory* study might ask: What factors increase or lower a patient's stress? Is a patient's stress related to nurses' behaviors or to the patient's age? Qualitative methods can be used to explore the nature of little understood phenomena and to shed light on the ways in which a phenomenon is expressed.

**Qualitative example of exploration:**
Overgaard and colleagues (2012) explored the illness experiences and vocational adjustments of patients with acute heart failure who had surgical implantation of a left ventricular assist device.

## Explanation

Explanatory research seeks to understand the underlying causes or full nature of a phenomenon. In quantitative research, *theories* or prior findings are used deductively to generate hypothesized explanations that are then tested. Qualitative researchers search for explanations about how or why a phenomenon exists or what a phenomenon means as a basis for *developing* a theory that is grounded in rich, in-depth, experiential evidence.

**Quantitative example of explanation:**
Liu et al. (2012) tested a theoretical model to explain family caregiving of older Chinese people with dementia. The model purported to explain how caregiving appraisal, coping, perceived social support, and familism influence the impact of caregiving stressors on the psychological health of caregivers.

## Prediction and Control

Many phenomena defy explanation, yet often it is possible to predict or control them based on research evidence. For example, research has shown that the incidence of Down syndrome in infants increases with maternal age. We can predict that a woman aged 40 years is at higher risk of bearing a child with Down syndrome than a woman aged 25 years. We can partially control the outcome by educating women about the risks and offering amniocentesis to women older than 35 years of age. The ability to predict and control in this example does not rely on an explanation of what *causes* older women to be at a higher risk. In many quantitative studies, prediction and control are key goals. Although explanatory studies are powerful, studies whose purpose is prediction and control are also critical to EBP.

**Quantitative example of prediction:**
Lilja and colleagues (2012) conducted a study to assess whether depressive mood in women at childbirth predicted their mood and quality of their relationship with their infant and partner at 12 months postpartum.

## Research Purposes Linked to EBP

Another system for classifying studies has emerged in efforts to communicate EBP-related purposes (e.g., DiCenso et al., 2005; Guyatt et al., 2008; Melnyk & Fineout-Overholt, 2011). Table 1.3 identifies some of the questions relevant for each EBP purpose, and offers an actual nursing research example. In this classification scheme, the various purposes can best be addressed with quantitative research, except the last category (meaning/process), which requires qualitative research.

**TABLE 1.3** **Research Purposes Linked to EBP, and Key Research Questions**

| EBP Purpose | Key Research Question | Nursing Research Example |
| --- | --- | --- |
| Therapy/ Intervention | What therapy or intervention will result in better health outcomes or prevent an adverse health outcome? | Hendrix and colleagues (2012) tested the effectiveness of an individualized caregiver intervention on caregivers' psychological well-being and cancer patients' physical symptoms. |
| Diagnosis/ Assessment | What test or assessment procedure will yield accurate diagnoses or assessments of critical patient conditions and outcomes? | Paulson-Conger and colleagues (2011) evaluated two methods of assessing pain in nonverbal critical care patients. |
| Prognosis | Does exposure to a disease or health problem increase the risk of subsequent adverse consequences? | Jalowiec and colleagues (2012) studied the prognosis of heart transplant recipients who had a sex-mismatched heart, compared to those with a sex-matched heart. |
| Etiology/ Cause/Harm | What factors cause or contribute to the risk of a health problem or disease? | Bowie and co-researchers (2012) studied whether parents' methods of regulating their children's emotions were associated with children's levels of anxiety and depression. |
| Meaning/ Process | What is the meaning of life experiences, and what is the process by which they unfold? | Wilkes and colleagues (2012) studied the meaning of impending fatherhood among prospective adolescent fathers. |

### Therapy, Treatment, or Intervention

Studies with a therapy purpose seek to identify effective treatments for ameliorating or preventing health problems. Such studies range from evaluations of highly specific treatments (e.g., comparing two types of cooling blankets for febrile patients) to complex multicomponent interventions designed to effect behavioral changes (e.g., nurse-led smoking cessation interventions). Intervention research plays a critical role in EBP.

### Diagnosis and Assessment

Many nursing studies concern the rigorous development and evaluation of formal instruments to screen, diagnose, and assess patients and to measure clinical outcomes. High-quality instruments with documented accuracy are essential both for clinical practice and for research.

### Prognosis

Studies of prognosis examine the consequences of a disease or health problem, explore factors that can modify the prognosis, and examine when (and for which types of people) the consequences are most likely. Such studies facilitate the development of long-term care plans for patients. They also provide valuable information for guiding patients to make beneficial lifestyle choices or to be vigilant for key symptoms.

### Etiology (Causation) and Harm

It is difficult to prevent harm or treat health problems if we do not know what causes them. For example, there would be no smoking cessation programs if research had not provided firm evidence that smoking cigarettes causes or contributes to a range of health problems. Thus, determining the factors and exposures that affect or cause illness, mortality, or morbidity is an important purpose of many studies.

## Meaning and Processes

Many health care activities (e.g., motivating people to comply with treatments, providing sensitive advice to patients, designing appealing interventions) can greatly benefit from understanding the clients' perspectives. Research that offers evidence about what health and illness mean to clients, what barriers they face to positive health practices, and what processes they experience in a transition through a health care crisis are important to evidence-based nursing practice.

> 👉 **TIP:** Most of these EBP-related purposes (except *diagnosis* and *meaning*) involve *cause-probing* research. For example, research on interventions focuses on whether an intervention *causes* improvements in key outcomes. Prognosis research asks if a disease or health condition *causes* subsequent adverse consequences. Etiology research seeks explanations about the underlying *causes* of health problems.

# ASSISTANCE FOR CONSUMERS OF NURSING RESEARCH

We hope that this book will help you develop skills that will allow you to read, appraise, and use nursing studies—and to appreciate nursing research. In each chapter, we present information relating to methods used by nurse researchers and provide guidance in several ways. First, we offer tips on what you can expect to find in actual research articles, identified by the icon ☞. There are also special "how-to-tell" tips (identified with the icon ☞) that help with some potentially confusing issues in research articles. Second, we include guidelines for critiquing various aspects of a study. The guiding questions in Box 1.1 are designed to assist you in using the information in this chapter in a preliminary assessment of a research article. And third, we offer opportunities to apply your new skills. The critical thinking activities at the end of each chapter guide you through appraisals of real research examples (some of which are presented in their entirety in the appendix) of both qualitative and quantitative studies. These activities also challenge you to think about how the findings from these studies could be used in nursing practice. Answers to many of these questions are available on thePoint website. The full journal article for studies identified with ⚙ are also available on thePoint website.

---

**BOX 1.1 Questions for a Preliminary Overview of a Research Report**

1. How relevant is the research problem to the actual practice of nursing?
2. Is the research quantitative or qualitative?
3. What is the underlying purpose (or purposes) of the study—identification, description, exploration, explanation, or prediction/control? Does the purpose correspond to an EBP focus such as therapy/treatment, diagnosis, prognosis, etiology/harm, or meaning?
4. What might be some clinical implications of this research? To what type of people and settings is the research most relevant? If the findings are accurate, how might *I* use the results of this study?

## RESEARCH EXAMPLES WITH CRITICAL THINKING EXERCISES

We conclude with a brief description of a quantitative and a qualitative nursing study.

Examples 1 and 2 below are also featured in our *Interactive Critical Thinking Activity* on thePoint website where you can easily record, print, and e-mail your responses to the related questions.

## EXAMPLE 1 ● Quantitative Research

**Study:** Improving hospice through systematic assessment (McMillan et al., 2011).

**Study Purpose:** The purpose of the study was to test whether providing information from systematic assessments about patient-caregiver hospice dyads to interdisciplinary teams (IDTs) (e.g., teams of nurses, physicians, social workers) is effective in improving hospice outcomes.

**Study Methods:** The IDTs planning care for newly admitted hospice dyads were assigned to one of two groups: (1) those caring for dyads after receiving information from standardized assessments regarding the patient's and caregiver's depression, symptoms and needs, and quality of life, and (2) those caring for dyads as usual, without routinely receiving assessment information. There were 338 dyads in the special group, and 371 in the usual care group. For all dyads, information regarding depression, quality of life, and symptom distress was obtained on admission, and then 1 week after the first two IDT meetings in which the dyads were discussed.

**Key Findings:** The researchers found that patients in the special intervention group had lower levels of depression than those in the usual care group at the end of the study. Quality of life improved over time in both the intervention and usual care groups.

**Conclusions:** McMillan and colleagues concluded that the IDT's knowledge regarding patient and caregiver depression assessments may have improved the care the team provided because depression is not normally a focus of hospice staff.

### CRITICAL THINKING EXERCISES
1. Answer the relevant questions from Box 1.1 on page 15 regarding this study.
2. Also consider the following targeted questions:
    a. Why do you think quality of life improved over time in both the intervention and usual-care groups?
    b. Could this study have been undertaken as a qualitative study? Why or why not?

## EXAMPLE 2 ● Qualitative Research

**Study:** Experiences of self-blame and stigmatization for self-infliction among individuals living with chronic obstructive pulmonary disease (COPD) (Halding et al., 2011).

**Study Purpose:** The purpose of this study was to understand how patients with COPD experience daily life in a society with strong messages about tobacco control.

**Study Methods:** Eighteen men and women with COPD were recruited from two Norwegian pulmonary rehabilitation units. Patients participated in two in-depth interviews, each lasting 40 to 90 minutes. Most interviews were conducted in the patients' homes. The interviews, which were audiotaped and then transcribed, focused on what the patients' day-to-day experiences with COPD were like.

**Key Findings:** Participants spontaneously brought up the topics of smoking, blame, and guilt. The overarching theme that emerged in the analysis of the interviews was *Exiled in the world of the healthy.* The participants experienced feelings of disgrace, self-blame, and lack of support from their social network and health care professionals, reflecting perceptions that COPD is self-inflicted.

**Conclusions:** The researchers noted the challenge of how to combine health advice on smoking cessation with nonblaming psychosocial support throughout the course of COPD.

### CRITICAL THINKING EXERCISES
1. Answer the relevant questions from Box 1.1 on page 15 regarding this study.
2. Also consider the following targeted questions, which may assist you in assessing aspects of the study's merit:
   a. Why do you think that the researchers audiotaped and transcribed their in-depth interviews with study participants?
   b. Do you think it would have been appropriate for the researchers to conduct this study using quantitative research methods? Why or why not?

## EXAMPLE 3 ● Quantitative Research in Appendix A
- Read the abstract and the introduction from Howell and colleagues' (2007) study ("Anxiety, anger, and blood pressure in children") in Appendix A on pages 395–402.

### CRITICAL THINKING EXERCISES
1. Answer the relevant questions from Box 1.1 on page 15 regarding this study.
2. Also consider the following targeted questions:
   a. Could this study have been undertaken as a qualitative study? Why or why not?
   b. Who helped to pay for this research? (This information appears at the end of the report.)

## EXAMPLE 4 ● Qualitative Research in Appendix B
- Read the abstract and the introduction from Beck and Watson's (2010) study ("Subsequent childbirth after a previous traumatic birth") in Appendix B on pages 403–412.

### CRITICAL THINKING EXERCISES
1. Answer the relevant questions from Box 1.1 on page 15 regarding this study.
2. Also consider the following targeted questions:
   a. What gap in the existing research was the study designed to fill?
   b. Was Beck and Watson's study conducted within the positivist paradigm or the constructivist paradigm? Provide a rationale for your choice.

---

**WANT TO KNOW MORE?** A wide variety of resources to enhance your learning and understanding of this chapter are available on thePoint.

- Interactive Critical Thinking Activity
- Chapter Supplement on The History of Nursing Research
- Answers to the Critical Thinking Exercises for Examples 3 and 4
- Student Review Questions
- Full-text online
- Internet Resources with useful websites for Chapter 1

Additional study aids including eight journal articles and related questions are also available in *Study Guide for Essentials of Nursing Research, 8e.*

# SUMMARY POINTS

- **Nursing research** is systematic inquiry to develop evidence on problems of importance to nurses.

- Nurses in various settings are adopting an **evidence-based practice (EBP)** that incorporates research findings into their decisions and interactions with clients.

- Knowledge of nursing research enhances the professional practice of all nurses—including both *consumers of research* (who read and evaluate studies) and *producers of research* (who design and undertake studies).

- Nursing research began with Florence Nightingale but developed slowly until its rapid acceleration in the 1950s. Since the 1980s, the focus has been on **clinical nursing research**—that is, on problems relating to clinical practice.

- The NINR, established at the U.S. NIH in 1993, affirms the stature of nursing research in the United States.

- Future emphases of nursing research are likely to include EBP projects, **replications** of research, research integration through **systematic reviews**, expanded dissemination efforts, and increased focus on health disparities.

- Disciplined research stands in contrast to other knowledge sources for nursing practice, such as tradition, authority, personal experience, and trial and error.

- Disciplined inquiry in nursing is conducted mainly within two broad **paradigms**—world views with underlying **assumptions** about reality: the positivist paradigm and the constructivist paradigm.

- In the **positivist paradigm**, it is assumed that there is an objective reality and that natural phenomena are regular and orderly. The related assumption of *determinism* refers to the belief that phenomena result from prior causes and are not haphazard.

- In the **constructivist paradigm**, it is assumed that reality is not a fixed entity but is rather a construction of human minds—and thus "truth" is a composite of multiple constructions of reality.

- **Quantitative research** (associated with positivism) involves the collection and analysis of numeric information. Quantitative research is typically conducted within the traditional **scientific method**, which is systematic and controlled. Quantitative researchers base their findings on **empirical evidence** (evidence collected by way of the human senses) and strive for **generalizability** beyond a single setting or situation.

- Constructivist researchers emphasize understanding human experience as it is lived through the collection and analysis of subjective, narrative materials using flexible procedures; this paradigm is associated with **qualitative research**.

- A fundamental distinction that is especially relevant in quantitative research is between studies whose primary intent is to *describe* phenomena and those that are **cause probing**—i.e., designed to illuminate underlying causes of phenomena. Specific purposes on the description/explanation continuum include identification, description, exploration, prediction/control, and explanation.

- Many nursing studies can also be classified in terms of a key EBP aim: therapy/treatment/intervention; diagnosis and assessment; prognosis; etiology and harm; and meaning and process.

# REFERENCES FOR CHAPTER 1

Bowie, B., Carrere, S., Cooke, C., Valdivia, G., McAllister, B., & Doohan, E. (2012). The role of culture in parents' socialization of children's emotional development. *Western Journal of Nursing Research*, PubMed ID 20500623.

Cong, X., Ludington-Hoe, S., McCain, G., & Fu, P. (2009). Kangaroo care modifies preterm infant heart rate variability in response to heel stick pain. *Early Human Development, 85*, 561–567.

Cong, X., Ludington-Hoe, S., & Walsh, S. (2011). Randomized crossover trial of kangaroo care to reduce biobehavioral pain responses in preterm infants. *Biological Research for Nursing, 13*, 204–216.

Covelli, M. M., Wood, C., & Yarandi, H. (2012). Biologic measures as epidemiological indicators of risk for the development of hypertension in an African American adolescent population. *Journal of Cardiovascular Nursing, 27*, 476–484.

DiCenso, A., Guyatt, G., & Ciliska, D. (2005). *Evidence-based nursing: A guide to clinical practice*. St. Louis, MO: Elsevier Mosby.

Gagnon, M. (2012). Understanding the experience of reconstructive treatments from the perspective of people who suffer from facial lipoatrophy: A qualitative study. *International Journal of Nursing Studies* 2012;49(5):539–548.

Gilbert, R., Salanti, G., Harden, M., & See, S. (2005). Infant sleeping position and the sudden infant death syndrome: Systematic review of observational studies and historical review of recommendations from 1940 to 2002. *International Journal of Epidemiology, 34*, 874–887.

Guyatt, G., Rennie, D., Meade, M., & Cook, D. (2008). *Users' guide to the medical literature: Essentials of evidence-based clinical practice* (2nd ed.). New York: McGraw Hill.

Halding, A., Heggad, K., & Wahl, A. (2011). Experiences of self-blame and stigmatisation for self-infliction among individuals living with COPD. *Scandinavian Journal of Caring Sciences, 25*, 100–107.

Hendrix, C., Landerman, R., & Abernathy, A. (2012). Effects of an individualized caregiver training intervention on self-efficacy of cancer caregivers. *Western Journal of Nursing Research*, PubMed ID 21949091.

Holman, E., Perisho, J., Edwards, A., & Mlakar, N. (2010). The myths of coping with loss in undergraduate psychiatric nursing books. *Research in Nursing & Health, 33*, 486–499.

Jalowiec, A., Grady, K., & White-Williams, C. (2012). First-year clinical outcomes in sex-mismatched heart transplant recipients. *Journal of Cardiovascular Nursing, 27*, 519–527.

Lilja, G., Edhborg, M., & Nissen, E. (2012). Depressive mood in women at childbirth predicts their mood and relationship with infant and partner during the first year postpartum. *Scandinavian Journal of Caring Science, 26*(2), 245–253.

Liu, Y., Insel, K., Reed, P., & Crist, J. (2012). Family caregiving of older Chinese people with dementia: Testing a model. *Nursing Research, 61*, 39–50.

Ludington-Hoe, S., Johnson, M., Morgan, K., Lewis, T., Gutman, J., Wilson, P., et al. (2006). Neurophysiologic assessment of neonatal sleep organization: Preliminary results of a randomized, controlled trial of skin contact with preterm infants. *Pediatrics, 117*, 909–923.

McMillan, S., Small, B., & Haley, W. (2011). Improving hospice through systematic assessment. *Cancer Nursing, 34*, 89–97.

Melnyk, B. M., & Fineout-Overhold, E. (2011). *Evidence-based practice in nursing and healthcare: A guide to best practice* (2nd ed.). Philadelphia, PA: Lippincott Williams & Wilkins.

Overgaard, D., Kjeldgaard, H., & Egerod, I. (2012). Life in transition: A qualitative study of the illness experience and vocational adjustment of patients with left ventricular assist device. *Journal of Cardiovascular Nursing*, PubMed ID 21912269.

Paulson-Conger, M., Leske, J., Maidl, C., Hanson, A., & Dziadulewicz, L. (2011). Comparison of two pain assessment tools in nonverbal critical care patients. *Pain Management Nursing, 12*, 218–224.

Rosedale, M. (2009). Survivor loneliness of women following breast cancer. *Oncology Nursing Forum, 36*, 175–183.

Spock, B. (1979). *Baby and child care*. New York: Dutton Publishing.

Wilkes, L., Mannix, J., & Jackson, D. (2012). "I am going to be a dad": Experiences and expectations of adolescent and young adult expectant fathers. *Journal of Clinical Nursing, 21*, 180–188.

Yu, F., Nelson, N., Savik, K., Wyman, J., Dyksen, M., & Bronas, U. (2012). Affecting cognition and quality of life via aerobic exercise in Alzheimer's disease. *Western Journal of Nursing Research*, PubMed ID 21911546.

# 2 Fundamentals of Evidence-Based Nursing Practice

## LEARNING OBJECTIVES

*On completing this chapter, you will be able to:*

- Distinguish research utilization (RU) and evidence-based practice (EBP), and discuss their current status within nursing
- Identify several resources available to facilitate EBP in nursing practice
- Identify several models for implementing EBP
- Discuss the five major steps in undertaking an EBP effort for individual nurses
- Identify the components of a well-worded clinical question and be able to frame such a question
- Discuss broad strategies for undertaking an EBP project at the organizational level
- Define new terms in the chapter

## KEY TERMS

Clinical practice guideline   Implementation potential   Research utilization
Cochrane Collaboration         Meta-analysis              Systematic review
Evidence hierarchy             Metasynthesis
Evidence-based practice        Pilot test

Learning about research methods provides a foundation for evidence-based nursing practice (EBP). The emphasis in EBP is on identifying the best available research evidence and *integrating* it with other factors in making clinical decisions. Advocates of EBP do not minimize the importance of clinical expertise. Rather, they argue that evidence-based decision making should integrate best research evidence with clinical expertise, patient preferences, and local circumstances. EBP involves efforts to personalize evidence to fit a specific patient's needs and a particular clinical situation.

This book will help you to develop methodologic skills for reading research articles and evaluating research evidence. Before we elaborate on methodologic techniques, we discuss key aspects of EBP to further help you understand the key role that research now plays in nursing.

## BACKGROUND OF EVIDENCE-BASED NURSING PRACTICE

This section provides a context for understanding EBP. Part of this context involves a closely related concept, research utilization.

## Research Utilization

**Research utilization** (RU) is the use of findings from disciplined research in a practical application that is unrelated to the original research. In RU, the emphasis is on translating research findings into real-world applications. The starting point in RU is new evidence or a research-based innovation.

EBP is broader than RU because it integrates research findings with other factors. Whereas RU begins with the research itself (how can I put this innovation to good use in my clinical setting?), EBP starts with a clinical question (what does the evidence say is the best approach to solving this problem?).

### The Research Utilization Continuum

RU begins with the emergence of new knowledge. Research is conducted and, over time, evidence on a topic accumulates. In turn, the evidence works its way into use—to varying degrees and at differing rates.

People who study the diffusion of ideas acknowledge a continuum in terms of the specificity of the use to which research findings are put. At one end of the continuum are clearly identifiable attempts to base specific actions on research findings (e.g., placing infants on their backs for sleeping to minimize the risk of sudden infant death syndrome). Yet, research findings can be used more diffusely, in a way that reflects cumulative awareness or understanding. Thus, a nurse may read a qualitative study describing *courage* among people with chronic illnesses as a dynamic process that includes efforts to accept reality and to develop problem-solving skills. The study may make the nurse more observant and sensitive in working with patients with chronic illnesses, but it may not lead to formal changes in clinical actions. The RU continuum suggests roles for both qualitative and quantitative research.

### The History of Research Utilization in Nursing Practice

During the 1980s, RU emerged as an important buzz word, and several changes in nursing education and research were prompted by the desire to develop a knowledge base for nursing practice. In education, nursing schools began to include courses on research methods so that students would become skillful research consumers. In the research arena, there was a shift in focus toward clinical nursing problems.

At the same time, there were growing concerns about how infrequently research findings were actually used in delivering nursing care. Some of these concerns were based on studies that found that practicing nurses were unaware of or ignored important research findings. Recognition of the gap between research and practice led to formal attempts to bridge the gap. The best-known of several early RU projects is the *Conduct and Utilization of Research in Nursing (CURN) Project*, which was awarded to the Michigan Nurses' Association by the Division of Nursing in the 1970s. CURN aimed to increase nurses' use of research findings by disseminating research findings, facilitating organizational changes, and encouraging collaborative clinical research. CURN project staff saw RU as an organizational process requiring commitment by organizations that employ nurses (Horsley, Crane, & Bingle, 1978). The CURN project team concluded that RU by practicing nurses was feasible, but only if the research is relevant to practice and if the results are broadly disseminated.

During the 1980s and 1990s, many RU projects were undertaken. These projects involved attempts to change nursing practices based on research findings, and to evaluate the effects of the changes. Although studies continued to document a gap between research and practice, the findings suggested some improvements in nurses' utilization of research. During the 1990s, however, the call for RU began to be superseded by the push for EBP.

## Evidence-Based Practice in Nursing

The EBP movement has had both advocates and critics. Supporters argue that EBP offers a solution for improving health care quality in a cost-constrained environment. In their view, a rational approach is needed to provide the best possible care to the most people, in the most cost-effective manner. Advocates also note that EBP provides a good framework for lifelong learning that is essential in an era of rapid clinical advances and the information explosion. Critics worry that EBP advantages are exaggerated and that clinical judgments and patient inputs are being devalued. They are also concerned that insufficient attention is being paid to qualitative research. Although there is a need for close scrutiny of how the EBP journey unfolds, health care professionals will likely follow an EBP path in the years ahead.

### Overview of the Evidence-Based Practice Movement

One keystone of the EBP movement is the Cochrane Collaboration, which was founded in the United Kingdom based on work by British epidemiologist Archie Cochrane. Cochrane published an influential book in the 1970s that drew attention to the dearth of solid evidence about the effects of health care. He called for efforts to make research summaries about interventions available to health care providers. This eventually led to the development of the Cochrane Center in Oxford in 1993, and the international **Cochrane Collaboration**, with centers now established in locations throughout the world. Its aim is to help providers make good health care decisions by preparing and disseminating systematic reviews of the effects of health care interventions.

At about the same time that the Cochrane Collaboration began, a group from McMaster Medical School in Canada developed a clinical learning strategy called *evidence-based medicine*. The evidence-based medicine movement, pioneered by Dr. David Sackett, has broadened to the use of best evidence by *all* health care practitioners. EBP has been considered a major paradigm shift in health care education and practice. With EBP, skillful clinicians can no longer rely on a repository of memorized information, but rather must be adept in accessing, evaluating, and using new research evidence.

### Types of Evidence and Evidence Hierarchies

There is no consensus about what constitutes usable evidence for EBP, but there is general agreement that findings from rigorous research are paramount. Yet, there is some debate about what constitutes "*rigorous*" research and what qualifies as "*best*" evidence.

Early in the EBP movement, there was a strong bias toward reliance on evidence from a type of study called a *randomized controlled trial* (RCT). This bias reflected the Cochrane Collaboration's initial focus on evidence about the effectiveness of therapies, rather than about broader health care questions. RCTs are especially well suited for drawing conclusions about the effects of health care interventions (see Chapter 9). The bias in ranking research approaches in terms of questions about effective therapies led to some resistance to EBP by nurses who felt that evidence from qualitative and non-RCT studies would be ignored.

Positions about the contribution of various types of evidence are less rigid than previously. Nevertheless, there are many published **evidence hierarchies** that purport to rank evidence sources according to the strength of the evidence they provide. We offer a modified evidence hierarchy that looks similar to others that are available in material on EBP, but ours illustrates that the ranking of evidence-producing strategies depends on the type of question being asked.

Figure 2.1 shows that systematic reviews are at the pinnacle of the hierarchy (level I), because the strongest evidence comes from careful syntheses of multiple studies. The next highest level (level II) depends on the nature of inquiry. For Therapy questions regarding the efficacy of a therapy or intervention (what works best for improving health outcomes?),

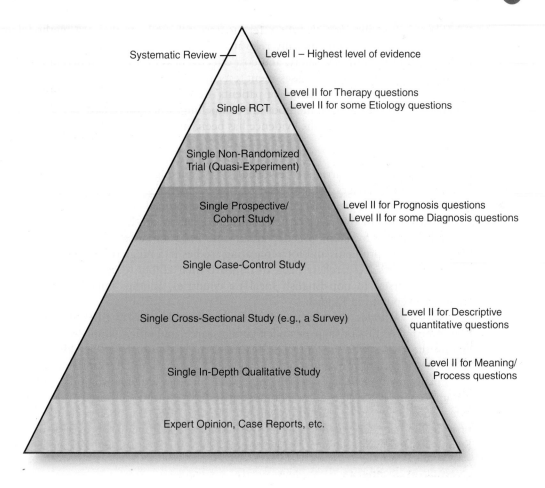

**FIGURE 2.1** ● Evidence hierarchy: levels of evidence.

individual RCTs constitute level II evidence (systematic reviews of multiple RCTs are level I). Going down the "rungs" of the evidence hierarchy for Therapy questions results in less reliable evidence—for example, level III evidence comes from a type of study called quasi-experiment. In-depth qualitative studies are near the bottom, in terms of evidence regarding intervention effectiveness. (Terms in Fig. 2.1 will be discussed in later chapters.)

For a Prognosis question, by contrast, level II evidence comes from a single prospective cohort study, and level III is from a type of study called case-control (level I evidence is from a systematic review of cohort studies). Thus, contrary to what is often implied in discussions of evidence hierarchies, multiple hierarchies are a reality. If one is interested in best evidence for questions about Meaning, an RCT would be a poor source of evidence, for example. We have tried to portray the notion of multiple hierarchies in Figure 2.1, with information on the right indicating the type of *individual study* that would offer the best evidence (level II) for different questions. In all cases, appropriate systematic reviews are at the pinnacle. Information about different hierarchies for different types of cause-probing questions is addressed in Chapter 9.

Of course, *within* any level in an evidence hierarchy, evidence quality can vary considerably. For example, an individual RCT could be well designed, yielding strong level II evidence for Therapy questions, or it could be so flawed that the evidence would be weak.

Thus, in nursing, *best evidence* refers to research findings that are methodologically appropriate, rigorous, and clinically relevant for answering pressing questions—questions not only about the efficacy, safety, and cost effectiveness of nursing interventions, but also about the reliability of nursing assessment tests, the causes and consequences of health problems, and the meaning and nature of patients' experiences. Confidence in the evidence is enhanced when the research methods are compelling, when there have been multiple confirmatory studies, and when the evidence has been carefully evaluated and synthesized.

### EBP Challenges

Studies that explored barriers to evidence-based nursing yielded similar results in many countries. Most barriers fall into one of three categories: (1) quality and nature of the research, (2) characteristics of nurses, and (3) organizational factors.

With regard to the research itself, one problem is the limited availability of strong research evidence for some practice areas. The need for research that directly addresses pressing clinical problems and for replicating studies in a range of settings remains a challenge. Also, nurse researchers need to improve their ability to communicate evidence to practicing nurses. In non-English speaking countries, another impediment is that most studies are reported in English.

Nurses' attitudes and education are also potential barriers to EBP. Studies have found that some nurses do not value or understand research, and others simply resist change. And, among the nurses who *do* appreciate research, many do not have the skills for accessing research evidence or for evaluating it for possible use in clinical decision making.

Finally, many challenges to using research in practice are organizational. "Unit culture" can undermine research use, and administrative or organizational barriers also play a major role. Although many organizations support the idea of EBP in theory, they do not always provide the necessary supports in terms of staff release time and provision of resources. Strong leadership in health care organizations is essential to making EBP happen.

# RESOURCES FOR EVIDENCE-BASED PRACTICE

In this section we describe some of the resources that are available to support EBP and to address some of the challenges.

## Preappraised Evidence

Research evidence comes in various forms, the most basic of which is from individual studies. *Primary studies* published in journals are not preappraised for quality and use in practice.

Preprocessed (preappraised) evidence is evidence that has been selected from primary studies and evaluated for use by clinicians. DiCenso and colleagues (2005) have described a hierarchy of preprocessed evidence. On the first rung above primary studies are synopses of single studies, followed by systematic reviews, and then synopses of systematic reviews. Clinical practice guidelines are at the top of the hierarchy. At each successive step in the hierarchy, there is greater ease in applying the evidence to clinical practice.

Synopses of systematic reviews and of single studies are available in evidence-based abstract journals. For example, *Evidence-Based Nursing*, published quarterly, presents critical summaries of studies and systematic reviews from hundreds of journals. The summaries include commentaries on the clinical implications of each reviewed study. Another journal-based resource is the "evidence digest" feature in each issue of *Worldviews on Evidence-Based Nursing*. In the remainder of this section, we focus on two important types of preappraised evidence: systematic reviews and clinical practice guidelines.

## Systematic Reviews

EBP relies on meticulous integration of all key evidence on a topic so that well-grounded conclusions can be drawn about EBP questions. A systematic review is not just a literature review. A systematic review is in itself a methodical, scholarly inquiry that follows many of the same steps as those for other studies.

Systematic reviews can take various forms. One form is a narrative (qualitative) integration that merges and synthesizes findings, much like a rigorous literature review. For integrating evidence from quantitative studies, narrative reviews increasingly are being replaced by a type of systematic review known as a meta-analysis.

**Meta-analysis** is a technique for integrating quantitative research findings statistically. In essence, meta-analysis treats the findings from a study as one piece of information. The findings from multiple studies on the same topic are combined and then all of the information is analyzed statistically in a manner similar to that in a usual study. Thus, instead of study participants being the *unit of analysis* (the most basic entity on which the analysis focuses), individual studies are the unit of analysis in a meta-analysis. Meta-analysis provides an objective method of integrating a body of findings and of observing patterns that might not have been detected.

**Example of a meta-analysis:**
Nam and colleagues (2012) conducted a meta-analysis to analyze evidence on the effectiveness of culturally tailored diabetes education interventions in ethnic minorities with Type 2 diabetes. Integrating results from 12 intervention studies, the researchers concluded that such interventions are effective for improving glycemic control among ethnic minorities. (This study appears in its entirety in *Study Guide for Essentials of Nursing Research, 8e*). 📖

For qualitative studies, integration may take the form of a **metasynthesis**. A metasynthesis, however, is distinct from a quantitative meta-analysis: a metasynthesis is less about reducing information and more about interpreting it.

**Example of a metasynthesis:**
Duggleby and colleagues (2012) undertook a metasynthesis of studies exploring the hope experience of older persons with chronic illness. Their metasynthesis of 20 qualitative studies identified five main themes that captured important concepts that emerged in the 20 studies.

Fortunately, systematic reviews are increasingly available. Such reviews are published in professional journals that can be accessed using standard literature search procedures (see Chapter 7), and are also available in databases that are dedicated to such reviews. In particular, the Cochrane Database of Systematic Reviews (CDSR) contains thousands of systematic reviews relating to health care interventions.

☞ **TIP:** Websites with useful content relating to EBP, including ones for locating systematic reviews, are in the Internet Resources file on thePoint for you to access simply by using the "Control/Click" feature. ✺

## Clinical Practice Guidelines

Evidence-based **clinical practice guidelines** distill a body of evidence into a usable form. Unlike systematic reviews, clinical practice guidelines (which often are *based* on systematic reviews) give specific recommendations for evidence-based decision making. Guideline development typically involves the consensus of a group of researchers, experts, and clinicians. The use or adaptation of a clinical practice guideline is often an ideal focus for an EBP project.

> **Example of a nursing clinical practice guideline:**
> In 2009, the Registered Nurses Association of Ontario issued an evidence-based practice guideline on the care and management of ostomies. Developed by an interdisciplinary panel under the leadership of Kathryn Kozell, the guideline provides nurses with an evidence-based summary of strategies to assess and manage people with various types of ostomy.

Finding clinical practice guidelines can be challenging, because there is no single guideline repository. A standard search in bibliographic databases such as MEDLINE (see Chapter 7) will yield many references—but could yield a mixture of citations to not only the actual guidelines, but also to commentaries, implementation studies, and so on.

A recommended approach is to search in guideline databases, or through specialty organizations that have sponsored guideline development. A few of the many possible sources deserve mention. In the United States, nursing and health care guidelines are maintained by the National Guideline Clearinghouse (www.guideline.gov). In Canada, the Registered Nurses Association of Ontario (RNAO) (www.rnao.org/bestpractices) maintains information about clinical practice guidelines. Two sources in the United Kingdom are the Translating Research into Practice (TRIP) database and the National Institute for Clinical Excellence (NICE).

There are many topics for which practice guidelines have not yet been developed, but the opposite problem is also true: sometimes there are multiple guidelines on the same topic. Worse yet, because of differences in the rigor of guideline development and interpretation of evidence, different guidelines sometimes offer different or even conflicting recommendations (Lewis, 2001). Thus, those who wish to adopt clinical practice guidelines should appraise them to identify ones that are based on the strongest evidence, have been meticulously developed, are user-friendly, and are appropriate for local use or adaptation.

Several appraisal instruments are available to evaluate clinical practice guidelines, but one with broad support is the Appraisal of Guidelines Research and Evaluation (AGREE) Instrument (AGREE Collaboration, 2001; www.agreecollaboration.org). The AGREE instrument has ratings for 23 dimensions within six domains (e.g., scope and purpose, rigor of development, presentation). As examples, a dimension in the Scope and Purpose domain is: "The patients to whom the guideline is meant to apply are specifically described"; and one in the Rigor of Development domain is: "The guideline has been externally reviewed by experts prior to its publication." The AGREE tool should be applied to a guideline by a team of two to four appraisers.

 **TIP:** Clinical decision support tools based on research evidence are becoming increasingly available in easily accessible forms like personal digital assistants or PDAs. Mechanisms for speedy guidance on best practice are likely to proliferate in the future.

## Models of the EBP Process

EBP models offer frameworks for designing and implementing EBP projects in practice settings. Some models focus on the use of research from the perspective of individual clinicians (e.g., the Stetler Model, one of the oldest models that originated as an RU model), but most focus on institutional EBP efforts (e.g., the Iowa Model). The many worthy EBP models are too numerous to list comprehensively, but include the following:

- ⊙ ACE Star Model of Knowledge Transformation (Academic Center for EBP, 2009)
- ⊙ Advancing Research and Clinical Practice Through Close Collaboration (ARCC) Model (Melnyk & Fineout-Overholt, 2011)
- ⊙ Clinical Nurse Scholar Model (Schultz, 2005)
- ⊙ Diffusion of Innovations Theory (Rogers, 2003)
- ⊙ Iowa Model of Evidence-Based Practice to Promote Quality Care (Titler et al., 2001)
- ⊙ Johns Hopkins Nursing EBP Model (Newhouse et al., 2005)
- ⊙ Model for Change to Evidence-Based Practice (Rosswurm & Larabee, 1999)
- ⊙ Promoting Action on Research Implementation in Health Services (PARiHS) Model, (Rycroft-Malone et al., 2002)
- ⊙ Stetler Model of Research Utilization (Stetler, 2001)

For those wishing to follow a formal EBP model, the cited references should be consulted. Several are also nicely synthesized by Melnyk and Fineout-Overholt (2011). Each model offers different perspectives on how to translate research findings into practice, but several steps and procedures are similar across the models. We provide an overview of key activities and processes in EBP efforts, based on a distillation of common elements from the various models, in a subsequent section of this chapter. We rely especially heavily on the Iowa Model, a diagram for which is shown in Figure 2.2.

☞ **TIP:** The most prominent of the EBP models have been the PARiHS model, the Stetler Model, the Johns Hopkins model, and the Iowa Model. Gawlinski and Rutledge (2008) offer suggestions for selecting an EBP model.

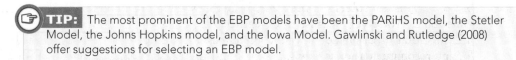

# EBP IN INDIVIDUAL NURSING PRACTICE

This and the following section provide an overview of how research can be put to use in clinical settings. We first discuss strategies and steps for individual clinicians and then describe activities used by organizations or teams of nurses.

## Clinical Scenarios and the Need for Evidence

Individual nurses make many decisions and are called upon to provide health care advice, and so they have ample opportunity to put research into practice. Here are four clinical scenarios that provide examples of such opportunities:

- ⊙ Clinical Scenario 1. You work on an intensive care unit and notice that *Clostridium difficile* infection has become more prevalent among surgical patients in your hospital. You want to know if there is a reliable screening tool for assessing the risk of infection so that preventive measures could be initiated in a more timely and effective manner.
- ⊙ Clinical Scenario 2. You work in an allergy clinic and notice how difficult it is for many children to undergo allergy scratch tests. You wonder if an interactive distraction intervention would help reduce children's pain when they are being tested for allergens.
- ⊙ Clinical Scenario 3. You work in a rehabilitation hospital and one of your elderly patients, who had total hip replacement, tells you she is planning a long airplane trip.

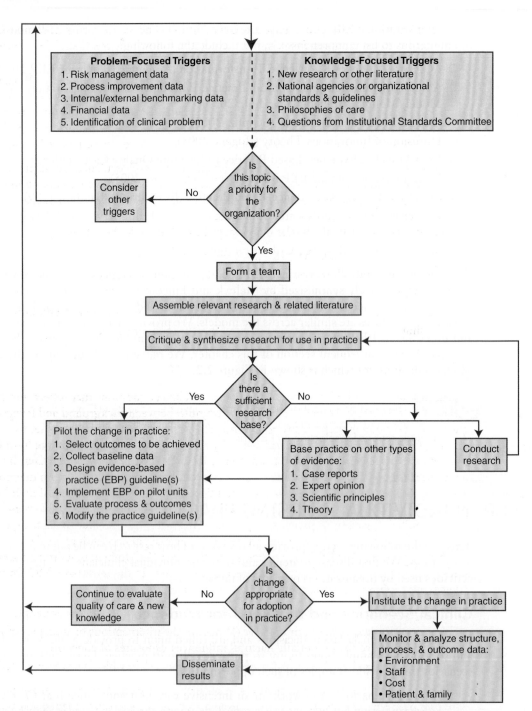

**FIGURE 2.2** ● Iowa model of evidence-based practice to promote quality care. (Adapted from Titler, M. G., Kleiber, C., Steelman, V., Rakel, B., Budreau, G., Everett, L., et al. (2001). The Iowa Model of Evidence-Based Practice to Promote Quality Care. *Critical Care Nursing Clinics of North America, 13,* 497–509.)

You know that a long plane ride will increase her risk of deep vein thrombosis and wonder if compression stockings are an effective in-flight treatment. You decide to look for the best possible evidence to answer this question.

○ Clinical Scenario 4. You are caring for a hospitalized cardiac patient who tells you that he has sleep apnea. He confides in you that he is reluctant to undergo continuous positive airway pressure (CPAP) treatment because he worries it will hinder intimacy with his wife. You wonder if there is any evidence about what it is like to undergo CPAP treatment so that you can better understand how to address your patient's concerns.

In these and thousands of other clinical situations, research evidence can be put to good use to improve nursing care. Some situations might lead to unit-wide or institution-wide scrutiny of current practices, but in other situations individual nurses can personally examine evidence to help address specific problems.

For individual EBP efforts, the major steps in EBP include the following:

1. Asking clinical questions that are answerable with research evidence
2. Searching for and collecting evidence that addresses the question
3. Appraising and synthesizing the evidence
4. Integrating the evidence with your own clinical expertise, patient preferences, and local context
5. Assessing the effectiveness of the decision, intervention, or advice

## Asking Clinical Questions: PIO and PICO

A crucial first step in EBP involves asking relevant clinical questions that reflect uncertainties in clinical practice. Some EBP writers distinguish between background and foreground questions. *Background questions* are foundational questions about a clinical issue, for example, what is cancer cachexia (progressive body wasting), and what is its pathophysiology? Answers to such questions are typically found in textbooks. *Foreground questions*, by contrast, are those that can be answered based on current best research evidence on diagnosing, assessing, or treating patients, or on understanding the meaning or prognosis of their health problems. For example, we may wonder, is a fish oil-enhanced nutritional supplement effective in stabilizing weight in patients with advanced cancer? The answer to such a question may provide guidance on how best to address the needs of patients with cachexia.

Most guidelines for EBP use the acronyms PIO or PICO to help practitioners develop well-worded questions that facilitate a search for evidence. In the most basic PIO form, the clinical question is worded to identify three components:

1. P: the *population* or *patients* (What are the characteristics of the patients or people?)
2. I: the *intervention, influence,* or *exposure* (What are the interventions or therapies of interest? or, What are the potentially harmful influences/exposures of concern?)
3. O: the *outcomes* (What are the outcomes or consequences in which we are interested?)

Applying this scheme to our question about cachexia, our *population* (P) is cancer patients with cachexia; the *intervention* (I) is fish oil-enhanced nutritional supplements; and the *outcome* (O) is weight stabilization. As another example, in the second clinical scenario about scratch tests cited earlier, the population is children being tested for allergies; the intervention is interactive distraction; and the outcome is pain.

For questions that can best be answered with qualitative information (e.g., about the meaning of an experience or health problem), two components are most relevant:

1. The *population* (What are the characteristics of the patients or clients?
2. The *situation* (What conditions, experiences, or circumstances are we interested in understanding?)

For example, suppose our question was, What is it like to suffer from cachexia? In this case, the question calls for rich qualitative information; the *population* is patients with advanced cancer and the *situation* is the experience of cachexia.

In addition to the basic PIO components, other components are sometimes important in an evidence search. In particular, a comparison (C) component may be needed, when the intervention or influence of interest is contrasted with a specific alternative. For example, we might be interested in learning whether fish oil-enhanced supplements (I) are better than melatonin (C) in stabilizing weight (O) in cancer patients (P). When a *specific* comparison is of interest, a PICO question is required, but if we were interested in uncovering evidence about *all* alternatives to the intervention of primary interest, then PIO components are sufficient. (By contrast, when asking questions to undertake an actual *study*, the "C" must always be specified).

> **TIP:** Other components may be relevant, such as a time frame or "T" (for PICOT questions) or a setting or "S" (for PICOS questions).

Table 2.1 offers templates for asking well-worded clinical questions for different types of foreground questions. The right hand column includes questions with an explicit comparison (PICO), while the middle column does not have a comparison (PIO). The questions are categorized in a manner similar to that discussed in Chapter 1 (EBP Purposes), as featured in Table 1.3 on page 14. One exception is that we have added Description as a category. Note that although there are some differences in components across question types, there is always a P component.

> **TIP:** It is crucial to practice asking clinical questions—it is the starting point for evidence-based nursing. Take some time to fill in the blanks in Table 2.1 for each question category. Do not be too self-critical at this point. Your comfort in developing questions will increase over time. Chapter 2 of *Study Guide for Essentials of Nursing Research, 8e* offers additional opportunities for you to practice asking well-worded questions.

## Finding Research Evidence

By wording clinical queries as PIO or PICO questions, you should be able to search the research literature for the information you need. Using the templates in Table 2.1, the information you insert into the blanks constitutes *key words* that can be used in an electronic search.

For an individual EBP endeavor, the best place to begin is by searching for evidence in a systematic review, clinical practice guideline, or other preprocessed sources because this approach leads to a quicker answer—and, if your methodologic skills are limited, potentially a superior answer as well. Researchers who prepare reviews and clinical guidelines typically are well trained in research methods and use rigorous standards in evaluating the evidence. Moreover, preprocessed evidence is often prepared by a team, which means that the conclusions are cross-checked and fairly objective. Thus, when preprocessed evidence is available to answer a clinical question, you may not need to look any farther—unless the review is outdated. When preprocessed evidence cannot be located or is old, you will need to look for best evidence in primary studies, using strategies we describe in Chapter 7.

> **TIP:** Searching for evidence for an EBP project has been greatly simplified in recent years. Guidance on doing an evidence-based search is available in the Chapter Supplement for Chapter 7 (the chapter on literature reviews) on the thePoint website.

**TABLE 2.1    Question Templates for Selected Clinical Foreground Questions: PIO and PICO**

| Type of Question | PIO Question Template (Questions Without an Explicit Comparison) | PICO Question Template (Questions With an Explicit Comparison) |
|---|---|---|
| Therapy/treatment/intervention | In _____ (**P**opulation), what is the effect of _____ (**I**ntervention) on _____ (**O**utcome)? | In _____ (**P**opulation), what is the effect of _____ (**I**ntervention), in comparison to _____ (**C**omparative/alternative intervention), on _____ (**O**utcome)? |
| Diagnosis/assessment | For _____ (**P**opulation), does _____ (**I**dentifying tool/procedure) yield accurate and appropriate diagnostic/assessment information about _____ (**O**utcome)? | For _____ (**P**opulation), does _____ (**I**dentifying tool/procedure) yield more accurate or more appropriate diagnostic/assessment information than _____ (**C**omparative tool/procedure) about _____ (**O**utcome)? |
| Prognosis | For _____ (**P**opulation), does _____ (**E**xposure to disease or condition) increase the risk of _____ (**O**utcome)? | For _____ (**P**opulation), does _____ (**E**xposure to disease or condition), relative to _____ (**C**omparative disease or condition) increase the risk of _____ (**O**utcome)? |
| Etiology/harm | In _____ (**P**opulation), does _____ (**I**nfluence, exposure, or characteristic) increase the risk of _____ (**O**utcome)? | Does _____ (**I**nfluence, exposure, or characteristic) increase the risk of _____ (**O**utcome) compared to _____ (**C**omparative influence, exposure or condition) in _____ (**P**opulation)? |
| Description (prevalence/incidence) | In _____ (**P**opulation), how prevalent is _____ (**O**utcome)? | *Explicit comparisons are not typical, except to compare different populations* |
| Meaning or process | What is it like for _____ (**P**opulation) to experience _____ (condition, illness, circumstance)?<br><br>**OR**<br><br>What is the process by which _____ (**P**opulation) cope with, adapt to, or live with _____ (condition, illness, circumstance)? | *Explicit comparisons are not typical in these types of questions* |

## Appraising the Evidence for EBP

Evidence should be appraised before clinical action is taken. The critical appraisal of evidence for the purposes of EBP may involve several types of assessments (Box 2.1), but often focuses primarily on evidence quality.

> ### BOX 2.1 Questions for Appraising the Evidence
>
> **1.** What is the quality of the evidence—i.e., how rigorous and reliable is it?
> **2.** What *is* the evidence—what is the magnitude of effects?
> **3.** How precise is the estimate of effects?
> **4.** What evidence is there of any side effects/side benefits?
> **5.** What is the financial cost of applying (and not applying) the evidence?
> **6.** Is the evidence relevant to my particular clinical situation?

## Evidence Quality

The overriding appraisal issue is the extent to which the findings are valid. That is, were the study methods sufficiently rigorous that the evidence can be believed? Ideally, you would find preappraised evidence, but a goal of this book is to help you evaluate research evidence yourself. If there are several primary studies and no existing systematic review, you would need to draw conclusions about the body of evidence taken as a whole. Clearly, you would want to put most weight on the most rigorous studies.

## Magnitude of Effects

You would also need to assess whether study findings are clinically important. This criterion considers not whether the results are "real," but how powerful the effects are. For example, consider clinical scenario 3 cited earlier, which suggests this question: Does the use of compression stockings lower the risk of flight-related deep vein thrombosis for high-risk patients? In our search, we found a relevant systematic review in the nursing literature—a meta-analysis of nine RCTs (Hsieh & Lee, 2005)—and another in the Cochrane database (Clarke et al., 2006). The conclusion of these reviews, based on reliable evidence, was that compression stockings are effective and the magnitude of the risk-reducing effect is fairly substantial. Thus, advice about using compression stockings may be appropriate, pending an appraisal of other factors. The magnitude of effects can be quantified in various ways, and several are described later in this book.

## Precision of Estimates

Another consideration, relevant when the evidence is quantitative, is how precise the estimate of effect is. This level of appraisal requires some statistical sophistication and so we postpone our discussion of *confidence intervals* to Chapter 12. Suffice it to say that research results provide only an *estimate* of effects and it may be useful to understand not only the exact estimate, but also the range within which the actual effect probably lies.

## Peripheral Effects

Even if the evidence is judged to be valid and the magnitude of effects is sizeable, peripheral benefits and costs may be important in guiding decisions. In framing your clinical question, you would have identified the outcomes (O) in which you were interested—for example, weight stabilization for an intervention to address cancer cachexia. Research on this topic, however, would likely have considered other outcomes that need to be taken into account—for example, quality of life, comfort, and side effects.

## Financial Costs

Another issue concerns the costs of applying the evidence. Costs sometimes may be small or nonexistent. For example, in clinical scenario 4 concerning the experience of CPAP treatment, nursing action would be cost-neutral because the evidence would be used to reassure and inform patients. When interventions and assessment protocols are costly, however, the resources needed to put best evidence into practice need to be estimated and factored into any decision. Of course, although the cost of a clinical decision needs to be considered, the cost of *not* taking action is equally important.

### Clinical Relevance

Finally, it is important to appraise the evidence in terms of its relevance for the clinical situation at hand—that is, for *your* patient in a specific clinical setting. Best practice evidence can most readily be applied to an individual patient in your care if he or she is sufficiently similar to people in the study or studies under review. Would your patient have qualified for participation in the study—or would some factor (e.g., age, illness severity, comorbidities) have disqualified him or her? DiCenso and colleagues (2005), who advised clinicians to ask whether there is a compelling reason to conclude that results may *not* be applicable in their clinical situation, have written some useful tips on applying evidence to individual patients.

### Actions Based on Evidence Appraisals

Appraisals of the evidence may lead you to different courses of action. You may reach this point on your EBP quest and conclude that the evidence base is not sufficiently sound, or that the likely effect is too small, or that the cost of applying the evidence is too high. The evidence appraisal may suggest that "usual care" is the best strategy. If, however, the initial appraisal of evidence suggests a promising clinical action, then you can proceed to the next step.

## Integrating Evidence in EBP

Research evidence needs to be integrated with other types of information, including your own clinical expertise and knowledge of your clinical setting. You may be aware of factors that would make implementation of the evidence, no matter how sound and how promising, inadvisable. Patient preferences and values are also important. A discussion with the patient may reveal strong negative attitudes toward a potentially beneficial course of action, or possible impediments (e.g., lack of health insurance).

One final issue is the desirability of integrating evidence from qualitative research. Qualitative research can provide rich insights about how patients experience a problem, or about barriers to complying with a treatment. A potentially beneficial intervention may fail to achieve desired outcomes if it is not implemented with sensitivity to the patients' perspectives. As Morse (2005) so aptly noted, evidence from an RCT may tell us whether a pill is effective, but qualitative research can help you understand why patients may not swallow the pill.

## Implementing the Evidence and Evaluating Outcomes

After the first four steps of the EBP process have been completed, you can use the integrated information to make an evidence-based decision or to provide evidence-based advice. Although the steps in the process, as just described, may seem complicated, in reality the process can be quite efficient—*if* there is adequate evidence, and especially if it has been skillfully preprocessed. EBP is most challenging when findings from research are contradictory, inconclusive, or "thin"—that is, when better quality evidence is needed.

One last step in an individual EBP effort concerns evaluation. Part of the evaluation process involves following up to determine if your actions achieved the desired outcome. Another part, however, concerns an evaluation of how well you are performing EBP. Sackett and colleagues (2000) offer self-evaluation questions that relate to the previous EBP steps, such as asking answerable questions (Am I asking any clinical questions at all? Am I asking well-worded questions?), and finding external evidence (Do I know the best sources of current evidence? Am I efficient in my searching?). A self-appraisal may lead to the conclusion that at least some of the clinical questions of interest to you are best addressed as a group effort.

# EBP IN AN ORGANIZATIONAL CONTEXT

For some clinical scenarios, individual nurses may be able to implement EBP strategies on their own (e.g., giving advice about compression stockings). Many situations, however, require decision making by an organization, or by a team of nurses working to solve a recurrent problem. This section describes some additional issues that are relevant to institutional efforts at EBP—efforts designed to result in a formal policy or protocol affecting the practice of many nurses.

Many of the steps in organizational EBP projects are similar to the ones described in the previous section. For example, gathering and appraising evidence are key activities in both, as shown in the Iowa Model in Figure 2.2 on page 28 (Assemble relevant research; critique and synthesize research). Additional issues are relevant at the organizational level, however, including the selection of a problem, an assessment of whether the topic is a priority for the organization, deciding whether the evidence is sufficiently sound to implement on a trial basis, and deciding, based on the trial, whether the innovation should be adopted into practice. We briefly discuss some of these topics.

## Selecting a Problem for an Institutional EBP Project

Some EBP projects originate in deliberations among clinicians who have encountered a recurrent problem and seek a resolution. Others, however, are "top-down" efforts in which administrators take steps to stimulate the use of research evidence among clinicians. This latter approach is increasingly likely to occur in United States hospitals as part of the Magnet recognition process.

Several models of EBP, such as the Iowa Model, have distinguished two types of stimulus ("triggers") for an EBP endeavor: (1) *problem-focused triggers*—the identification of a clinical practice problem in need of solution, or (2) *knowledge-focused triggers*—readings in the research literature. Problem-focused triggers may arise in the course of clinical practice (as in the case of the clinical scenarios described earlier) or in the context of quality-assessment or quality-improvement efforts. The problem-identification approach is likely to be clinically relevant and to have staff support if the problem is one that numerous nurses have encountered.

A second catalyst for an EBP project is the research literature—knowledge-focused triggers, which is the origin akin to RU. The catalyst might be a new clinical guideline or a research article discussed in a journal club. With knowledge-focused triggers, the clinical relevance and applicability of the research might need to be assessed. The central issue is whether a problem of significance to nurses in that particular setting will be solved by making a change or introducing an innovation. Using concepts from Rogers' Diffusion of Innovations Model, Titler and Everett (2001) offer suggestions for selecting interventions to test.

## Appraising Implementation Potential

With either type of trigger, an important issue concerns the feasibility of undertaking an EBP project in a particular organizational setting. In the Iowa Model (Fig. 2.2), the first major decision point involves determining whether the topic is a priority for the organization considering practice changes. Titler and colleagues (2001) advised considering the following issues before finalizing a topic for EBP: the topic's fit with the organization's strategic plan; the magnitude of the problem; the number of people invested in the problem; support of nurse leaders and of those in other disciplines; costs; and possible barriers to change.

Some EBP models recommend a formal assessment of organizational "fit," often called **implementation potential** (or, *environmental readiness*). In determining the implementation potential of an innovation in a particular setting, several issues should be considered, particularly the transferability of the innovation (i.e., the extent to which the innovation might be appropriate in new settings), the feasibility of implementing it, and its cost-benefit ratio.

> **☞ TIP:** For those interested in learning more about assessments of implementation potential, we offer an expanded summary in the Chapter Supplements on thePoint website. ☀

If the implementation assessment suggests that there might be problems in testing the innovation in that particular practice setting, then the team can either identify a new problem and begin the process anew or consider adopting a plan to improve the implementation potential (e.g., seeking external resources if costs are prohibitive).

## Evidence Appraisals and Subsequent Actions

In the Iowa Model, the second major decision relies on the synthesis and appraisal of research evidence. The crux of the decision concerns whether the research base is sufficient to justify an evidence-based change—for example, whether an existing clinical practice guideline is of sufficiently high quality that it can be used or adapted, or whether the research evidence is sufficiently rigorous to recommend a practice innovation.

Assessments about the adequacy of the evidence can lead to different action paths. If the research evidence is weak or inconclusive, the team could assemble nonresearch evidence (e.g., through consultation with experts or client surveys) to determine the benefit of a practice change. Another option is to conduct an original study to address the practice question, thereby gathering new evidence. This course of action may be impractical, and would result in years of delay.

If, on the other hand, there is a solid research base or a high-quality clinical practice guideline, then the team would develop plans for moving forward with implementing a practice innovation. A key activity usually involves developing or adapting a local evidence-based clinical practice protocol or guideline. Strategies for developing clinical practice guidelines are suggested in DiCenso et al. (2005) and Melnyk and Fineout-Overholt (2011). Whether a guideline is developed "from scratch" or adapted from an existing one, independent peer review is advisable to ensure that the guidelines are clear, comprehensive, and congruent with best existing evidence.

## Implementing and Evaluating the Innovation

Once the EBP product has been developed, the next step is to **pilot test** it (give it a trial run) and evaluate the outcome. Building on the Iowa Model, this phase of the project likely would involve the following activities:

1. Developing an evaluation plan (e.g., identifying outcomes to be achieved, determining how many clients to include, deciding when and how often to measure outcomes).
2. Measuring client outcomes prior to implementing the innovation, so that there is a comparison against which the outcomes of the innovation can be assessed.

3. Training relevant staff in the use of the new guideline and, if necessary, "marketing" the innovation to users.

4. Trying the guideline out on one or more units or with a group of clients.

5. Evaluating the pilot project, in terms of both process (e.g., how was the innovation received, what problems were encountered?) and outcomes (e.g., how were client outcomes affected, what were the costs?).

A fairly informal evaluation may be adequate, but formal efforts are often appropriate and provide opportunities for dissemination to others at conferences or in professional journals.

---

 **TIP:** Every nurse can play a role in using research evidence. Here are some strategies:

○ *Read widely and critically.* Professionally accountable nurses keep abreast of important developments and read journals relating to their specialty, including research reports in them.

○ *Attend professional conferences.* Studies with clinical relevance are presented at many nursing conferences. Conference attendees get opportunities to meet researchers and to explore practice implications.

○ *Become involved in a journal club.* Many hospitals sponsor journal clubs that review studies with potential relevance to practice. Online journal clubs that acknowledge time constraints and the inability of nurses from all shifts to come together at one time are increasingly common.

○ *Pursue and participate in EBP projects.* Several studies have found that nurses who are involved in research-related activities (e.g., an EBP project or data collection activities) develop more positive attitudes toward research and better research skills.

---

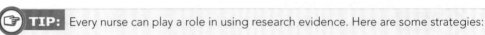

## RESEARCH EXAMPLES WITH CRITICAL THINKING EXERCISES

Example 1 below is also featured in our *Interactive Critical Thinking Activity* on thePoint website where you can easily record, print, and e-mail your responses to the related questions.

### EXAMPLE 1 ● **Research Translation Project**

Hundreds of projects to translate research evidence into nursing practice are underway worldwide. Those that have been described in the nursing literature offer good information about planning and implementing such an endeavor. In this section we summarize such a project.

**Study:** Care of the patient with enteral tube feeding: An evidence-based protocol (Kenny & Goodman, 2010)

**Purpose:** The TriService Nursing Research Program sought to create a culture of incorporating best evidence into nursing practices in military hospitals throughout the United States. Kenny and Goodman's article described a protocol development and testing project that was implemented at a large military medical center under that initiative. The project's purpose was to understand the evidence for managing enteral tube feedings in adult patients, to develop and implement an evidence-based protocol, and to evaluate its effects. A secondary aim was to educate the nursing staff about the EBP process.

**Framework:** The project used the Iowa Model as its guiding framework. The team's decision to select enteral feedings was based on a sentinel event.

*(continues on page 37)*

**Protocol Development:** When the project began, nursing practice relating to enteral feedings in the medical center was based on tradition, and varied from nurse to nurse. The topic had support from clinical nursing staff and administrators, and fit with organizational priorities. The project team included nurses, a physician, a clinical nurse specialist, and a nutrition care specialist. The team met for about 6 months to review evidence and develop a protocol. The work began with a thorough review and evaluation of existing evidence on managing enteral tube feedings. The evidence was not especially strong, but the team identified many practices with sufficient research support to craft a set of recommendations. The team developed relevant educational materials (e.g., one-page *Nursing Cliff Notes*, tabletop education in acrylic sign holders), and offered inservice sessions on each ward to explain the new protocol.

**Evaluation:** Project outcomes were assessed at three levels: patient, nursing, and organization. Patient outcomes were assessed using anecdotal reports of tube clogging incidents. Nursing outcomes included knowledge of the evidence base (measured before and after protocol implementation), and process measures to examine compliance with the new protocol. The organizational outcome was actions by executives demonstrating support of the EBP model.

**Findings and Conclusions:** Anecdotal data supported a tentative conclusion of better patient outcomes (e.g., a decrease in clogged tubes). There was a significant increase in staff knowledge and implementation of evidence-based processes. The authors concluded that "The project has infused the creation of a culture of value for EBP from the level of the clinical staff nurse to the nursing executive level" (p. S29).

## CRITICAL THINKING EXERCISES

1. Of the EBP-focused research purposes (Table 1.3, p. 14), which purpose was the central focus of this project?
2. Using the template in Table 2.1 on page 31, phrase a clinical question that the EBP team might have asked when they were searching for evidence for their project. The questions might be about tube placement, tube management, prevention of aspiration, and so on.
3. Would you say that this project had a knowledge-focused or problem-focused trigger?

## EXAMPLE 2 ● Quantitative Research in Appendix A
- Read the abstract and the introduction from the Howell and colleagues' (2007) study ("Anxiety, anger, and blood pressure in children") in Appendix A on pages 395–402.

## CRITICAL THINKING EXERCISES

1. Identify one or more clinical foreground questions that, if posed, would be addressed by this study. Which PIO or PICO components do your questions capture?
2. How, if at all, might evidence from this study be used in an EBP project (individual or organizational)?

## EXAMPLE 3 ● Qualitative Research in Appendix B
- Read the abstract and the introduction from Beck and Watson's (2010) study ("Subsequent childbirth after a previous traumatic birth") in Appendix B on pages 403–412.

## CRITICAL THINKING EXERCISES

1. Identify one or more clinical foreground questions that, if posed, would be addressed by this study. Which PIO or PICO components do your questions capture?
2. How, if at all, might evidence from this study be used in an EBP project (individual or organizational)?

**WANT TO KNOW MORE?** A wide variety of resources to enhance your learning and understanding of this chapter are available on the**Point**.

- Interactive Critical Thinking Activity
- Chapter Supplement on Assessing Implementation Potential for EBP Projects
- Answers to the Critical Thinking Exercises for Examples 2 and 3
- Student Review Questions
- Full-text online
- Internet Resources with useful websites for Chapter 2

Additional study aids including eight journal articles and related questions are also available in *Study Guide for Essentials of Nursing Research, 8e.*

## SUMMARY POINTS

- **Evidence-based practice (EBP)** is the conscientious use of current best evidence in making clinical decisions about patient care; it is a clinical problem-solving strategy that de-emphasizes decision making based on custom and emphasizes the integration of research evidence with clinical expertise and patient preferences.

- **Research utilization (RU)** and EBP are overlapping concepts that concern efforts to use research as a basis for clinical decisions, but RU *starts* with a research-based innovation that gets evaluated for possible use in practice.

- Nurse researchers have undertaken several major utilization projects, such as the *Conduct and Utilization of Research in Nursing* or *CURN* project.

- Two underpinnings of the EBP movement are the **Cochrane Collaboration** (which is based on the work of British epidemiologist Archie Cochrane), and the clinical learning strategy developed at the McMaster Medical School called *evidence-based medicine.*

- EBP involves evaluating evidence to determine *best evidence*; often an **evidence hierarchy** is used to rank study findings according to the strength of evidence provided, but different hierarchies are appropriate for different types of questions. In all evidence hierarchies, however, *systematic reviews* are at the pinnacle.

- **Systematic reviews** are rigorous integrations of research evidence from multiple studies on a topic. Systematic reviews can involve either narrative approaches to integration (including **metasynthesis** of qualitative studies), or quantitative methods (**meta-analysis**) that integrate findings statistically.

- Evidence-based **clinical practice guidelines** combine an appraisal of research evidence with specific recommendations for clinical decisions.

- Many models of EBP have been developed, including models that provide a framework for individual clinicians (e.g., the *Stetler model*) and others for organizations or teams of clinicians (e.g., the *Iowa Model*).

- Individual nurses have opportunities to put research into practice. The five basic steps for individual EBP are: (1) asking an answerable clinical question; (2) searching for relevant research-based evidence; (3) appraising and synthesizing the evidence; (4) integrating evidence with other factors; and (5) assessing effectiveness.

- One scheme for asking well-worded clinical questions involves four primary components, an acronym for which is PICO: Population (P), Intervention or influence (I), Comparison (C), and Outcome (O). When there is no explicit comparison, the acronym is PIO.

- An appraisal of the evidence involves such considerations as the validity of study findings; their clinical importance; the magnitude and precision of effects; associated costs and risks; and utility in a particular clinical situation.

- EBP in an organizational context involves many of the same steps as individual EBP efforts, but is more formalized and must take organizational factors into account.

- *Triggers* for an organizational project include both pressing clinical problems (*problem-focused*) and existing knowledge (*knowledge-focused*).

- Before an EBP-based guideline or protocol can be tested, there should be an assessment of its **implementation potential**, which includes the issues of transferability, feasibility, and the cost–benefit ratio of implementing a new practice in a clinical setting.

- Once an evidence-based protocol or guideline has been developed and deemed worthy of implementation, the EBP team can move forward with a **pilot test** of the innovation and an assessment of the outcomes prior to widespread adoption.

# REFERENCES FOR CHAPTER 2

Academic Center for Evidence-Based Practice (2009). ACE Star Model of Knowledge Transformation. Retrieved October 8, 2009, from http://www.acestar.uthscsa.edu

AGREE Collaboration (2001). *Appraisal of guidelines for research and evaluation: AGREE instrument*. Retrieved July, 2012, from www.agreecollaboration.org

Clarke, M., Hopewell, S., Juszczak, E., Eisinga, A., & Kjeldstrom, M. (2006). Compression stockings for preventing deep vein thrombosis in airline passengers. *Cochrane Database of Systematic Reviews*, CD004002.

DiCenso, A., Guyatt, G., & Ciliska, D. (2005). *Evidence-based nursing: A guide to clinical practice*. St. Louis, MO: Elsevier Mosby.

Duggleby, W., Hicks, D., Nekolaichuk, C., Holtslander, L. Williams, A., Chambers, T., et al. (2012). Hope, older adults, and chronic illness: A metasynthesis of qualitative research. *Journal of Advanced Nursing, 68*(6), 1211–1223.

Gawlinksi, A., & Rutledge, D. (2008). Selecting a model for evidence-based practice changes. *AACN Advanced Critical Care, 19*, 291–300.

Horsley, J. A., Crane, J., & Bingle, J. D. (1978). Research utilization as an organizational process. *Journal of Nursing Administration, 8*, 4–6.

Hsieh, H. F., & Lee, F. P. (2005). Graduated compression stockings as prophylaxis for flight-related venous thrombosis: Systematic literature review. *Journal of Advanced Nursing, 51*, 83–98.

Kenny, D. J., & Goodman, P. (2010). Care of the patient with enteral tube feeding: An evidence-based practice protocol. *Nursing Research, 59*, S22–S31.

Lewis, S. (2001). Further disquiet on the guidelines front. *Canadian Medical Association Journal, 154*, 180–181.

Melnyk, B. M., & Fineout-Overhold, E. (2011). *Evidence-based practice in nursing and healthcare: A guide to best practice* (2nd ed.). Philadelphia, PA: Lippincott Williams & Wilkins.

Morse, J. (2005). Beyond the clinical trial: Expanding criteria for evidence. *Qualitative Health Research, 15*, 3–4.

Nam, S., Janson, S., Stotts, N., Chesla, C., & Kroon. L. (2012). Effect of culturally tailored diabetes education in ethnic minorities with Type 2 diabetes: A meta-analysis. *Journal of Cardiovascular Nursing 27*, 505–518.

Newhouse, R., Dearholt, S., Poe, S., Pugh, L. C., & White, K. M. (2005). Evidence-based practice: A practical approach to implementation. *Journal of Nursing Administration, 35*, 35–40.

Rogers, E. M. (2003). *Diffusion of innovations* (5th ed.). New York: Free Press.

Rosswurm, M. A., & Larrabee, J. H. (1999). A model for change to evidence-based practice. *Image: The Journal of Nursing Scholarship, 31*, 317–322.

Rycroft-Malone, J., Seers, K., Titchen, A., Harvey, G., Kitson, A., & McCormack, B. (2002). Getting evidence into practice: Ingredients for change. *Nursing Standard, 16*, 38–43.

Sackett, D. L., Straus, S. E., Richardson, W. S., Rosenberg, W., & Haynes, R. B. (2000). *Evidence-based medicine: How to practice and teach EBM* (2nd ed.). Edinburgh, UK: Churchill Livingstone.

Schultz, A. (2005). Clinical scholars at the bedside. An EBP mentorship model for how nurses work today. Nursing Knowledge International, Sigma Theta Tau International, retrieved April 6, 2011, from http://www.nursingknowledge.org

Stetler, C. B. (2001). Updating the Stetler model of research utilization to facilitate evidence-based practice. *Nursing Outlook, 49*, 272–279.

Titler, M. G., & Everett, L. Q. (2001). Translating research into practice. Considerations for critical care investigators. *Critical Care Nursing Clinics of North America, 13*, 587–604.

Titler, M. G., Kleiber, C., Steelman, V., Rakel, B., Budreau, G., Everett, L., et al. (2001). The Iowa model of evidence-based practice to promote quality care. *Critical Care Nursing Clinics of North America, 13*, 497–509.

# 3 Key Concepts and Steps in Qualitative and Quantitative Research

## LEARNING OBJECTIVES

*On completing this chapter, you will be able to:*

● Define new terms presented in the chapter, and distinguish terms associated with quantitative and qualitative research

● Distinguish experimental and nonexperimental research

● Identify the three main disciplinary traditions for qualitative nursing research

● Describe the flow and sequence of activities in quantitative and qualitative research, and discuss why they differ

## KEY TERMS

| | | |
|---|---|---|
| Cause-and-effect (causal) relationship | Grounded theory | Quantitative data |
| Clinical trial | Hypothesis | Relationship |
| Concept | Independent variable | Research design |
| Conceptual definition | Informant | Sample |
| Construct | Intervention protocol | Saturation |
| Data | Literature review | Statistical analysis |
| Dependent variable | Nonexperimental research | Study participant |
| Emergent design | Observational research | Subject |
| Ethnography | Operational definition | Theme |
| Experimental research | Outcome variable | Variable |
| Gaining entrée | Phenomenology | |
| | Qualitative data | |

# THE BUILDING BLOCKS OF RESEARCH

Research, like any discipline, has its own language—its own *jargon*—and that jargon can sometimes be intimidating. We readily admit that the jargon is abundant and is sometimes confusing. A lot of research jargon used in nursing research has its roots in the social sciences, but sometimes different terms for the same concepts are used in medical research. Also, some terms are used by both qualitative and quantitative researchers, but others are used mainly by one or the other group. Please bear with us as we cover key terms that you will need to understand to read other chapters of this book.

## The Faces and Places of Research

When researchers answer a question through disciplined research—regardless of whether it is qualitative or quantitative—they are doing a **study** (or an *investigation*). Studies with

**TABLE 3.1  Key Terms in Quantitative and Qualitative Research**

| Concept | Quantitative Term | Qualitative Term |
|---|---|---|
| Person contributing information | Subject<br>Study participant<br>— | —<br>Study participant<br>Informant, key informant |
| Person undertaking the study | Researcher<br>Investigator | Researcher<br>Investigator |
| That which is being investigated | —<br>Concepts<br>Constructs<br>Variables | Phenomena<br>Concepts<br>—<br>— |
| Information gathered | Data (numerical values) | Data (narrative descriptions) |
| Connections between concepts | Relationships (cause-and-effect, associative) | Patterns of association |
| Logical reasoning processes | Deductive reasoning | Inductive reasoning |

humans involve two sets of people: those who do the research and those who provide the information. In a quantitative study, the people being studied are called **subjects** or **study participants**, as shown in Table 3.1. In a qualitative study, the people cooperating in the study are called study participants or **informants**. The person who conducts the research is the *researcher* or *investigator*. Studies are often undertaken by a research team rather than by a single researcher.

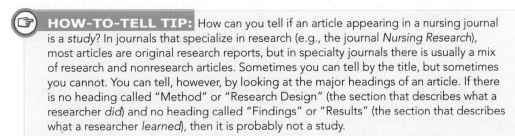

**HOW-TO-TELL TIP:** How can you tell if an article appearing in a nursing journal is a *study*? In journals that specialize in research (e.g., the journal *Nursing Research*), most articles are original research reports, but in specialty journals there is usually a mix of research and nonresearch articles. Sometimes you can tell by the title, but sometimes you cannot. You can tell, however, by looking at the major headings of an article. If there is no heading called "Method" or "Research Design" (the section that describes what a researcher *did*) and no heading called "Findings" or "Results" (the section that describes what a researcher *learned*), then it is probably not a study.

Research can be undertaken in a variety of *settings* (the types of place where information is gathered), for example, hospitals, homes, or other community settings. A *site* is the specific location for the research—it could be an entire community (e.g., a Haitian neighborhood in Miami) or an institution (e.g., a clinic in Seattle). Researchers sometimes do *multisite studies* because the use of multiple sites offers a larger and often more diverse sample of participants.

## Concepts, Constructs, and Theories

Research involves real-world problems, but studies are conceptualized in abstract terms. For example, *pain*, *fatigue*, and *resilience* are all abstractions of particular aspects of human behavior and characteristics. These abstractions are called *phenomena* (especially in qualitative studies) or **concepts**.

Researchers sometimes use the term **construct**, which also refers to an abstraction, but often one that is deliberately invented (or constructed). For example, *self-care* in Orem's model of health maintenance is a construct. The terms *construct* and *concept* are sometimes used interchangeably, but by convention a construct often refers to a slightly more complex abstraction than a concept.

A **theory** is an explanation of some aspect of reality. In a theory, concepts are knitted together into a coherent system to describe or explain some aspect of the world. Theories play a role in both qualitative and quantitative research. In a quantitative study, researchers often start with a theory and, using deductive reasoning, make predictions about how phenomena would behave in the real world *if the theory were true*. The specific predictions are then tested in a study, and the results are used to support or challenge the theory. In qualitative studies, theory often is the *product* of the research: The investigators use information from study participants inductively to develop a theory rooted in the participants' experiences.

> **☞ TIP:** The reasoning process of *deduction* is associated with quantitative research, and *induction* is associated with qualitative research. See the Chapter Supplement located on thePoint website for a full discussion of these terms.

## Variables

In quantitative studies, concepts are usually called **variables**. A variable, as the name implies, is something that varies. Weight, anxiety, and fatigue are all variables—they vary from one person to another. Most human characteristics are variables. If everyone weighed 150 pounds, weight would not be a variable, it would be a *constant*. But it is precisely because people and conditions *do* vary that most research is conducted. Quantitative researchers seek to understand how or why things vary, and to learn how differences in one variable relate to differences in another. For example, in lung cancer research, lung cancer is a variable because not everybody has this disease. Researchers have studied factors that might be linked to lung cancer, such as cigarette smoking. Smoking is also a variable because not everyone smokes. A variable, then, is any quality of a person, group, or situation that varies or takes on different values. Variables are the central building blocks of quantitative studies.

> **☞ TIP:** Every study focuses on one or more phenomena, concepts, or variables, but these terms per se are not necessarily used in research reports. For example, a report might say: "The purpose of this study is to examine the effect of nurses' workload on hand hygiene compliance." Although the researcher did not explicitly label anything a variable, the variables under study are *workload* and *hand hygiene compliance*. Key concepts or variables are often indicated in the study title.

Variables are often inherent human characteristics, such as age or weight, but sometimes researchers *create* a variable. For example, if a researcher tests the effectiveness of patient-controlled analgesia compared to intramuscular analgesia in relieving pain after surgery, some patients would be given one type of analgesia and some would receive the other. In the context of this study, the method of pain management is a variable because different patients are given different analgesics.

Some variables take on a wide range of values than can be represented on a continuum (e.g., a person's age or weight). Other variables take on only a few values; sometimes such variables convey quantitative information (e.g., number of children) but others simply involve placing people into categories (e.g., male, female, or blood type A, B, AB, or O).

## Dependent and Independent Variables

As noted in Chapter 1, many studies seek to understand causes of phenomena. Does a nursing intervention *cause* improvements in patient outcomes? Does smoking *cause* lung cancer? The presumed cause is the **independent variable**, and the presumed effect is the **dependent or outcome variable**. In terms of the PICO scheme discussed in Chapter 2, the dependent variable corresponds to the "O" (outcome). The independent variable corresponds to the "I" (the intervention, influence, or exposure), plus the "C" (the comparison).

> 👉 **TIP:** In searching for evidence, a nurse might want to learn about the effects of an intervention or influence, compared to *any* alternative, on a designated outcome. In a study, however, researchers must always specify what the comparative intervention or influence (the "C") is.

Variation in the dependent variable is presumed to *depend on* variation in the independent variable. For example, researchers investigate the extent to which lung cancer (the dependent variable) depends on smoking (the independent variable). Or, investigators might examine the extent to which patients' pain (the dependent variable) depends on different nursing actions (the independent variable). The dependent variable is the outcome that researchers want to understand, explain, or predict.

The terms *independent variable* and *dependent variable* also can be used to indicate *direction of influence* rather than cause and effect. For example, suppose we compared levels of depression among men and women diagnosed with pancreatic cancer and found men to be more depressed. We could not conclude that depression was *caused* by gender. Yet the direction of influence clearly runs from gender to depression: it makes no sense to suggest that patients' depression influenced their gender. Although it may not make sense to infer a cause-and-effect connection, it is appropriate to consider depression as the outcome variable and gender as the independent variable.

> 👉 **TIP:** Few research reports explicitly label variables as dependent and independent. Moreover, variables (especially independent variables) are sometimes not fully spelled out. Take the following research question: What is the effect of exercise on heart rate? In this example, heart rate is the dependent variable. Exercise, however, is not in itself a variable. Rather, exercise versus something else (e.g., no exercise) is a variable; "something else" is implied rather than stated in the research question.

Many outcomes have multiple causes or influences. If we were studying factors that influence people's body mass index, the independent variables might be height, physical activity, and diet. And, two or more outcome variables may be of interest. For example, a researcher may compare two alternative dietary interventions in terms of participants' weight, lipid profile, and self esteem. It is common to design studies with multiple independent and dependent variables.

Variables are not *inherently* dependent or independent. A dependent variable in one study could be an independent variable in another. For example, a study might examine the effect of an exercise intervention (the independent variable) on osteoporosis (the dependent variable) to answer a therapy question. Another study might investigate the effect of osteoporosis (the independent variable) on bone fracture incidence (the dependent variable) to address a prognosis question. In short, whether a variable is independent or dependent is a function of the role that it plays in a particular study.

**Example of independent and dependent variables:**
*Research question (Etiology/Harm question)*: Is low cognitive functioning associated with reduced instrumental activities of daily living (e.g., medication management, driving) in people with heart failure (Alosco et al., 2012)?
  *Independent variable*: Level of cognitive functioning
  *Dependent variables*: Instrumental activities of daily living

## Conceptual and Operational Definitions

The concepts of interest to researchers are abstractions of observable phenomena, and researchers' world view shapes how those concepts are defined. A **conceptual definition** is the abstract or theoretical meaning of a concept. Researchers need to conceptually define even seemingly straightforward terms. A classic example is the concept of *caring*. Morse and colleagues (1990) examined how researchers and theorists defined *caring*, and identified five categories of conceptual definitions: as a human trait; a moral imperative; an affect; an interpersonal relationship; and a therapeutic intervention. Researchers undertaking studies of caring need to clarify which conceptual definition they have adopted.

In qualitative studies, conceptual definitions of key phenomena may be a major end product, reflecting an intent to have the meaning of concepts defined by those being studied. In quantitative studies, however, researchers must define concepts at the outset, because they must decide how the variables will be observed and measured. An **operational definition** indicates what the researchers specifically must do to measure the concept and collect needed information.

Variables differ in the ease with which they can be operationalized. The variable weight, for example, is easy to define and measure. We might operationally define weight as the amount that a person weighs in pounds, to the nearest full pound. This definition designates that weight will be measured using one measuring system (pounds) rather than another (grams). We could also specify that weight will be measured using a digital scale with subjects fully undressed after 10 hours of fasting. This operational definition clearly indicates what the variable *weight* means.

Few variables are operationalized as easily as weight, however. Most variables can be measured several ways, and researchers must choose a method that best captures the variables as they conceptualize them. Take, for example, *anxiety*, which can be defined in terms of both physiologic and psychological functioning. For researchers emphasizing physiologic aspects of anxiety, the operational definition might involve a measure such as pulse rate. If, on the other hand, anxiety is conceptualized as a psychological state, the operational definition might be scores on a paper-and-pencil test such as the State Anxiety Scale. Readers of research articles may not agree with how researchers conceptualized and operationalized variables, but definitional precision is important in communicating what concepts mean within the context of the study.

**Example of conceptual and operational definitions:**
Fogg and colleagues (2011) developed a scale to measure people's beliefs and intentions about HIV screening. The scale relied on constructs from a theory called the Theory of Planned Behavior (see Chapter 8). The article provided examples of both conceptual and operational definitions of key constructs. For example, "Subjective norm" was conceptually defined as "The overall perception of social pressure to perform or not perform the behavior" and a scale item used to measure this construct was "The people in my life whose opinions I value are regularly tested for HIV" (p. 76).

---

**BOX 3.1 Example of Quantitative Data**

**Question:** Thinking about the past week, how depressed would you say you have been on a scale from 0 to 10, where 0 means "not at all" and 10 means "the most possible"?

| | |
|---|---|
| **Data:** 9 | (Subject 1) |
| 0 | (Subject 2) |
| 4 | (Subject 3) |

---

## Data

Research **data** (singular, datum) are the pieces of information gathered in a study. In quantitative studies, researchers identify and define their variables, and then collect relevant data from subjects. The actual *values* of the study variables constitute the data. Quantitative researchers collect primarily **quantitative data**—information in numeric form. For example, if we conducted a quantitative study in which a key variable was *depression*, we would need to measure how depressed participants were. We might ask, "Thinking about the past week, how depressed would you say you have been on a scale from 0 to 10, where 0 means 'not at all' and 10 means 'the most possible'?" Box 3.1 presents quantitative data from three fictitious respondents. The subjects provided a number along the 0 to 10 continuum corresponding to their degree of depression—9 for subject 1 (a high level of depression), 0 for subject 2 (no depression), and 4 for subject 3 (little depression). The numeric values for all subjects, collectively, would comprise the data on depression.

In qualitative studies, researchers collect primarily **qualitative data**, that is, narrative descriptions. Narrative data can be obtained by conversing with participants, by making notes about their behavior in naturalistic settings, or by obtaining narrative records, such as diaries. Suppose we were studying depression qualitatively. Box 3.2 presents qualitative data for three participants responding conversationally to the question, "Tell me about how you've been feeling lately—have you felt sad or depressed at all, or have you generally been in good spirits?" Here, the data consist of rich narrative descriptions of participants' emotional state.

---

**BOX 3.2 Example of Qualitative Data**

**Question:** Tell me about how you've been feeling lately—have you felt sad or depressed at all, or have you generally been in good spirits?

**Data:** "Well, Actually, I've been pretty depressed lately, to tell you the truth. I wake up each morning and I can't seem to think of anything to look forward to. I mope around the house all day, kind of in despair. I just can't seem to shake the blues and I've begun to think I need to go see a shrink." (Participant 1)

"I can't remember ever feeling better in my life. I just got promoted to a new job that makes me feel like I can really get ahead in my company. And I've just gotten engaged to a really great guy who is very special." (Participant 2)

"I've had a few ups and downs the past week but basically things are on a pretty even keel. I don't have too many complaints." (Participant 3)

## Relationships

Researchers usually study phenomena in relation to other phenomena—they examine relationships. A **relationship** is a bond or connection between two or more phenomena; for example, researchers repeatedly have found that there is a *relationship* between cigarette smoking and lung cancer. Qualitative and quantitative studies examine relationships in different ways.

In quantitative studies, researchers are interested in the relationship between independent variables and outcomes. Variation in the outcome variable is presumed to be systematically related to variation in the independent variable. Relationships are often explicitly expressed in quantitative terms, such as *more than*, *less than*, and so on. For example, consider a person's weight as our dependent variable. What variables are related to (associated with) a person's weight? Some possibilities include height, caloric intake, and exercise. For each of these independent variables, we can make a prediction about its relationship to the outcome variable:

*Height*: Taller people will weigh more than shorter people.
*Caloric intake*: People with higher caloric intake will be heavier than those with lower caloric intake.
*Exercise*: The lower the amount of exercise, the greater will be the person's weight.

Each statement expresses a predicted relationship between weight (the outcome) and a measurable independent variable. Most quantitative research is conducted to assess whether relationships exist among variables and to measure how strong the relationship is.

> **TIP:** Relationships are expressed in two basic forms. First, relationships can be expressed as "if more of Variable X, then more of (or less of) Variable Y." For example, there is a relationship between height and weight: With greater height, there tends to be greater weight, i.e., taller people tend to weigh more than shorter people. The second form involves relationships expressed as group differences. For example, there is a relationship between gender and height: men tend to be taller than women.

Variables can be related to one another in different ways. One type of relationship is a **cause-and-effect** (or **causal**) **relationship**. Within the positivist paradigm, natural phenomena are assumed to have antecedent causes that are discoverable. In our example about a person's weight, we might speculate that there is a causal relationship between caloric intake and weight: all else being equal, eating more calories causes weight gain. As noted in Chapter 1, many quantitative studies are *cause-probing*—they seek to illuminate the causes of phenomena.

**Example of a study of causal relationships:**
Chuang and co-researchers (2012) studied whether a structured relaxation program caused lower stress in hospitalized pregnant women with preterm labor.

Not all relationships between variables can be interpreted as cause-and-effect. There is a relationship, for example, between a person's pulmonary artery and tympanic temperatures: people with high readings on one tend to have high readings on the other. We cannot say, however, that pulmonary artery temperature *caused* tympanic temperature, nor that tympanic temperature *caused* pulmonary artery temperature, despite the relationship that exists between the two variables. This type of relationship is sometimes referred to as an *associative* (or *functional*) *relationship* rather than a causal one.

**Example of a study of associative relationships:**
Kelly and colleagues (2012) studied the relationship between social support networks and adherence to antiretroviral therapy among HIV-infected substance abusers.

Qualitative researchers are not concerned with quantifying relationships, nor in testing and confirming causal relationships. Rather, qualitative researchers may seek patterns of association as a way of illuminating the underlying meaning and dimensionality of phenomena of interest. Patterns of interconnected concepts are identified as a means of understanding the whole.

**Example of a qualitative study of patterns:**
Stålkrantz and colleagues (2012) studied everyday life for the spouses of patients with untreated obstructive sleep apnea syndrome. They found that the spouses differed on two key dimensions: social adjustment (circumstances limited or unchanged) and new feelings (against the partner or supporting the partner).

# MAJOR CLASSES OF QUANTITATIVE AND QUALITATIVE RESEARCH

Researchers usually work within a paradigm that is consistent with their world view, and that gives rise to the types of question that excite their curiosity. In this section, we briefly describe broad categories of quantitative and qualitative research.

## Quantitative Research: Experimental and Nonexperimental Studies

A basic distinction in quantitative studies is the difference between experimental and nonexperimental research. In **experimental research**, researchers actively introduce an intervention or treatment—most often, to address therapy questions. In **nonexperimental research**, on the other hand, researchers are bystanders—they collect data without introducing treatments or making changes (most often, to address etiology, prognosis, or diagnosis questions). For example, if a researcher gave bran flakes to one group of subjects and prune juice to another to evaluate which method facilitated elimination more effectively, the study would be experimental because the researcher intervened in the normal course of things. If, on the other hand, a researcher compared elimination patterns of two groups whose regular eating patterns differed, the study would be nonexperimental because there is no intervention. In medical and epidemiological research, experimental studies usually are called **clinical trials**, and nonexperimental inquiries are called **observational studies**.

> ☞ **TIP:**  There are many different strategies and designs for experimental and nonexperimental research, as we discuss in Chapter 9. On the evidence hierarchy shown in Figure 2.1 on page 23, the two rungs below systematic reviews (Randomized Controlled Trials and quasi-experiments) involve interventions and are experimental. The four rungs below that are nonexperimental.

Experimental studies are explicitly designed to test causal relationships—to test whether an intervention *caused* changes in the outcome variable. Sometimes nonexperimental studies also explore causal relationships, but causal inferences in nonexperimental research are tricky and less conclusive, for reasons explained in a later chapter.

**Example of experimental research:**
Yang and colleagues (2011) tested the effectiveness of a home-based walking intervention in improving symptom and mood distress in women following surgery for breast cancer. Some study participants received the moderate-intensity intervention while others did not.

In this example, the researchers intervened by designating that some patients would receive the special walking intervention, and that others would not be given this opportunity. In other words, the researcher *controlled* the independent variable, which in this case was the walking intervention.

**Example of nonexperimental research:**
Enderlin and co-researchers (2012) compared sleep quality and daytime sleepiness in women with nonmetastatic breast cancer versus those without cancer. The two groups differed with regard to several sleep outcomes, such as sleep onset latency and insomnia severity.

In this nonexperimental study to address a prognosis question, the researchers did not intervene in any way. They were interested in a similar population as in the previous example (women with breast cancer), but their intent was to explore existing relationships rather than to test a potential solution to a problem.

## Qualitative Research: Disciplinary Traditions

The majority of qualitative studies can best be described as **qualitative descriptive research.** Many qualitative studies, however, are rooted in research traditions that originated in anthropology, sociology, and psychology. Three such traditions, prominent in qualitative nursing research, are briefly described here. Chapter 14 provides a fuller discussion of these and other traditions, and the methods associated with them.

The **grounded theory** tradition seeks to describe and understand the key social psychological processes that occur in a social setting. Grounded theory was developed in the 1960s by two sociologists, Glaser and Strauss (1967). The focus of most grounded theory studies is on a developing social experience—the social and psychological phases that characterize a particular event or episode. A major component of grounded theory is the discovery of a *core variable* that is central in explaining what is going on in that social scene. Grounded theory researchers strive to generate explanations of phenomena that are grounded in reality.

**Example of a grounded theory study:**
Neill and colleagues (2012) studied how families manage acute childhood illnesses at home, and the role that felt or enacted criticism play in parents' help-seeking behaviors.

**Phenomenology,** rooted in a philosophical tradition developed by Husserl and Heidegger, is concerned with the lived experiences of humans. Phenomenology is an approach to thinking about what life experiences of people are like and what they mean.

The phenomenological researcher asks the questions: What is the *essence* of this phenomenon as experienced by these people? Or, What is the meaning of the phenomenon to those who experience it?

> **Example of a phenomenological study:**
> McCloud and colleagues (2012) studied the lived experience of undergoing vitreoretinal day surgery in an Australian public hospital.

**Ethnography**, the primary research tradition in anthropology, provides a framework for studying the patterns, lifeways, and experiences of a defined cultural group in a holistic fashion. Ethnographers typically engage in extensive *fieldwork*, often participating to the extent possible in the life of the culture under study. Ethnographers strive to learn from members of a cultural group, to understand their world view, and to describe their customs and norms.

> **Example of an ethnographic study:**
> Emilsdóttir and Gústafsdóttir (2011) conducted extensive ethnographic fieldwork in a nursing home in Iceland to examine nurses' care of the dying elderly.

## Major Steps in a Quantitative Study

In quantitative studies, researchers move from the beginning point of a study (posing a question) to the end point (obtaining an answer) in a reasonably linear sequence of steps that is broadly similar across studies (see Fig. 3.1). This section describes that flow, and the next section describes how qualitative studies differ.

## Phase 1: The Conceptual Phase

The early steps in a quantitative study typically involve activities with a strong conceptual element. During this phase, researchers call on such skills as creativity, deductive reasoning, and a grounding in existing research evidence on the topic of interest.

### Step 1: Formulating and Delimiting the Problem

Quantitative researchers begin by identifying an interesting, significant research problem and formulating good **research questions**. In developing their questions, nurse researchers must attend to substantive issues (Is this problem important?); theoretical issues (Is there a conceptual context to enrich understanding of this problem?); clinical issues (Will study findings be useful in clinical practice?); methodologic issues (How can this question be answered to yield high-quality evidence?); and ethical issues (Can this question be addressed in an ethical manner?).

### Step 2: Reviewing the Related Literature

Quantitative research is conducted within the context of previous knowledge. Quantitative researchers typically strive to understand what is already known about a topic by undertaking a thorough **literature review** before any data are collected.

### Step 3: Undertaking Clinical Fieldwork

Researchers embarking on a clinical study often benefit from spending time in relevant clinical settings (in the *field*), discussing the topic with clinicians and observing

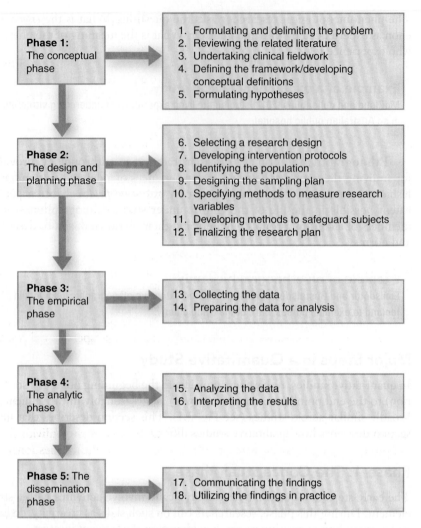

**Phase 1:**
The conceptual phase

1. Formulating and delimiting the problem
2. Reviewing the related literature
3. Undertaking clinical fieldwork
4. Defining the framework/developing conceptual definitions
5. Formulating hypotheses

**Phase 2:**
The design and planning phase

6. Selecting a research design
7. Developing intervention protocols
8. Identifying the population
9. Designing the sampling plan
10. Specifying methods to measure research variables
11. Developing methods to safeguard subjects
12. Finalizing the research plan

**Phase 3:**
The empirical phase

13. Collecting the data
14. Preparing the data for analysis

**Phase 4:**
The analytic phase

15. Analyzing the data
16. Interpreting the results

**Phase 5:** The dissemination phase

17. Communicating the findings
18. Utilizing the findings in practice

**FIGURE 3.1** ● Flow of steps in a quantitative study.

current practices. Such clinical fieldwork can provide insights into clinicians' and clients' perspectives.

### Step 4: Defining the Framework and Developing Conceptual Definitions

When quantitative research is performed within the context of a theoretical framework, the findings may have broader significance and utility. Even when the research question is not embedded in a theory, researchers should have a conceptual rationale and a clear vision of the concepts under study.

### Step 5: Formulating Hypotheses

**Hypotheses** state researchers' deductively derived expectations about relationships between study variables. Hypotheses are predictions of the relationships researchers expect to observe in the study data. The research question identifies the concepts of interest and asks how the concepts might be related; a hypothesis is the predicted answer. Most quantitative studies are designed to test hypotheses through statistical analysis.

## Phase 2: The Design and Planning Phase

In the second major phase of a quantitative study, researchers make decisions about the methods and procedures to be used to address the research question. Researchers typically have flexibility in designing a study, and make many methodologic decisions that have crucial implications for the integrity and generalizability of the study findings.

### Step 6: Selecting a Research Design

The **research design** is the overall plan for obtaining answers to the research questions and for handling challenges that can undermine the study evidence. Quantitative research designs tend to be highly structured and controlled, with the goal of minimizing bias. Research designs also indicate other aspects of the research—for example, how often data will be collected, what types of comparisons will be made, and where the study will take place. The research design is the architectural backbone of the study.

### Step 7: Developing Protocols for the Intervention

In experimental research, researchers create the independent variable, which means that participants are exposed to different treatments. An **intervention protocol** for the study must be developed, specifying exactly what the intervention will entail (e.g., who would administer it, how frequently and over how long a period the treatment would last, and so on) *and* what the alternative condition would be. In nonexperimental research, this step is not necessary.

### Step 8: Identifying the Population

Quantitative researchers need to know what characteristics the study participants should possess, and clarify the group to whom study results can be generalized—that is, they must identify the population to be studied. A **population** is *all* the individuals or objects with common, defining characteristics (the "P" component in PICO questions).

### Step 9: Designing the Sampling Plan

Researchers typically collect data from a **sample**, which is a subset of the population. Using samples is more practical than collecting data from an entire population, but the risk is that the sample might not adequately reflect the population's traits. The researcher's *sampling plan* specifies how the sample will be selected and how many subjects there will be.

### Step 10: Specifying Methods to Measure Variables

Quantitative researchers must find methods to measure the research variables accurately. A variety of quantitative data collection approaches exist; the primary methods are *self-reports* (e.g., interviews and questionnaires), *observations* (e.g., watching and recording people's behavior), and *biophysiologic measurements*. The task of measuring research variables and developing a *data collection plan* is complex and challenging.

### Step 11: Developing Methods to Safeguard Human/Animal Rights

Most nursing research involves human subjects, although some involve animals. In either case, procedures need to be developed to ensure that the study adheres to ethical principles.

### Step 12: Reviewing and Finalizing the Research Plan

Before collecting data, researchers often perform a number of "tests" to ensure that procedures will work smoothly. For example, they may evaluate the *readability* of written materials to see if participants with low reading skills can comprehend them. Researchers usually have their research plan critiqued by reviewers to obtain clinical or methodologic feedback before implementing it. Researchers seeking financial support submit a *proposal* to a funding source, and reviewers usually suggest improvements.

## Phase 3: The Empirical Phase

The third phase of quantitative studies involves collecting the research data. This phase is often the most time-consuming part of the study. Data collection may require months of work.

### Step 13: Collecting the Data

The actual collection of data in a quantitative study often proceeds according to a pre-established plan. The plan typically spells out procedures for training data collection staff; for actually collecting data (e.g., where and when the data will be gathered); and for recording information.

### Step 14: Preparing the Data for Analysis

Data collected in a quantitative study must be prepared for analysis. For example, one preliminary step is *coding*, which involves translating verbal data into numeric form (e.g., coding gender information as "1" for females and "2" for males). Another step may involve transferring the data from written documents onto computer files for analysis.

## Phase 4: The Analytic Phase

Quantitative data gathered in the empirical phase must be subjected to analysis and interpretation, which occurs in the fourth major phase of a project.

### Step 15: Analyzing the Data

To answer research questions and test hypotheses, researchers analyze their data in an orderly fashion. Quantitative data are analyzed through **statistical analyses**, which include some simple procedures (e.g., computing an average) as well as more complex, sophisticated methods.

### Step 16: Interpreting the Results

*Interpretation* involves making sense of study results and examining their implications. Researchers attempt to explain the findings in light of prior evidence, theory, and clinical experience—and in light of the adequacy of the methods they used in the study.

## Phase 5: The Dissemination Phase

In the analytic phase, researchers come full circle: the questions posed at the outset are answered. The researchers' job is not completed, however, until the study results are disseminated.

### Step 17: Communicating the Findings

A study cannot contribute evidence to nursing practice if the results are not communicated. Another—and often final—task of a research project is the preparation of a *research report* that can be shared with others. We discuss research reports in the next chapter.

### Step 18: Putting the Evidence into Practice

Ideally, the concluding step of a high-quality study is to plan for its use in practice settings. Although nurse researchers may not themselves be able to implement a plan for using research findings, they can contribute to the process by developing recommendations on how the evidence could be used in practice, by ensuring that adequate information has been provided for a meta-analysis, and by pursuing opportunities to disseminate the findings to practicing nurses.

# ACTIVITIES IN A QUALITATIVE STUDY

Quantitative research involves a fairly linear progression of tasks—researchers plan the steps to be taken and then follow those steps as faithfully as possible. In qualitative studies, by contrast, the progression is closer to a circle than to a straight line. Qualitative researchers are continually examining and interpreting data and making decisions about how to proceed based on what has already been discovered (Fig. 3.2).

Because qualitative researchers have a flexible approach to collecting and analyzing data, we cannot show the flow of activities precisely—the flow varies from one study to another, and researchers themselves do not know in advance exactly how the study will unfold. We try to provide a sense of how qualitative studies are conducted by describing some major activities and indicating how and when they might be performed.

## Conceptualizing and Planning a Qualitative Study

### Identifying the Research Problem

Qualitative researchers usually begin with a broad topic, often focusing on an aspect about which little is known. Qualitative researchers often proceed with a fairly broad initial

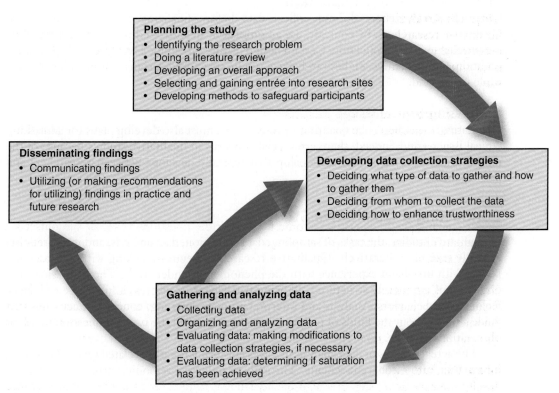

**FIGURE 3.2** ● Flow of activities in a qualitative study.

question that allows the focus to be sharpened and delineated more clearly once the study is underway.

### Doing a Literature Review

Not all qualitative researchers agree about the value of doing an upfront literature review. Some believe that researchers should not consult the literature before collecting data. They worry that prior studies might influence the conceptualization of the phenomenon under study, which they believe should be elucidated based on participants' viewpoints rather than on prior findings. Others believe that researchers should conduct at least a brief literature review at the outset. In any case, qualitative researchers typically find a relatively small body of relevant previous work because of the type of questions they ask.

### Selecting and Gaining Entrée Into Research Sites

Before going into the field, qualitative researchers must identify an appropriate site. For example, if the topic is the health beliefs of the urban poor, an inner-city neighborhood with a concentration of low-income residents must be identified. In some cases, researchers may have access to the selected site, but in others they need to **gain entrée** into it. Gaining entrée typically involves negotiations with **gatekeepers** who have the authority to permit entry into their world.

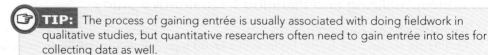

**TIP:** The process of gaining entrée is usually associated with doing fieldwork in qualitative studies, but quantitative researchers often need to gain entrée into sites for collecting data as well.

### Developing an Overall Approach

Quantitative researchers do not collect data before finalizing their research design. Qualitative researchers, by contrast, use an **emergent design**—a design that emerges during the course of data collection. Certain design features are guided by the study's qualitative tradition, but qualitative studies rarely have rigidly structured designs that prohibit changes while in the field.

### Addressing Ethical Issues

Qualitative researchers, like quantitative researchers, must also develop plans for addressing ethical issues—and, indeed, there are special concerns in qualitative studies because of the more intimate nature of the relationship that typically develops between researchers and participants.

## Conducting a Qualitative Study

In qualitative studies, the tasks of sampling, data collection, data analysis, and interpretation typically take place iteratively. Qualitative researchers begin by talking with or observing people with first-hand experience with the phenomenon under study. The discussions and observations are loosely structured, allowing participants to express a full range of beliefs, feelings, and behaviors. Analysis and interpretation are ongoing, concurrent activities that guide choices about the kinds of people to question next and the types of question to ask or observations to make.

The actual process of data analysis involves clustering together related types of narrative information into a coherent scheme. Through an inductive reasoning process, researchers begin to identify **themes** and categories, which are used to build a rich description or theory of the phenomenon. The kinds of data gathered become increasingly purposeful as the theory emerges. Concept development and verification shape sampling choices—as conceptualizations develop, the researcher seeks participants who can confirm and enrich theoretical understandings, as well as participants who can potentially challenge them and lead to further insights.

Quantitative researchers decide in advance how many subjects to include in the study, but qualitative researchers' sampling decisions are guided by the data. Many qualitative researchers use the principle of **saturation**, which occurs when themes and categories in the data become repetitive and redundant, such that no new information can be gleaned by further data collection.

Quantitative researchers seek to collect high-quality data by measuring their variables with instruments that have been demonstrated to be accurate and valid. Qualitative researchers, by contrast, *are* the main data collection instrument and must take steps to demonstrate the *trustworthiness* of the data. The central feature of these efforts is to confirm that the findings accurately reflect the experiences and viewpoints of participants, rather than researchers' perceptions. One confirmatory activity, for example, involves going back to participants, sharing preliminary interpretations with them, and asking them to evaluate whether the researcher's thematic analysis is consistent with their experiences.

Qualitative nursing researchers also strive to share their findings at conferences and in journal articles. Qualitative studies help to shape nurses' perceptions of a problem or situation, their conceptualizations of potential solutions, and their understanding of patients' concerns and experiences.

# GENERAL QUESTIONS IN REVIEWING A STUDY

Box 3.3 presents some further suggestions for performing a preliminary overview of a research report, drawing on concepts explained in this chapter. These guidelines supplement those presented in Box 1.1, Chapter 1 on page 15.

---

**BOX 3.3  Additional Questions for a Preliminary Review of a Study**

1. What is the study all about? What are the main phenomena, concepts, or constructs under investigation?
2. If the study is quantitative, what are the independent and dependent variables?
3. Did the researchers examine relationships or patterns of association among variables or concepts? Does the report imply the possibility of a causal relationship?
4. Are key concepts defined, both conceptually and operationally?
5. What type of study does it appear to be, in terms of types described in this chapter—experimental or nonexperimental/observational, grounded theory, phenomenology, or ethnography?
6. Does the report provide information to suggest how long the study took to complete?

## RESEARCH EXAMPLES WITH CRITICAL THINKING EXERCISES

In this section, we illustrate the progression of activities and discuss the time schedule of two studies (one quantitative and the other qualitative) conducted by the second author of this book.

☀–Examples 1 and 2 below are also featured in our *Interactive Critical Thinking Activity* on thePoint☀ website where you can easily record, print, and e-mail your responses to the related questions.

### EXAMPLE 1 ● Project Schedule for a Quantitative Study

**Study:** Further validation of the Postpartum Depression Screening Scale (PDSS) (Beck & Gable, 2001)

**Study Purpose:** Beck and Gable undertook a study to assess the PDSS, an instrument designed for use by clinicians and researchers to screen mothers for postpartum depression. The scale is currently in wide use throughout the world.

**Study Methods:** This study required nearly 3 years to complete. Key activities and methodological decisions included the following:

**Phase 1. Conceptual Phase: 1 Month.** This phase was short, because much of the conceptual work had been done in a prior study, in which Beck and Gable actually developed the scale. The literature had already been reviewed, so they only needed to update it. The framework and conceptual definitions that had been used in the first study were used in the new study.

**Phase 2. Design and Planning Phase: 6 Months.** The second phase was time-consuming. It included developing the research design for the study, gaining entrée into the hospital from which subjects were recruited, and obtaining approval from the hospital's human subjects review committee. During this period, Beck met with statistical consultants and with Gable, an instrument development specialist, numerous times to finalize the study design.

**Phase 3. Empirical Phase: 11 Months.** Data collection took almost a year to complete. The design called for administering the PDSS to 150 mothers who were 6 weeks postpartum, and then scheduling them for a psychiatric diagnostic interview to evaluate if they were suffering from postpartum depression. Women were recruited into the study during prepared childbirth classes. Recruitment began 4 months before data collection, and then the researchers gathered their data 6 weeks after delivery. The nurse psychotherapist, who had her own practice, was able to come to the hospital only 1 day a week to conduct the diagnostic interviews; this contributed to the time required to achieve the desired sample size.

**Phase 4. Analytic Phase: 3 Months.** Statistical tests were performed to determine a cut-off score on the PDSS above which mothers would be identified as having screened positive for postpartum depression. Data analysis also was undertaken to determine the accuracy of the PDSS in predicting diagnosed postpartum depression. The scale was found to be highly accurate. During this phase, Beck met with Gable and other statisticians to interpret results.

**Phase 5. Dissemination Phase: 18 Months.** The researchers prepared and submitted their report to the journal *Nursing Research* for possible publication. It was accepted within 4 months, but it was "in press" (awaiting publication) for 14 months before being published. During this period, the authors presented their findings at regional and international conferences. The researchers also prepared a summary report for the agency that funded the research.

### CRITICAL THINKING EXERCISES

1. Answer the relevant questions from Box 3.3 on page 55 regarding this study.
2. Also consider the following targeted questions:
   a. Who do you think is the *population* for this study?
   b. Would you describe the method of data collection as *self-report* or *observation*?
   c. How would you evaluate Beck and Gable's dissemination plan?

   d. Do you think an appropriate amount of time was allocated to the various phases and steps in this study?

   e. Would it have been appropriate for the researchers to address the research question using qualitative research methods? Why or why not?

3. If the results of this study are valid and generalizable, in what ways do you think the findings could be used in clinical practice?

## EXAMPLE 2 ● Project Schedule for a Qualitative Study

**Study:**  The Arm: There is no escaping the reality for mothers of children with obstetric brachial plexus injuries (OBPIs) (Beck, 2009).

**Study Purpose:**  The purpose of this study was to understand the experience of mothers' caring for their children with OBPIs.

**Study Methods:**  The total time required to complete this study was nearly 4 years. Beck's key activities included the following:

**Phase 1. Conceptual Phase: 3 Months.**  One of the participants in Beck's earlier study on traumatic childbirth was a member of the Board of Directors of the United Brachial Plexus Network (UBPN). This mother had experienced a traumatic birth due to shoulder dystocia, which resulted in her infant suffering an OBPI. Every 2 years the UBPN holds a camp for families of children with OBPIs, and the camps include educational sessions for parents. Beck was invited to present her findings on traumatic childbirth at the camp in 2005. At camp Beck discussed with some UBPN Board members the possibility of conducting research on mothers' experiences caring for their children with OBPIs. She obtained their enthusiastic support.

**Phase 2. Design and Planning Phase: 3 Months.**  Beck selected a phenomenological approach for this research in the fall of 2005. She corresponded by email with the UBPN Board of Directors to obtain formal approval to post a recruitment notice on the organization's website www.ubpn.org. Once the basic design was finalized, Beck obtained approval from the human subjects review committee at her university.

**Phase 3. Empirical/Analytic Phases: 30 months.**  Data were collected from October 2005 to December 2007. During this period, 11 women participated in the study via the Internet by sending Beck stories of their experiences of caring for their children with OBPIs. In 2007 Beck was invited to present her research findings about the anniversary of birth trauma at the UPBN camp in Auburn, WA. Beck interviewed 12 mothers individually at the camp, for a total of 23 study participants. For an additional 4 months Beck analyzed the mothers' stories. Six themes emerged from data analysis: (1) In an instant: dreams shattered, (2) The arm: No escaping the reality, (3) Tormented: Agonizing worries and questions, (4) Therapy and surgeries: Consuming mothers' lives, (5) Anger: Simmering pot inside, and (6) So much to bear: enduring heartbreak.

**Phase 4. Dissemination Phase: 10 Months.**  A manuscript describing this study was submitted to the journal *Nursing Research* on September 9, 2008. On December 2, 2008 Beck received a letter from the journal's editor indicating that reviewers recommended she revise and resubmit the paper. On January 6, 2009, Beck submitted a revised manuscript that incorporated the reviewers' recommendations. On February 23, 2009, Beck was notified that the paper had been accepted for publication, and the article was published in the July/August issue. Beck has presented the findings at national conferences. Also, Beck was interviewed regarding her findings, and parts of this interview were featured in UBPN's DVD entitled: "Newborn injuries: The untold story: Preventing the tragedy of unnecessary birth trauma." The DVD has been aired on Public Broadcasting System television stations and is on the UBPN website.

## CRITICAL THINKING EXERCISES

1. Answer the questions from Box 3.3 on page 55 regarding this study.

2. Also consider the following targeted questions:

   a. Given the study purpose, was a phenomonological approach appropriate for this study?

   b. Do you think an appropriate amount of time was allocated to the various phases and steps in this study?

    c. How would you evaluate the Beck dissemination plan?

    d. Would it have been appropriate for Beck to address the research question using quantitative research methods? Why or why not?

## EXAMPLE 3 ● Quantitative Research in Appendix A

• Read the abstract and the introduction from Howell and colleagues' (2007) study ("Anxiety, anger, and blood pressure in children") in Appendix A on pages 395–402.

### CRITICAL THINKING EXERCISES

1. Answer the relevant questions in Box 3.3 on page 55.
2. Also consider the following targeted questions:
    a. Could any of the variables in this study be considered *constructs*?
    b. Did this report present any actual *data* from the study participants?
    c. Would it have been possible for the researchers to use an experimental design for this study?

## EXAMPLE 4 ● Qualitative Research in Appendix B

• Read the abstract and the introduction from Beck and Watson's (2010) study ("Subsequent childbirth after a previous traumatic birth") in Appendix B on pages 403–412.

### CRITICAL THINKING EXERCISES

1. Answer the relevant questions in Box 3.3 on page 55.
2. Also consider the following targeted questions, which may further sharpen your critical thinking skills and assist you in assessing aspects of the study's merit:
    a. Find an example of actual *data* in this study. (You will need to look at the "Results" section of this study.)
    b. How long did it take Beck and Watson to collect the data for this study? (You will find this information in the "Procedure" section.)
    c. How much time elapsed between when the paper was accepted for publication and when it was actually published? (You will find relevant information at the end of the paper.)

**WANT TO KNOW MORE?** A wide variety of resources to enhance your learning and understanding of this chapter are available on thePoint.

• Interactive Critical Thinking Activity
• Chapter Supplement on Deductive and Inductive Reasoning
• Answers to the Critical Thinking Exercises for Examples 3 and 4
• Student Review Questions
• Full-text online
• Internet Resources with useful websites for Chapter 3

Additional study aids including eight journal articles and related questions are also available in *Study Guide for Essentials of Nursing Research, 8e.*

# SUMMARY POINTS

- The people who provide information to the researchers in a **study** are referred to as **subjects** or **study participants** in quantitative research, or study participants or **informants** in qualitative research; collectively they comprise the **sample**.

- The *site* is the location for the research; researchers sometimes engage in *multisite studies*.

- Researchers investigate **concepts** and *phenomena* (or **constructs**), which are abstractions inferred from people's behavior or characteristics.

- Concepts are the building blocks of **theories**, which are systematic explanations of some aspect of the real world.

- In quantitative studies, concepts are called variables. A **variable** is a characteristic or quality that takes on different values (i.e., varies from one person or object to another).

- The **dependent** (or **outcome**) **variable** is the behavior, characteristic, or outcome the researcher is interested in explaining, predicting, or affecting (the "O" in the PICO scheme). The **independent variable** is the presumed cause of or influence on the dependent variable. The independent variable corresponds to the "I" and the "C" components in the PICO scheme.

- A **conceptual definition** describes the abstract or theoretical meaning of a concept being studied. An **operational definition** specifies how the variable will be measured.

- **Data**—the information collected during the course of a study—may take the form of narrative information (**qualitative data**) or numeric values (**quantitative data**).

- A **relationship** is a bond or connection (or pattern of association) between variables. Quantitative researchers study the relationship between the independent variables and outcome variables.

- When the independent variable causes or affects the outcome, the relationship is a **cause-and-effect** (or **causal**) **relationship**. In an *associative relationship*, variables are related in a noncausal way.

- A key distinction in quantitative studies is between **experimental research**, in which researchers actively intervene to test an intervention or therapy, and **nonexperimental** (or **observational) research**, in which researchers collect data about existing phenomena without intervening.

- Qualitative research often is rooted in research traditions that originate in other disciplines. Three such traditions are grounded theory, phenomenology, and ethnography.

- **Grounded theory** seeks to describe and understand key social psychological processes that occur in a social setting.

- **Phenomenology** focuses on the lived experiences of humans and is an approach to gaining insight into what the life experiences of people are like and what they mean.

- **Ethnography** provides a framework for studying the meanings, patterns, and lifeways of a culture in a holistic fashion.

- In a quantitative study, researchers usually progress in a linear fashion from asking research questions to answering them. The main phases in a quantitative study are the conceptual, planning, empirical, analytic, and dissemination phases.

- The *conceptual phase* involves (1) defining the problem to be studied; (2) doing a **literature review**; (3) engaging in **clinical fieldwork** for clinical studies; (4) developing a framework and conceptual definitions; and (5) formulating **hypotheses** to be tested.

- The *planning phase* entails (6) selecting a **research design**; (7) developing **intervention protocols** if the study is experimental; (8) specifying the **population**; (9) developing a plan to select a **sample**; (10) specifying a **data collection plan** and methods to measure the research variables; (11) developing strategies to safeguard subjects' rights; and (12) finalizing the research plan.

- The *empirical phase* involves (13) collecting data and (14) preparing data for analysis (e.g., *coding* data).

- The *analytic phase* involves (15) analyzing data through **statistical analysis** and (16) interpreting the results.

- The *dissemination phase* entails (17) communicating the findings and (18) efforts to promote the use of the study evidence in nursing practice.

- The flow of activities in a qualitative study is more flexible and less linear. Qualitative studies typically involve an **emergent design** that evolves during data collection.

- Qualitative researchers begin with a broad question regarding a phenomenon of interest, often focusing on a little-studied aspect. In the early phase of a qualitative study, researchers select a site and seek to **gain entrée** into it, which typically involves enlisting the cooperation of **gatekeepers** within the site.

- Once in the field, researchers select informants, collect data, and then analyze and interpret them in an iterative fashion; experiences during data collection help in an ongoing fashion to shape the design of the study.

- Early analysis in qualitative research leads to refinements in sampling and data collection, until **saturation** (redundancy of information) is achieved. Analysis typically involves a search for critical **themes**.

- Both qualitative and quantitative researchers disseminate their findings, most often by publishing their research reports in professional journals.

# REFERENCES FOR CHAPTER 3

Alosco, M., Spitznagel, M., Cohen, R., Sweet, S., Colbert, L., Josephson, R., et al. (2012). Cognitive impairment is independently associated with reduced instrumental activities of daily living in persons with heart failure. *Journal of Cardiovascular Nursing, 27*, 44–50.

Beck, C. T. (2009). The arm: There is no escaping the reality for mothers of children with obstetric brachial plexus injuries. *Nursing Research, 58*, 237–245.

Beck, C. T., & Gable, R. K. (2001). Further validation of the Postpartum Depression Screening Scale. *Nursing Research, 50*, 155–164.

Chuang, L. L., Lin, L., Cheng, C., Wu, S., & Chang, C. (2012). Effects of a relaxation training programme on immediate and prolonged stress responses in women with preterm labour. *Journal of Advanced Nursing, 68*, 170–180.

Emilsdóttir, A., & Gústafsdóttir, M. (2011). End of life in an Icelandic nursing home: An ethnographic study. *International Journal of Palliative Nursing, 17*, 405–411.

Enderlin, C., Coleman, E., Cole, C., Richards, K., Kennedy, R., Goodwin, J., et al. (2012). Subjective sleep quality, objective sleep characteristics, insomnia symptom severity, and daytime sleepiness in women aged 50 and older with nonmetastatic breast cancer. *Oncology Nursing Forum, 38*, E314–E325.

Fogg, C., Mawn, B., & Powell, F. (2011). Development of the Fogg Intent-to-screen for HIV Questionnaire. *Research in Nursing & Health, 34*, 73–84.

Glaser, B. G., & Strauss, A. (1967). *The discovery of grounded theory.* New York: Aldine de Gruyter.

Kelly, P., Ramaswamy, M., Li, X., Litwin, A., Berg, K., & Arnsten, J. (2012). Social networks of substance users with HIV infection. *Western Journal of Nursing Research, 34*, 621–634.

McCloud, C., Harrington, A., & King, L. (2012). Understanding people's experience of vitreo-retinal day surgery. *Journal of Advanced Nursing, 68*, 94–103.

Morse, J. M., Solberg, S., Neander, W., Bottorff, J., & Johnson, J. (1990). Concepts of caring and caring as a concept. *Advances in Nursing Science, 13*, 1–14.

Neill, S., Cowley, S., & Williams, C. (2012). The role of felt or enacted criticism in understanding parents' help seeking in acute childhood illness at home: A grounded theory study. *International Journal of Nursing Studies,*.

Stålkrantz, A., Brostrom, A., Wiberg, J., Svnborg, E., & Malm, D. (2012). Everyday life for the spouses of patients with untreated OSA syndrome. *Scandinavian Journal of Caring Sciences, 26*(2), 324–332.

Yang, C., Tsai, J., Huang, Y., & Lin, C. (2011). Effects of a home-based walking program on perceived symptom and mood status in postoperative breast cancer women receiving adjuvant chemotherapy. *Journal of Advanced Nursing, 67*, 158–168.

# 4 Reading and Critiquing Research Articles

## LEARNING OBJECTIVES

*On completing this chapter, you will be able to:*

- Identify and describe the major sections in a research journal article
- Characterize the style used in quantitative and qualitative research reports
- Read a research article and broadly grasp its "story"
- Describe aspects of a research critique
- Understand the many challenges researchers face and identify some tools for addressing methodologic challenges
- Define new terms in the chapter

## KEY TERMS

| | | |
|---|---|---|
| Abstract | Inference | Research control |
| Bias | Journal article | Scientific merit |
| Blinding | Level of significance | Statistical significance |
| Confounding variable | *p* | Statistical test |
| Credibility | Placebo | Transferability |
| Critique | Randomness | Triangulation |
| Findings | Reflexivity | Trustworthiness |
| IMRAD format | Reliability | Validity |

E̶vidence from nursing studies is communicated through research reports that describe what was studied, how it was studied, and what was found. Research reports are often daunting to readers without research training. This chapter aims to make research reports more accessible, and also provides some guidance regarding critiques of research reports.

## TYPES OF RESEARCH REPORTS

Nurses are most likely to encounter research evidence in journals or at professional conferences. Research **journal articles** are descriptions of studies published in professional journals. Competition for journal space is keen, and so the typical research article is brief—generally only 15 to 20 double-spaced pages. This means that researchers must condense a lot of information about the study into a short report.

Usually, manuscripts are reviewed by two or more *peer reviewers* (other researchers) who make recommendations about whether to accept or reject the manuscript, or to suggest revisions. Reviews are usually *"blind"*—reviewers are not told researchers' names, and authors are not told reviewers' names. As a result of peer review, consumers have some assurance that journal articles have been critiqued by other nurse researchers. Nevertheless, publication does not mean that findings can be uncritically accepted. Research method courses help nurses to evaluate the quality of evidence reported in journal articles.

At conferences, research findings are presented as oral presentations or poster sessions. *Oral presentations* follow a format similar to that used in journal articles, which we discuss next. The presenter is typically allotted 10 to 20 minutes to describe key features of the study. In *poster sessions*, many researchers simultaneously present visual displays summarizing their studies, and conference attendees walk around the room looking at these displays.

Conferences also offer an opportunity for dialogue between attendees. Attendees can ask questions to help them better understand what the findings mean; moreover, they can offer the researchers suggestions relating to clinical implications of the study. Thus, professional conferences are a valuable forum for clinical audiences.

# THE CONTENT OF RESEARCH JOURNAL ARTICLES

Many research articles follow a conventional organization called the **IMRAD format**. This format organizes content into four main sections—**I**ntroduction, **M**ethod, **R**esults, and **D**iscussion. The paper is preceded by a title and an abstract, and concludes with references.

## The Title and Abstract

Research reports have a title that succinctly conveys key information. In qualitative studies, the title normally includes the central phenomenon and group under investigation. In quantitative studies, the title communicates key variables and the population (in other words, the PICO components described in Chapter 2).

The **abstract** is a brief description of the study placed at the beginning of the article. The abstract answers questions like the following: What were the research questions? What methods were used to address those questions? What were the findings? What are the implications for nursing practice? Readers can review an abstract to judge whether to read the full report.

Some journals have moved from having traditional abstracts—single paragraphs summarizing the study's main features—to slightly longer, structured abstracts with headings. For example, *Nursing Research* suggests the following abstract heading: Background, Objectives, Method, Results, and Conclusions. Beck and Watson's (2010) qualitative study in Appendix B of this book exemplifies this longer abstract style, whereas the abstract in Appendix A (Howell et al., 2007) illustrates the traditional one-paragraph format.

## The Introduction

The introduction to a research article acquaints readers with the research problem and its context. This section usually describes the following:

- The central phenomena, concepts, or variables under study
- The study purpose and the research questions or hypotheses
- A review of the related literature

- The theoretical or conceptual framework
- The significance of and need for the study.

Thus, the introduction sets the stage for presenting what the researcher did and what was learned.

> **Example of an introductory paragraph:**
> As the aging population increases, the demand grows for technologies to enhance quality of life and ameliorate physical decline....Yet few practitioners and researchers have asked older persons their opinions of technological devices..., including traditional technologies like canes and walkers....Our purpose was to elaborate on what it was like for 40 older homebound women...to negotiate reliance on a cane or walker as a walking device (Porter et al., 2011, p. 534).

In this paragraph, the researchers described the concepts of interest (experiences of relying on canes and walkers among older persons), the need for the study (the fact that little is known about the experience directly from elders), and the study purpose.

☞ **TIP:** The introduction section of many journal articles is not specifically labeled "Introduction." The report's introduction immediately follows the abstract.

## The Method Section

The method section describes the methods used to answer the research questions. In a quantitative study, the method section usually describes the following, which may be presented in labeled subsections:

- The research design
- The sampling plan
- Methods of measuring variables and collecting data
- Study procedures, including procedures to protect human rights
- Data analysis methods

Qualitative researchers discuss many of the same issues, but with different emphases. For example, a qualitative researchers often provide more information about the study setting and context than quantitative researchers, and less information on sampling and data collection. Increasingly, reports of qualitative studies describe the researchers' efforts to enhance the integrity of the study.

## The Results Section

The results section presents the **findings** that were obtained by analyzing the study data. The text presents a narrative summary of key findings, often accompanied by more detailed tables. Virtually all results sections contain basic descriptive information, including a description of the participants (e.g., average age, percent male and female).

In quantitative studies, the results section also reports the following information relating to any statistical tests performed:

- *The names of statistical tests used.* Researchers use **statistical tests** to test their hypotheses and assess the probability that the results are accurate. For example, if the researcher finds that the average birth weight of drug-exposed infants in the sample is lower than the birth weight of infants not exposed to drugs, how probable is it that the same would be true for other infants not in the sample? A statistical test helps answer the question, Is the relationship between prenatal drug exposure and infant birth weight *real*, and would it likely be observed with a new sample from the same population? Statistical tests are based on common principles; you do not have to know the names of all statistical tests to comprehend the findings.

○ *The value of the calculated statistic.* Computers are used to calculate a numeric value for the particular statistical test used. The value allows researchers to reach conclusions about their hypotheses. The *actual* value of the statistic, however, is not inherently meaningful and need not concern you.

○ *The significance.* A critical piece of information is whether the statistical tests were significant (not to be confused with clinically important). If a researcher reports that the results are **statistically significant,** it means the findings are probably true and replicable with a new sample. Research reports also indicate the **level of significance,** which is an index of how *probable* it is that the findings are reliable. For example, if a report indicates that a finding was significant at the .05 level, this means that only 5 times out of 100 (5/100 = .05) would the obtained result be spurious. In other words, 95 times out of 100, similar results would be obtained with a new sample. Readers can thus have a high degree of confidence—but not total assurance—that the results are accurate.

> **Example from the results section of a quantitative study:**
> Li and colleagues (2011) tested the effectiveness of implementing sleep care guidelines for improving sleep quality among patients in a surgical ICU. Half the patients were in a usual care group, and the other half were cared for by nurses who followed guidelines for noise and light reduction. Here is a sentence adapted from the reported results: Sleep interruptions from care-related activities ($t = 5.28$, $p < .001$) were significantly lower in the special intervention group than in the usual care control group.

In this example, the researchers stated that sleep interruptions were *significantly* lower among those cared for by nurses who followed sleep care guidelines. The group differences in sleep interruptions were not likely to have been haphazard, and would probably be replicated with a new sample of patients. This finding is highly reliable: less than one time in 1,000 ($p < .001$) could a difference of the magnitude obtained occur as a fluke. Note that to comprehend this finding, you do not need to understand what a *t* statistic is, nor do you need to concern yourself with the actual value of the statistic, 5.28.

👉 **TIP:** Be alert to *p* values (probabilities) when reading statistical results. If a *p* value is $>.05$ (e.g., $p = .08$), the results are *not* statistically significant, by convention. Also, be aware that results are *more* reliable if the *p* value is *smaller*. For example, there is a higher probability that the results are accurate when $p = .01$ (1 in 100 chance of a spurious result) than when $p = .05$ (5 in 100 chances of a spurious result). Researchers either report an exact probability (e.g., $p = .03$) or a probability below conventional threshholds (e.g., $p < .05$).

In qualitative reports, researchers often organize findings according to the major themes, processes, or categories that were identified in the data. The results section of qualitative reports sometimes has several subsections, the headings of which correspond to the researcher's labels for the themes. Excerpts from the *raw data* (the actual words of participants) are presented to support and provide a rich description of the thematic analysis. The results section of qualitative studies may also present the researcher's emerging theory about the phenomenon under study.

> **Example from the results section of a qualitative study:**
> Murdoch and Franck (2012) conducted a phenomenological study of mothers' experiences caring for infants at home after neonatal unit discharge. Six themes formed the mothers' experiences, one of which was *apprehension*. Here is an excerpt illustrating that theme: "Obviously when she did come home it was obviously a big shock from coming from this big support network, in terms of the nurses and doctors around you, to suddenly not having anything at all" (p. 2014).

## The Discussion Section

In the discussion, the researcher presents conclusions about the meaning and implications of the findings, i.e., what the results mean, why things turned out the way they did, how the findings fit with other evidence, and how the results can be used in practice. The discussion in both qualitative and quantitative reports may include the following elements:

- An interpretation of the results
- Clinical and research implications
- Study limitations and ramifications for the believability of the results

Researchers are in the best position to point out deficiencies in their studies. A discussion section that presents the researcher's grasp of study limitations demonstrates to readers that the authors were aware of the limitations and probably took them into account in interpreting the findings.

## References

Research articles conclude with a list of the books and articles that were referenced. If you are interested in pursuing additional reading on a topic, the reference list of a recent study is an excellent place to begin.

# THE STYLE OF RESEARCH JOURNAL ARTICLES

Research reports tell a story. However, the style in which many research journal articles are written—especially reports of quantitative studies—makes it difficult for some readers to figure out or become interested in the story.

## Why Are Research Articles So Hard to Read?

To unaccustomed audiences, research reports may seem stuffy and bewildering. Four factors contribute to this impression:

1. *Compactness.* Journal space is limited, so authors compress a lot of information into a short space. Interesting, personalized aspects of the investigation cannot be reported, and, in qualitative studies, only a handful of supporting quotes can be included.
2. *Jargon.* The authors of research articles use research terms that may seem esoteric.
3. *Objectivity.* Quantitative researchers tend to avoid any impression of subjectivity, and so they tell their research stories in a way that makes them sound impersonal. Most quantitative research articles are written in the passive voice, which tends to make the articles less inviting and lively. Qualitative reports, by contrast, are often written in a more conversational style.

4. *Statistical information.* In quantitative reports, numbers and statistical symbols may intimidate readers who do not have statistical training.

A goal of this textbook is to assist you in understanding the content of research reports and in overcoming anxieties about jargon and statistical information.

 **HOW-TO-TELL TIP:** How can you tell if the voice is active or passive? In the active voice, the article would say what the researchers *did* (e.g., "We used a mercury sphygmomanometer to measure blood pressure"). In the passive voice, the article indicates what *was done*, without indicating who did it, although it is implied that the researchers were the agents ("e.g., a mercury sphygmomanometer *was used* to measure blood pressure").

## Tips on Reading Research Articles

As you progress through this book, you will acquire skills for evaluating research articles, but the skills involved in critical appraisal take time to develop. The first step is to comprehend research articles. Your first few attempts to read a research article might be overwhelming, and you may wonder whether being able to understand them, let alone appraise them, is a realistic goal. Here are some hints on digesting research reports.

- Grow accustomed to the style of research articles by reading them frequently, even though you may not yet understand all the technical points.
- Read from a report that has been photocopied (or downloaded and printed) so that you can highlight or underline portions, and write questions or notes in the margins.
- Read journal articles slowly. It may be useful to skim the article first to get the major points and then read the article more carefully a second time.
- On the second reading, train yourself to become an *active* reader. Reading actively means that you constantly monitor yourself to verify that you understand what you are reading. If you have difficulty, you can ask someone for help. In most cases, that "someone" will be your instructor, but also consider contacting the researchers themselves.
- Keep this textbook with you as a reference when you read articles so that you can look up unfamiliar terms in the glossary or the index.
- Try not to get bogged down in (or scared away by) statistical information. Try to grasp the gist of the story without letting symbols and numbers frustrate you.
- Until you become accustomed to the style and jargon of research articles, you may want to "translate" them. You can do this by translating jargon into more familiar words, by recasting the report into an active voice, and by summarizing findings with words rather than numbers. As an example, Box 4.1 presents a summary of a fictitious study about the psychological consequences of having an abortion, written in a style that is typical for a journal article. Terms that can be looked up in the glossary of this book are underlined, and marginal notes indicate the type of information being communicated. Box 4.2 on page 68 presents a "translation" of this summary into more digestible language.

# CRITIQUING RESEARCH REPORTS

A critical reading of a research article involves a careful appraisal of the researcher's major conceptual and methodologic decisions. You may find it difficult to criticize these decisions at this point, but your skills will improve as you progress through this book.

| | | |
|---|---|---|
| **BOX 4.1** | **Summary of a Fictitious Study for Translation** | |

| | | |
|---|---|---|
| **Purpose of the study** | The potentially negative sequelae of having an abortion on the psychological adjustment of adolescents have not been adequately studied. The present study sought to examine whether alternative pregnancy resolution decisions have different long-term effects on the psychological functioning of young women. | **Need for the study** |
| **Research design** | Three groups of low-income pregnant teenagers attending an inner-city clinic were the <u>subjects</u> in this study: those who delivered and kept the baby; those who delivered and relinquished the baby for adoption; and those who had an abortion. The <u>sample</u> included 25 subjects in each group. | **Study population** |
| **Research instruments** | The study <u>instruments</u> included a self-administered <u>questionnaire</u> and a battery of psychological tests measuring depression, anxiety, and psychosomatic symptoms. The instruments were administered upon entry into the study (when the subjects first came to the clinic) and then 1 year after termination of the pregnancy. | **Research sample** |
| **Data analysis procedure** | The <u>data</u> were analyzed using <u>analysis of variance (ANOVA)</u>. The ANOVA tests indicated that the three groups did not differ significantly in terms of depression, anxiety, or psychosomatic symptoms at the initial testing ($p = .36$). At the <u>post-test</u>, however, the abortion group had significantly higher scores on the depression scale, and these girls were significantly more likely than the two delivery groups to report severe tension headaches (both $p < .01$). There were no <u>significant</u> differences on any of the <u>dependent variables</u> for the two delivery groups. | **Results** |
| **Implications** | The results of this study suggest that young women who elect to have an abortion may experience a number of long-term negative consequences. It would appear that appropriate efforts should be made to follow up abortion patients to determine their need for suitable treatment. | **Interpretation** |

## What Is a Research Critique?

A research **critique** is an objective assessment of a study's strengths and limitations. Critiques usually conclude with the reviewer's summary of the study's merits, recommendations regarding the value of the evidence, and suggestions about improving the study or the report.

Research critiques of individual studies are prepared for various reasons, and they vary in scope. Peer reviewers who are asked to prepare a written critique for a journal considering publication of a manuscript may evaluate the strengths and weaknesses in terms of substantive issues (Was the research problem significant to nursing?); theoretical issues (Were the conceptual underpinnings sound?); methodologic decisions (Were the methods rigorous, yielding believable evidence?); interpretive (Did the researcher reach defensible conclusions?); ethics (Were participants' rights protected?); and style (Is the report clear, grammatical, and well organized?). In short, peer reviewers do a comprehensive review to provide feedback to the researchers and to journal editors about the merit of both the study and the report, and typically offer suggestions for revisions.

Students taking a research methods course also may be asked to critique a study. Such critiques are usually expected to be comprehensive, encompassing the various dimensions just described. The purpose of such a thorough critique is to cultivate critical thinking and to induce students to apply newly acquired skills in research methods.

---

**BOX 4.2  Translated Version of Fictitious Research Study**

As researchers, we wondered whether young women who had an abortion had any emotional problems in the long run. It seemed to us that not enough research had been done to know whether any psychological harm resulted from an abortion.

We decided to study this question ourselves by comparing the experiences of three types of teenagers who became pregnant—first, girls who delivered and kept their babies; second, those who delivered the babies but gave them up for adoption; and third, those who elected to have an abortion. All teenagers that we recruited were poor, and all were patients at an inner-city clinic. Altogether, we studied 75 girls—25 in each of the three groups. We evaluated the teenagers' emotional states by asking them to fill out a questionnaire and to take several psychological tests. These tests allowed us to assess things such as the girls' degree of depression and anxiety and whether they had any complaints of a psychosomatic nature. We asked them to fill out the forms twice: once when they came into the clinic, and then again a year after the abortion or the delivery.

We learned that the three groups of teenagers looked pretty much alike in terms of their emotional states when they first filled out the forms. Yet, when we compared how the three groups looked a year later, we found that the teenagers who had abortions were more depressed and were more likely to say they had severe tension headaches than teenagers in the other two groups. The teenagers who kept their babies and those who gave their babies up for adoption looked pretty similar 1 year after their babies were born, at least in terms of depression, anxiety, and psychosomatic complaints.

Thus, it seems that we might be right in having some concerns about the emotional effects of having an abortion. Nurses should be aware of these long-term emotional effects, and it even may be advisable to institute some type of follow-up procedure to find out if these young women need additional help.

---

Note, however, that critiques designed to inform evidence-based nursing practice are seldom comprehensive. For example, it is of little consequence to evidence-based practice (EBP) that a research article is ungrammatical. A critique of the clinical utility of a study focuses on whether the evidence is accurate, believable, and clinically relevant. These narrower critiques focus more squarely on appraising the research methods and the findings themselves.

## Critiquing Support in This Textbook

We provide several types of support for research critiques. First, detailed critiquing suggestions relating to chapter content are included at the end of most chapters. Second, it is always illuminating to have a good model, so we prepared comprehensive critiques of two studies, one quantitative, the other qualitative. The two studies in their entirety and the critiques are in Appendixes C and D.

Third, we offer an abbreviated set of key critiquing guidelines for quantitative and qualitative reports in this chapter, in Tables 4.1 and 4.2, respectively. These guidelines are appropriate for a more focused critique designed to assess evidence quality. The questions in the guidelines concern the rigor with which the researchers dealt with critical research challenges, some of which are outlined in the next section.

☞ **TIP:** For those undertaking a comprehensive critique, such as the ones included in Appendixes C and D, we offer more inclusive critiquing guidelines in the Chapter Supplement on thePoint website.

The second column of Tables 4.1 and 4.2 lists some key critiquing questions, and the third column cross-references the more detailed guidelines in the various chapters of the book.

*(Text continued on page 71)*

**TABLE 4.1 Guide to a Focused Critique of Evidence Quality in a Quantitative Research Report**

| Aspect of the Report | Critiquing Questions | Detailed Critiquing Guidelines |
|---|---|---|
| **Method** Research design | • Was the most rigorous possible design used, given the purpose of the research? <br> • Were appropriate comparisons made to enhance interpretability of the findings? <br> • Was the number of data collection points appropriate? <br> • Did the design minimize biases and threats to the internal, construct, and external validity of the study (e.g., was blinding used, was attrition minimized)? | Box 9.1, page 170 |
| Population and sample | • Was the population identified and described? Was the sample described in sufficient detail? <br> • Was the best possible sampling design used to enhance the sample's representativeness? Were sample biases minimized? <br> • Was the sample size adequate? Was a power analysis used to estimate sample size needs? | Box 10.1, page 183 |
| Data collection and measurement | • Were key variables operationalized using the best possible method (e.g., interviews, observations, and so on)? <br> • Are the specific instruments adequately described and were they good choices, given the study purpose and study population? <br> • Does the report provide evidence that the data collection methods yielded data that were high on reliability and validity? | Box 10.2, pages 193–94 <br> Box 11.1, page 209 |
| Procedures | • If there was an intervention, is it adequately described, and was it properly implemented? Did most participants allocated to the intervention group actually receive it? Was there evidence of intervention fidelity? <br> • Were data collected in a manner that minimized bias? Was the staff who collected data appropriately trained? | Box 9.1, page 170 <br> Box 10.2, pages 193–94 |
| **Results** Data analysis | • Were appropriate statistical methods used? <br> • Was the most powerful analytic method used? (e.g., did the analysis control for confounding variables)? <br> • Were Type I and Type II errors avoided or minimized? | Box 12.1, page 243 |
| Findings | • Was information about statistical significance presented? <br> • Was information about effect size and precision of estimates (confidence intervals) presented? | Box 13.1, page 261 |
| Summary assessment | • Despite any limitations, do the study findings appear to be valid—do you have confidence in the *truth* value of the results? <br> • Does the study contribute any meaningful evidence that can be used in nursing practice or that is useful to the nursing discipline? | |

**TABLE 4.2 Guide to a Focused Critique of Evidence Quality in a Qualitative Research Report**

| Aspect of the Report | Critiquing Questions | Detailed Critiquing Guidelines |
|---|---|---|
| **Method** Research design and research tradition | • Is the identified research tradition (if any) congruent with the methods used to collect and analyze data? <br>• Was an adequate amount of time spent in the field or with study participants? <br>• Was there evidence of reflexivity in the design? | Box 14.1, page 278 |
| Sample and setting | • Was the group or population of interest adequately described? Were the setting and sample described in sufficient detail? <br>• Was the best possible method of sampling used to enhance information richness and address the needs of the study? <br>• Was the sample size adequate? Was saturation achieved? | Box 15.1, page 289 |
| Data collection | • Were the methods of gathering data appropriate? Were data gathered through two or more methods to achieve triangulation? <br>• Did the researcher ask the right questions or make the right observations? <br>• Was there a sufficient amount of data? Were they of sufficient depth and richness? | Box 15.3, page 296 |
| Procedures | • Do data collection and recording procedures appear appropriate? <br>• Were data collected in a manner that minimized bias? Were the people who collected data appropriately trained? | Box 15.3, page 296 |
| Enhancement of trustworthiness | • Did the researchers use strategies to enhance the trustworthiness/integrity of the study, and were those strategies adequate? <br>• Do the researchers' clinical, substantive, or methodologic qualifications and experience enhance confidence in the findings and their interpretation? | Box 17.1, page 334 |
| **Results** Data analysis | • Was the data analysis strategy compatible with the research tradition and with the nature and type of data gathered? <br>• Did the analysis yield an appropriate "product" (e.g., a theory, taxonomy, thematic pattern, etc.)? <br>• Did the analytic procedures suggest the possibility of biases? | Box 16.2, page 316 |
| Findings | • Were the findings effectively summarized, with good use of excerpts and supporting arguments? <br>• Do the themes adequately capture the meaning of the data? Does it appear that the researcher satisfactorily conceptualized the themes or patterns in the data? <br>• Did the analysis yield an insightful, provocative, authentic, and meaningful picture of the phenomenon under investigation? | Box 16.2, page 316 |
| Summary assessment | • Do the study findings appear to be trustworthy—do you have confidence in the *truth* value of the results? <br>• Does the study contribute any meaningful evidence that can be used in nursing practice or that is useful to the nursing discipline? | |

We know that most of the critiquing questions are too difficult for you to answer at this point, but your methodologic and critiquing skills will develop as you progress through this book.

The wording of questions in these guidelines calls for a yes or no answer (although it may well be that the answer sometimes will be, "Yes, *but*…"). In all cases, the desirable answer is *yes*, that is, a *no* suggests a possible limitation and a *yes* suggests a strength. Therefore, the more *yeses* a study gets, the stronger it is likely to be. Cumulatively, then, these guidelines can suggest a global assessment: a report with 10 *yeses* is likely to be superior to one with only two. However, these guidelines are not intended to yield a formal quality "score."

We acknowledge that our critiquing guidelines have some shortcomings. In particular, they are generic even though critiquing cannot use a one-size-fits-all list of questions. Important critiquing questions that are relevant to certain studies (e.g., those that have a Therapy purpose) do not fit into a set of general questions for all quantitative studies. Thus, you need to use some judgment about whether the guidelines are sufficiently comprehensive for the type of study you are critiquing. We also note that there are questions in these guidelines for which there are no totally objective answers. Even experts sometimes disagree about methodologic strategies.

> **☞ TIP:** An important thing to remember is that it is appropriate to assume the posture of a skeptic when you are critiquing research reports. Just as a careful clinician seeks research evidence that certain practices are or are not effective, you as a reviewer should demand evidence that the researchers' methodologic decisions were sound.

## Critiquing With Key Research Challenges in Mind

In critiquing a study, it is useful to be aware of the challenges that confront researchers. For example, they face ethical challenges (e.g., Can the study achieve its goals without infringing on human rights?); practical challenges (Will I be able to recruit enough study participants?); and methodologic challenges (Will the adopted methods yield results that can be trusted and applied to other settings?). Most of this book provides guidance relating to the last question, and this section highlights key methodologic challenges as a way of introducing important terms and concepts that are relevant in a critique. Keep in mind that the worth of a study's evidence for nursing practice relies on how well researchers deal with these challenges.

### Inference

Inference is an integral part of doing and critiquing research. An **inference** is a conclusion drawn from the study evidence using logical reasoning and taking into account the methods used to generate that evidence.

Inference is necessary because researchers use proxies that "stand in" for things that are fundamentally of interest. A sample of participants is a proxy for an entire population. A study site is a proxy for all relevant sites in which the phenomena of interest could unfold. A measuring scale yields proxy information about constructs that can only be captured through approximations. A control group that does not receive an intervention is a proxy for what would happen to the *same* people if they simultaneously received *and* did not receive an intervention.

Researchers face the challenge of using methods that yield good and persuasive evidence in support of inferences that they wish to make. Readers must draw their own inferences based on a critique of methodologic decisions.

### Reliability, Validity, and Trustworthiness

Researchers want their inferences to correspond to the *truth*. Research cannot contribute evidence to guide clinical practice if the findings are inaccurate, biased, or fail to represent the experiences of the target group.

Quantitative researchers use several criteria to assess the quality of a study, sometimes referred to as its **scientific merit**. Two especially important criteria are reliability and validity. **Reliability** refers to the accuracy and consistency of information obtained in a study. The term is most often associated with the methods used to measure variables. For example, if a thermometer measured Alan's temperature as 98.1°F one minute and as 102.5°F the next minute, the thermometer would be unreliable. The concept of reliability is also important in interpreting statistical analyses. *Statistical reliability* refers to the probability that the same results would be obtained with a new sample of subjects—that is, that the results are an accurate reflection of a wider group than just the particular people who participated in the study.

**Validity** is a more complex concept that broadly concerns the *soundness* of the study's evidence. Like reliability, validity is an important criterion for evaluating methods to measure variables. In this context, the validity question is whether the methods are really measuring the concepts that they purport to measure. Is a paper-and-pencil measure of depression *really* measuring depression? Or is it measuring something else, such as loneliness or stress? Researchers strive for solid conceptual definitions of research variables and valid methods to operationalize them.

Another aspect of validity concerns the quality of evidence about the relationship between the independent variable and the dependent variable. Did a nursing intervention *really* bring about improvements in patients' outcomes—or were other confounding factors responsible for patients' progress? Researchers make numerous methodologic decisions that can influence this type of study validity.

Qualitative researchers use different criteria (and different terminology) in evaluating a study's quality. In general, qualitative researchers discuss methods of enhancing the **trustworthiness** of the study's data and findings (Lincoln & Guba, 1985). Trustworthiness encompasses several different dimensions—credibility, transferability, confirmability, dependability, and authenticity—which are described in Chapter 17.

**Credibility** is an especially important aspect of trustworthiness. Credibility is achieved to the extent that the research methods inspire confidence that the results and interpretations are truthful and accurate. Credibility in a qualitative study can be enhanced through various approaches, but one strategy merits early discussion because it has implications for the design of all studies, including quantitative ones. **Triangulation** is the use of multiple sources or referents to draw conclusions about what constitutes the truth. In a quantitative study, this might mean having two ways to measure a dependent variable, to assess whether predicted effects are consistent. In a qualitative study, triangulation might involve efforts to understand the complexity of a phenomenon by using multiple data collection methods to converge on the truth (e.g., having in-depth discussions with participants, as well as watching their behavior in natural settings). Nurse researchers are also beginning to triangulate across paradigms—that is, to integrate both qualitative and quantitative data in a single study to offset the shortcomings of each approach and enhance the validity of the conclusions.

**Example of triangulation:**
Carlsson and colleagues (2012) conducted a study to describe the accuracy of discharge information for patients with eating difficulties after stroke. They triangulated information from hospital records, interviews with nurses, and observations of patients' eating.

Nurse researchers need to design their studies in such a way that threats to the reliability, validity, and trustworthiness of their studies are minimized, and users of research must evaluate the extent to which they were successful.

**TIP:** In reading and critiquing research articles, it is appropriate to have a "show me" attitude—that is, to expect researchers to build and present a solid case for the merit of their inferences. They do this by providing evidence that the findings are reliable and valid or trustworthy.

## Bias

Bias can threaten a study's validity and trustworthiness. A **bias** is an influence that results in an error in an inference or estimate. Biases can affect the quality of evidence in both qualitative and quantitative studies. Bias can result from various factors, including study participants' lack of candor or desire to please, researchers' preconceptions, or faulty methods of collecting data.

Bias can never be avoided totally because the potential for its occurrence is so pervasive. Some bias is haphazard and affects only small segments of the data. As an example of such *random bias*, a few study participants might provide inaccurate information because they were tired at the time of data collection. *Systematic bias* results when the bias is consistent or uniform. For example, if a spring scale consistently measured people's weight as being 2 pounds heavier than their true weight, there would be systematic bias in the data on weight. Rigorous research methods aim to eliminate or minimize bias.

Researchers adopt a variety of strategies to address bias. Triangulation is one such approach, the idea being that multiple sources of information or points of view help to counterbalance biases and offer avenues to identify them. In quantitative research, methods to combat bias often entail research control.

## Research Control

One of the central features of quantitative studies is that they typically involve efforts to control aspects of the research. **Research control** usually involves holding constant influences on the outcome variable so that the true relationship between the independent and outcome variables can be understood. In other words, research control attempts to eliminate contaminating factors that might cloud the relationship between the variables that are of central interest.

Contaminating factors, often called **confounding** (or *extraneous*) **variables**, can best be illustrated with an example. Suppose we were studying whether urinary incontinence (UI) leads to depression. Prior evidence suggests that this is the case, but previous studies have not clarified whether it is UI per se or other factors that contribute to risk of depression. The question is whether UI itself (the independent variable) contributes to higher levels of depression, or whether there are other factors that can account for the relationship between UI and depression. We need to design a study so as to control other determinants of the outcome—determinants that are also related to the independent variable, UI.

One confounding variable here is age. Levels of depression tend to be higher in older people; and, people with UI tend to be older than those without this problem. In other words, perhaps age is the *real* cause of higher depression in people with UI. If age is not controlled, than any observed relationship between UI and depression could be caused by UI, or by age.

Three possible explanations might be portrayed schematically as follows:

1. UI→depression
2. Age→UI→depression

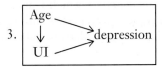

The arrows here symbolize a causal mechanism or an influence. In model 1, UI directly affects depression, independently of any other factors. In model 2, UI is a *mediating variable*—the effect of age on depression is *mediated* by UI. According to this representation, age affects depression *through* the effect that age has on UI. In model 3, both age and UI have separate effects on depression, and age also increases the risk of UI. Some research is specifically designed to test paths of mediation and multiple causation, but in the present example age is extraneous to the research question. We want to design a study so that the first explanation can be tested. Age must be controlled if our goal is to explore the validity of model 1, which posits that, no matter what a person's age, having UI makes a person more vulnerable to depression.

How can we impose such control? There are a number of ways, as we discuss in Chapter 9, but the general principle underlying each alternative is that the confounding variables must be *held constant*. The confounding variable must somehow be handled so that, in the context of the study, the confounding variable is not related to the independent variable or the outcome. As an example, let us say we wanted to compare the average scores on a depression scale for those with and without UI. We would want to design a study in such a way that the ages of those in the UI and non-UI groups are comparable, even though, in general, the groups are not comparable in terms of age.

By exercising control over age in this example, we would be taking a step toward explaining the relationship between variables. The world is complex, and many variables are interrelated in complicated ways. When studying a problem within the positivist paradigm, researchers usually analyze a couple of relationships at a time. Modest quantitative studies can contribute evidence, but the value of the evidence is often related to how well researchers control confounding influences.

Research rooted in the constructivist paradigm does not impose controls. With their emphasis on holism and individual human experience, qualitative researchers typically believe that imposing controls removes some of the meaning of reality.

## Bias Reduction: Randomness and Blinding

For quantitative researchers, a powerful tool for eliminating bias involves **randomness**—having certain features of the study established by chance rather than by design or researcher preference. When people are selected *at random* to participate in a study, for example, each person in the initial pool has an equal chance of being selected. This in turn means that there are no systematic biases in the make-up of the sample. Men and women have an equal chance of being selected, for example. Similarly, if participants are allocated *at random* to groups that will be compared (e.g., a special intervention and "usual care" group), then there can be no systematic biases in the groups' composition. Randomness is a compelling method of controlling confounding variables and reducing bias.

**Example of randomness:**
Lindseth and colleagues (2012) studied the effect of alternative diets on sleep outcomes. Their sample of 44 healthy adults was randomly assigned to different orderings of four diets—a normal diet, high-protein diet, high-fat diet, and high-carbohydrate diet. Sleep efficiency and other measures of sleep were monitored under the different diets.

Another bias-reducing strategy is called **blinding** (or *masking*), which is used in some quantitative studies to prevent biases stemming from people's awareness. Blinding involves concealing information from participants, data collectors, care providers, or data analysts to enhance objectivity. For example, if study participants are aware of whether they are getting an experimental drug or a sham drug (a **placebo**), then their outcomes could be influenced by their expectations of the new drug's efficacy. Blinding involves disguising or withholding information about participants' status in the study (e.g., whether they are in a certain group), or about the study hypotheses.

Qualitative researchers do not consider randomness or blinding desirable tools for understanding phenomena. A researcher's judgment is viewed as an indispensable vehicle for uncovering the complexities of the phenomena of interest.

## Reflexivity

Qualitative researchers are also interested in discovering the truth about human experience. Qualitative researchers often rely on reflexivity to guard against personal bias. **Reflexivity** is the process of reflecting critically on the self, and of analyzing and making note of personal values that could affect data collection and interpretation. Qualitative researchers are trained to explore these issues, to be reflective about decisions made during the inquiry, and to record their thoughts in personal diaries and memos.

**Example of reflexivity:**
Frisvold and colleagues (2012) explored nurses' perceptions of having participated in a stress-reduction course a year earlier. The researchers used reflexive journaling and reflexive tape recording: "the investigator's reactions to certain observations were immediately documented to identify personal bias and preconceived notions that may affect the analysis of data" (p. 271).

**TIP:** Reflexivity can be a useful tool in quantitative as well as qualitative research—self-awareness and introspection can enhance the quality of any study.

## Generalizability and Transferability

Nurses increasingly rely on evidence from disciplined research as a guide in their clinical practice. EBP is based on the assumption that study findings are not unique to the people, places, or circumstances of the original research.

As noted in Chapter 1, *generalizability* is the criterion used in quantitative studies to assess the extent to which the findings can be applied to other groups and settings. How do researchers enhance the generalizability of a study? First and foremost, they must design studies strong in reliability and validity. There is little point in wondering whether results are generalizable if they are not accurate or valid. In selecting participants, researchers must also give thought to the types of people to whom results might be generalized—and then select subjects in such a way that a representative sample is obtained. If a study is intended to have implications for male and female patients, then men and women should be included as participants.

Qualitative researchers do not specifically aim for generalizability, but they do want to generate knowledge that might be useful in other situations. Lincoln and Guba (1985), in their influential book on naturalistic inquiry, discuss the concept of **transferability**, the extent to which qualitative findings can be transferred to other settings, as another aspect of trustworthiness. An important mechanism for promoting transferability is the amount of rich descriptive information qualitative researchers provide about the contexts of their studies.

# RESEARCH EXAMPLES WITH CRITICAL THINKING EXERCISES

Abstracts for a quantitative and a qualitative nursing study are presented below, followed by some questions to guide critical thinking.

Examples 1 and 2 below are also featured in our *Interactive Critical Thinking Activity* on thePoint website where you can easily record, print, and e-mail your responses to the related questions.

## EXAMPLE 1 ● Quantitative Research

**Study:** Effect on pain of changing the needle prior to administering medicine intramuscularly (Ağac & Günes, 2011, p. 563)

**Aim:** This paper is the report of a study to determine whether changing the needle before administering an intramuscular injection could reduce pain, and to investigate gender differences in pain perception.

**Background:** A skilled injection technique can make the patient's experience less painful and avoid unnecessary complications, and the use of separate needles to draw up and administer medication ensures that the tip of the needle is sharp and free from medication residue.

**Method:** A randomized controlled trial was carried out between January 2009 and May 2009 with 100 patients receiving diclofenac sodium intramuscularly in an emergency and traffic hospital in Izmir, Turkey. The primary outcome was pain intensity measured on a numerical rating scale. Each patient received two injections by the same investigator using two different techniques. The two techniques were randomly allocated and the patients were blinded to the injection technique being administered. After each injection, another investigator who had no prior knowledge of which injection technique was used immediately assessed pain intensity using a numerical rating scale. Descriptive statistics, paired t-test, and t-test were used to evaluate the data.

**Findings:** Findings demonstrated that changing the needle prior to intramuscular medication administration significantly reduced pain intensity. A statistical difference in pain intensity was observed between the two injection techniques.

**Conclusions:** The results supported the hypothesis that changing the needle prior to administering the medicine significantly reduced pain intensity.

### CRITICAL THINKING EXERCISES

1. "Translate" the abstract into a summary that is more consumer friendly. Underline any technical terms and look them up in the glossary.
2. Also consider the following targeted questions:
   a. What were the independent and dependent variables in this study?
   b. Is this study experimental or nonexperimental?
   c. How, if at all, was *randomness* used in this study?
   d. How, if at all, was *blinding* used in this study?
3. If the results of this study are valid and generalizable, in what ways do you think the findings could be used in clinical practice?

## EXAMPLE 2 ● Qualitative Research

**Study:** "How should I touch you?": A qualitative study of attitudes on intimate touch in nursing care (O'Lynn & Krauscheid, 2011, p. 24)

**Objective:** Although touch is essential to nursing practice, few studies have investigated patients' preferences for how nurses should perform tasks involving touch, especially intimate touch involving private and sometimes anxiety-provoking areas of patients' bodies. Some studies suggest that patients have more concerns about intimate touch from male than female nurses. This study sought to elicit the attitudes of laypersons on intimate touch provided by nurses in general and male nurses in particular.

**Methods:** A maximum-variation sample of 24 adults was selected and semi-structured interviews were conducted in four focus groups. Interviews were recorded and transcribed; thematic analysis was performed.

**Results:** Four themes emerged from the interviews: "Communicate with me," "Give me choices," "Ask me about gender," and "Touch me professionally, not too fast and not too slow." Participants said they want to contribute to decisions about whether intimate touch is necessary, and when it is, they want information from and rapport with their nurses. Participants varied in their responses to questions on the nurse's gender. They said they want a firm but not rough touch and for nurses to ensure their privacy.

**Conclusion:** These findings suggest that nurses and other clinicians who provide intimate care should be more aware of patients' attitudes on touch. Further research on the patient's perspective is warranted.

## CRITICAL THINKING EXERCISES
1. "Translate" the abstract into a summary that is more consumer friendly. Underline any technical terms and look them up in the glossary.
2. Also consider the following targeted questions:
   a. On which qualitative research tradition, if any, was this study based?
   b. Is this study experimental or nonexperimental?
   c. How, if at all, was *randomness* used in this study?
   d. Is there any indication in the abstract that *triangulation* was used? What about *Reflexivity*?
3. If the results of this study are trustworthy and transferable, what might be some of the uses to which the findings could be put in clinical practice?
4. Compare the headings used in the two abstracts in Examples 1 and 2. Which do you prefer?

## EXAMPLE 3 ● Quantitative Research in Appendix A
- Read the abstract for Howell and colleagues' (2007) study ("Anxiety, anger, and blood pressure in children") in Appendix A on pages 395–402.

## CRITICAL THINKING EXERCISES
1. "Translate" the abstract into a summary that is more consumer friendly. Underline any technical terms and look them up in the glossary.
2. Also consider the following targeted questions:
   a. Where does the introduction to this article begin and end?
   b. How, if at all, was *randomness* used in this study?
   c. How, if at all, was *blinding* used?
   d. Comment on the possible generalizability of the study findings.

## EXAMPLE 4 ● Qualitative Research in Appendix B
- Read the abstract for Beck and Watson's (2010) study ("Subsequent childbirth after a previous traumatic birth") in Appendix B on pages 403–412.

## CRITICAL THINKING EXERCISES
1. "Translate" the abstract into a summary that is more consumer-friendly. Underline any technical terms and look them up in the glossary.
2. Also consider the following targeted questions, which may assist you in assessing aspects of the study's merit:
   a. Where does the introduction to this article begin and end?
   b. How, if at all, was *randomness* used in this study?
   c. Is there any indication in the abstract that *triangulation* was used? What about *Reflexivity*?
   d. Comment on the possible transferability of the study findings.

**WANT TO KNOW MORE?** A wide variety of resources to enhance your learning and understanding of this chapter are available on thePoint.

- Interactive Critical Thinking Activity
- Chapter Supplement on Critiquing Guidelines for Quantitative and Qualitative Research Reports
- Answers to the Critical Thinking Exercises for Examples 3 and 4
- Student Review Questions
- Full-text online

Additional study aids including eight journal articles and related questions are also available in *Study Guide for Essentials of Nursing Research, 8e.*

## SUMMARY POINTS

- Both qualitative and quantitative researchers disseminate their findings, most often by publishing reports of their research as **journal articles**, which concisely communicate what the researcher did and what was found.

- Journal articles often consist of an **abstract** (a synopsis of the study) and four major sections that often follow the **IMRAD format**: an **I**ntroduction (the research problem and its context); **M**ethod section (the strategies used to answer research questions); **R**esults (study findings); and **D**iscussion (interpretation of the findings).

- Research reports are often difficult to read because they are dense, concise, and contain jargon. Quantitative research reports may be intimidating at first because, compared to qualitative reports, they are more impersonal and report on statistical tests.

- **Statistical tests** are used to test hypotheses and to evaluate the reliability of the findings. Findings that are **statistically significant** have a high probability of being "real."

- A goal of this book is to help students to prepare a research **critique**, which is a critical appraisal of the strengths and limitations of a study, often to assess the worth of the evidence for nursing practice.

- Researchers face numerous challenges, the solutions to which must be considered in critiquing a study because they affect the inferences that can be made.

- An **inference** is a conclusion drawn from the study evidence, taking into account the methods used to generate that evidence. Researchers strive to have their inferences correspond to the *truth*.

- **Reliability** (a key challenge in quantitative research) refers to the accuracy and consistency of information obtained in a study. **Validity** is a more complex concept that broadly concerns the *soundness* of the study's evidence—that is, whether the findings are cogent, convincing, and well grounded.

- **Trustworthiness** in qualitative research encompasses several different dimensions, including credibility, dependability, confirmability, transferability and authenticity.

- **Credibility** is achieved to the extent that the methods engender confidence in the truth of the data and in the researchers' interpretations. **Triangulation**, the use of multiple sources or referents to draw conclusions about what constitutes the truth, is one approach to enhancing credibility.

- A **bias** is an influence that produces a distortion in the study results. In quantitative studies, research control is an approach to addressing bias. **Research control** is used to *hold constant* outside influences on the dependent variable so that the relationship between the independent and dependent variables can be better understood.

- Researchers seek to control **confounding** (or *extraneous*) **variables**—variables that are extraneous to the purpose of a specific study.

- For quantitative researchers, **randomness**—having certain features of the study established by chance rather than by design or personal preference—is a powerful tool to eliminate bias.

- **Blinding** (or *masking*) is sometimes used to avoid biases stemming from participants' or research agents' awareness of study hypotheses or research status.

- **Reflexivity**, the process of reflecting critically on the self and of scrutinizing personal values that could affect data collection and interpretation, is an important tool in qualitative research.

- **Generalizability** in a quantitative study concerns the extent to which the findings can be applied to other groups and settings.

- A similar concept in qualitative studies is **transferability**, the extent to which qualitative findings can be transferred to other settings. One mechanism for promoting transferability is a rich and thorough description of the research context so that others can make inferences about contextual similarities.

# REFERENCES FOR CHAPTER 4

Ağac, E., & Günes, U. (2011). Effect on pain of changing the needle prior to administering medicine intramuscularly. *Journal of Advanced Nursing, 67*, 563–568.

Carlsson, E., Ehnfors, M., Aldh, A., & Ehrenberg, A. (2012). Accuracy and continuity in discharge information for patients with eating difficulties after stroke. *Journal of Clinical Nursing, 21*, 21–31.

Frisvold, M., Lindquist, R., & McAlpine, C. (2012). Living life in the balance at midlife: Lessons learned from mindfulness. *Western Journal of Nursing Research, 34*(2), 265–278.

Li, S., Wang, T., Vivienne Wu, S., Liang, S., & Tung, H. (2011). Efficacy of controlling night-time noise and activities to improve paitents' sleep quality in a surgical intensive care unit. *Journal of Clinical Nursing, 20*, 396–407.

Lincoln, Y. S., & Guba, E. G. (1985). *Naturalistic inquiry.* Newbury Park, CA: Sage.

Lindseth, G., Lindseth, P., & Thompson, M. (2012). Nutritional effects on sleep. *Western Journal of Nursing Research*, PubMed ID 21816963.

Murdoch, M., & Franck, L. (2012). Gaining confidence and perspective: A phenomenological study of mothers' lived experiences caring for infants at home after neonatal unit discharge. *Journal of Advanced Nursing, 68*, 2008–2020.

O'Lynn, C., & Krautscheid, L. (2011). "How should I touch you?": A qualitative study of attitudes on intimate touch in nursing care. *American Journal of Nursing, 111*, 24–31.

Porter, E., Benson, J., & Matsuda, S. (2011). Older homebound women: Negotiating reliance on a cane of walker. *Qualitative Health Research, 21*, 534–548.

# 5 Ethics in Research

## LEARNING OBJECTIVES

*On completing this chapter, you will be able to:*

- Discuss the historical background that led to the creation of various codes of ethics
- Understand the potential for ethical dilemmas stemming from conflicts between ethics and research demands
- Identify the three primary ethical principles articulated in the *Belmont Report* and the important dimensions encompassed by each
- Identify procedures for adhering to ethical principles and protecting study participants
- Given sufficient information, evaluate the ethical dimensions of a research report
- Define new terms in the chapter

## KEY TERMS

| | | |
|---|---|---|
| Anonymity | Confidentiality | Minimal risk |
| Assent | Debriefing | Process consent |
| *Belmont Report* | Ethical dilemma | Research misconduct |
| Beneficence | Full disclosure | Risk/benefit assessment |
| Certificate of confidentiality | Implied consent | Stipend |
| Code of ethics | Informed consent | Vulnerable population |
| Consent form | Institutional Review Board (IRB) | |

This chapter discusses some of the major ethical principles relevant to health care research. It also describes procedures that researchers can use to address these principles.

# ETHICS AND RESEARCH

In any research with human beings or animals, researchers must address ethical issues. Ethical concerns are especially prominent in nursing research because the line between what constitutes the expected practice of nursing and the collection of research data sometimes gets blurred.

## Historical Background

We might like to think that violations of moral principles among researchers occurred centuries ago rather than recently, but this is not the case. The Nazi medical experiments of the

1930s and 1940s are the most famous example of recent disregard for ethical conduct. The Nazi program of research involved using prisoners of war and racial "enemies" in experiments designed to test human endurance and reactions to untested drugs. The studies were unethical not only because they exposed people to harm and even death, but because subjects could not refuse participation. Similar wartime experiments that raised ethical concerns were conducted in Japan and Australia.

There are more recent examples. For instance, between 1932 and 1972, the Tuskegee Syphilis Study, sponsored by the U.S. Public Health Service, investigated the effects of syphilis among 400 poor African-American men. Medical treatment was deliberately withheld to study the course of the untreated disease. Similarly, Dr. Herbert Green in Auckland, New Zealand, studied women with cervical cancer in the 1980s; patients with carcinoma *in situ* were not given treatment so that researchers could study the natural progression of the disease.

In Willowbrook, an institution for the mentally retarded on Staten Island, children were deliberately infected with the hepatitis virus during the 1960s. It was revealed in 1993 that U.S. federal agencies had sponsored radiation experiments since the 1940s on hundreds of people, many of them prisoners or elderly hospital patients. And, in 2010 it was revealed that a United States doctor who worked on the Tuskegee study inoculated prisoners in Guatemala with syphilis in the 1940s. Other examples of studies with ethical transgressions have emerged to give ethical concerns the high visibility they have today.

## Codes of Ethics

In response to human rights violations, various **codes of ethics** have been developed. One of the first international set of ethical standards was the Nuremberg Code, developed in 1949 in response to the Nazi atrocities. Several other international standards have subsequently been developed, including the Declaration of Helsinki, which was adopted in 1964 by the World Medical Association and most recently revised in 2008.

Most disciplines, such as medicine and psychology, have established their own code of ethics. Nurses also have developed ethical guidelines. In the United States, the American Nurses Association (ANA) issued *Ethical Guidelines in the Conduct, Dissemination, and Implementation of Nursing Research* in 1995 (Silva, 1995). ANA (2001) also published a revised *Code of Ethics for Nurses with Interpretive Statements*, a document that covers ethical issues for practicing nurses primarily but also includes principles that apply to nurse researchers. In Canada, the Canadian Nurses Association published its *Ethical Research Guidelines for Registered Nurses* in 2002. And, the International Council of Nurses (ICN) has developed the *ICN Code of Ethics for Nurses*, which was most recently updated in 2006.

> **TIP:** There are many useful websites devoted to ethical principles, some of which are listed in the Internet Resources on thePoint website, for you. to click on directly.

## Government Regulations for Protecting Study Participants

Governments throughout the world fund research and establish rules for adhering to ethical principles. In the United States, an important code of ethics was adopted by the National Commission for the Protection of Human Subjects of Biomedical and Behavioral Research. The commission issued a report in 1978, known as the *Belmont Report*, which provided a model for many guidelines adopted by disciplinary organizations in the

United States. The Belmont Report also served as the basis for regulations affecting research sponsored by the U.S. government, including studies supported by the National Institute of Nursing Research (NINR). The United States ethical regulations have been codified at Title 45 Part 46 of the Code of Federal Regulations, and were revised most recently in 2005.

## Ethical Dilemmas in Conducting Research

Research that violates ethical principles typically occurs out of a researcher's conviction that knowledge is potentially life-saving or beneficial in the long run. There are research problems in which participants' rights and study demands are put in direct conflict, posing **ethical dilemmas** for researchers. Here are examples of research problems in which the desire for rigor conflicts with ethical considerations:

1. *Research question*: Are nurses equally empathic in their treatment of ICU patients from different ethnic backgrounds?

   *Ethical dilemma*: Ethics require that participants be informed of their role in a study. Yet if the researcher tells participating nurses that their degree of empathy in treating different patients will be scrutinized, will their behavior be "normal?" If the nurses' usual behavior is altered because of the presence of research observers, then the findings will not be valid.

2. *Research question*: What are the coping mechanisms of parents whose children have a terminal illness?

   *Ethical dilemma*: To answer this question, the researcher may need to probe into parents' psychological state at a vulnerable time; such probing could be painful, and yet knowledge of the parents' coping mechanisms might help to design more effective ways of addressing parents' grief and stress.

3. *Research question*: Does a new medication prolong life in patients with cancer?

   *Ethical dilemma*: The best way to test the effectiveness of an intervention is to administer it to some people but withhold it from others to see if the groups have different outcomes. Yet, if the intervention is untested (e.g., a new drug), the group receiving the intervention may be exposed to harmful side effects. On the other hand, the group *not* receiving the drug may be denied a beneficial treatment.

4. *Research question*: What is the process by which adult children adapt to the day-to-day stresses of caring for a parent with Alzheimer's disease?

   *Ethical dilemma*: In a qualitative study, which would be appropriate for this question, participants may get so closely involved with the researcher that they become willing to share "secrets." Interviews can become confessions. In this example, suppose a woman admitted to physically abusing her mother—how can the researcher report such information to authorities without breaking a pledge of confidentiality? And, if the researcher divulges the information to authorities, how can a pledge of confidentiality be given in good faith to other participants?

As these examples suggest, researchers are sometimes in a bind. Their goal is develop high-quality evidence for practice, but they must also adhere to rules for protecting human rights. Another type of dilemma may arise if nurse researchers face conflict-of-interest situations, in which their expected behavior as nurses conflicts with standard research behavior (e.g., deviating from a research protocol to assist a patient). It is precisely because of such dilemmas that codes of ethics have been developed to guide researchers' efforts.

# ETHICAL PRINCIPLES FOR PROTECTING STUDY PARTICIPANTS

The *Belmont Report* articulated three primary ethical principles on which standards of ethical research conduct are based: beneficence, respect for human dignity, and justice. We briefly discuss these principles and then describe methods researchers use to comply with them.

## Beneficence

A fundamental ethical principle in research is that of **beneficence**, the duty to minimize harm and maximize benefits. Human research should produce benefits for participants themselves or—a situation that is more common—for other individuals or society as a whole.

### The Right to Freedom From Harm and Discomfort

Researchers have an obligation to prevent or minimize harm in studies with humans. Participants must not be subjected to unnecessary risks of harm or discomfort, and their participation in research must be essential to achieving societally important aims. In research with humans, *harm* and *discomfort* can be physical (e.g., injury), emotional (e.g., stress), social (e.g., loss of social support), or financial (e.g., loss of wages). Ethical researchers must use strategies to minimize all types of harms and discomforts, even ones that are temporary.

Protecting human beings from physical harm is often straightforward, but it is not as easy to address the psychological aspects of study participation, which can be subtle. For example, participants may be asked questions about their personal views, weaknesses, or fears. Such queries might lead people to reveal deeply personal information. The need for sensitivity may be greater in qualitative studies, which often involve in-depth exploration into highly personal areas. The point is not that researchers should refrain from asking questions but rather that they need to be aware of the nature of the intrusion on people's psyches.

### The Right to Protection From Exploitation

Involvement in a study should not place participants at a disadvantage. Participants need to be assured that their participation, or information they provide, will not be used against them in any way. For example, people describing their economic situation should not risk loss of public health benefits; people reporting drug abuse should not fear exposure to criminal authorities.

Study participants enter into a special relationship with researchers, and this relationship should not be exploited. Exploitation may be overt and malicious (e.g., sexual exploitation), but it might also be more subtle (e.g., getting people to complete a 1-year follow-up interview, without having warned them of this possibility at the outset). Because nurse researchers may have a nurse–patient (in addition to a researcher–participant) relationship, special care may be needed to avoid exploiting that bond. Patients' consent to participate in a study may result from their understanding of the researcher's role as *nurse*, not as *researcher*.

In qualitative research, the risk of exploitation may become high because the psychological distance between investigators and participants typically declines as the study progresses. The emergence of a pseudo-therapeutic relationship is not uncommon, which could create additional risks that exploitation could inadvertently occur. On the other hand, qualitative researchers typically are in a better position than quantitative researchers to *do good*, rather than just to avoid doing harm, because of the close relationships they often develop with participants.

> **Example of therapeutic research experiences:**
> Participants in Beck's (2005) studies on birth trauma and posttraumatic stress disorder (PTSD) expressed a range of benefits they derived from e-mail exchanges with Beck. Here is what one informant voluntarily shared: "You thanked me for everything in your e-mail, and I want to THANK YOU for caring. For me, it means a lot that you have taken an interest in this subject and are taking the time and effort to find out more about PTSD. For someone to even acknowledge this condition means a lot for someone who has suffered from it" (p. 417).

## Respect for Human Dignity

Respect for human dignity is the second ethical principle articulated in the *Belmont Report*. This principle includes the right to self-determination and the right to full disclosure.

## The Right to Self-Determination

The principle of *self-determination* means that prospective participants have the right to decide voluntarily whether to participate in a study, without risking penalty or prejudicial treatment. It also means that people have the right to ask questions, to refuse to give information, and to withdraw from the study.

A person's right to self-determination includes freedom from coercion. *Coercion* involves explicit or implicit threats of penalty from failing to participate in a study or excessive rewards from agreeing to participate. The issue of coercion requires careful thought when researchers are in a position of authority or influence over potential participants, as might be the case in a nurse–patient relationship. The issue of coercion may require scrutiny in other situations as well. For example, a generous monetary incentive (or **stipend**) offered to encourage the participation of a low-income group (e.g., the homeless) might be considered mildly coercive because such incentives may place undue pressure on prospective participants.

## The Right to Full Disclosure

Respect for human dignity encompasses people's right to make informed, voluntary decisions about study participation, which requires full disclosure. **Full disclosure** means that the researcher has fully described the study, the person's right to refuse participation, and possible risks and benefits. The right to self-determination and the right to full disclosure are the two major elements on which informed consent—discussed later in this chapter—is based.

Achieving full disclosure is not always straightforward because it can sometimes create two types of bias: biases affecting the accuracy of the data and biases from sample recruitment problems. Suppose we were testing the hypothesis that high school students with a high absentee rate are more likely to be substance abusers than students with good attendance. If we approached potential participants and fully explained the study's purpose, some students might refuse to participate, and nonparticipation likely would be biased; students who are substance abusers—the group of primary interest—might be least likely to participate. Moreover, by knowing the study purpose, those who participate might not give candid responses. In such a situation, full disclosure could undermine the study.

In such situations, researchers sometimes use *covert data collection* or *concealment—* collecting data without participants' knowledge and thus without their consent. This might happen if a researcher wanted to observe people's behavior and was concerned that doing so openly would change the behavior of interest. Researchers might choose to obtain needed information through concealed methods, such as by videotaping with hidden equipment or observing while pretending to be engaged in other activities.

A more controversial technique is the use of deception. *Deception* can involve deliberately withholding information about the study, or providing participants with false information. For example, in studying high school students' use of drugs we might describe the research as a study of students' health practices, which is a mild form of misinformation.

Deception and concealment are problematic ethically because they interfere with people's right to make truly informed decisions about personal costs and benefits of participation. Some people think that deception is never justified, but others believe that if the study involves minimal risk yet offers great benefits to society, then deception may be justified.

Full disclosure has emerged as a concern in connection with data collected over the Internet (e.g., analyzing the content of messages posted to chat rooms). The issue is whether such messages can be used as data without the authors' consent. Some researchers believe that anything posted electronically is in the public domain, but others feel that the same ethical standards must apply in cyberspace research and that researchers must carefully protect the rights of individuals who are participants in "virtual" communities.

## Justice

The third broad principle articulated in the *Belmont Report* concerns justice, which includes participants' right to fair treatment and their right to privacy.

### The Right to Fair Treatment

One aspect of justice concerns the equitable distribution of benefits and burdens of research. The selection of participants should be based on research requirements and not on people's vulnerabilities. Historically, subject selection has been a key ethical concern, with many researchers selecting groups deemed to have lower social standing (e.g., poor people, prisoners, the mentally disabled) as study participants. The principle of justice imposes particular obligations toward individuals who are unable to protect their own interests (e.g., dying patients) to ensure that they are not exploited for the advancement of knowledge.

Distributive justice also imposes duties to not discriminate against those who may benefit from advances in research. During the early 1990s, there was evidence that women and minorities were being *ex*cluded from many clinical studies in the United States. This led to the promulgation of regulations requiring that researchers who seek funding from the National Institutes of Health (NIH) (including NINR) include women and minorities as study participants.

The right to fair treatment encompasses other obligations. For example, researchers must treat people who decline to participate in a study or who withdraw from it in a nonprejudicial manner; they must honor all agreements made with participants; they must show respect for the beliefs and lifestyles of people from different backgrounds; and they must treat participants courteously and tactfully at all times.

### The Right to Privacy

Virtually all research with humans involves intruding into personal lives. Researchers should ensure that their research is not more intrusive than it needs to be and that privacy is maintained. Participants have the right to expect that any data they provide will be kept in strict confidence.

Privacy issues have become even more salient in the U.S. health care community since the passage of the Health Insurance Portability and Accountability Act of 1996 (HIPAA), which articulates federal standards to protect patients' medical records and health information. For health care providers who transmit health information electronically, compliance with HIPAA regulations (the Privacy Rule) has been required since 2003.

>  **TIP:** Here are two websites that offer information about the implications of HIPAA for research: http://privacyruleandresearch.nih.gov/ and www.hhs.gov/ocr/hipaa/guidelines/research.pdf. ⚫ See the Internet Resources on thePoint website.

# PROCEDURES FOR PROTECTING STUDY PARTICIPANTS

Now that you are familiar with ethical principles for conducting research, you need to understand the procedures researchers use to adhere to them. It is these procedures that should be evaluated in critiquing the ethical aspects of a study.

> **TIP:** Information about ethical considerations is usually presented in the method section of a research report, often in a subsection labeled Procedures.

## Risk/Benefit Assessments

One strategy that researchers use to protect participants is to conduct a **risk/benefit assessment**. Such an assessment is designed to evaluate whether the benefits of participating in a study are in line with the costs, be they financial, physical, emotional, or social—i.e., whether the *risk/benefit ratio* is acceptable. Box 5.1 summarizes major costs and benefits of research participation.

---

### BOX 5.1 Potential Benefits and Risks of Research to Participants

**Major Potential Benefits to Participants**

- Access to a potentially beneficial intervention that might otherwise be unavailable
- Comfort in being able to discuss their situation or problem with a friendly, objective person
- Increased knowledge about themselves or their conditions, either through opportunity for self-reflection or through direct interaction with researchers
- Escape from normal routine, excitement of being part of a study
- Satisfaction that information they provide may help others with similar problems
- Direct monetary or material gains through stipends or other incentives

**Major Potential Risks to Participants**

- Physical harm, including unanticipated side effects
- Physical discomfort, fatigue, or boredom
- Emotional distress resulting from self-disclosure, fear of the unknown or repercussions, discomfort with strangers, and embarrassment at the type of questions being asked
- Social risks, such as the risk of stigma, adverse effects on personal relationships, or loss of status
- Loss of privacy
- Loss of time
- Monetary costs (e.g., for transportation, child care, time lost from work)

The risk/benefit ratio should also be considered in terms of whether risks to participants are commensurate with benefits to society and to nursing. The degree of risk by participants should never exceed the potential humanitarian benefits of the knowledge to be gained. Thus, the selection of a significant topic that has the potential to improve patient care is the first step in ensuring that research is ethical.

 **TIP:** In evaluating the risk/benefit ratio of a study design, you might want to consider how comfortable *you* would have felt about being a study participant.

In some cases, the risks may be negligible. **Minimal risk** is a risk expected to be no greater than those ordinarily encountered in daily life or during routine tests or procedures. When the risks are not minimal, researchers must proceed with caution, taking every step possible to reduce risks and maximize benefits.

In quantitative studies, most details of the study are spelled out in advance, and so a reasonably accurate risk/benefit assessment can be developed. Qualitative studies, however, usually evolve as data are gathered, and so assessing all risks at the outset may be more difficult. Qualitative researchers must remain sensitive to potential risks throughout the study.

## Informed Consent

An important procedure for safeguarding participants involves obtaining their informed consent. **Informed consent** means that participants have adequate information about the study, comprehend the information, and have the power of free choice, enabling them to consent to or decline participation voluntarily.

Researchers usually document informed consent by having participants sign a **consent form**, an example of which is shown in Figure 5.1. This form includes information about the study purpose, specific expectations regarding participation (e.g., how much time will be required), the voluntary nature of participation, and potential costs and benefits.

 **TIP:** Information on the content of informed consent is available in the Chapter Supplements located on thePoint website.

**Example of informed consent:**
Zhang and coresearchers (2012) tested the effectiveness of preoperative education on postoperative anxiety symptoms and complications for patients undergoing coronary artery bypass grafting. Written informed consent was obtained from all participants. Six patients who were otherwise eligible for the study were excluded because they were unable to give written consent.

Researchers may not obtain written informed consent when data collection is through self-administered questionnaires. Researchers often assume **implied consent** (i.e., the return of a completed questionnaire reflects the person's voluntary consent to participate). This assumption may not always be warranted, however (e.g., if patients believe that their care might be affected by failure to cooperate).

In some qualitative studies, especially those requiring repeated contact with participants, it is difficult to obtain meaningful informed consent at the outset. Because the design emerges during data collection and analysis, researchers may not know the exact nature of the data to be collected, what the risks and benefits will be, or how much time will be required. Thus, in a qualitative study, consent may be an ongoing process, called **process consent**, in which consent is continuously renegotiated.

I understand that I am being asked to participate in a research study at Saint Francis Hospital and Medical Center. This research study will evaluate: What it is like being a mother of multiples during the first year of the infants' lives. If I agree to participate in the study, I will be interviewed for approximately 30 to 60 minutes about my experience as a mother of multiple infants. The interview will be tape-recorded and take place in a private office at St. Francis Hospital. No identifying information will be included when the interview is transcribed. I understand I will receive $25.00 for participating in the study. There are no known risks associated with this study.

I realize that I may not participate in the study if I am younger than 18 years of age or I cannot speak English.

I realize that the knowledge gained from this study may help either me or other mothers of multiple infants in the future.

I realize that my participation in this study is entirely voluntary, and I may withdraw from the study at any time I wish. If I decide to discontinue my participation in this study, I will continue to be treated in the usual and customary fashion.

I understand that all study data will be kept confidential. However, this information may be used in nursing publications or presentations.

I understand that if I sustain injuries from my participation in this research project, I will not be automatically compensated by Saint Francis Hosptal and Medical Center.

If I need to, I can contact Dr. Cheryl Beck, University of Connecticut, School of Nursing, any time during the study.

The study has been explained to me. I have read and understand this consent form, all of my questions have been answered, and I agree to participate. I understand that I will be given a copy of this signed consent form.

| | |
|---|---|
| Signature of Participant | Date |
| Signature of Witness | Date |
| Signature of Investigator | Date |

**FIGURE 5.1** ● Example of an informed consent form.

> **Example of process consent:**
> Beech and coresearchers (2012) conducted a longitudinal grounded theory study of the process of restoring a sense of wellness following colorectal cancer. In-depth interviews were conducted with 12 patients at four points in time for 1 year following surgery. Written informed consent was completed at the first interview and process consent was used at later interviews by confirming participant agreement at each contact.

## Confidentiality Procedures

Study participants have the right to expect that any data they provide will be kept in strict confidence. Participants' right to privacy is protected through confidentiality procedures.

## Anonymity

**Anonymity**, the most secure means of protecting confidentiality, occurs when the researcher cannot link participants to their data. For example, if questionnaires were distributed to a group of nursing home residents and were returned without any identifying information, responses would be anonymous.

**Example of anonymity:**

Farrell and Belza (2012) conducted a study to examine whether older patients are comfortable discussing sexuality and sexual health with nurses. The researchers distributed anonymous questionnaires to elders in fitness classes and in retirement communities. Respondents returned the questionnaires in a secure drop box or by mail using preaddressed stamped envelopes.

## Confidentiality in the Absence of Anonymity

When anonymity is impossible, appropriate confidentiality procedures need to be implemented. A promise of **confidentiality** is a pledge that any information participants provide will not be publicly reported in a manner that identifies them and will not be made accessible to others.

Researchers may develop elaborate confidentiality procedures. These include securing confidentiality assurances from everyone with access to research data; maintaining identifying information in locked files; substituting *identification (ID) numbers* for participants' names on records and files, to prevent an accidental breach of confidentiality; and reporting only aggregate data for groups of participants, or taking steps to disguise a person's identity in a research report.

Confidentiality is especially salient in qualitative studies because of their in-depth nature, yet anonymity is rarely possible. Another challenge that many qualitative researchers face is adequately disguising participants in their reports to avoid a breach of confidentiality. Because the number of respondents is small and because rich descriptive information is presented, qualitative researchers need to take extra precautions to safeguard participants' identity.

**TIP:** As a means of enhancing individual and institutional privacy, research articles frequently avoid giving information about the locale of the study. For example, a report might say that data were collected in a 200-bed, private nursing home, without mentioning its name or location.

Confidentiality sometimes creates tension between researchers and legal authorities, especially if participants are involved in criminal activity like substance abuse. To avoid the risk of forced disclosure of sensitive information (e.g., through a court order), researchers in the United States can apply for a **Certificate of Confidentiality** from the NIH. The certificate allows researchers to refuse to disclose information on study participants in any civil, criminal, administrative, or legislative proceeding.

**Example of confidentiality procedures:**

Mallory and Hesson-McInnis (2012) tested an HIV prevention intervention with incarcerated and other high-risk women. To enhance confidentiality, data were collected using computer-assisted self-interviewing. A federal Certificate of Confidentiality was obtained.

## Debriefings and Referrals

Researchers should show their respect for participants during the interactions they have with them. For example, researchers should be polite and tactful, and should make evident their acceptance of cultural, linguistic, and lifestyle diversity.

There are also more formal strategies for communicating respect and concern for participants' well-being. For example, it is sometimes advisable to offer **debriefing** sessions following data collection so that participants can ask questions or air complaints. Debriefing is especially important when the data collection has been stressful or when ethical guidelines had to be "bent" (e.g., if any deception was used).

Researchers can also demonstrate their interest in participants by offering to share study findings with them after the data have been analyzed. Finally, researchers may need to assist participants by making referrals to appropriate health, social, or psychological services.

> **Example of referrals:**
> Wong and colleagues (2011) studied depression among Chinese women who experienced intimate partner violence. The interviewers were nonjudgmental and supportive during the interviews and, if deemed necessary, asked participants if they needed referral to community resources or a call to the police.

## Treatment of Vulnerable Groups

Adherence to ethical standards is often straightforward. The rights of special vulnerable groups, however, may need extra protections. **Vulnerable populations** may be incapable of giving fully informed consent (e.g., developmentally delayed people) or may be at high risk of unintended side effects (e.g., pregnant women). You should pay particular attention to the ethical dimensions of a study when people who are vulnerable are involved. Among the groups that should be considered as being vulnerable are the following:

- *Children.* Legally and ethically, children do not have the competence to give informed consent and so the consent of children's parents or guardians should be obtained. However, it is appropriate—especially if the child is at least 7 years of age—to obtain the child's assent as well. **Assent** refers to the child's affirmative agreement to participate.

- *Mentally or emotionally disabled people.* Individuals whose disability makes it impossible for them to make informed decisions (e.g., people affected by cognitive impairment, coma, and so on) also cannot legally provide informed consent. In such cases, researchers should obtain the written consent of a legal guardian.

- *Severely ill or physically disabled people.* For patients who are very ill or undergoing certain treatments (e.g., mechanical ventilation), it might be necessary to assess their ability to make reasoned decisions about study participation. For certain disabilities, special consent procedures may be required. For example, with people who cannot read or who have a physical impairment preventing them from writing, alternative procedures for documenting informed consent (e.g., videotaping) should be used.

- *The terminally ill.* Terminally ill people can seldom expect to benefit personally from research, and thus the risk/benefit ratio needs to be carefully assessed.

- *Institutionalized people.* Nurses often conduct studies with hospitalized or institutionalized people who might feel that their care would be jeopardized by failure to cooperate. Inmates of prisons and correctional facilities may similarly feel constrained in their ability to give free consent. Researchers studying institutionalized groups need to emphasize the voluntary nature of participation.

○ *Pregnant women*. The U.S. government has issued additional requirements governing research with pregnant women and fetuses. These requirements reflect a desire to safeguard both the pregnant woman, who may be at heightened physical or psychological risk, and the fetus, who cannot give informed consent. The regulations stipulate that a pregnant woman cannot be involved in a study unless risks are minimal.

**Example of research with a vulnerable group:**
Baggott and colleagues (2012) studied how symptoms clustered in a sample of 131 pediatric oncology patients aged 10 to 18, children and adolescents. Parents or guardians of the patients, if they were younger than 18, signed written informed consent forms. All children provided consent or assent.

## External Reviews and the Protection of Human Rights

Researchers may not be objective in developing procedures to protect participants' rights. Biases may arise from their commitment to an area of knowledge and their desire to conduct a rigorous study. Because of the risk of a biased evaluation, the ethical dimensions of a study are usually subjected to external review.

Most hospitals, universities, and other institutions where research is conducted have established formal committees for reviewing research plans. These committees are sometimes called *human subjects committees* or (in Canada) *Research Ethics Boards*. In the United States, the committee is often called an **Institutional Review Board (IRB)**. Before undertaking a study, researchers must submit research plans to the IRB, and must also undergo formal IRB training. An IRB can approve the proposed plans, require modifications, or disapprove them.

**Example of IRB approval:**
Dickson and Flynn (2012) explored nurses' clinical reasoning regarding safe practices of medication administration. The procedures and protocols for the study were approved by the university IRB where the researchers worked, as well as by the hospital ethics review boards of the 10 hospitals where the data were collected.

# OTHER ETHICAL ISSUES

In discussing research ethics, we have given primary consideration to protecting human study participants. Two other ethical issues also deserve mention: the treatment of animals in research and research misconduct.

## Ethical Issues in Using Animals in Research

Some nurse researchers who focus on biophysiologic phenomena use animals as their subjects. Ethical considerations are clearly different for animals and humans; for example, *informed consent* is not relevant for animals. In the United States, the Public Health Service has issued a policy statement on the humane care and use of animals. The guidelines articulate principles for the proper care and treatment of animals used in research, covering such issues as the transport of research animals, pain and distress in animal subjects, the use of appropriate anesthesia, and euthanizing animals under certain conditions during or after the study.

Holtzclaw and Hanneman (2002), in discussing the use of animals in nursing research, noted several important considerations. For example, there must be a compelling reason to use an animal model—not simply convenience or novelty. Also, the study procedures should be humane, well planned, and well funded. Animal studies are not necessarily less costly than those with human participants, and they require serious scientific consideration to justify their use.

> **Example of research with animals:**
> Akase and colleagues (2011) studied skin changes induced by ultraviolet radiation using an animal model (mice). Animal care included careful attention to temperature, humidity, and lighting. All animals were handled in accordance with ethical guidelines, and the procedures were reviewed by animal ethics committees at two universities.

## Research Misconduct

Ethics in research involves not only the protection of the rights of human and animal subjects, but also protection of the public trust. **Research misconduct** has received increasing attention in recent years as incidents of researcher fraud and misrepresentation have come to light.

Research misconduct, as defined by a U.S. Public Health Service regulation, is fabrication, falsification, or plagiarism in proposing, conducting, or reviewing research, or in reporting results. *Fabrication* involves making up data or study results. *Falsification* involves manipulating research materials or processes; it also involves changing or omitting data, or distorting results. *Plagiarism* involves the appropriation of someone's ideas, results, or words without giving due credit. Although the official definition focuses on only these three types of misconduct, there is widespread agreement that research misconduct covers many other issues including improprieties of authorship, conflicts of interest, inappropriate financial arrangements, failure to comply with governmental regulations, and unauthorized use of confidential information.

> **Example of research misconduct:**
> In 2008, the U.S. Office of Research Integrity ruled that a nurse in Missouri engaged in scientific misconduct in research supported by the National Cancer Institute. The nurse falsified and fabricated data that were reported to the National Surgical Adjuvant Breast and Bowel Project (NIH Notice Number NOT-OD-08-096).

# CRITIQUING THE ETHICAL ASPECTS OF A STUDY

Guidelines for critiquing the ethical aspects of a study are presented in Box 5.2. Members of an IRB or human subjects committee are provided with sufficient information to answer all these questions, but research articles do not always include detailed information about ethics because of space constraints in journals. Thus, it may be difficult to critique researchers' adherence to ethical guidelines. Nevertheless, we offer a few suggestions for considering ethical issues.

Many research reports do acknowledge that the study procedures were reviewed by an IRB or human subjects committee. When a report mentions a formal review, it is usually safe to assume that a panel of concerned people thoroughly reviewed ethical issues raised by the study.

---

**BOX 5.2   Guidelines for Critiquing the Ethical Aspects of a Study**

1. Was the study approved and monitored by an Institutional Review Board, Research Ethics Board, or other similar ethics review committee?
2. Were study participants subjected to any physical harm, discomfort, or psychological distress? Did the researchers take appropriate steps to remove or prevent harm?
3. Did the benefits to participants outweigh any potential risks or actual discomfort they experienced? Did the benefits to society outweigh the costs to participants?
4. Was any type of coercion or undue influence used to recruit participants? Did they have the right to refuse to participate or to withdraw without penalty?
5. Were participants deceived in any way? Were they fully aware of participating in a study and did they understand the purpose and nature of the research?
6. Were appropriate informed consent procedures used with all participants? If not, were the reasons valid and justifiable?
7. Were adequate steps taken to safeguard participants' privacy? How was confidentiality maintained? Was a Certificate of Confidentiality obtained—and, if not, should one have been obtained?
8. Were vulnerable groups involved in the research? If yes, were special precautions instituted because of their vulnerable status?
9. Were groups omitted from the inquiry without a justifiable rationale, such as women (or men), or minorities?

---

You can also come to some conclusions based on a description of the study methods. There may be sufficient information to judge, for example, whether study participants were subjected to harm or discomfort. Reports do not always state whether informed consent was secured, but you should be alert to situations in which the data could not have been gathered as described if participation were purely voluntary (e.g., if data were gathered unobtrusively).

In thinking about the ethical aspects of a study, you should also consider who the study participants were. For example, if the study involves vulnerable groups, there should be more information about protective procedures. You might also need to attend to who the study participants were *not*. For example, there has been considerable concern about the omission of certain groups (e.g., minorities) from clinical research.

## RESEARCH EXAMPLES WITH CRITICAL THINKING EXERCISES

Brief summaries of a quantitative and a qualitative nursing study are presented below, followed by some questions to guide critical thinking about the ethical aspects of these studies.

⁌ Examples 1 and 2 below are also featured in our *Interactive Critical Thinking Activity* on thePoint. website where you can easily record, print, and e-mail your responses to the related questions.

### EXAMPLE 1 ● Quantitative Research

**Study:** Parenting and feeding behaviors associated with school-aged African American and white children (Polfuss & Frenn, 2012)

**Study Purpose:** The purpose of the study was to examine the relationship between parenting and feeding behaviors on the one hand and children's body mass index on the other hand in families of African American and white children aged 9 to 15.

*(continues on page 94)*

**Research Methods:** A total of 176 parent/child dyads were recruited into the study. Parents completed questionnaires about their own parenting behavior, their perceptions and concerns about childhood obesity, and their feeding practices. The children also completed a questionnaire, and both parents and children were measured for height and weight.

**Ethics-Related Procedures:** The families were recruited through flyers and personal contact at several locations (e.g., clinics, boys and girls clubs). To be eligible, participants had to be alert and oriented, able to speak and read English, and willing to be measured for height and weight. Parents were asked to complete written informed consent forms, and children were asked to give their verbal assent. Data were collected in private areas, and parent and child questionnaires were completed independently. A research assistant was available to help children with reading the questionnaires or to answer any questions. All participants (parents and children) were offered a $10 gift certificate to a local department store. The entire consent and data collection process took 30 minutes. IRBs of a children's hospital and a university granted approval for this study.

**Key Findings:** Parents who were concerned about their children's weight exhibited greater authoritarian (controlling) parenting and feeding behavior.

## CRITICAL THINKING EXERCISES

1. Answer the relevant questions from Box 5.2 on page 93 regarding this study.
2. Also consider the following targeted questions:
    a. Could the data for this study have been collected anonymously?
    b. Comment on the appropriateness of the participant stipend in this study.
3. If the results of this study are valid and generalizable, in what ways do you think the findings could be used in clinical practice?

## EXAMPLE 2 ● Qualitative Research

**Study:** "Grief interrupted: The experience of loss among incarcerated women" (Harner et al., 2011)

**Study Purpose:** The purpose of the study was to explore the experiences of grief among incarcerated women following the loss of a loved one.

**Study Methods:** The researchers used phenomenological methods in this study. They recruited 15 incarcerated women who had experienced the loss of a loved one during their confinement. In-depth interviews about the women's experience of loss lasted 1 to 2 hours.

**Ethics-Related Procedures:** The researchers recruited women by posting flyers in the prison's dayroom. The flyers were written at the 4.5 grade level. Because the first author was a nurse practitioner at the prison, the researchers used several strategies to "diffuse any perceived coercion" (p. 457), such as not posting flyers near the health services unit and not offering any monetary or work-release incentives to participate. Written informed consent was obtained, but because of high rates of illiteracy, the informed consent document was read aloud to all potential participants. During the consent process, and during the interviews, the women were given opportunities to ask questions. They were informed that participation would have no effect on sentence length, sentence structure, parole, or access to health services. They were also told they could end the interview at any time without fear of reprisals. Furthermore, they were told that the researcher was a mandated reporter and would report any indication of suicidal or homicidal ideation. Participants were not required to give their names to the research team. During the interview, efforts were made to create a welcoming and nonthreatening environment. The research team received approval for the study from a university IRB and from the Department of Corrections Research Division.

**Key Findings:** The researchers revealed four themes, which they referred to as existential life-worlds: Temporality: frozen in time; Spatiality: no place, no space to grieve; Corporeality: buried emotions; and Relationality: never alone, yet feeling so lonely.

## CRITICAL THINKING EXERCISES

1. Answer the relevant questions from Box 5.2 on page 93 regarding this study.
2. Also consider the following targeted questions:
   a. The reseachers did not offer any stipend—was this ethically appropriate?
   b. Might the researchers have benefited from obtaining a Certificate of Confidentiality for this research?
3. If the results of this study are trustworthy and transferable, in what ways do you think the findings could be used in clinical practice?

## EXAMPLE 3 ● Quantitative Study in Appendix A

- Read the method section from Howell and colleagues' (2007) study ("Anxiety, anger, and blood pressure in children") in Appendix A on page 395–402.

## CRITICAL THINKING EXERCISES

1. Answer relevant questions from Box 5.2 on page 93 regarding this study.
2. Also consider the following targeted questions:
   a. Where was information about ethical issues located in this report?
   b. What additional information regarding the ethical aspects of their study could the researchers have included in this article?
   c. If you had a school-aged sibling or child of your own, how would you feel about him or her participating in the study?

## EXAMPLE 4 ● Qualitative Study in Appendix B

- Read the method section from Beck and Watson's (2010) study ("Subsequent childbirth after a previous traumatic birth") in Appendix B on page 403–412.

## CRITICAL THINKING EXERCISES

1. Answer the relevant questions from Box 5.2 on page 93 regarding this study.
2. Also consider the following targeted questions:
   a. Where was information about the ethical aspects of this study located in the report?
   b. What additional information regarding the ethical aspects of Beck and Watson's study could the researchers have included in this article?

**WANT TO KNOW MORE?** A wide variety of resources to enhance your learning and understanding of this chapter are available on thePoint.

- Interactive Critical Thinking Activity
- Chapter Supplement on Elements of Informed Consent
- Answers to the Critical Thinking Exercises for Examples 3 and 4
- Student Review Questions
- Full-text online
- Internet Resources with useful websites for Chapter 5

Additional study aids including eight journal articles and related questions are also available in *Study Guide for Essentials of Nursing Research, 8e.*

# SUMMARY POINTS

- Because research has not always been conducted ethically, and because of genuine **ethical dilemmas** that researchers face in designing studies that are both ethical and rigorous, **codes of ethics** have been developed to guide researchers.

- Three major ethical principles from the *Belmont Report* are incorporated into many guidelines: beneficence, respect for human dignity, and justice.

- **Beneficence** involves the performance of some good and the protection of participants from physical and psychological harm and exploitation.

- Respect for human dignity involves the participants' right to self-determination, which includes participants' right to participate in a study voluntarily.

- **Full disclosure** means that researchers have fully described to prospective participants their rights and the costs and benefits of the study. When full disclosure poses the risk of biased results, researchers sometimes use *concealment* (the collection of information without participants' knowledge or consent) or *deception* (either withholding information from participants or providing false information).

- Justice includes the right to fair treatment and the right to privacy. In the United States, privacy has become a major issue because of the Privacy Rule regulations that resulted from the Health Insurance Portability and Accountability Act (HIPAA).

- Procedures have been developed to safeguard study participants' rights, including the performance of a risk/benefit assessment, the implementation of informed consent procedures, and taking steps to safeguard participants' confidentiality.

- In a **risk/benefit assessment**, the potential benefits of the study to individual participants and to society are weighed against the costs to individuals.

- **Informed consent** procedures, which provide prospective participants with information needed to make a reasoned decision about participation, normally involve signing a **consent form** to document voluntary and informed participation.

- In qualitative studies, consent may need to be continually renegotiated with participants as the study evolves, through **process consent** procedures.

- Privacy can be maintained through **anonymity** (wherein not even researchers know participants' identities) or through formal **confidentiality procedures** that safeguard the information participants provide.

- Some United States researchers obtain a **Certificate of Confidentiality** that protects them against the forced disclosure of confidential information through a court order.

- Researchers sometimes offer **debriefing** sessions after data collection to provide participants with more information or an opportunity to air complaints.

- **Vulnerable populations** require additional protection. These people may be vulnerable because they are not able to make an informed decision about study participation (e.g., children); because of diminished autonomy (e.g., prisoners); or because their circumstances heighten the risk of harm (e.g., pregnant women, the terminally ill).

- External review of the ethical aspects of a study by a human subjects committee or **Institutional Review Board (IRB)** is highly desirable and is often required by universities and organizations from which participants are recruited.

- Ethical conduct in research involves not only protecting the rights of human and animal subjects, but also efforts to maintain high standards of integrity and avoid such forms of **research misconduct** as plagiarism, fabrication of results, or falsification of data.

# REFERENCES FOR CHAPTER 5

Akase, T., Nagase, T., Huang, L., Ibuki, A., Minematsu, T., & Sanada, S. (2011). Aging-like skin changes induced by ultraviolet irradiation in an animal model of metabolic syndrome. *Biological Research for Nursing, 14*(2), 180–187.

American Nurses' Association. (2001). *Code for nurses with interpretive statements.* Kansas City, MO: Author.

Baggott, C., Cooper, B., Marina, N., Matthay, K., & Maiskowski, C. (2012). Symptom cluster analyses based on symptom occurrence and severity ratings among pediatric oncology patients during myelosuppressive chemotherapy. *Cancer Nursing, 35*, 18–28.

Beck, C. T. (2005). Benefits of participating in internet interviews: Women helping women. *Qualitative Health Research, 15*, 411–422.

Beech, N., Arber, A., & Faithful, S. (2012). Restoring a sense of wellness following colorectal cancer: A grounded theory. *Journal of Advanced Nursing, 68*(5), 1134–1144.

Canadian Nurses Association. (2002). *Ethical guidelines for nurses in research involving human subjects.* Ottawa, ON: Author.

Dickson, G., & Flynn, L. (2012). Nurses' clinical reasoning: Processes and practices of medication safety. *Qualitative Health Research, 22*, 3–16.

Farrell, J., & Belza, B. (2012). Are older patients comfortable discussing sexual health with nurses? *Nursing Research, 61*, 51–67.

Harner, H., Hentz, P., & Evangelista, M. (2011). Grief interrupted: The experience of loss among incarcerated women. *Qualitative Health Research, 21*, 454–464.

Holtzclaw, B. J., & Hanneman, S. K. (2002). Use of non-human biobehavioral models in critical care nursing research. *Critical Care Nursing Quarterly, 24*(4), 30–40.

Mallory, C., & Hesson-McInnis, M. (2012). Pilot test results of an HIV prevention intervention for high-risk women. *Western Journal of Nursing Research.*

Polfuss, M. L., & Frenn, M. (2012). Parenting and feeding behaviors associated with school-aged African American and white children. *Western Journal of Nursing Research, 34*, 677–696.

Silva, M. C. (1995). *Ethical guidelines in the conduct, dissemination, and implementation of nursing research.* Washington, DC: American Nurses' Association.

Wong, J., Tiwari, A., Fong, D., Humphreys, J., & Bullock, L. (2011). Depression among women experiencing intimate partner violence in a Chinese community. *Nursing Research, 60*, 58–65.

Zhang, C., Jiang, Y., Yin, Q., Chen, F., Ma, L., & Wang, L. (2012). Impact of nurse-initiated preoperative education on postoperative anxiety symptoms and complications after coronary artery bypass grafting. *Journal of Cardiovascular Nursing, 27*, 84–88.

# Preliminary Steps in Research

## 6 Research Problems, Research Questions, and Hypotheses

### LEARNING OBJECTIVES

*On completing this chapter, you will be able to:*

- Describe the process of developing and refining a research problem
- Distinguish the functions and forms of statements of purpose and research questions for quantitative and qualitative studies
- Describe the function and characteristics of research hypotheses and distinguish different types of hypotheses (directional vs. nondirectional, research vs. null)
- Critique statements of purpose, research questions, and hypotheses in research reports with respect to their placement, clarity, wording, and significance
- Define new terms in the chapter

### KEY TERMS

| | | |
|---|---|---|
| Directional hypothesis | Null hypothesis | Research problem |
| Hypothesis | Problem statement | Research questions |
| Nondirectional hypothesis | Research hypothesis | Statement of purpose |

## OVERVIEW OF RESEARCH PROBLEMS

Studies to generate new research evidence begin in much the same fashion as an evidence-based practice (EBP) effort—as problems that need to be solved or questions that need to be answered. This chapter discusses the formulation and evaluation of research problems. We begin by clarifying some relevant terms.

**TABLE 6.1  Terms Relating to Research Problems, With Examples**

| Term | Example |
| --- | --- |
| Topic | Side effects of chemotherapy |
| Research problem (Problem statement) | Nausea and vomiting are common side effects among patients on chemotherapy, and interventions to date have been only moderately successful in reducing these effects. New interventions that can reduce or prevent these side effects need to be identified. |
| Statement of purpose | The purpose of the study is to test an intervention to reduce chemotherapy-induced side effects—specifically, to compare the effectiveness of patient-controlled and nurse-administered antiemetic therapy for controlling nausea and vomiting in patients on chemotherapy. |
| Research question | What is the relative effectiveness of patient-controlled antiemetic therapy versus nurse-controlled antiemetic therapy with regard to (a) medication consumption and (b) control of nausea and vomiting in patients on chemotherapy? |
| Hypotheses | Subjects receiving antiemetic therapy by a patient-controlled pump will (1) be less nauseated, (2) vomit less, and (3) consume less medication than subjects receiving nurse-administered therapy. |

## Basic Terminology

At the most general level, a researcher selects a *topic* on which to focus. Examples of research topics are claustrophobia during MRI tests and pain management for sickle cell disease. Within broad topic areas are many possible research problems. In this section, we illustrate various terms using the topic *side effects of chemotherapy*.

A **research problem** is an enigmatic or troubling condition. The purpose of research is to "solve" the problem—or to contribute to its solution—by gathering relevant data. A **problem statement** articulates the problem and an *argument* that explains the need for a study. Table 6.1 presents a simplified problem statement related to the topic of side effects of chemotherapy.

Many reports include a **statement of purpose** (or purpose statement), which is the researcher's summary of the overall goal. Sometimes the words *aim* or *objective* are used in lieu of purpose, but these alternatives sometimes encompass broader goals (e.g., developing recommendations for changes to nursing practice based on the study evidence).

**Research questions** are the specific queries researchers want to answer, which guide the types of data to be collected in a study. Researchers who make specific predictions about answers to research questions pose **hypotheses** that are then tested.

These terms are not always consistently defined in research textbooks. Table 6.1 illustrates the interrelationships among terms as we define them.

## Research Problems and Paradigms

Some research problems are better suited to qualitative versus quantitative inquiry. Quantitative studies usually involve concepts that are fairly well developed and for which reliable methods of measurement have been (or can be) developed. For example, a quantitative study might be undertaken to assess whether people with chronic illness who continue working past age 62 are less (or more) depressed than those who retire. There are relatively accurate measures of depression that would yield quantitative data about the level of depression in employed and retired chronically ill seniors.

Qualitative studies are often undertaken because a researcher wants to develop a rich and context-bound understanding of a poorly understood phenomenon. Qualitative methods would not be well suited to comparing levels of depression among employed and retired seniors, but they would be ideal for exploring, for example, the *meaning* of depression among chronically ill retirees. In evaluating a research report, one consideration is whether the research problem is suitable for the chosen paradigm and its associated methods.

## Sources of Research Problems

Where do ideas for research problems come from? At the most basic level, research topics originate with researchers' interests. Because research is a time-consuming enterprise, curiosity about and interest in a topic are essential to a project's success.

Research reports rarely indicate the source of researchers' inspiration for a study, but a variety of explicit sources can fuel their curiosity, including the following:

- *Clinical experience*. Nurses' everyday experience is a rich source of ideas for research topics.
- *Nursing literature*. Ideas for studies often come from reading the nursing literature.
- *Social issues*. Topics are sometimes suggested by global social or political issues of relevance to the health care community (e.g., health disparities).
- *Theories*. Theories from nursing and other disciplines sometime suggest a research problem.
- *Ideas from external sources*. External sources can sometimes provide the impetus for a study (e.g., a funding agency's research priorities).

Additionally, researchers who have developed a *program of research* may get inspiration for "next steps" from their own findings, or from a discussion of those findings with others.

> **Example of a problem source for a quantitative study:**
> Beck (one of this book's authors) developed a strong research program on postpartum depression (PPD). Beck was approached by Dr. Carol Lanni Keefe, a professor in nutritional sciences, who had studied the effect of DHA (docosahexaemoic acid, a fat found in cold-water marine fish) on fetal brain development. Evidence suggested that DHA might play a role in reducing the severity of PPD, and so the two researchers collaborated in a study to test the effects of dietary DHA supplements on the incidence and severity of PPD. Their clinical trial has recently been completed and analyses are underway.

## Development and Refinement of Research Problems

Developing a research problem is a creative process. Researchers often begin with interests in a broad topic area, and then develop a more specific researchable problem. For example, suppose a hospital nurse begins to wonder why some patients complain about having to wait for pain medication when certain nurses are assigned to them. The general topic is discrepancy in patient complaints about pain medications administered by different nurses. The nurse might ask, What accounts for this discrepancy? This broad question may lead to other questions, such as, How do the two groups of nurses differ? or What characteristics do the complaining patients share? The nurse may then observe that the ethnic background of the patients and nurses could be a relevant factor. This may direct the nurse to review the literature on nursing behaviors and ethnicity, or it may provoke a discussion of these observations with peers. These efforts may result in several research questions, such as the following:

- What is the essence of patient complaints among patients of different ethnic backgrounds?
- Is the ethnic background of nurses related to the frequency with which they dispense pain medication?
- Is the ethnic background of patients related to the frequency of complaints of having to wait for pain medication?
- Does the number of patient complaints increase (or do nurses' dispensing behaviors change) when the patients are of dissimilar ethnic backgrounds as opposed to when they are of the same ethnic background as the nurse?

These questions stem from the same general problem, yet each would be studied differently; for example, some suggest a qualitative approach, and others suggest a quantitative one. A quantitative researcher might become curious about nurses' dispensing behaviors, based on some evidence in the literature regarding ethnic differences. Both ethnicity and nurses' dispensing behaviors are variables that can be measured reliably. A qualitative researcher would be more interested in understanding the *essence* of patients' complaints, patients' *experience* of frustration, or the *process* by which the problem got resolved. These aspects of the research problem would be difficult to measure quantitatively. Researchers choose a problem to study based on its inherent interest to them, and on its fit with a paradigm of preference.

# COMMUNICATING RESEARCH PROBLEMS AND QUESTIONS

Every study needs a problem statement that articulates what is problematic and what is driving the research. Most research reports also present either a statement of purpose, research questions, or hypotheses, and often combinations of these three elements are included.

Many students do not really understand problem statements and may even have trouble identifying them in a research article. A problem statement is presented early in a research article and often begins with the first sentence after the abstract. Research questions, purpose statements, or hypotheses appear later in the introduction.

## Problem Statements

A good problem statement is a well-structured declaration of what it is that is problematic, what it is that "needs fixing," or what it is that is poorly understood. Problem statements, especially for quantitative studies, often have most of the following six components:

1. *Problem identification*: What is wrong with the current situation?
2. *Background*: What is the nature of the problem, or the context of the situation, that readers need to understand?
3. *Scope of the problem*: How big a problem is it, and how many people are affected?
4. *Consequences of the problem*: What is the cost of *not* fixing the problem?
5. *Knowledge gaps*: What information about the problem is lacking?
6. *Proposed solution*: How will the new study contribute to the solution of the problem?

---

**BOX 6.1 Draft Problem Statement on Humor and Stress**

A diagnosis of cancer is associated with high levels of stress. Sizeable numbers of patients who receive a cancer diagnosis describe feelings of uncertainty, fear, anger, and loss of control. Interpersonal relationships, psychological functioning, and role performance have all been found to suffer following cancer diagnosis and treatment.

A variety of alternative/complementary therapies have been developed in an effort to decrease the harmful effects of cancer-related stress on psychological and physiological functioning, and resources devoted to these therapies (money and staff) have increased in recent years. However, many of these therapies have not been carefully evaluated to assess their efficacy, safety, or cost effectiveness. For example, the use of humor has been recommended as a therapeutic device to improve quality of life, decrease stress, and perhaps improve immune functioning, but the evidence to justify its advocacy is scant.

---

Let us suppose that our topic was humor as a complementary therapy for reducing stress in hospitalized patients with cancer. One research question (discussed later in this section) might be, "What is the effect of nurses' use of humor on stress and natural killer cell activity in hospitalized cancer patients?" Box 6.1 presents a rough draft of a problem statement for such a study. This problem statement is a reasonable draft, but it could be improved.

Box 6.2 illustrates how the problem statement could be made stronger by adding information about scope (component 3), long-term consequences (component 4), and possible solutions (component 6). This second draft builds a more compelling *argument* for new research: millions of people are affected by cancer, and the disease has adverse consequences not only for patients and their families, but also for society. The revised problem statement also suggests a basis for the new study by describing a possible solution on which the new study might build.

---

**BOX 6.2 Some Possible Improvements to Problem Statement on Humor and Stress**

Each year, more than 1 million people are diagnosed with cancer, which remains one of the top causes of death among both men and women (reference citations).* Numerous studies have documented that a diagnosis of cancer is associated with high levels of stress. Sizeable numbers of patients who receive a cancer diagnosis describe feelings of uncertainty, fear, anger, and loss of control (citations). Interpersonal relationships, psychological functioning, and role performance have all been found to suffer following cancer diagnosis and treatment (citations). These stressful outcomes can, in turn, adversely affect health, long-term prognosis, and medical costs among cancer survivors (citations).

A variety of alternative/complementary therapies have been developed in an effort to decrease the harmful effects of cancer-related stress on psychological and physiological functioning, and resources devoted to these therapies (money and staff) have increased in recent years (citations). However, many of these therapies have not been carefully evaluated to determine their efficacy, safety, or cost effectiveness. For example, the use of humor has been recommended as a therapeutic device to improve quality of life, decrease stress, and perhaps improve immune functioning (citations), but the evidence to justify its advocacy is scant. Preliminary findings from a recent small-scale endocrinology study with a healthy sample exposed to a humorous intervention (citation), however, hold promise for further inquiry with immunocompromised populations.

---

*Reference citations would be inserted to support the statements.

☞ **HOW-TO-TELL TIP:** How can you tell a problem statement? Problem statements are rarely explicitly labeled and must therefore be ferreted out. The first sentence of a research report is often the starting point of a problem statement. The problem statement is usually interwoven with findings from the research literature. Prior findings provide the evidence backing up assertions in the problem statement and suggest gaps in knowledge. In many articles it is difficult to disentangle the problem statement from the literature review, unless there is a subsection specifically labeled "Literature Review" or something similar.

Problem statements for a qualitative study similarly express the nature of the problem, its context, its scope, and information needed to address it, as in the study in Appendix B on page 403. Qualitative studies embedded in a research tradition often incorporate terms and concepts that foreshadow the tradition in their problem statements. For example, the problem statement in a grounded theory study might mention the need to generate a theory relating to social processes. A problem statement for a phenomenological study might note the need to know more about people's experiences or meanings they attribute to those experiences. An ethnographer might indicate the desire to describe how cultural forces influence people's behavior.

## Statements of Purpose

Many researchers articulate their research goals as a statement of purpose. The purpose statement establishes the general direction of the inquiry and captures, usually in one or two sentences, the study's substance. It is usually easy to identify a purpose statement because the word *purpose* is explicitly stated: "The purpose of this study was…"—although sometimes the words *aim*, *goal*, or *objective* are used instead, as in "The aim of this study was to…."

In a quantitative study, a statement of purpose identifies the key study variables and their possible interrelationships, as well as the population of interest (i.e., all the PICO elements).

**Example of a statement of purpose from a quantitative study:**
The purpose of this study was to investigate the effectiveness of chilled and unchilled baby oil therapy for treating uremic pruritus in hemodialysis patients (Lin et al., 2012).

This purpose statement identifies the population of interest as patients on hemodialysis. The key study variables were the patients' exposure to chilled or unchilled baby oil therapy (the independent variable), and the patients' severity of itchiness (the dependent variable).

In qualitative studies, the statement of purpose indicates the nature of the inquiry, the key concept or phenomenon, and the group, community, or setting under study.

**Example of a statement of purpose from a qualitative study:**
The purpose of this study was to explore the experiences of Latina mothers who immigrated to the United States without legal documentation, and without their children (Sternberg & Barry, 2011).

This statement indicates that the group under study is Latina mothers, and the central phenomenon is the experience of illegally immigrating to the United States without their children.

In the statement of purpose researchers also communicate the manner in which they sought to solve the problem, or the state of knowledge on the topic, through their choice of verbs. A study whose purpose is to *explore* or *describe* some phenomenon is likely to be an investigation of a little-researched topic, often involving a qualitative approach, such as phenomenology or ethnography. A statement of purpose for a qualitative study—especially a grounded theory study—may also use verbs such as *understand, discover, develop,* or *generate.* The statements of purpose in qualitative studies often "encode" the tradition of inquiry not only through the researcher's choice of verbs but also through the use of certain terms or "buzz words" associated with those traditions, as follows:

- *Grounded theory*: Processes; social structures; social interactions
- *Phenomenological studies*: Experience; lived experience; meaning; essence
- *Ethnographic studies*: Culture; roles; lifeways; cultural behavior

Quantitative researchers also use verbs to communicate the nature of the inquiry. A statement indicating that the study purpose is to *test* or *evaluate* something (e.g., an intervention) suggests an experimental design, for example. A study whose purpose is to *examine* or *explore* the relationship between two variables is more likely to involve a nonexperimental design. Sometimes the verb is ambiguous: if a purpose statement states that the researcher's intent is to *compare* two things, the comparison could involve alternative treatments (using an experimental design) or two preexisting groups (using a nonexperimental design). In any event, verbs such as *test, evaluate,* and *compare* suggest quantifiable variables and designs with scientific controls.

The verbs in a purpose statement should connote objectivity. A statement of purpose indicating that the study goal was to *prove, demonstrate,* or *show* something suggests a bias.

## Research Questions

Research questions are, in some cases, direct rewordings of statements of purpose, phrased interrogatively rather than declaratively, as in the following example:

- The purpose of this study is to assess the relationship between the dependency level of renal transplant recipients and their rate of recovery.
- What is the relationship between the dependency level of renal transplant recipients and their rate of recovery?

Direct and simple questions invite an answer and help to focus attention on the kinds of data needed to answer them. Some research articles omit a statement of purpose and state only research questions. Other researchers use research questions to clarify or add greater specificity to a global purpose statement.

### Research Questions in Quantitative Studies

In Chapter 2, we discussed clinical foreground questions to guide an EBP inquiry. Many of the EBP question templates in Table 2.1 on page 31 could yield questions to guide a research project as well, but *researchers* tend to conceptualize their questions in terms of their *variables.* Take, for example, the first question in Table 2.1: "In (population), what is the effect of (intervention) on (outcome)?" A researcher would be more likely to think of the question in these terms: "In (population), what is the effect of (independent variable) on (dependent variable)?" Thinking in terms of variables helps to guide researchers' decisions about how to operationalize them. Thus, in quantitative studies research questions identify the population (P) under study, the key study variables (I, C, and O components), and relationships among the variables.

> **TIP:** As noted in Chapter 3, the independent variable in a study captures both the I and C components of PICO questions because researchers must be explicit about what the comparison is. Those pursuing an evidence-based practice (EBP) question are often interested in the "I" component in contrast to *any* comparison that has been made by researchers.

Most research questions concern relationships among variables, and thus many quantitative research questions could be articulated using a general question template: "In (population), what is the relationship between (independent variable or IV) and (dependent variable or DV)?" Examples of variations include the following:

○ *Treatment, intervention*: In (population), what is the effect of (IV: intervention versus an alternative) on (DV)?

○ *Prognosis*: In (population), does (IV: disease or illness versus its absence) affect or increase the risk of (DV)?

○ *Etiology/harm*: In (population), does (IV: exposure versus nonexposure) cause or increase risk of (DV)?

Not all research questions are about relationships—some are primarily descriptive. As examples, here are some descriptive questions that could be answered in a quantitative study on nurses' use of humor:

○ What is the frequency with which nurses use humor as a complementary therapy with hospitalized cancer patients?

○ What are the characteristics of nurses who use humor as a complementary therapy with hospitalized cancer patients?

○ Is my *Use of Humor Scale* a reliable and valid measure of nurses' use of humor with patients in clinical settings?

Answers to such questions might, if addressed in a methodologically sound study, be useful in developing effective strategies for reducing stress in patients with cancer.

**Example of research questions from a quantitative study:**
Ryan-Wenger and Gardner (2012) studied the perspectives of 496 hospitalized children regarding their nursing care. Their research questions included: (1) What nurse behaviors matter most to hospitalized pediatric patients? And (2) What physical or emotional characteristics of the children are related to their perceptions of nurses' behaviors?

In this example, the first question is descriptive, and the second asks about the relationship between independent variables (children's characteristics) and a dependent variable (their perception of nurses' behavior).

## Research Questions in Qualitative Studies

Research questions in qualitative studies include the phenomenon and the group of interest. Researchers in the various qualitative traditions vary in their views of what types of question are important. Grounded theory researchers are likely to ask *process* questions, phenomenologists tend to ask *meaning* questions, and ethnographers generally ask *descriptive* questions about cultures. The terms associated with the various traditions, discussed previously in connection with purpose statements, are likely to be incorporated into the research questions.

**Example of a research question from a phenomenological study:**
What is the lived experience and personal meaning of hereditary breast cancer risk and surveillance? (Underhill & Dickerson, 2011)

Not all qualitative studies are rooted in a specific research tradition. Many researchers use constructivist methods to describe or explore phenomena without focusing on cultures, meaning, or social processes.

> **Example of a research question from a descriptive qualitative study:**
> In their descriptive qualitative study, Weng and co-researchers (2012) asked, What is the nature of distress among family caregivers of children with a rare genetic disorder, Russell-Silver Syndrome?

In qualitative studies, research questions sometimes evolve during the study. Researchers begin with a *focus* that defines the broad boundaries of the inquiry, but the boundaries are not cast in stone. Constructivists are often sufficiently flexible that the question can be modified as new information makes it relevant to do so.

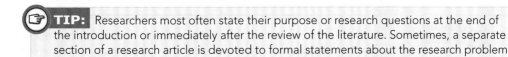 **TIP:** Researchers most often state their purpose or research questions at the end of the introduction or immediately after the review of the literature. Sometimes, a separate section of a research article is devoted to formal statements about the research problem and might be labeled "Purpose," "Statement of Purpose," "Research Questions," or, in quantitatve studies, "Hypotheses."

# RESEARCH HYPOTHESES

Some quantitative researchers explicitly state their hypotheses. A hypothesis is a prediction, almost always involving a predicted relationship between two or more variables. Qualitative researchers do not have formal hypotheses, because qualitative researchers want the inquiry to be guided by participants' viewpoints rather than by their own hunches. Thus, our discussion here focuses on hypotheses in quantitative research.

## Function of Hypotheses in Quantitative Research

Many research questions are queries about relationships between variables, and hypotheses are predicted answers to these queries. For instance, the research question might ask: Does sexual abuse in childhood affect the development of irritable bowel syndrome in women? The researcher might predict the following: Women (P) who were sexually abused in childhood (I) have a higher incidence of irritable bowel syndrome (O) than women who were not abused (C).

Hypotheses sometimes emerge from a theory. Scientists reason from theories to hypotheses and test those hypotheses in the real world; the soundness of a theory is evaluated through hypothesis testing. For example, the theory of reinforcement posits that behavior that is positively reinforced (rewarded) tends to be learned (repeated). The theory is too abstract to test directly, but predictions based on it can be tested. For instance, we could test the following hypothesis, deduced from reinforcement theory: Pediatric patients who are given a reward (e.g., permission to watch television) for cooperating during nursing procedures tend to be more cooperative than nonrewarded peers. This proposition can be put to a test, and the theory gains support if the hypotheses are supported with real data.

Even in the absence of a theory, well-conceived hypotheses offer direction and suggest explanations. For example, suppose we hypothesized that the incidence of desaturation in low-birth-weight infants undergoing intubation and ventilation would be lower using the closed tracheal suction system (CTSS) than using partially ventilated endotracheal suction (PVETS). Our hypothesis might be based on studies or clinical observations. *The development of predictions forces researchers to think logically and to exercise critical judgment.*

Now let us suppose the preceding hypothesis is not confirmed in a study; that is, we find that rates of desaturation are similar for both the PVETS and CTSS methods. *The failure of data to support a prediction forces researchers to analyze theory or previous research critically, to review study limitations, and to explore alternative explanations for the findings.* The use of hypotheses tends to induce critical thinking and to facilitate interpretation of the data.

To illustrate further the utility of hypotheses, suppose we conducted the study guided only by the question, Is there a relationship between suction method and rates of desaturation? Without a hypothesis, the researcher is seemingly prepared to accept any results. The problem is that it is almost always possible to explain something superficially after the fact, no matter what the findings are. Hypotheses reduce the possibility that spurious results will be misconstrued.

👉 **TIP:** Some quantitative research articles explicitly state the hypotheses that guided the study, but many do not. The absence of a hypothesis may indicate that researchers have failed to consider critically the existing evidence or theory, or have failed to disclose their hunches.

## Characteristics of Testable Hypotheses

Research hypotheses usually state the expected relationship between the independent variable (the presumed cause or influence) and the dependent variable (the presumed outcome or effect) within a population.

**Example of a research hypothesis:**
Liu and colleagues (2011) studied quality of life in community-dwelling patients with heart failure in Taiwan. They hypothesized that sleep quality and daytime sleepiness were factors influencing the patients' quality of life.

In this example, the population is community-dwelling Taiwanese patients with heart failure. The independent variables are sleep quality and daytime sleepiness, and the outcome variable is the patients' quality of life. The hypothesis predicts that, in the population, sleep quality and daytime sleepiness are related to (affects) quality of life.

Hypotheses that do not make a relational statement are problematic. Take the following example: *Pregnant women who receive prenatal instruction about postpartum experiences are not likely to experience postpartum depression.* This statement expresses no anticipated relationship, and cannot be tested using standard statistical procedures. In our example, how would we decide whether to accept or reject the hypothesis?

To illustrate more concretely, suppose we asked a group of new mothers who had received prenatal instruction the following question: On the whole, how depressed have you been since you gave birth? Would you say (1) extremely depressed, (2) moderately depressed, (3) a little depressed, or (4) not at all depressed? Based on their responses, how could we compare the actual outcome with the predicted outcome? Would *all* the women have to say they were "not at all depressed?" Would the prediction be supported if 51% of the women said they were "not at all depressed" *or* "a little depressed?" It is difficult to test the accuracy of the original prediction.

We could, however, modify the prediction as follows: Pregnant women who receive prenatal instruction are less likely than those who do not to experience postpartum depression. Here, the outcome variable (O) is postpartum depression, and the independent variable is receipt (I) versus nonreceipt (C) of prenatal instruction. The relational aspect of the prediction is embodied in the phrase *less than*. If a hypothesis lacks a phrase such as *more than, less than, different from, related to,* or something similar, it is not readily testable. To test the revised hypothesis, we could ask two groups of women with different prenatal instruction experiences to respond to the question on depression and then compare the groups' responses. The absolute degree of depression of either group would not be at issue.

Hypotheses should be based on justifiable rationales. Hypotheses often follow from previous research findings or are deduced from a theory. When a new area is being investigated, researchers may have to rely on logical reasoning or clinical experience to justify the predictions.

 **TIP:** Hypotheses are typically fairly easy to identify because researchers make statements such as, "The study tested the hypothesis that ..." or, "It was predicted that ...".

## Wording of Hypotheses

Hypotheses can be stated in various ways, as in the following example:

1. Older patients are more likely to fall than younger patients.
2. There is a relationship between a patient's age and the likelihood of falling.
3. The older the patient, the greater the likelihood that she or he will fall.
4. Older patients differ from younger ones with respect to their risk of falling.
5. Younger patients are at lower risk of falling than older patients.
6. The risk of falling increases with the age of the patient.

In all six examples, the hypotheses state the population (patients), the independent variable (age), the outcome variable (falling), and an anticipated relationship between them.

Hypotheses can be either directional or nondirectional. A **directional hypothesis** specifies not only the existence but the expected direction of the relationship between variables. In the six versions of the hypothesis, versions 1, 3, 5, and 6 are directional because they explicitly predict that older patients are more likely to fall than younger ones. A **nondirectional hypothesis** does not stipulate the direction of the relationship (versions 2 and 4). These hypotheses predict that a patient's age and falling are related, but they do not specify whether *older* patients or *younger* ones are predicted to be at greater risk. Note that in all six examples, the hypotheses are worded in the present tense. Researchers make a prediction about a relationship that exists in the population—not just about a relationship for a particular sample of study participants.

 **TIP:** Hypotheses can be either simple hypotheses (with a single independent variable and dependent variable) or complex (multiple independent or dependent variables). Supplementary information about this differentiation is available in the Chapter Supplement on thePoint website.

Another distinction is between research and null hypotheses. **Research hypotheses** are statements of expected relationships between variables. All the hypotheses presented thus far are research hypotheses that indicate actual expectations.

Statistical inference operates on a logic that may be confusing. This logic requires that hypotheses be expressed as an expected *absence* of a relationship. **Null hypotheses** state that there is no relationship between the independent and dependent variables. The null form of the hypothesis in our preceding example would be: "Older patients are just as likely as younger patients to fall." The null hypothesis might be compared with the assumption of innocence in English-based systems of criminal justice: the variables are assumed to be "innocent" of any relationship until they can be shown "guilty" through statistical procedures. The null hypothesis is the formal statement of this assumption of innocence.

Research articles typically state research rather than null hypotheses. In statistical testing, the underlying null hypotheses are assumed, without being stated. If the researcher's *actual* research hypothesis is that no relationship among variables exists, the hypothesis cannot be adequately tested using traditional statistical procedures, as explained in Chapter 13.

> ☞ **TIP:** If a researcher uses statistical tests (which is true in most quantitative studies), it means that there are underlying hypotheses—regardless of whether the researcher explicitly stated them—because statistical tests are designed to test hypotheses.

## Hypothesis Testing and Proof

Hypotheses are formally tested through statistical analysis. Researchers use statistics to test whether their hypotheses have a high probability of being correct (i.e., has a probability <.05). Statistical analysis does not provide proof, it only supports inferences that a hypothesis is *probably* correct (or not). Hypotheses are never *proved* (or disproved); rather, they are *accepted* or *supported* (or rejected). Findings are always tentative. Hypotheses come to be increasingly supported with evidence from multiple studies.

To illustrate why this is so, suppose we hypothesized that height and weight are related. We predict that, on average, tall people weigh more than short people. Suppose we happened by chance to get a sample of short, heavy people, and tall, thin people. Our results might indicate that there is no relationship between a person's height and weight. Would we be justified in stating that this study *proved* or *demonstrated* that height and weight are unrelated?

As another example, suppose we hypothesized that tall nurses are more effective than short ones. In reality, we would expect no relationship between height and job performance. But suppose that, by chance again, we drew a sample of nurses in which tall nurses received better job evaluations than short ones. Could we conclude definitively that height is related to a nurse's performance? These two examples illustrate the difficulty of using observations from a sample to generalize to a population. Other issues, such as the accuracy of the measures and the effects of uncontrolled variables prevent researchers from concluding that hypotheses are proved.

# CRITIQUING RESEARCH PROBLEMS, RESEARCH QUESTIONS, AND HYPOTHESES

In a comprehensive critique of a research article, you would evaluate whether researchers have adequately communicated their research problem. The problem statement, purpose, research questions, and hypotheses set the stage for describing what was done and what was learned. You should not have to dig too deeply to decipher the research problem or to discover the questions.

A critique of the research problem involves multiple dimensions. Substantively, you need to consider whether the problem has significance for nursing. Studies that build on existing evidence in a meaningful way are well-poised to make contributions to evidence-based nursing practice. Also, research problems stemming from established research priorities (see Chapter 1) have a high likelihood of yielding important new evidence for nurses because they reflect expert opinion about areas of needed research.

Another dimension in critiquing the research problem concerns methodologic issues—in particular, whether the research problem is compatible with the chosen research paradigm

---

**BOX 6.3   Guidelines for Critiquing Research Problems, Research Questions, and Hypotheses**

1. What is the research problem? Is the problem statement easy to locate and is it clearly stated? Does the problem statement build a cogent and persuasive argument for the new study?
2. Does the problem have significance for nursing? How might the research contribute to nursing practice, administration, education, or policy?
3. Is there a good fit between the research problem and the paradigm within which the research was conducted? Is there a good fit with the qualitative research tradition (if applicable)?
4. Does the report formally present a statement of purpose, research question, and/or hypotheses? Is this information communicated clearly and concisely, and is it placed in a logical and useful location?
5. Are purpose statements or research questions worded appropriately (e.g., are key concepts/ variables identified and the population specified? Are verbs used appropriately to suggest the nature of the inquiry and/or the research tradition?
6. If there are no formal hypotheses, is their absence justified? Are statistical tests used in analyzing the data despite the absence of stated hypotheses?
7. Do hypotheses (if any) flow from a theory or previous research? Is there a justifiable basis for the predictions?
8. Are hypotheses (if any) properly worded? Do they state a predicted relationship between two or more variables? Are they presented as research or as null hypotheses?

---

and its associated methods. You should also evaluate whether the statement of purpose or research questions have been properly worded and lend themselves to empirical inquiry.

If a research article describing a quantitative study does not state hypotheses, you should consider whether their absence is justified. If there are hypotheses, you should evaluate whether the hypotheses are sensible and consistent with existing evidence or relevant theory. Also, hypotheses are valid guideposts in scientific inquiry only if they are testable. To be testable, hypotheses must predict a relationship between two or more measurable variables.

Specific guidelines for critiquing research problems, research questions, and hypotheses are presented in Box 6.3.

## RESEARCH EXAMPLES WITH CRITICAL THINKING EXERCISES

This section describes how the research problem and research questions were communicated in two nursing studies, one quantitative and one qualitative.

⸙–Examples 1 and 2 below are also featured in our *Interactive Critical Thinking Activity* on thePoint website where you can easily record, print, and e-mail your responses to the related questions.

### EXAMPLE 1 ● Quantitative Research

**Study:** "Randomized clinical trial testing efficacy of a nurse-coached intervention (NCI) in arthroscopy patients" (Jones, Duffy, & Flanagan, 2011)

**Problem Statement (excerpt):** "Ambulatory surgical patients experience many symptoms such as pain, nausea and vomiting, fatigue, and unexpected limitations in daily living, isolation, and suffering. Collectively, findings show that patients have many distressing symptoms after ambulatory surgery, and these constitute major problems during recovery for patients and their families.

There is a lack of data about nursing interventions aimed at assisting ambulatory surgical patients with the management of postoperative symptoms at home." (pp. 92–93) (Citations were omitted to streamline the presentation).

**Statement of Purpose:** "The purpose of this study was to determine the efficacy of a NCI in relieving symptom distress and in improving functional health state" (p. 93).

**Hypotheses:** Arthroscopy patients who receive the NCI intervention (NCI group) when compared with a similar group who receive usual practice (UP group) will significantly have: (Hypothesis 1) less symptom distress at 72 hours and 1 week postsurgery; and (Hypothesis 2) better functional health status as measured by perceived physical health status and mental health status at 1 week postsurgery.

**Intervention:** The NCI focused on giving information, interpreting the experience, and validating and clarifying responses and actions related to the surgical experience. The NCI was delivered by telephone, beginning on the first surgical evening and at 24, 48, and 72 hours postarthroscopic surgery.

**Study Methods:** A sample of 102 arthroscopy patients at an academic medical center was assigned at random to either the NCI group or the UP group. Symptom distress was measured using the Symptom Distress Scale, and functional health was measured using the Medical Outcomes Study Short Form Health Survey (widely referred to as the SF-36). Data were collected from all participants three times: at baseline when patients enrolled in the study, 72 hours postsurgery, and 1 week postsurgery.

**Key Findings:** Participants in the intervention group had significantly less symptom distress at 72 hours and 1 week postsurgery, and significantly better physical and mental health status scores at 1 week postsurgery than those in the usual practice group.

## CRITICAL THINKING EXERCISES

1. Answer the relevant questions from Box 6.3 on page 111 regarding this study.
2. Also consider the following targeted questions:
   a. Where in the research report do you think the researchers would have presented the hypotheses? Where in the report would the results of the hypothesis tests be placed?
   b. The report did not state research questions. What might some research questions be?
   c. Were the hypotheses directional or nondirectional?
3. If the results of this study are valid and generalizable, what are some of the uses to which the findings might be put in clinical practice?

## EXAMPLE 2 ● Qualitative Research

**Study:** Andropause syndrome in men treated for metastatic prostate cancer (Grunfeld et al., 2012)

**Problem Statement (excerpt):** "Prostate cancer is the most common cancer among men in the United Kingdom, with more than 36,000 new cases per year. The incidence rate has increased threefold in the last 30 years, mainly due to improvements in detection of the disease. Outcomes are good, with a 5-year survival rate of 77% in the United Kingdom. Androgen deprivation therapy (ADT) has become the cornerstone of treatment for men with metastatic prostate cancer… However, treatments are associated with a number of adverse effects. Adverse effects vary according to the type of treatment but include erectile dysfunction, decreased libido, infertility, loss in bone mineral density, gynecomastia, depressed mood, and hot flashes. Collectively, these symptoms in healthy men are referred to as andropause syndrome… Previous studies have neglected to examine the impact of these symptoms or the cognitive and behavioral responses used to reduce the impact of the symptoms." (p. 64). (Citations were omitted to streamline the presentation.)

**Statement of Purpose:** "The aim of this study was to explore, through in-depth interviews, the experiences and impact of andropause symptoms (particularly hot flashes) among men being treated with ADT for metastatic prostate cancer" (p. 64). (The researchers did not state specific research questions in this article.)

**Method:** The researchers recruited 21 men who were identified from a clinic database at a large London teaching hospital. The researchers conducted in-depth interviews with the men, mostly in face-to-face interviews at the hospital. Participants were asked several conversational questions, such as, What have been the main effects of your symptoms on your daily life?

**Key Findings:** Hot flashes and night sweats were among the most frequently mentioned adverse effects of ADT. These symptoms disturbed the men's sleep patterns and led to irritability and fatigue. The men expressed reluctance to disclose their symptoms to others.

## CRITICAL THINKING EXERCISES
1. Answer the relevant questions from Box 6.3 on page 111 regarding this study.
2. Also consider the following targeted questions:
   a. Where in the research report do you think the researchers would have presented the statement of purpose?
   b. Does it appear that this study was conducted within one of the three main qualitative traditions? If so, which one?
3. If the results of this study are trustworthy, what are some of the uses to which the findings might be put in clinical practice?

## EXAMPLE 3 ● Quantitative Research in Appendix A
- Read the abstract and the introduction from Howell and colleagues' (2007) study ("Anxiety, anger, and blood pressure in children") in Appendix A on page 395–402.

## CRITICAL THINKING EXERCISES
1. Answer the relevant questions from Box 6.3 on page 111 regarding this study.
2. Also consider the following targeted questions:
   a. Based on the review of the literature, it would be possible to state several research hypotheses. State one or two.
   b. If your hypothesis in exercise 2.a was a directional hypothesis, state it as a nondirectional hypothesis (or vice versa). Also state it as a null hypothesis.

## EXAMPLE 4 ● Qualitative Research in Appendix B
- Read the abstract and introduction from Beck and Watson's (2010) study ("Subsequent childbirth after a previous traumatic birth") in Appendix B on page 403–412.

## CRITICAL THINKING EXERCISES
1. Answer the relevant questions from Box 6.3 on page 111 regarding this study.
2. Also consider the following targeted questions:
   a. Do you think that Beck and Watson provided a sufficient rationale for the significance of their research problem?
   b. In their argument for their study, did Beck and Watson say anything about the fourth element of an argument identified in the book—i.e., the consequences of the problem?

**WANT TO KNOW MORE?** A wide variety of resources to enhance your learning and understanding of this chapter are available on the**Point**.

- Interactive Critical Thinking Activity
- Chapter Supplement on Simple and Complex Hypotheses
- Answers to the Critical Thinking Exercises for Examples 3 and 4
- Student Review Questions
- Full-text online

Additional study aids including eight journal articles and related questions  are also available in *Study Guide for Essentials of Nursing Research, 8e.*

## SUMMARY POINTS

- A **research problem** is a perplexing or troubling situation that a researcher wants to address through disciplined inquiry.

- Researchers usually identify a broad *topic*, narrow the scope of the problem, and then identify research questions consistent with a paradigm of choice.

- Common sources of ideas for nursing research problems are clinical experience, relevant literature, social issues, theory, and external suggestions.

- Researchers communicate their aims in research articles as problem statements, statements of purpose, research questions, or hypotheses.

- The **problem statement** articulates the nature, context, and significance of a problem to be studied and an *argument* explaining the need for the study. Problem statements typically include several components: problem identification; background, scope, and consequences of the problem; knowledge gaps; and possible solutions to the problem.

- A **statement of purpose**, which summarizes the overall study goal, identifies the key concepts (variables) and the study group or population. Purpose statements often communicate, through the choice of verbs and other key terms, aspects of the research design or the research tradition.

- **Research questions** are the specific queries researchers want to answer in addressing the research problem.

- A **hypothesis** states predicted relationships between two or more variables—that is, the anticipated association between independent and dependent variables.

- **Directional hypotheses** predict the direction of a relationship; **nondirectional hypotheses** predict the existence of relationships, not their direction.

- **Research hypotheses** predict the existence of relationships; **null hypotheses**, which express the absence of a relationship, are the hypotheses subjected to statistical testing.

- Hypotheses are never proved or disproved in an ultimate sense—they are accepted or rejected, supported or not supported by the data.

# REFERENCES FOR CHAPTER 6

Jones, D., Duffy, M., & Flanagan, J. (2011). Randomized clinical trial testing efficacy of a nurse-coached intervention in arthroscopy patients. *Nursing Research, 60*, 92–99.

Grunfeld, E., Halliday, A., Martin, P., & Drudge-Coates, L. (2012). Andropause syndrome in men treated for metastatic prostate cancer: A qualitative study of the impact of symptoms. *Cancer Nursing, 35*, 63–72.

Lin, T. C., Lai, Y., Guo, S., Liu, C., Tsai, J., Guo, H., (2012). Baby oil therapy for uremic pruritus in haemodialysis patients. *Journal of Clinical Nursing, 21*, 139–148.

Liu, J. C., Hung, H., Shyu, Y., & Tsai, P. (2011). The impact of sleep quality and daytime sleepiness on global quality of life in community-dwelling patients with heart failure. *Journal of Cardiovascular Nursing, 26*, 99–105.

Ryan-Wenger, N., & Gardner, W. (2012). Hospitalized children's perspectives on the quality and equity of their nursing care. *Journal of Nursing Care Quality, 27*, 35–42.

Sternberg, R., & Barry, C. (2011). Transnational mothers crossing the border and bringing their health care needs. *Journal of Nursing Scholarship, 43*, 64–71.

Underhill, M., & Dickerson, S. (2011). Engaging in medical vigilance: Understanding the personal meaning of breast surveillance. *Oncology Nursing Forum, 38*, 686–694.

Weng, H. J., Niu, D., Turale, S., Tsao, L., Shih, F., Yamamoto-Mitani, N., et al. (2012). Family caregiver distress with children having rare genetic disorders. *Journal of Clinical Nursing, 21*, 160–169.

# Finding and Reviewing Research Evidence in the Literature

## LEARNING OBJECTIVES

*On completing this chapter, you will be able to:*

- Understand the steps involved in doing a literature review
- Identify bibliographic aids for retrieving nursing research reports, and locate references for a research topic
- Understand the process of screening, abstracting, critiquing, and organizing research evidence
- Evaluate the style, content, and organization of a literature review
- Define new terms in the chapter

## KEY TERMS

| | | |
|---|---|---|
| Bibliographic database | Literature review | PubMed |
| CINAHL database | MEDLINE® database | Secondary source |
| Keyword | Primary source | |

A literature review is a written summary of the state of evidence on a research problem. Both consumers and producers of nursing research need to acquire skills for reading, critiquing, and preparing written evidence summaries.

# BASIC ISSUES RELATING TO LITERATURE REVIEWS

Before discussing the activities involved in undertaking a research-based literature review, we briefly discuss some general issues. The first concerns the purposes of doing a literature review.

## Purposes of Research Literature Reviews

The primary purpose of literature reviews is to integrate research evidence to sum up what is known and what is not known. Literature reviews are sometimes stand-alone documents intended to share the state of evidence with interested readers, but reviews are also used to lay the foundation for new studies. A literature review undertaken for a quantitative study can help to shape research questions, suggest appropriate methods, and point to a conceptual framework. Literature reviews also help researchers to interpret their findings.

In qualitative research, opinions about literature reviews vary. Grounded theory researchers typically begin to collect data before examining the literature. As the grounded theory emerges, researchers then turn to the literature, seeking to relate prior findings to the theory. Phenomenologists, by contrast, often undertake a preliminary literature search at the outset of a study. Ethnographers often familiarize themselves with the literature to help shape their choice of a cultural problem before going into the field.

Regardless of when they perform the review, researchers usually include brief summaries of relevant literature in their introductions. The literature review tells readers about current knowledge on a topic and illuminates the significance of the new study. Literature reviews are often intertwined with the problem statement as part of the argument for the study.

## Types of Information to Seek for a Research Review

Findings from prior studies are the most important type of information for a research review. If you are preparing a literature review, you should rely mostly on **primary sources**, which are descriptions of studies written by the researchers who conducted them. **Secondary source** research documents are descriptions of studies prepared by someone else. Literature reviews, then, are secondary sources. Recent reviews may be a good place to start because they offer a quick overview of the literature and a valuable bibliography. If you are doing your own literature review, however, secondary sources should not be considered substitutes for primary sources because secondary sources are not sufficiently detailed and are seldom completely objective.

> ☞ **TIP:** For an evidence-based practice (EBP) project, a recent, high-quality systematic review may be sufficient to provide the needed information about the evidence base, although it is usually wise to search for studies published after the review. We provide more explicit guidance on searching for evidence for an EBP query in the Chapter Supplements on thePoint website. ☀–

A literature search may yield nonresearch references, including opinion articles, case reports, and clinical anecdotes. Such materials may broaden understanding of a problem, demonstrate a need for research, or describe aspects of clinical practice. These writings, however, usually have limited utility in research reviews because they do not address the central question of written reviews: What is the current state of *evidence* on this research problem?

## Major Steps and Strategies in Doing a Literature Review

Conducting a literature review is a little bit like doing a full-fledged study: a reviewer must start with a question, such as an evidence-based practice (EBP) question (Chapter 2) or a question for a new study (Chapter 6). The reviewer then must gather, analyze, and interpret the information, and summarize the "findings" in a written product. Figure 7.1 depicts the literature review process, and shows that there are potential feedback loops, with opportunities to go back to earlier steps in search of more information.

Conducting a literature review is an art and a science. A high-quality review should be unbiased, thorough, and up-to-date. Also, a high-quality review is systematic. Decision rules for including or excluding a study should be explicit because a good review should be reproducible. This means that another diligent reviewer would be able to apply the same decision rules and come to similar conclusions about the state of evidence on the topic.

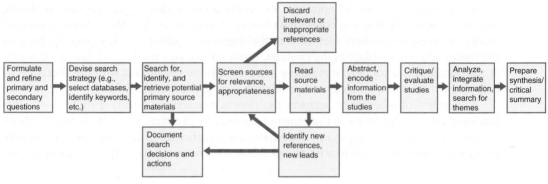

**FIGURE 7.1** ● Flow of tasks in a literature review.

> 👉 **TIP:** Locating all relevant information on a research question is like being a detective. The literature retrieval tools we discuss in this chapter are helpful, but there inevitably needs to be some digging for, and sifting of, the clues to evidence on a topic. Be prepared for sleuthing!

Doing a literature review is in some ways similar to undertaking a qualitative study. This means that it is useful to have a flexible approach to "data collection" and to think creatively about opportunities for new sources of information. It also means that the analysis of the "data" typically involves a search for important themes.

# LOCATING RELEVANT LITERATURE FOR A RESEARCH REVIEW

An early step in a literature review is devising a strategy to locate relevant studies. The ability to locate evidence on a topic is an important skill that requires adaptability—rapid technological changes mean that new methods of searching the literature are introduced continuously. We urge you to consult with librarians or faculty at your institution for updated suggestions.

## Developing a Search Strategy

Having good search skills is critically important for EBP and for researchers. A particular important approach is to search for evidence in bibliographic databases, which we discuss next. Another strategy is the *ancestry approach* ("footnote chasing"), in which citations from relevant studies are used to track down earlier research on which the studies are based (the "ancestors"). A third method, called the *descendancy approach*, is to find a pivotal early study and to search forward in citation indexes to find more recent studies ("descendants") that cited the key study.

> 👉 **TIP:** You may be tempted to begin a literature search through an Internet search engine, such as Google or Yahoo. Such a search is likely to provide you with a lot of "hits" on your topic, including information about support groups, advocacy organizations, commercial products, and the like. Internet searches are not likely to give you comprehensive bibliographic information on the *research* literature on your topic.

Decisions must also be made about delimiting the search. For example, many reviewers constrain their search to reports written in their own language. You may also want to limit your search to studies conducted within a certain time frame (e.g., within the past 15 years).

## Searching Bibliographic Databases

Bibliographic databases are accessed by computer, often through software made available by commercial vendors. These programs are user-friendly, offering menu-driven systems with on-screen support so that minimal instruction is needed to retrieve articles. Your university or hospital library probably has a subscription to these services.

### Getting Started With an Electronic Search

Before searching a bibliographic database electronically, you should become familiar with the features of the software you are using to access it. The software has options for restricting or expanding your search, for combining two searches, for saving your search, and so on. Most programs have tutorials, and most also have Help buttons.

An early task in an electronic search is identifying keywords to launch the search (although an *author search* for prominent researchers in a field is also possible). A **keyword** is a word or phrase that captures the key concepts in your question. For quantitative studies, the keywords are usually the independent or dependent variables (i.e., at a minimum, the "I" and "O" of the PICO components), and perhaps the population. For qualitative studies, the keywords are the central phenomenon and the population. If you use the question templates for asking clinical questions in Table 2.1 on page 31, the words you enter in the blanks are likely to be good keywords.

> **TIP:** If you want to identify all research reports on a topic, you need to be flexible and to think broadly about keywords. For example, if you are interested in anorexia nervosa, you might look up *anorexia, eating disorders,* and *weight loss,* and perhaps *appetite, eating behavior, food habits, bulimia,* and *body weight changes.*

There are various search approaches for a bibliographic search. All citations in a database have to be coded so they can be retrieved, and databases and programs use their own system of categorizing entries. The indexing systems have specific *subject headings* (subject codes) and a hierarchical organizational structure with subheadings.

You can undertake a *subject* search by entering a subject heading into the search field. You do not have to worry about knowing the subject codes because most software has mapping capabilities. *Mapping* is a feature that allows you to search for topics using your own keywords, rather than the exact subject heading used in the database. The software translates ("maps") your keywords into the most plausible subject heading, and then retrieves citation records that have been coded with that subject heading.

Keyword searches and subject heading searches yield overlapping but nonidentical search results, so it is a good idea to identify relevant subject headings. Subject headings for databases can be accessed in the database's thesaurus or other reference tools.

When you enter a keyword into the search field, the program likely will launch both a subject search, as just described, and a textword search. A *textword search* looks for your keyword in the text fields of the records, that is, in the title and the abstract. Thus, if you searched for *lung cancer* in the MEDLINE® database (which we describe in a subsequent section), the search would retrieve citations coded for the subject code of *lung neoplasms* (the MEDLINE® subject heading used to code entries), and also any entries in which the phrase *lung cancer* appeared, even if it had not been coded for the *lung neoplasm* subject heading.

Although it is beyond the scope of this book to offer extensive guidance on doing an electronic search, we offer a few suggestions. One widely available tool is wildcard characters. A **wildcard character**—which is a symbol, such as "*" or "$," depending on the search program—allows you to search for multiple words with the same root. The wildcard character typically is inserted after a truncated root. For example, if we entered nurs* in the search field for a MEDLINE® search, the software would search for any word that begins with "nurs," such as *nurse*, *nurses*, and *nursing*. This can be efficient, but the use of a wildcard character may turn off mapping and result in a textword search exclusively.

One way to force a textword search is to use quotation marks around a phrase, which yields citations in which the exact phrase appears in text fields. In other words, *lung cancer* and "lung cancer" might yield different results. A thorough search strategy might entail doing a search with and without wildcard characters and with and without quotation marks.

**Boolean operators** can be used to expand or restrict a search. For example, if you wanted citations on *lung cancer* and *smoking*, you could enter the following: *lung cancer AND smoking*. The Boolean operator AND would restrict the search to citations with both lung cancer and smoking as textwords or subject headings. The Boolean operator "OR" expands a search—if you entered *lung cancer OR smoking*, you would retrieve all references with either term.

Two especially useful electronic databases for nurses are **C**umulative **I**ndex to **N**ursing and **A**llied **H**ealth **L**iterature (CINAHL) and MEDLINE® (**M**edical **L**iterature **On-L**ine), which we discuss in the next sections. Other useful bibliographic databases for nurses include the Cochrane Database of Systematic Reviews, Web of Knowledge, Scopus, and EMBASE (the Excerpta Medica database). The Web of Knowledge database is useful for a descendancy search strategy because of its strong citation indexes.

> **☞ TIP:** If your goal is to conduct a *systematic* review, you will need to establish an explicit formal plan about your search strategy and keywords, as discussed in Chapter 19.

## The CINAHL Database

**CINAHL** is an important electronic database for nurses. It covers references to hundreds of nursing and allied health journals, as well as to books, book chapters, and dissertations. CINAHL contains more than 1 million records.

CINAHL provides information for locating references (i.e., the author, title, journal, year of publication, volume, and page numbers), and abstracts for most citations. Documents identified as potentially useful can often be ordered electronically. We illustrate some basic features of CINAHL, but note that changes are introduced periodically.

A "basic search" in CINAHL involves entering keywords in the search field (more options for expanding and limiting the search are available in the "Advanced Search" mode). You can restrict your search to records with certain features (e.g., only ones with abstracts); to specific publication dates (e.g., only those after 2005); to those published in English; or to those coded as being in a certain subset (e.g., nursing). The basic search screen also allows you to expand the search by clicking the option "Apply related words."

To illustrate with a concrete example, suppose we were interested in research on the effect of music on agitation in people with dementia.

We entered the following terms in the search field, and placed only one limit on the search—only records with abstracts:

---

## Search Terms

> music AND agitat* AND (dementia OR Alzheimer)    [ Search ] [ Clear ]  (?)

---

By clicking the "Search" button, we got 47 "hits" (citations). Note that we used two Boolean operators. The use of "AND" ensured that retrieved records had to include all three keywords, and the use of "OR" allowed either dementia or Alzheimer to be the third keyword. Also, we used a wildcard character* in the second keyword. This instructed the computer to search for any word that begins with "agitat" such as agitated or agitation. (Note that a search without the Boolean operators—that is, searching for the keywords music, agitat*, dementia, Alzheimer—yielded nearly 800 records).

By clicking the Search button, the 47 references would be displayed on the monitor, and we could view and print full information for ones that seemed promising. An example of an abridged CINAHL record entry for a report identified through this search is presented in Figure 7.2. The title of the article and author information is displayed, followed by source information. The source indicates the following:

- Name of the journal (*Pain Management Nursing*)
- Year and month of publication (2010 September)

| | |
|---|---|
| Title: | Effect of music on pain for home-dwelling persons with dementia. |
| Authors: | Park H. |
| Affiliation: | College of Nursing, Keimyung University, South Korea, hparknursing@yahoo.co.kr |
| Source: | Pain Management Nursing (PAIN MANAGE NURS), 2010 Sep; 11(3): 141-7 (37 ref) |
| Language: | English |
| Major Subjects: | Music Therapy -- In Old Age; Pain -- Prevention and Control -- In Old Age; Dementia; Community Living; Comfort -- In Old Age |
| Minor Subjects: | Human; Aged; Pilot Studies; Quasi-Experimental Studies; Clinical Nursing Research; Male; Female; South Korea; Nonprobability Sample; Convenience Sample; Pain Measurement; Home Environment; Effect Size; Prospective Studies; Analysis of Variance; Descriptive Statistics; Patient Attitudes -- Evaluation; Time Factors; Scales |
| Abstract: | The purpose of this study was to investigate the effect of **music** on pain for home-dwelling persons with **dementia**. A quasiexperimental design was used. Fifteen subjects listened to their preferred **music** for 30 minutes before peak **agitation** time, for 2 days per week, followed by no **music** for 2 weeks. The process was repeated once. The findings of this study showed that mean pain levels after listening to **music** were significantly lower than before listening to the **music** (t=2.21, df=28; p < .05). The findings of this pilot study suggest the importance of **music** intervention to control pain for home-dwelling persons with **dementia**. |
| Instrumentation: | Mini-Mental Status Examination (MMSE) (Folstein et al) Assessment of Personal **Music** Preference (APMP) Modified Cohen-Mansfield **Agitation** Inventory (M-CMAI) Modified Pain Assessment in the Dementing Elderly (M-PADE) |
| MEDLINE Info: | *PMID: 20728063 NLM UID: 100890606* |
| Accession Number: | 2010767993 |

**FIGURE 7.2** ● Example of a printout from a Cumulative Index to Nursing and Allied Health Literature search (CINAHL).

○ Volume (11)

○ Issue (3)

○ Page numbers (141–147)

○ Number of cited references (37)

Figure 7.2 also shows the CINAHL major and minor subject headings that were coded for this particular study. Any of these headings could have been used in a subject heading search to retrieve this reference. Note that the subject headings include substantive headings, such as *Music Therapy in Old Age*, as well as methodologic (e.g., *Quasi-Experimental Studies*) and sample characteristic headings (e.g., *Male; Female*). The subject names have hyperlinks so that we could expand the search by clicking on them (we could also click on the author's name or on the journal). The abstract for the study is then presented, with the search terms appearing in boldface. Next, the names of any formal instruments are printed under Instrumentation. Each entry shows an accession number that is the unique identifier for each record in the database, as well as other identifying numbers. Based on the abstract, we would then decide whether this reference was pertinent to our inquiry.

### The MEDLINE® Database

The MEDLINE® database, developed by the U.S. National Library of Medicine, is the premier source for bibliographic coverage of the biomedical literature. MEDLINE® covers about 5,000 medical, nursing, and health journals and has more than 21 million records. MEDLINE® can be accessed for free on the Internet at the **PubMed** website (http://www. ncbi.nlm.nih.gov/PubMed). PubMed is a lifelong resource regardless of your institution's access to bibliographic databases.

MEDLINE® uses a controlled vocabulary called **MeSH** (Medical Subject Headings) to index articles. MeSH terminology provides a consistent way to retrieve information that may use different terminology for the same concepts. Once you have begun a search, a field on the right side of the screen labeled "Search Details" lets you see how keywords you entered mapped onto MeSH terms, which might lead you to pursue other leads. You can also search for references using the MeSH database directly by clicking on "MeSH database" on the PubMed home page. MeSH subject headings may overlap with, but are not identical to, subject headings in CINAHL.

When we did a PubMed search of MEDLINE® analogous to the one we described earlier for CINAHL, using the same keywords and restrictions, 40 records were retrieved. The list of records in the two PubMed and CINAHL searches overlapped considerably, but new references were found in each search. Both searches, however, retrieved the study by Park—the CINAHL record for which was shown in Figure 7.2. The PubMed record for the same reference is presented in Figure 7.3. (To get MeSH codes, you would need to click on the link for "Publication Types, MeSH terms" that appears after the abstract). As you can see, the MeSH terms in Figure 7.3 are different from the CINAHL subject headings in Figure 7.2.

> **TIP:** After you have found a study that is a good exemplar of what you are looking for, you usually can search for similar studies in the database. In PubMed, for example, after identifying a key study, you could click on "Related Citations" on the right of the screen to locate similar studies. In Cumulative Index to Nursing and Allied Health Literature, you would click on "Find Similar Results."

Pain Manag Nurs. 2010 Sep;11(3):141-7. Epub 2009 Sep 8.

## Effect of music on pain for home-dwelling persons with dementia.

Park H. College of Nursing, Florida State University, Tallahassee, FL, USA. hparknursing@yahoo.co.kr

The purpose of this study was to investigate the effect of music on pain for home-dwelling persons with dementia. A quasiexperimental design was used. Fifteen subjects listened to their preferred music for 30 minutes before peak agitation time, for 2 days per week, followed by no music for 2 weeks. The process was repeated once. The findings of this study showed that mean pain levels after listening to music were significantly lower than before listening to the music (t=2.21, df=28; p < .05). The findings of this pilot study suggest the importance of music intervention to control pain for home-dwelling persons with dementia.

PMID: 20728063

**MeSH Terms**

- Aged, 80 and over
- Analysis of Variance
- Assisted Living Facilities
- Attitude to Health*
- Dementia/complications*
- Dementia/psychology
- Factor Analysis, Statistical
- Female
- Home Care Services*/organization & administration
- Humans
- Male
- Mental Status Schedule
- Music Therapy/methods*
- Nursing Evaluation Research
- Pain/diagnosis
- Pain/etiology
- Pain/prevention & control*
- Pain Measurement
- Pilot Projects
- Severity of Illness Index
- Treatment Outcome

**FIGURE 7.3** ● Example of printout from PubMed search.

## Screening, Documentation, and Abstracting

After searching for and retrieving references, several important steps remain before a synthesis can begin.

### Screening and Gathering References

References that have been identified in the search need to be screened for accessibility (will I be able to retrieve the article?) and relevance. You can usually surmise a reference's relevance by reading the abstract. When you find a relevant article, try to obtain a copy rather than taking notes about its content. Each article should be organized in a manner that permits easy retrieval. We find that alphabetical filing, using the first author's last name, is a good method.

### Documentation in Literature Retrieval

Search strategies are often complex, so it is wise to document your search actions and results. You should make note of databases searched, keywords used, limits instituted, studies used to launch a "descendancy" search, and any other information that would help you keep track of what you did. Part of your strategy can be documented by printing your search history from the electronic databases. Documentation will help you to conduct a more efficient search by preventing unintended duplication, and will also help you to assess what else needs to be tried.

### Abstracting and Recording Information

Once you have retrieved useful articles, you need a strategy to organize and make sense of the information in the articles. For simple literature reviews, it may be sufficient to make notes about key features of the retrieved studies, and to base your review on these notes. When a literature review is complex or involves a large number of studies, a formal system of recording information from each study may be needed. One mechanism that we recommend for very complex reviews is to code the characteristics of each study and then record codes in a set of matrices, a system that we describe in detail elsewhere (Polit & Beck, 2012).

**Example of a Mini Protocol for a Literature Review (Therapy Question)**

Citation and Abstract    (copy and paste information from bibliographic database)

| | |
|---|---|
| Variables: | Intervention (Independent Variable): _____ |
| | Outcome Variable: _____ |
| Framework/Theory: | _____ |
| Design Type: | ☐ Experimental    ☐ Quasi-experimental |
| | Specific Design: _____ |
| | Control for confounding variables: _____ |
| | Blinding? ☐ No   ☐ Yes  Who blinded? _____ |
| | Intervention description: _____ |
| | Control group condition: _____ |
| Sample: | Size: ____ Sampling method: _____ |
| | Sample characteristics: _____ |
| Data Sources: | ☐ Self-report ☐ Observational ☐ Biophysiologic ☐ Other |
| | Description of measures: _____ |
| | Data Quality: _____ |
| Key Findings: | _____ |

**FIGURE 7.4** ● Example of a mini protocol for a literature review (therapy question).

Another approach is to "copy and paste" each abstract and citation information from the bibliographic database into a word processing document. Then, the bottom of each page could have a "miniprotocol" for recording important information that you want to record consistently across studies. There is no fixed format for such a protocol—you must decide what elements are important to record systematically to help you organize and analyze information. We present an example for a half-page protocol in Figure 7.4, with entries that would be most suitable for Therapy/Intervention questions. Although many of the terms on this protocol are probably not familiar to you at this point, you will learn their meaning in subsequent chapters.

# EVALUATING AND ANALYZING THE EVIDENCE

In drawing conclusions about a body of research, reviewers must make judgments about the worth of the studies' evidence. Thus, an important part of doing a literature review is evaluating the body of completed studies and integrating the evidence across studies.

## Evaluating Studies for a Review

In reviewing the literature, you typically would not undertake a comprehensive critique of each study, but you would need to evaluate the quality of each study so that you could draw conclusions about the overall evidence and about gaps in the evidence base. Critiques for a literature review tend to focus on methodological aspects, and so the critiquing guidelines in Table 4.1 on page 69 and Table 4.2 on page 70 might be useful.

In literature reviews, methodological features of the studies under review need to be assessed with an eye to answering a broad question: To what extent do the findings reflect the *truth* (the true state of affairs) or, conversely, to what extent do flaws undermine the believability of the evidence? The "truth" is most likely to be discovered when researchers use powerful designs, good sampling plans, high-quality data collection procedures, and appropriate analyses.

## Analyzing and Synthesizing Information

Once relevant studies have been retrieved, abstracted, and critiqued, the information has to be analyzed and synthesized. As previously noted, we find the analogy between doing a literature review and doing a qualitative study useful, and this is particularly true with respect to the analysis of the "data" (i.e., the information from the retrieved studies). In both, the focus is on the identification of important *themes*.

A thematic analysis essentially involves detecting patterns and regularities—as well as inconsistencies. A number of different types of themes can be identified in a literature review analysis, three of which are as follows:

○ *Substantive themes*: What is the pattern of evidence—what findings predominate? How much evidence is there? How consistent is the body of evidence? What gaps are there in the evidence?

○ *Methodologic themes*: What methods have been used to address the question? What strategies have *not* been used? What are major methodologic deficiencies and strengths?

○ *Generalizability/transferability themes*: To what types of people or settings does the evidence apply? Do the findings vary for different types of people (e.g., men vs. women) or setting (e.g., urban vs. rural)?

In preparing a review, you would need to determine which themes are most relevant for the purpose at hand. Most often substantive themes are of greatest interest.

# PREPARING A WRITTEN LITERATURE REVIEW

Writing literature reviews can be challenging, especially when voluminous information and thematic analyses must be condensed into a small number of pages. We offer a few suggestions, but we acknowledge that skills in writing literature reviews develop over time.

## Organizing the Review

Organization is crucial in preparing a written review. When literature on a topic is extensive, it is useful to summarize information in a table. The table could include columns with headings such as Author, Sample Characteristics, Design, and Key Findings. Such a table provides a quick overview that allows you to make sense of a mass of information.

Most writers find an outline helpful. Unless the review is very simple, it is important to have an organizational plan so that the review has a meaningful and understandable flow. Lack of organization is a common weakness in first attempts at writing a research literature review. Although the specifics of the organization differ from topic to topic, the goal is to structure the review to lead logically to a conclusion about the state of evidence on the topic.

After finalizing an organizing structure, you should review your notes or protocols to decide where a particular reference fits in the outline. If some references do not seem to fit anywhere, they may need to be omitted. Remember that the number of references is less important than their relevance.

## Writing a Literature Review

It is beyond the scope of this textbook to offer detailed guidance on writing research reviews, but we offer a few comments on their content and style. Additional assistance is provided in books such as those by Fink (2010) and Garrard (2011).

## Content of the Written Literature Review

A written research review should provide readers with an objective, well-organized synthesis of current evidence on a topic. A literature review should be neither a series of quotes nor a series of abstracts. The central tasks are to summarize and critically evaluate the evidence to reveal the current state of knowledge on a topic—not simply to describe what researchers have done.

Although key studies may be described in detail, it is not necessary to provide particulars for every reference. Studies with comparable findings often can be summarized together, as illustrated in the third paragraph of Example 1 at the end of this chapter.

Findings should be summarized in your own words. The review should demonstrate that you have considered the cumulative worth of the body of research. Stringing together quotes from articles fails to show that previous research has been assimilated and understood.

The review should be as unbiased as possible. The review should not omit a study because its findings contradict those of other studies or if they conflict with your ideas. Inconsistent results should be analyzed and the supporting evidence evaluated objectively.

A literature review typically concludes with a summary of current evidence on the topic. The summary should recap key findings, assess their credibility, and point out gaps in the evidence. When the literature review is conducted for a new study, the summary should demonstrate the need for the research and clarify the context for any hypotheses.

As you read this book, you will become increasingly proficient in critically evaluating the research literature. We hope you will understand the mechanics of doing a research review once you have completed this chapter, but we do not expect that you will be in a position to write a state-of-the-art review until you have acquired more skills in research methods.

## Style of a Research Review

Students preparing research reviews often have trouble writing in an acceptable, tentative style. Hypotheses cannot be proved or disproved by statistical testing, and no question can be definitely answered in a single study. The problem is partly semantic: hypotheses are not proved or verified, they are *supported* by research findings.

> **☞ TIP:** Phrases indicating the tentativeness of research results, such as the following, are appropriate:
> - Several studies have *found*...
> - Findings thus far *suggest*...
> - The results *are consistent* with the conclusion that...
> - Results from a landmark study *imply* that ...
> - There *appears* to be fairly strong evidence that...

A related stylistic problem concerns the expression of opinions. A literature review should include opinions sparingly, and should explicitly reference the source. Reviewers' own opinions do not belong in a review, with the exception of assessments of study quality.

The left-hand column of Table 7.1 presents several examples of stylistic flaws. The right-hand column offers rewordings that are more acceptable for a research literature review. Many alternative wordings are possible.

**TABLE 7.1 Examples of Stylistic Difficulties for Research Literature Reviews**

| Problematic Style or Wording | Improved Style or Wording |
|---|---|
| Women who do not participate in childbirth preparation classes manifest a high degree of anxiety during labor. | *Studies have found that* women who participate in childbirth preparation classes *tend to* manifest less anxiety than those who do not (Giblin, 2012; Tucker, 2012; Finnerty, 2013). |
| Studies have proved that doctors and nurses do not fully understand the psychobiologic dynamics of recovery from a myocardial infarction. | Studies by Fortune (2012) and Crampton (2013) *suggest that many* doctors and nurses do not fully understand the psychobiologic dynamics of recovery from a myocardial infarction. |
| Attitudes cannot be changed quickly. | Attitudes *have been found to be* relatively stable attributes that do not change quickly (Nicolet, 2011; Carroll, 2012). |
| It is known that uncertainty engenders stress. | *According to* Dr. A. Cassard (2011), an expert on stress and anxiety, uncertainty is a stressor. |

Note: Italicized words in the improved version indicate key alterations.

# CRITIQUING RESEARCH LITERATURE REVIEWS

Some nurses never prepare a written research review, and perhaps you will never be required to do one. Most nurses, however, do *read* research reviews (including the literature review sections of research reports) and they should be prepared to evaluate such reviews critically.

It is often difficult to critique a research review if you are not familiar with the topic. You may not be able to judge whether the author has included all relevant literature and has adequately summarized knowledge on that topic. Some aspects of a research review, however, are amenable to evaluation by readers who are not experts on the topic. A few suggestions for critiquing research reviews are presented in Box 7.1. Extra critiquing questions are relevant for systematic reviews, as we discuss in Chapter 19.

---

**BOX 7.1 Guidelines for Critiquing Literature Reviews**

1. Does the review seem thorough and up-to-date? Does it include major studies on the topic? Does it include recent research?
2. Does the review rely on appropriate materials (e.g., mainly on research reports, using primary sources)?
3. Is the review merely a summary of existing work, or does it critically appraise and compare key studies? Does the review identify important gaps in the literature?
4. Is the review well organized? Is the development of ideas clear?
5. Does the review use appropriate language, suggesting the tentativeness of prior findings? Is the review objective? Does the author paraphrase, or is there an overreliance on quotes from original sources?
6. If the review is in the introduction for a new study, does the review support the need for the study?
7. If it is a review designed to summarize evidence for clinical practice, does the review draw appropriate conclusions about practice implications?

In assessing a literature review, the overarching question is whether it summarizes the current state of research evidence. If the review is written as part of an original research report, an equally important question is whether the review lays a solid foundation for the new study.

> 👉 **TIP:** Literature reviews in the introductions of research articles are unlikely to present a thorough critique of existing studies, but are likely to identify gaps in what has been studied.

## RESEARCH EXAMPLES WITH CRITICAL THINKING EXERCISES

The best way to learn about the style, content, and organization of a research literature review is to read reviews that appear in the nursing literature. We present an excerpt from a review for a mixed methods study—one involving the collection and analysis of both qualitative and quantitative data.

⚡ Example 1 below is also featured in our *Interactive Critical Thinking Activity* on thePoint website where you can easily record, print, and e-mail your responses to the related questions.

### EXAMPLE 1 ● Literature Review from a Mixed Methods Study

**Study:** "Adherence to leg ulcer lifestyle advice; qualitative and quantitative outcomes associated with a nurse-led intervention" (Van Hecke et al., 2011)

**Statement of Purpose:** The purpose of this study was to examine changes associated with a nursing intervention to enhance adherence to leg ulcer lifestyle advice.

**Literature Review (excerpt):** "A venous leg ulcer is a chronic problem that mainly occurs as a consequence of chronic venous insufficiency (Brem et al., 2004). Prevalence in adult populations is estimated at 0.63% to 1.9% in Europe, the UK, the USA, and Australia (Briggs & Closs, 2003)... Venous leg ulcers indicate a lifelong treatment plan (Reichardt, 1999) including compression therapy (Nelson et al., 2000, O'Meara et al., 2009), leg exercises, and leg elevation (Heinen et al., 2004). Nonadherence to leg ulcer treatment frequently occurs. However, few studies report the development and testing of nursing interventions to enhance adherence to leg ulcer treatment.

Several authors report the problem of nonadherence among patients with venous leg ulcers. Jull et al. (2004) found that only 52% of the included patients (*n* = 129) reported wearing compression stockings daily for the first 6 months after leg ulcer healing. About one fifth (22%) of the patients had not worn compression stockings at all. In the study of Raju et al. (2007), only 37% of the patients with chronic venous disease (including leg ulcers) reported full or partial adherence and 63% did not use compression stockings at all or abandoned them after a trial period in the past... Few studies examined nonadherence to leg exercises and leg elevation. Twenty percent of the patients with venous leg ulcers elevated their legs when sitting and they walked for 1.7 hours per day (Johnson 1995). Heinen et al. (2007b) described less positive results regarding physical activity: 56% of the 150 patients were physically active <2.5 hours per week, 13% of the patients walked for 30 minutes at least 5 days of the week and 35% performed lower leg exercises...

Published research concerning the determinants of nonadherence to leg ulcer treatment is limited. Pain, discomfort and inadequate lifestyle advice by health care professionals are the main reasons for nonadherence, as reported by leg ulcer patients (Van Hecke et al., 2009). Additional reasons for nonadherence are difficulties in applying compression, skin problems, uncomfortable footwear, poor cosmetic appearance of compression bandages, and financial restrictions (Van Hecke et al., 2009).... Heinen et al. (2007a) report that pain, comorbidity, difficulties in finding appropriate footwear, compression bandages, incorrect health beliefs, low self-efficacy, and lack of social support are linked to insufficient activity in leg ulcer patients. The fear that physical activity will cause injury and aggravate pain has also been documented as a reason for nonadherence (Walshe, 1995; Chase et al., 1997; Hyde et al., 1999; Ebbeskog & Ekman, 2001).

Nonadherence has a negative impact on the outcomes of venous leg ulcers. It increases the time to complete healing (Mayberry et al., 1991; Erickson et al., 1995; Moffatt et al., 2009). Recurrence rates also increase when patients do not wear compression stockings (Mayberry et al., 1991; Erickson et al., 1995; Harper et al., 1999; Finlayson et al., 2009; Moffatt etal., 2009). Nonadherence is also associated with increased costs (Korn et al., 2002). Therefore, adherence to leg ulcer treatment is important. The need to improve patient adherence to maximize therapeutic benefits is highlighted in the literature. However, few comprehensive programs to optimize patient adherence to leg ulcer lifestyle advice have been initiated (Van Hecke et al., 2008)."

## CRITICAL THINKING EXERCISES

1. Answer the relevant questions from Box 7.1 on page 127 regarding this literature review.
2. Also consider the following targeted questions, which may further sharpen your critical thinking skills and assist you in understanding this study:
   a. In performing the literature review, what keywords might the researchers have used to search for prior studies?
   b. Using the keywords, perform a computerized search to see if you can find a recent relevant study to augment the review.

## EXAMPLE 2 ● Quantitative Research in Appendix A

- Read the abstract and the introduction from Howell and colleagues' (2007) study ("Anxiety, anger, and blood pressure in children") in Appendix A on page 395–402.

## CRITICAL THINKING EXERCISES

1. Answer the relevant questions from Box 7.1 on page 127 regarding this study.
2. Also consider the following targeted questions:
   a. What do you think the independent variable was in this study? Did the literature review cover findings from prior studies about this variable?
   b. What were the dependent variables in this study? Did the literature review cover findings from prior studies about these variables and their relationship with the independent variable?
   c. In performing the literature review, what keywords might have been used to search for prior studies?

## EXAMPLE 3 ● Qualitative Research in Appendix B

- Read the abstract and introduction from Beck and Watson's (2010) study ("Subsequent childbirth after a previous traumatic birth") in Appendix B on page 403–412.

## CRITICAL THINKING EXERCISES

1. Answer the relevant questions in Box 7.1 on page 127 regarding this study.
2. Also consider the following targeted questions:
   a. What was the central phenomenon in this study? Was that phenomenon adequately covered in the literature review?
   b. In performing their literature review, what keywords might Beck and Watson have used to search for prior studies?

**WANT TO KNOW MORE?** A wide variety of resources to enhance your learning and understanding of this chapter are available on thePoint.

- Interactive Critical Thinking Activity
- Chapter Supplement on Finding Evidence for an EBP Inquiry in PubMed
- Answers to the Critical Thinking Exercises for Examples 2 and 3
- Student Review Questions
- Full-text online
- Internet Resources with useful websites for Chapter 7

Additional study aids including eight journal articles and related questions are also available in *Study Guide for Essentials of Nursing Research, 8e.*

## SUMMARY POINTS

- A research **literature review** is a written summary of the state of evidence on a research problem.

- The major steps in preparing a written research review include formulating a question, devising a search strategy, searching and retrieving relevant sources, abstracting and encoding information, critiquing studies, analyzing and integrating the information, and preparing a written synthesis.

- Research reviews rely primarily on findings in research reports. Information in nonresearch references (e.g., opinion articles, case reports) may broaden understanding of a problem, but has limited utility in summarizing evidence.

- A **primary source** is the original description of a study prepared by the researcher who conducted it; a **secondary source** is a description of a study by another person. Literature reviews should be based on primary source material.

- Strategies for finding studies on a topic include the use of bibliographic tools, but also include the *ancestry approach* (tracking down earlier studies cited in a reference list of a report) and the *descendancy approach* (using a pivotal study to search forward to subsequent studies that cited it.)

- Key resources for a research literature search are the **bibliographic databases** that can be searched electronically. For nurses, the **CINAHL** and **MEDLINE®** databases are especially useful.

- In searching a bibliographic database, users can do a keyword search that looks for terms in *text fields* of a database record (or that *maps* keywords onto the database's subject codes), or can search according to the *subject heading* codes themselves.

- Retrieved references must be screened for relevance, and then pertinent information can be abstracted and encoded for subsequent analysis. Studies must also be critiqued to assess the strength of evidence in existing research.

- The analysis of information from a literature search essentially involves the identification of important *themes*—regularities and patterns in the information.

- In preparing a written review, it is important to organize materials coherently. Preparation of an outline is recommended. The reviewers' role is to point out what has been studied, how adequate and dependable the studies are, and what gaps exist in the body of research.

# REFERENCES FOR CHAPTER 7

Fink, A. (2010). *Conducting research literature reviews: From paper to the Internet* (3rd ed.). Thousand Oaks, CA: Sage.

Garrard, J. (2011). *Health sciences literature review made easy: The matrix method* (3rd ed.). Boston, MA: Jones and Bartlett Publishers.

Polit, D., & Beck, C. (2012). *Nursing research: Generating and appraising evidence for nursing practice* (9th ed.) Philadelphia, PA: Lippincott Williams & Wilkins.

Van Hecke, A., Grypdonck, M., Beele, H., Vanderwee, K., & Defloor, T. (2011). Adherence to leg ulcer lifestyle advice; Qualitative and quantitative outcomes associated with a nurse-led intervention. *Journal of Clinical Nursing, 20,* 429–443.

# 8 Theoretical and Conceptual Frameworks

## LEARNING OBJECTIVES

**On completing this chapter, you will be able to:**

● Identify major characteristics of theories, conceptual models, and frameworks
● Identify several conceptual models or theories frequently used by nurse researchers
● Describe how theory and research are linked in quantitative and qualitative studies
● Critique the appropriateness of a theoretical framework—or its absence—in a study
● Define new terms in the chapter

## KEY TERMS

| | | |
|---|---|---|
| Conceptual framework | Framework | Theoretical framework |
| Conceptual map | Middle-range theory | Theory |
| Conceptual model | Model | |
| Descriptive theory | Schematic model | |

High-quality studies typically achieve a high level of *conceptual integration*. This means that the research questions fit the chosen methods, that the questions are consistent with existing evidence, and that there is a plausible conceptual rationale for expected outcomes—including a rationale for any hypotheses or interventions. For example, suppose a research team hypothesized that a nurse-led smoking cessation intervention would reduce smoking among patients with cardiovascular disease. Why would they make this prediction—what is the "theory" about how the intervention might change people's behavior? Is it predicted that the intervention will change patients' knowledge? their attitudes? their motivation? or their sense of control over decision making? The researchers' view of how the intervention would "work" should drive the design of the intervention and the study.

Design decisions cannot be developed in a vacuum—there must be an underlying conceptualization of people's behaviors and characteristics, and how these affect and are affected by internal, interpersonal, and environmental forces. In some studies the underlying conceptualization is fuzzy or unstated, but in good research, a clear and defensible conceptualization is made explicit. This chapter discusses theoretical and conceptual contexts for nursing research problems.

# THEORIES, MODELS, AND FRAMEWORKS

Many terms are used in connection with conceptual contexts for research, such as theories, models, frameworks, schemes, and maps. These terms are interrelated but are used differently by different writers. We offer guidance in distinguishing these terms, but our definitions are not universal.

## Theories

In nursing education, the term *theory* is used to refer to content covered in classrooms, as opposed to actual nursing practice. In both lay and scientific language, *theory* connotes an *abstraction*.

Classically, **theory** is defined as an abstract generalization that explains how phenomena are interrelated. The traditional definition requires a theory to embody at least two concepts that are systematically related in a manner that the theory claims to explain. As classically defined, theories consist of concepts and a set of propositions that form a logically interrelated system, providing a mechanism for deducing hypotheses from the original propositions. To illustrate, consider *reinforcement theory*, which posits that behavior that is reinforced (i.e., rewarded) tends to be repeated and learned. The proposition is that one concept (reinforcement) affects the other (learning). The proposition lends itself to hypothesis generation. For example, if reinforcement theory is valid, we could deduce that hyperactive children who are rewarded when they engage in quiet play will exhibit less acting-out behaviors than unrewarded children. This prediction, as well as others based on reinforcement theory, could then be tested in a study.

The term *theory* is also used less restrictively to refer to a broad characterization of a phenomenon. A **descriptive theory** accounts for and thoroughly describes a phenomenon. Descriptive theories are inductive, observation-based abstractions that describe or classify characteristics of individuals, groups, or situations by summarizing their commonalities. Such theories are important in qualitative studies.

Both classical and descriptive theories help to make research findings meaningful and interpretable. Theories may guide researchers' understanding not only of the "what" of natural phenomena but also of the "why" of their occurrence. Theories can also help to stimulate research by providing both direction and impetus.

Theories vary in their level of generality. *Grand theories* (or *macrotheories*) claim to explain large segments of human experience. In nursing, there are grand theories that offer explanations for the whole of nursing and that address the nature and mission of nursing practice, as distinct from the discipline of medicine. Parse's Theory of Human Becoming (Parse, 1999), for example, has been called a nursing grand theory. Theories of relevance to researchers are often less abstract than grand theories. **Middle-range theories** attempt to explain such phenomena as stress, comfort, and health promotion. Middle-range theories, compared to grand theories, are more specific and more amenable to empirical testing.

## Models

A **conceptual model** deals with abstractions (concepts) that are assembled because of their relevance to a common theme. Conceptual models provide a conceptual perspective regarding interrelated phenomena, but they are more loosely structured than theories and do not link concepts in a logically derived deductive system. A conceptual model broadly presents an understanding of the phenomenon of interest and reflects the assumptions and philosophical views of the model's designer. Like theories, conceptual models can serve as springboards for generating hypotheses.

Some writers use the term **model** to designate a method of representing phenomena with a minimal use of words. Words can convey different meanings to different people; thus, a visual or symbolic representation of a phenomenon can sometimes help to express abstract ideas more clearly. Two types of models that are used in research contexts are schematic models and statistical models. *Statistical models*, not discussed here, are equations that mathematically express relationships among a set of variables. These models are tested using sophisticated statistical methods.

**Schematic models** (or **conceptual maps**) visually represent relationships among phenomena, and are used in both qualitative and quantitative research. Concepts and linkages between them are depicted graphically through boxes, arrows, or other symbols. As an example of a schematic model, Figure 8.1 shows **Pender's Health Promotion Model**

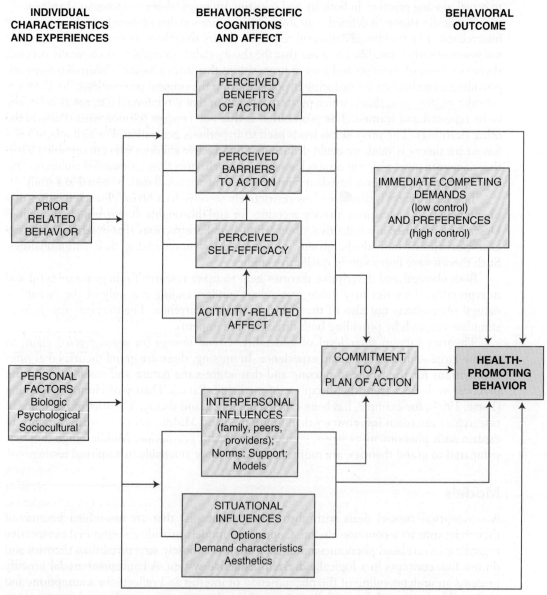

| INDIVIDUAL CHARACTERISTICS AND EXPERIENCES | BEHAVIOR-SPECIFIC COGNITIONS AND AFFECT | BEHAVIORAL OUTCOME |

**FIGURE 8.1** ● The Health Promotion Model (HPM). (From: The University of Michigan website: http://sitemaker.umich.edu/pender.health.promotion.model/files/chart.gif, retrieved July 25, 2012).

(HPM), which is a model for explaining and predicting the health-promotion component of lifestyle (Pender et al., 2011). Schematic models are appealing as visual summaries of complex ideas.

## Frameworks

A **framework** is the conceptual underpinning of a study. Not every study is based on a theory or conceptual model, but every study has a framework. In a study based on a theory, the framework is called the **theoretical framework**; in a study that has its roots in a specified conceptual model, the framework may be called the **conceptual framework**. However, the terms *conceptual framework*, *conceptual model*, and *theoretical framework* are often used interchangeably.

A study's framework is often implicit (i.e., not formally acknowledged or described). World views shape how concepts are defined, but researchers often fail to clarify the conceptual foundations of their variables. Researchers who clarify conceptual definitions of key variables provide important information about the study's framework.

Quantitative researchers are generally more guilty of failing to identify their frameworks than qualitative researchers. In qualitative research, the framework is part of the research tradition in which the study is embedded. For example, ethnographers generally begin within a theory of culture. Grounded theory researchers incorporate sociological principles into their framework and approach. The questions that qualitative researchers ask and the methods they use to address those questions often inherently reflect certain theoretical formulations.

In recent years, *concept analysis* has become an important enterprise among students and nurse scholars. Several methods have been proposed for undertaking a concept analysis and clarifying conceptual definitions (e.g., Walker & Avant, 2010). Efforts to analyze concepts of relevance to nursing should facilitate greater conceptual clarity among nurse researchers.

> **Example of developing a conceptual definition:**
> Hodges (2009) did a concept analysis of the concept of *life purpose*. She considered philosophical underpinnings, theoretical frameworks, and research evidence. She proposed this conceptual definition of *life purpose* as it applies to older adults in critical care settings: "The degree to which a person realizes his/her own interpersonal, intrapersonal, and psychological uniqueness on the basis of life experiences that correspond with spiritual values and goals at a specific time in life" (p. 169).

## The Nature of Theories and Conceptual Models

Theories, conceptual frameworks, and models are not *discovered*; they are created. Theory building depends not only on observable evidence, but also on a theorist's ingenuity in pulling evidence together and making sense of it. Theory construction is a creative enterprise that can be done by anyone who is insightful, understands existing evidence, and can knit evidence together into a lucid pattern. Because theories are not just "out there" waiting to be discovered, it follows that theories are tentative. A theory cannot be proved—a theory represents a theorist's best efforts to describe and explain phenomena. Through research, theories evolve and are sometimes discarded. This may happen if new evidence undermines a previously accepted theory. Or, a new theory might integrate new observations with an existing theory to yield a more parsimonious explanation of a phenomenon.

Theory and research have a reciprocal relationship. Theories are built inductively from observations, and research is an excellent source for those observations. The theory, in turn, must be tested by subjecting deductions from it (hypotheses) to systematic inquiry. Thus, research plays a dual and continuing role in theory building and testing. Theory guides and generates ideas for research; research assesses the worth of the theory and provides a foundation for new theories.

**Example of theory development:**

Jean Johnson (1999) developed the middle-range Self-Regulation Theory that explicates relationships between health care experiences, coping, and health outcomes. Here is how she described theory development: "The theory was developed in a cyclic process. Research was conducted using the self-regulation theory of coping with illness. Propositions supported by data were retained, and other propositions were altered when they were not supported. And new theoretical propositions were added when research produced unexpected findings. This cycle has been repeated many times over three decades leading to the present stage of development of the theory" (pp. 435 to 436). Several researchers have developed and tested interventions based on Self-Regulation Theory.

# CONCEPTUAL MODELS AND THEORIES USED IN NURSING RESEARCH

Nurse researchers have used both nursing and nonnursing frameworks to provide a conceptual context for their studies. This section briefly discusses several frameworks that have been found useful by nurse researchers.

## Conceptual Models of Nursing

Several nurses have formulated conceptual models representing formal explanations of what the nursing discipline is and what the nursing process entails, in the view of the model developer. Four concepts are central to models of nursing (Fawcett, 2005): *human beings, environment, health*, and *nursing*. The various conceptual models define these concepts differently, link them in diverse ways, and emphasize different relationships among them. Moreover, the models emphasize different processes as being central to nursing. For example, Sister Calista Roy's Adaptation Model identifies adaptation of patients as a critical phenomenon (Roy & Andrews, 1999). Martha Rogers (1994), by contrast, emphasized the centrality of the individual as a unified whole, and her model views nursing as a process in which clients are aided in achieving maximum well-being within their potential.

The conceptual models were not developed primarily as a base for nursing research. Indeed, most models have had more impact on nursing education and clinical practice than on nursing research. Nevertheless, nurse researchers have turned to these conceptual frameworks for inspiration in formulating research questions and hypotheses.

**TIP:** The Chapter Supplement for Chapter 8 on the thePoint website includes a table of 10 prominent conceptual models in nursing. The table describes the model's key features and identifies a study that claimed the model as its framework.

Let us consider one conceptual model of nursing that has received considerable research attention, **Roy's Adaptation Model**. In this model, humans are viewed as biopsychosocial adaptive systems who cope with environmental change through the process of adaptation (Roy & Andrews, 1999). Within the human system, there are four subsystems: physiologic/physical, self-concept/group identity, role function, and interdependence. These subsystems constitute adaptive modes that provide mechanisms for coping with environmental stimuli and change. Health is viewed as both a state and a process of being and becoming integrated and whole that reflects the mutuality of persons and environment. The goal of nursing, according to this model, is to promote client adaptation; nursing also regulates stimuli affecting adaptation. Nursing interventions usually take the form of increasing, decreasing, modifying, removing, or maintaining internal and external stimuli that affect adaptation. Roy's Adaptation Model has been the basis for several middle-range theories and dozens of studies.

**Research example using Roy's adaptation model:**
Fawcett and colleagues (2011) used Roy's adaptation model as a basis for their international study of the relationship between a woman's perception of and responses to caesarean birth on the one hand and type of caesarean (planned or unplanned) and prior preparation for caesarean birth on the other.

## Middle-Range Theories Developed by Nurses

In addition to conceptual models that describe and characterize the nursing process, nurses have developed middle-range theories and models that focus on more specific phenomena of interest to nurses. Examples of middle-range theories that have been used in research include Beck's (2012) Theory of Postpartum Depression, the Theory of Unpleasant Symptoms (Lenz et al., 1997), Kolcaba's (2003) Comfort Theory, Pender's Health Promotion Model, and Mishel's (1990) Uncertainty in Illness Theory. The latter two are briefly described here.

Nola Pender's (2006) **Health Promotion Model** (HPM) focuses on explaining health-promoting behaviors, using a wellness orientation. According to the revised model (Fig 8.1, p.134), *health promotion* entails activities directed toward developing resources that maintain or enhance a person's well-being. The model embodies a number of propositions that can be used in developing and testing interventions and understanding health behaviors. For example, one HPM proposition is that people commit to engaging in behaviors from which they anticipate deriving valued benefits, and another is that perceived competence or self-efficacy relating to a given behavior increases the likelihood of commitment to action and actual performance of the behavior.

**Example using the HPM:**
Mohamadian and colleagues (2011) used the HPM as the basis for a study of the determinants of health-related quality of life among Iranian adolescent girls.

Mishel's **Uncertainty in Illness Theory** (Mishel, 1990) focuses on the concept of uncertainty—the inability of a person to determine the meaning of illness-related events. According to this theory, people develop subjective appraisals to assist them in interpreting the experience of illness and treatment. Uncertainty occurs when people are unable to recognize and categorize stimuli. Uncertainty results in the inability to obtain a clear conception of the situation, but a situation appraised as uncertain will mobilize individuals to use their resources to adapt to the situation. Mishel's conceptualization of uncertainty and her Uncertainty in Illness Scale have been used in many nursing studies.

> **Example using Uncertainty in Illness Theory:**
> Stewart, Mishel, Lynn, and Terhorst (2010) tested a model of uncertainty and psychological distress in children and adolescents with cancer.

## Other Models Used by Nurse Researchers

Many concepts in which nurse researchers are interested are not unique to nursing, and therefore their studies are sometimes linked to frameworks that are not models from the nursing profession. Several of these alternative models have gained special prominence in the development of nursing interventions to promote health-enhancing behaviors and life choices. Five non-nursing theories that have frequently been used in nursing are briefly described in this section.

- **Social Cognitive Theory** (Bandura, 1985, 2001), which is sometimes called *self-efficacy theory*, offers an explanation of human behavior using the concepts of self-efficacy, outcome expectations, and incentives. Self-efficacy concerns people's belief in their own capacity to carry out particular behaviors (e.g., smoking cessation). Self-efficacy expectations determine the behaviors a person chooses to perform, their degree of perseverance, and the quality of the performance. As a research example, Poomsrikaew, Berger, Kim, and Zerwic (2012) examined age and gender differences in social cognitive factors linked to exercise behavior in Thai adults.

> **☞ TIP:** Bandura's self-efficacy is a key construct in several models discussed in this chapter. Self-efficacy has repeatedly been found to affect people's behaviors and to be amenable to change, and so self-efficacy enhancement is often a goal in interventions designed to change people's health-related actions and behaviors.

- In the **Transtheoretical Model** (Prochaska et al., 2002), the core construct is *stages of change*, which conceptualizes a continuum of motivational readiness to change problem behavior. The five stages of change are precontemplation, contemplation, preparation, action, and maintenance. Studies have shown that successful self-changers use different processes at each particular stage, thus suggesting the desirability of interventions that are individualized to the person's stage of readiness for change. For example, Plow, Finlayson, and Cho (2011) studied stages of change for physical activity behavior in a sample of people with multiple sclerosis in relation to their health symptoms, self-efficacy, and behavioral and cognitive processes.
- Becker's **Health Belief Model** (HBM) is a framework for explaining people's health-related behavior, such as health care use and compliance with a medical regimen. According to the model, health-related behavior is influenced by a person's perception of a threat posed by a health problem as well as by the value associated with actions aimed at reducing the threat (Becker, 1976). A revised HBM (RHBM) has incorporated the concept of self-efficacy (Rosenstock et al., 1988). Nurse researchers have used the HBM extensively. For example, Chen and colleagues (2011) used the HBM as a guiding framework in their study of factors affecting parents' decision to vaccinate their children for influenza.
- Ajzen's (2005) **Theory of Planned Behavior** (TPB), which is an extension of another theory called the Theory of Reasoned Action, offers a framework for understanding people's behavior and its psychological determinants. According to the theory, behavior that is volitional is determined by people's intention to perform that behavior. Intentions, in turn, are affected by attitudes toward the behavior, subjective norms

(i.e., perceived social pressure to perform or not perform the behavior), and perceived behavioral control (i.e., anticipated ease or difficulty of engaging in the behavior). Ben Natan and Gorkov (2011), for example, tested the utility of TBP for explaining blood donations among Israelis.

⊙ Lazarus and Folkman's (1984, 2006) **Theory of Stress and Coping** offers an explanation of people's methods of dealing with stress, i.e., environmental and internal demands that tax or exceed a person's resources and endanger his or her well-being. The theory posits that coping strategies are learned and deliberate responses to stressors, and are used to adapt to or change the stressors. According to this model, people's perception of mental and physical health is related to the ways they evaluate and cope with the stresses of living. As a research example, Street and colleagues (2010) studied psychosocial adaptation over time in female partners of men with prostate cancer, and used the Lazarus and Folkman theory for interpreting their findings.

Although the use of theories and models from other disciplines such as psychology (*borrowed theories*) has stirred some controversy, nursing research is likely to continue on its current path of conducting studies within a multidisciplinary perspective. A borrowed theory that is tested and found to be empirically adequate in health-relevant situations of interest to nurses becomes *shared theory*.

> ☞ **TIP:** There are websites devoted to many of the theories and models mentioned in this chapter. Several specific websites are listed in the Internet Resources for this chapter on thePoint website. ☼

# USING A THEORY OR FRAMEWORK IN RESEARCH

The manner in which theory and conceptual frameworks are used by qualitative and quantitative researchers is elaborated on in this section. In the discussion, the term *theory* is used in its broadest sense to include conceptual models, formal theories, and frameworks.

## Theories and Qualitative Research

Theory is almost always present in studies that are embedded in a qualitative research tradition such as ethnography or phenomenology. However, different traditions involve theory in different ways.

Sandelowski (1993) distinguished between *substantive theory* (conceptualizations of a specific phenomenon under study) and theory reflecting a conceptualization of human inquiry. Some qualitative researchers insist on an atheoretical stance vis-a-vis the phenomenon of interest, with the goal of suspending prior conceptualizations (substantive theories) that might bias their inquiry. For example, phenomenologists are committed to theoretical naiveté, and try to hold preconceived views of the phenomenon in check. Nevertheless, phenomenologists are guided by a framework that focuses their inquiry on certain aspects of a person's lifeworld—i.e., lived experiences.

Ethnographers bring a cultural perspective to their studies, and this perspective shapes their fieldwork. Fetterman (2010) has observed that most ethnographers adopt one of two cultural theories: *ideational theories*, which suggest that cultural conditions and adaptation stem from mental activity and ideas, or *materialistic theories*, which view material conditions (e.g., resources, money, production) as the source of cultural developments.

Grounded theory is a general inductive method that is not attached to a particular theoretical perspective. Grounded theorists can use various theoretical perspectives, such as systems theory or social organization theory. A popular theoretical underpinning of grounded theory research is *symbolic interaction* (or *interactionism*), which has three underlying premises (Blumer, 1986). First, humans act toward things based on the meanings that the things have for them. Second, the meaning of things is derived from the interaction humans have with fellow humans. And third, meanings are handled in, and modified through, an interpretive process.

**Example of a grounded theory study:**
Thomas (2011) did a grounded theory study within a symbolic interaction framework to explore older adults' experience managing diabetes in the workplace and maintaining employment.

Despite this theoretical perspective, grounded theory researchers, like phenomenologists, try to hold prior substantive theory about the phenomenon in abeyance until their own substantive theory begins to emerge. The goal of grounded theory is to develop a conceptually dense understanding of a phenomenon that is *grounded* in actual observations. The intent is to use the data, grounded in reality, to describe or explain processes as they occur in reality, not as they have been conceptualized previously. Once the theory starts to take shape, grounded theorists use previous literature for comparison with the emerging categories of the theory. Grounded theory researchers, who focus on social or psychological processes, often develop conceptual maps to illustrate how a process unfolds. Figure 8.2 illustrates such a conceptual map for a study of women controlling urinary tract symptoms (Wang et al., 2011); this study is described at the end of this chapter.

In recent years, a growing number of qualitative nurse researchers have adopted a perspective known as *critical theory* as a framework in their research. Critical theory is a paradigm that involves a critique of society and societal processes and structures, as we discuss in Chapter 14.

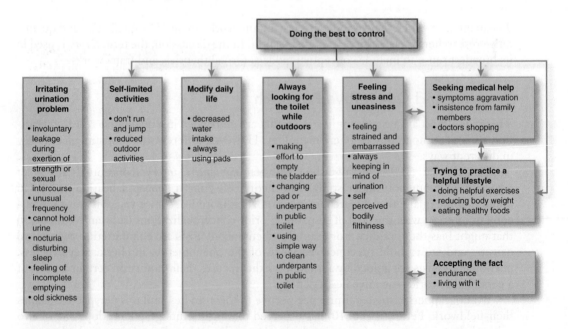

**FIGURE 8.2** ● Model for a grounded theory, "Doing the Best to Control." (From: Wang, Y., Chen, S., Jou, H., & Tsao, L. (2011). Doing the best to control: The experience of Taiwanese women with lower urinary tract symptoms. *Nursing Research, 60,* 66–72, Figure 1, with permission.)

Qualitative researchers sometimes use conceptual models of nursing or theories as interpretive frameworks. For example, a number of qualitative nurs acknowledge that the philosophic roots of their studies lie in conceptual models such as those developed by Newman (1997), Parse (1999), and Rogers (1994).

> **Example of using nursing theory in a qualitative study:**
> Rosa (2011) based her study of the process of transformative nursing practice in caring for patients with a chronic illness in Margaret Newman's (1997) Theory of Health as Expanding Consciousness.

Another strategy that can lead to substantive theory development relies on a systematic review of qualitative studies on a specific topic. In such metasyntheses, qualitative studies are combined to identify their essential elements. The findings from different sources are then used for theory building. Metasyntheses are discussed in Chapter 19.

## Theories in Quantitative Research

Quantitative researchers link research to theory or models in various ways. The classic approach is to test hypotheses deduced from an existing theory. For example, a nurse might read about Pender's HPM (Fig. 8.1, p.134) and might reason as follows: If the HPM is valid, then I would expect that patients with osteoporosis who perceive the benefit of a calcium-enriched diet would be more likely to alter their eating patterns than those who perceived no benefits.

In testing a theory, quantitative researchers deduce implications (as in the preceding example) and develop hypotheses, which are predictions about the manner in which variables would be interrelated if the theory were correct. Key variables in the theory would be measured, data would be collected, and the hypotheses would be tested through statistical analysis. The testing process involves a comparison between observed outcomes with those predicted in the hypotheses. Repeated acceptance of hypotheses derived from a theory lends support to the theory.

> **TIP:** When a quantitative study is based on a theory or conceptual model, the research article typically states this fact fairly early—often in the first paragraph, or even in the title. Some studies also have a subsection of the introduction called "Conceptual Framework" or "Theoretical Framework." The report usually includes a brief overview of the theory so that all readers can understand, in a broad way, the conceptual context of the study.

Tests of a theory also take the form of testing theory-based interventions. Theories have implications for influencing people's health-related attitudes or behavior, and hence their health outcomes. If an intervention is developed based on an explicit conceptualization of human behavior, then it likely has a better chance of being effective than if it is developed in a conceptual vacuum. Interventions rarely affect outcomes directly—there are mediating factors that play a role in the causal pathway between the intervention and the outcomes. For example, interventions based on Social Cognitive Theory posit that improvements to a person's self-efficacy will in turn result in positive changes in health behavior.

> **Example of theory testing in an intervention study:**
> Wambach and colleagues (2011) developed an educational and counseling intervention designed to promote breast-feeding in adolescent mothers, and designed their intervention elements on the basis of the TPB.

Many researchers who cite a theory or model as their framework are not directly *testing* the theory. One older study found, for example, that when nursing models were used in research, they most often were used to provide an *organizing structure* (Silva, 1986). In such an approach, researchers begin with a broad conceptualization of nursing (or stress, and so on) that is consistent with the model. The researchers *assume* that the model they espouse is valid, and then use its constructs or schemas to provide a broad interpretive context. To our knowledge, Silva's study has not been replicated with a more recent sample of studies. We suspect that, even today, a high percentage of quantitative studies that cite theories as their conceptual frameworks are using them primarily as organizational or interpretive tools, not as tests of the theory.

Quantitative researchers also use another approach to creating a conceptual context, and that involves using findings from prior research to develop an original model, usually presented in a conceptual map. In some cases the model incorporates elements or constructs from a theory, but the research is not a direct test of the theory.

**Example using an original conceptual framework:**
Chang and Mark (2011) studied whether a hospital's learning climate moderates the relationship between error-producing conditions in the hospital and medication errors. They developed an original framework based on theoretical writings by organizational learning researchers, and on studies of factors affecting patient safety. Their conceptual framework is shown in Figure 8.3.

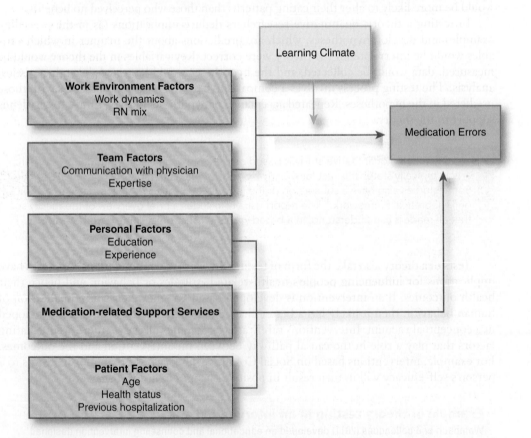

**FIGURE 8.3** ● Theoretical framework to explain medication errors. (From: Chang, Y., & Mark, B. (2011). Effects of learning climate and registered nurse staffing on medication errors. *Nursing Research, 60,* 32–39, Figure 1, with permission.)

# CRITIQUING FRAMEWORKS IN RESEARCH REPORTS

You will find references to theories and conceptual frameworks in some (but not all) of the studies you read. It is often challenging to critique the theoretical context of a published research report—or its absence—but we offer a few suggestions.

In a qualitative study in which a grounded theory is developed and presented, you may not be given enough information to refute the proposed theory because only evidence supporting the theory is presented. You can, however, assess whether the theory seems logical, whether conceptualizations are truly insightful, and whether the evidence is convincing. In a phenomenological study you should look to see if the researcher discusses the philosophical underpinnings of the study, that is, the philosophy of phenomenology.

Critiquing a theoretical framework in a quantitative report is also difficult, especially because you are not likely to be familiar with the theories and models that might be relevant. Some suggestions for evaluating the conceptual basis of a quantitative study are offered in the following discussion and in Box 8.1.

The first task is to determine whether the study does, in fact, have a conceptual framework. If there is no mention of a theory, model, or framework (and often there is not), you should consider whether this absence diminishes the value of the study. Research often benefits from an explicit conceptual context, but some studies are so pragmatic that the lack of a theory has no effect on its usefulness. For example, research designed to test the optimal frequency of turning patients has a utilitarian goal; a theory might not enhance the value of the findings. If, however, the study involves the test of a hypothesis or a complex intervention, the absence of a formal framework suggests conceptual fuzziness and perhaps interpretive problems.

If the study does have an explicit framework, you can examine its appropriateness. You may not be able to challenge the researcher's use of a particular theory or to recommend an

---

**BOX 8.1  Guidelines for Critiquing Theoretical and Conceptual Frameworks**

1. Does the report describe an explicit theoretical or conceptual framework for the study? If not, does the absence of a framework detract from the study's significance or its conceptual integration?
2. Does the report adequately describe the major features of the theory or model so that readers can understand the conceptual basis of the study?
3. Is the theory or model appropriate for the research problem? Does the purported link between the problem and the framework seem contrived?
4. Is the theory or model used as the basis for generating hypotheses, or is it used as an organizational or interpretive framework? Was this appropriate? Do the hypotheses (if any) naturally flow from the framework?
5. Are the concepts defined in a way that is consistent with the theory? If there is an intervention, are intervention components consistent with the theory?
6. Did the framework guide the study methods? For example, was the appropriate research tradition used if the study was qualitative? If quantitative, do the operational definitions correspond to the conceptual definitions?
7. Does the researcher tie the study findings back to the framework at the end of the report? Are the findings interpreted within the context of the framework?

alternative, but you can evaluate the logic of using a particular framework and assess whether the link between the problem and the theory is genuine. Does the researcher present a convincing rationale for the framework used? In quantitative studies, do the hypotheses flow from the theory? Will the findings contribute to theory validation? Does the researcher interpret the findings within the context of the framework? If the answer to such questions is no, you may have grounds for criticizing the study's framework, even though you may not be able to suggest ways to improve the conceptual basis of the study.

> **TIP:** Some studies claim theoretical linkages that are not justified. This is most likely to occur when researchers first formulate the research problem and then later find a theoretical context to fit it. An after-the-fact linkage of theory to a research question is usually problematic because the researcher will not have taken the nuances of the theory into consideration in designing the study. If a research problem is truly linked to a conceptual framework, then the design of the study, the measurement of key constructs, and the analysis and interpretation of data will *flow* from that conceptualization.

## RESEARCH EXAMPLES WITH CRITICAL THINKING EXERCISES

This section presents two examples of studies that have a strong theoretical link. Read the summaries and then answer the critical thinking questions, referring to the full research report if necessary.

Examples 1 and 2 below are also featured in our *Interactive Critical Thinking Activity* on thePoint website where you can easily record, print, and e-mail your responses to the related questions.

### EXAMPLE 1 ● The Health Promotion Model in a Quantitative Study

**Study:** "The effects of coping skills training (CST) among teens with asthma" (Srof et al., 2012)

**Statement of Purpose:** The purpose of the study was to evaluate the effects of a school-based intervention, CST, for teenagers with asthma.

**Theoretical Framework:** The HPM, shown in Figure 8.1 on page 134, was the guiding framework for the intervention. The authors noted that within the HPM, various behavior-specific cognitions (e.g., perceived barriers to behavior, perceived self-efficacy) influence health-promoting behavior *and* are modifiable through an intervention. In this study, the overall behavior of interest was asthma self-management. The CST Training intervention was a five-session small-group strategy designed to promote problem solving, cognitive–behavior modification, and conflict resolution using strategies to improve self-efficacy and reduce perceived barriers. The researchers hypothesized that participation in CST would result in improved outcomes: asthma self-efficacy, asthma-related quality of life, social support, and peak expiratory flow rate (PEFR).

**Method:** In this pilot study, 39 teenagers with asthma were randomly assigned to one of two groups—one that participated in the intervention, and the other that did not. The researchers collected data about the outcomes from all participants at two points in time, before the start of the intervention and 6 weeks later.

**Key Findings:** Teenagers in the treatment group scored significantly higher at the end of the study on self-efficacy, activity-related quality of life, and social support than those in the control group.

**Conclusions:** The researchers noted that the self-efficacy and social support effects of the intervention were consistent with the HPM model. They recommended that, although the findings were promising, replication of the study and an extension to specifically examine asthma self-management behavior would be useful.

*(continues on page 145)*

## CRITICAL THINKING EXERCISES

1. Answer the relevant questions from Box 8.1 on page 143 regarding this study.
2. Also consider the following targeted questions:
   a. In the model shown in Figure 8.1 on page 134, which factors did the researchers predict that the intervention would affect, according to the abbreviated description in the textbook?
   b. Is there another model or theory that was described in this chapter that could have been used to study the effect of this intervention?
3. If the results of this study are valid and generalizable, in what ways do you think the findings could be used in clinical practice?

## EXAMPLE 2 ● A Grounded Theory Study

**Study:** "Doing the best to control: The experiences of Taiwanese women with lower urinary tract symptoms (LUTS)" (Wang et al., 2011)

**Statement of Purpose:** The purpose of the study was to generate descriptive theory of the experiences in controlling urinary tract symptoms among Taiwanese women.

**Theoretical Framework:** A grounded theory approach was chosen because an explicit goal of the study was to develop a substantive theory based on the first-hand experiences of women with LUTS. Grounded theory methods enabled the researchers to explore the "multilayered and interconnected experiences of women living with LUTS" (p. 71).

**Method:** Data were collected through individual interviews with 16 Taiwanese women with LUTS. Women were recruited to participate through diverse social and medical connections. Each interview lasted between 40 and 90 minutes. The interviewer asked broad questions, such as "Would you talk about what urination symptoms you have now?" "What do you think causes your urination symptoms?" "How have these symptoms affected your life?" Interviewing continued until no new information was revealed—that is, until data saturation occurred. All interviews were audiotaped and transcribed for analysis.

**Key Findings:** Based on their analysis of the in-depth interviews, Wang and colleagues identified a core category to describe the process of women's finding unique ways to control urination problems: Doing the best to control. A schematic model for the substantive theory is shown in Figure 8.2 on page 140.

## CRITICAL THINKING EXERCISES

1. Answer the relevant questions from Box 8.1 on page 143 regarding this study.
2. Also consider the following targeted questions:
   a. In what way was the use of theory different in Wang et al.'s study than in the previous study by Srof and colleagues?
   b. Comment on the utility of the schematic model shown in Figure 8.2 on page 140.
3. If the results of this study are trustworthy, in what ways do you think the findings could be used in clinical practice?

## EXAMPLE 3 ● Quantitative Research in Appendix A

- Read the introduction of Howell and colleagues' (2007) study ("Anxiety, anger, and blood pressure in children") in Appendix A on page 395–402.

## CRITICAL THINKING EXERCISES

1. Answer relevant questions from Box 8.1 on page 143 regarding this study.
2. Also consider the following targeted questions:
   a. Develop a simple schematic model that captures the hypothesized relationships that were implied in this study.
   b. Would any of the theories or models described in this chapter have provided an appropriate conceptual context for this study?

## EXAMPLE 4 ● Qualitative Research in Appendix B

- Read the introduction of Beck and Watson's (2010) study ("Subsequent childbirth after a previous traumatic birth") in Appendix B on page 403–412.

### CRITICAL THINKING EXERCISES

1. Answer relevant questions from Box 8.1 on page 143 regarding this study.
2. Also consider the following targeted questions:
    a. Do you think that a schematic model would have helped to present the findings in this report?
    b. Did Beck and Watson present convincing evidence to support their use of the philosophy of phenomenology?

**WANT TO KNOW MORE?** A wide variety of resources to enhance your learning and understanding of this chapter are available on thePoint.

- Interactive Critical Thinking Activity
- Chapter Supplement on Prominent Conceptual Models of Nursing Used by Nurse Researchers
- Answers to the Critical Thinking Exercises for Examples 3 and 4
- Student Review Questions
- Full-text online
- Internet Resources with useful websites for Chapter 8

Additional study aids including eight journal articles and related questions are also available in *Study Guide for Essentials of Nursing Research, 8e.*

## SUMMARY POINTS

- High-quality research requires *conceptual integration*, one aspect of which is having a defensible theoretical rationale for the study. Researchers demonstrate conceptual clarity through the delineation of a theory, model, or framework on which the study is based.

- As classically defined, a **theory** is an abstract generalization that systematically explains relationships among phenomena. **Descriptive theory** thoroughly describes a phenomenon.

- *Grand theories* (or *macrotheories*) attempt to describe large segments of the human experience. **Middle-range theories** are specific to certain phenomena.

- Concepts are also the basic elements of **conceptual models**, but concepts are not linked in a logically ordered, deductive system.

- In research, the overall objective of theories and models is to make findings meaningful, to integrate knowledge into coherent systems, to stimulate new research, and to explain phenomena and relationships among them.

- **Schematic models** (or **conceptual maps**) are graphic representations of phenomena and their interrelationships using symbols or diagrams and a minimal use of words.

- A **framework** is the conceptual underpinning of a study, including an overall rationale and conceptual definitions of key concepts. In qualitative studies, the framework often springs from distinct research traditions.

(continues on page 147)

- Several conceptual models of nursing have been used in nursing research. The concepts central to models of nursing are *human beings, environment, health,* and *nursing.* An example of a model of nursing used by nurse researchers is Roy's Adaptation Model.

- Nonnursing models used by nurse researchers (e.g., Bandura's Social Cognitive Theory) are referred to as *borrowed theories;* when the appropriateness of borrowed theories for nursing inquiry is confirmed, the theories become *shared theories.*

- In some qualitative research traditions (e.g., phenomenology), the researcher strives to suspend previously held *substantive theories* of the specific phenomena under study, but each tradition has rich theoretical underpinnings.

- Some qualitative researchers seek to develop *grounded theories,* data-driven explanations to account for phenomena under study through inductive processes.

- In the classical use of theory, quantitative researchers test hypotheses deduced from an existing theory. An emerging trend is the testing of theory-based interventions.

- In both qualitative and quantitative studies, researchers sometimes use a theory or model as an organizing framework, or as an interpretive tool.

# REFERENCES FOR CHAPTER 8

Ajzen, I. (2005). *Attitudes, personality, and behavior.* (2nd ed.). Milton Keynes: Open University Press/McGraw Hill.

Bandura, A. (1985). *Social foundations of thought and action: A social cognitive theory.* Englewood Cliffs: Prentice Hall.

Bandura, A. (2001). Social cognitive theory: An agentic perspective. *Annual review of psychology, 52,* 1–26.

Beck, C. T. (2012).Exemplar: Teetering on the edge: A second grounded theory modification (pp. 257–284). In P. L. Munhall (Ed.). *Nursing research: A qualitative perspective* (5th ed).Sudbury: Jones & Bartlett Learning.

Becker, M. (1976). *Health Belief Model and personal health behavior.* Thorofare: Slack, Inc.

Ben Natan, M., & Gorkov, L. (2011). Investigating the factors affecting blood donation among Israelis. *International Emergency Nursing, 19,* 37–43.

Blumer, H. (1986). *Symbolic interactionism: Perspective and method.* Berkeley: University of California Press.

Chang, Y., & Mark, B. (2011). Effects of learning climate and registered nurse staffing on medication errors. *Nursing Research, 60,* 32–39.

Chen, M., Wang, R., Schneider, J., Tsai, C., Jiang, D., Hung, M., et al. (2011). Using the Health Belief Model to understand caregiver factors influencing childhood influenza vaccinations. *Journal of Community Health Nursing, 28,* 29–40.

Fawcett, J. (2005). *Contemporary nursing knowledge: Analysis and evaluation of nursing models and theories.* Philadelphia: F.A. Davis Company.

Fawcett, J., Aber, C., Haussler, S., Weiss, M., Myers, S., Hall, J., et al. (2011). Women's perceptions of caesarean birth: A Roy international study. *Nursing Science Quarterly, 24,* 352–362.

Fetterman, D. M. (2010). *Ethnography: Step by step.* (3rd ed.). Newbury Park: Sage.

Hodges, P. J. (2009). The essence of life purpose. *Critical Care Nursing Quarterly, 32,* 163–170.

Johnson, J. E. (1999). Self-Regulation Theory and coping with physical illness. *Research in Nursing & Health, 22,* 435–448.

Kolcaba, K. (2003). *Comfort theory and practice.* New York: Springer Publishing Co.

Lazarus, R. (2006). *Stress and emotion: A new synthesis.* New York: Springer Publishing.

Lazarus, R., & Folkman, S. (1984). *Stress, appraisal, and coping.* New York: Springer Publishing.

Lenz, E. R., Pugh, L. C., Milligan, R. A., Gift, A., & Suppe, F. (1997). The middle-range theory of unpleasant symptoms. *Advances in Nursing Science, 19,* 14–27.

Mishel, M. H. (1990). Reconceptualization of the uncertainty in illness theory. *Image: Journal of Nursing Scholarship, 22*(4), 256–262.

Mohamadian, H., Eftekhar, H., Rahimi, A., Mohamad, H., Shojaiezade, D., & Montazeri, A. (2011). Predicting health-related quality of life by using a health promotion model among Iranian adolescent girls. *Nursing & Health Sciences, 13,* 141–148.

Newman, M. (1997). Evolution of the theory of health as expanding consciousness. *Nursing Science Quarterly, 10,* 22–25.

Parse, R. R. (1999). *Illuminations: The human becoming theory in practice and research.* Sudbury: Jones & Bartlett.

Pender, N. J., Murdaugh, C., & Parsons, M. A. (2011). *Health promotion in nursing practice* (6th ed.). Upper Saddle River: Prentice Hall.

Plow, M., Finlayson, M., & Cho, C. (2011). Correlates of stages of change for physical activity in adults with multiple sclerosis. *Research in Nursing & Health, 34,* 378–388.

Poomsrikaew, O., Berger, B., Kim, M., & Zerwic, J. (2012). Age and gender differences in social cognitive factors and exercise behavior among Thais. *Western Journal of Nursing Research, 34*(2), 245–264.

Prochaska, J. O., Redding, C. A., & Evers, K. E. (2002). The Transtheoretical Model and stages of changes. In F.M. Lewis (Ed.). *Health behavior and health education: Theory, research and practice* (pp. 99–120). San Francisco: Jossey Bass.

Rogers, M. E. (1994). The science of unitary human beings: current perspectives. *Nursing Science Quarterly, 7,* 33–35.

Rosa, K. C. (2011). The process of healing transformations. *Journal of Holistic Nursing, 29,* 292–301.

Rosenstock, I., Stretcher, V., & Becker, M. (1988). Social learning theory and the Health Belief Model. *Health Education Quarterly, 15*, 175–183.

Roy, C., Sr., & Andrews, H. (1999). *The Roy Adaptation Model.* (2nd ed.). Norwalk: Appleton & Lange.

Sandelowski, M. (1993). Theory unmasked: The uses and guises of theory in qualitative research. *Research in Nursing & Health, 16*, 213–218.

Silva, M. C. (1986). Research testing nursing theory: State of the art. *Advances in Nursing Science, 9*, 1–11.

Srof, B., Velsor-Friedrich, B., & Penckofer, S. (2012). The effects of coping skills training among teens with asthma. *Western Journal of Nursing Research*, PubMed ID 21511980.

Stewart, J., Mishel, M., Lynn, M., & Terhorst, L. (2010). Test of a conceptual model of uncertainty in children and adolescents with cancer. *Research in Nursing & Health, 33*, 179–191.

Street, A., Couper, J., Love, A., Bloch, S., Kissane, D., & Street, B. (2010). Psychosocial adaptation in female partners of men with prostate cancer. *European Journal of Cancer Care, 19*, 234–242.

Thomas, E. A. (2011). Diabetes at work: A grounded theory pilot study. *AAOHN Journal, 59*, 213–220.

Walker, L., & Avant, K. (2010). *Strategies for theory construction in nursing* (5th ed.). Upper Saddle River: Prentice-Hall.

Wambach, K., Aronson, L., Breedlove, G., Domian, E., Roijanasrirat, W., & Yeh, H. (2011). A randomized controlled trial of breastfeeding support and education for adolescent mothers. *Western Journal of Nursing Research, 33*, 486–505.

Wang, Y., Chen, S., Jou, H., & Tsao, L. (2011). Doing the best to control: The experience of Taiwanese women with lower urinary tract symptoms. *Nursing Research, 60*, 66–72.

# part 3

# Quantitative Research

# 9 Quantitative Research Design

## LEARNING OBJECTIVES

*On completing this chapter, you will be able to:*

● Discuss key research design decisions for a quantitative study

● Discuss the concepts of causality and counterfactuals, and identify criteria for causal relationships

● Describe and evaluate experimental, quasi-experimental, and nonexperimental designs

● Distinguish between and evaluate cross-sectional and longitudinal designs

● Identify and evaluate alternative methods of controlling confounding variables

● Understand various threats to the validity of quantitative studies

● Evaluate a quantitative study in terms of its overall research design and methods of controlling confounding variables

● Define new terms in the chapter.

## KEY TERMS

Attrition
Baseline data
Case–control design
Cohort design
Control (comparison) group
Correlational study
Crossover design
Cross-sectional design
Counterfactual
Experiment
External validity
History threat

Homogeneity
Internal validity
Intervention fidelity
Longitudinal design
Matching
Maturation threat
Mortality threat
Nonequivalent control group design
Nonexperimental study
Posttest-only design
Pretest–posttest design

Prospective design
Quasi-experiment
Random assignment (randomization)
Randomized controlled trial (RCT)
Retrospective design
Selection threat (self-selection)
Time-series design

F or quantitative studies, no aspect of a study's methods has a bigger impact on the validity and accuracy of the results than the research design—particularly if the inquiry is *cause probing*. Thus, this chapter has important information about how you can draw appropriate conclusions about the worth of evidence in a quantitative study.

# OVERVIEW OF RESEARCH DESIGN ISSUES

The research design of a study spells out the strategies that researchers adopt to answer their questions and test their hypotheses. This section describes some basic design issues.

## Key Research Design Features

Table 9.1 describes seven key design features that are typically addressed in the design of a quantitative study. The design decisions that researchers must make include the following:

- *Will there be an intervention?* A basic design issue is whether or not researchers will actively introduce an intervention and test its effects—the distinction between experimental and nonexperimental research.
- *What types of comparisons will be made?* Quantitative researchers often make comparisons to provide a context for interpreting results. Sometimes the *same* people are compared under different conditions or at different points in time (e.g., preoperatively

**TABLE 9.1  Key Design Features**

| Feature | Key Questions | Design Options |
|---------|---------------|----------------|
| Intervention | Will there be an intervention? What specific design will be used? | Experimental (RCT), quasi-experimental, nonexperimental (observational) design |
| Comparisons | What type of comparisons will be made to illuminate key relationships? | Same participants (at different times or conditions); different participants |
| Control over confounding variables | How will confounding variables be controlled? Which confounding variables will be controlled? | Randomization, crossover, homogeneity, matching, statistical control |
| Blinding | From whom will critical information be withheld to avert bias? | Blinding participants, family members, interventionists, other staff, data collectors |
| Time frames | How often will data be collected? When, relative to other events, will data be collected? | Cross-sectional, longitudinal design |
| Relative timing | When will information on independent and dependent variables be collected—looking backward or forward? | Retrospective (case control), prospective (cohort) |
| Location | Where will the study take place? | Setting choice: single site versus multisite |

versus postoperatively), but often different people are compared (e.g., those getting versus not getting an intervention).

○ *How will confounding variables be controlled?* In quantitative research, efforts typically are made to control factors extraneous to the research question. This chapter discusses techniques for controlling confounding variables.

○ *Will blinding be used?* Researchers must decide if information about the study—e.g., who is getting an intervention—will be withheld from data collectors, study participants, or others to minimize the risk of *expectation bias* or *awareness bias*—i.e., the risk that such knowledge could influence study outcomes.

○ *How often will data be collected?* Data sometimes are collected from participants at a single point in time *(cross-sectionally)*, but other studies involve multiple points of data collection *(longitudinally)*.

○ *When will "effects" be measured, relative to potential causes?* Some studies collect information about outcomes and then look back *retrospectively* for potential causes. Other studies, however, begin with a potential cause and then see what outcomes ensue, in a *prospective* fashion.

○ *Where will the study take place?* Data for quantitative nursing studies are collected in various settings, such as in hospitals or people's homes. Another design decision concerns how many different sites will be involved in the study—a decision that could affect the generalizability of the results.

Many design decisions are independent of the others. For example, both experimental and nonexperimental studies can compare different people or the same people at different times. This chapter describes the implications of design decisions on the study's rigor.

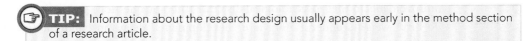

**TIP:** Information about the research design usually appears early in the method section of a research article.

## Causality

Many research questions—and questions for evidence-based practice (EBP)—are about *causes* and *effects*. For example, does turning patients cause reductions in pressure ulcers? Does exercise cause improvements in heart function? Causality is a hotly debated issue, but we all understand the general concept of a **cause**. For example, we understand that failure to sleep *causes* fatigue and that high caloric intake *causes* weight gain. Most phenomena are multiply determined. Weight gain, for example, can reflect high caloric intake *or* other factors. Most causes are not *deterministic*; they only increase the likelihood that an effect will occur. For example, smoking is a cause of lung cancer, but not everyone who smokes develops lung cancer, and not everyone with lung cancer smoked.

While it might be easy to grasp what researchers mean when they talk about a *cause*, what exactly is an **effect**? One way to understand an effect is by conceptualizing a counterfactual (Shadish et al., 2002). A **counterfactual** is what would happen to people if they were exposed to a causal influence and were simultaneously *not* exposed to it. An effect represents the difference between what actually did happen with the exposure and what would have happened without it. A counterfactual clearly can never be realized, but it is a good model to keep in mind in thinking about research design.

Three criteria for establishing causal relationships are attributed to John Stuart Mill.

1. *Temporal*: a cause must precede an effect in time. If we test the hypothesis that smoking causes lung cancer, we need to show that cancer occurred *after* the smoking behavior.
2. *Relationship*: there must be an association between the presumed cause and the effect. In our example, we have to demonstrate an association between smoking behavior and cancer—that is, that a higher percentage of smokers than nonsmokers get lung cancer.
3. *Confounders*: the relationship cannot be explained as being *caused by a third variable*. Suppose that smokers were especially likely to live in urban environments. There would then be a possibility that the relationship between smoking and lung cancer reflects an underlying causal connection between the environment and lung cancer.

Other criteria for causality have been proposed. One important criterion in health research is *biologic plausibility*—evidence from basic physiologic studies that a causal pathway is credible. Researchers investigating casual relationships must provide persuasive evidence regarding these criteria through their research design.

## Research Questions and Research Design

Quantitative research is used to address different types of research questions (Chapters 1 and 2), and different designs are appropriate for different questions. In this chapter, we focus primarily on designs for therapy, prognosis, etiology/harm, and description questions (meaning questions require a qualitative approach, and diagnosis questions are discussed in Chapter 11).

Except for description questions, questions that call for a quantitative approach usually concern causal relationships:

- Does a telephone counseling intervention for patients with prostate cancer *cause* improvements in their psychological distress? (therapy question)
- Do birth weights under 1,500 g *cause* developmental delays in children? (prognosis question)
- Does salt *cause* increases in blood pressure? (etiology/harm question)

Some designs are better at revealing cause-and-effect relationships than others. In particular, experimental designs (randomized controlled trials or RCTs) are the best possible designs for illuminating causal relationships—but it is not always possible to use such designs. Table 9.2 summarizes a "hierarchy" of designs for answering different types of causal questions and augments the evidence hierarchy presented in Figure 2.1 on page 23.

## TABLE 9.2 Hierarchy of Designs for Different Cause-Probing Research Questions

| Type of Question | Hierarchy of Designs |
|---|---|
| Therapy | RCT/Experimental > Quasi-experimental > Cohort > Case control > Descriptive correlational |
| Prognosis | Cohort > Case control > Descriptive correlational |
| Etiology/harm (prevention) | RCT/Experimental > Quasi-experimental > Cohort > Case control > Descriptive correlational |

# EXPERIMENTAL, QUASI-EXPERIMENTAL, AND NONEXPERIMENTAL DESIGNS

This section describes designs that differ with regard to whether or not there is an intervention.

## Experimental Design: Randomized Controlled Trials

Early physical scientists learned that complexities occurring in nature often made it difficult to understand relationships through pure observation. This problem was addressed by isolating phenomena and controlling the conditions under which they occurred. These experimental procedures have been profitably adopted by researchers interested in human physiology and behavior.

### Characteristics of True Experiments

A true experimental design or RCT is characterized by the following properties:

- *Intervention*—the experimenter *does* something to some participants by manipulating the independent variable.
- *Control*—the experimenter introduces controls into the study, including devising a good approximation of a counterfactual—usually a control group that does not receive the intervention.
- *Randomization*—the experimenter assigns participants to a control or experimental condition on a random basis.

By introducing an **intervention** or treatment, experimenters consciously vary (manipulate) the independent variable and then observe its effect on the outcome. To illustrate, suppose we were investigating the effect of physical exertion (I) on mood (O) in healthy young adults (P). One experimental design for this research problem is a **pretest–posttest design**, which involves observation of the outcome (mood) at two points in time: before and after the intervention. Participants in the experimental group undergo a physically demanding exercise routine, whereas those in the control group undergo a sedentary activity. This design permits us to examine what changes in mood were *caused* by the exertion because only some people were subjected to it, providing an important comparison. In this example, we met the first criterion of a true experiment by varying physical exertion, the independent variable.

This example also meets the second requirement for experiments, use of a control group. Inferences about causality require a comparison, but not all comparisons yield equally persuasive evidence. For example, if we were to supplement the diet of premature babies (P) with special nutrients (I) for 2 weeks, their weight (O) at the end of 2 weeks would tell us nothing about the intervention's effectiveness. At a minimum, we would need to compare their posttreatment weight with their pretreatment weight to determine whether their weights had increased. But suppose we find an average weight gain of one pound. Does this finding support an inference of a causal connection between the nutritional intervention (the independent variable) and weight gain (the outcome)? No, because infants normally gain weight as they mature. Without a control group—a group that does not receive the supplements (C)—it is impossible to separate the effects of maturation from those of the treatment. The term **control group** refers to a group of participants whose performance on an outcome variable is used to evaluate the performance of the **experimental group** (the group getting the intervention) on the same outcome. A control group used for comparative purposes represents a proxy for the ideal counterfactual.

Experimental designs also involve placing participants in groups at random. Through **randomization** (or *random assignment*), every participant has an equal chance of being included in any group. If people are randomly assigned, there is no systematic bias in the groups with regard to attributes that may affect the dependent variable. *Randomly assigned groups are expected to be comparable, on average, with respect to an infinite number of biologic, psychological, and social traits at the outset of the study.* Group differences on outcomes observed *after* randomization can therefore be inferred as being caused by the treatment.

Random assignment can be accomplished by flipping a coin or pulling names from a hat. Researchers typically either use computers to perform the randomization or rely on a *table of random numbers*, a table displaying hundreds of digits arranged in random order.

> **TIP:** There is a lot of confusion about random assignment versus random sampling. Random assignment is a *signature* of an experimental design (RCT). If subjects are not randomly assigned to intervention groups, then the design is not a true experiment. Random *sampling*, by contrast, refers to a method of selecting people for a study, as we discuss in Chapter 10. Random sampling is *not* a signature of an experimental design. In fact, most RCTs do *not* involve random sampling.

## Experimental Designs

The most basic experimental design involves randomizing people to different groups and then measuring the outcome. This design is sometimes called a **posttest-only design**. A more widely used design, discussed previously, is the pretest–posttest design, which involves collecting *pretest data* (also called **baseline data**) on the outcome before the intervention and **posttest** (outcome) **data** after it.

> **Example of a pretest–posttest design:**
> Carter and colleagues (2012) evaluated the effectiveness of a brief postanesthesia care unit (PACU) visit on reducing family members' anxiety. Participants were randomly assigned to a PACU visit or usual care. The family members' anxiety was measured before and after the visit, and changes in anxiety levels were used as the outcome variable.

> **TIP:** Experimental designs can be depicted graphically using symbols to represent features of the design. In these diagrams, the convention is that R stands for randomization to treatment groups, X represents receipt of the intervention, and O is the measurement of outcomes. So, for example, a pretest–posttest design would be depicted as follows:
>
> $$R\ O_1\ X\ O_2$$
> $$R\ O_1\ \ \ O_2$$
>
> Space does not permit us to present these diagrams for all designs, but many are shown in the Chapter Supplement on thePoint website.

In a standard design, the people who are randomly assigned to different conditions are different people. For example, if we were testing the effect of music on agitation (O) on patients with dementia (P), we could give some patients music (I) and others no music (C). A **crossover design**, by contrast, involves exposing people to more than one treatment. Such studies are true experiments only if people are randomly assigned to different orderings of treatment. For example, if a crossover design were used to compare the effects of music on patients with dementia, some would be randomly assigned to receive music first followed by a period of no music, and others would receive no music first. In such a study, the three conditions for an experiment have been met: there is intervention, randomization, and control—with *subjects serving as their own control group*.

A crossover design has the advantage of ensuring the highest possible equivalence among the people exposed to different conditions. Such designs are inappropriate for certain research questions, however, because of possible *carryover effects*. When subjects are exposed to two different treatments, they may be influenced in the second condition by their experience in the first. However, when carryover effects are implausible, as when intervention effects are immediate and short-lived, a crossover design is extremely powerful.

**Example of a crossover design:**

Liaw and colleagues (2012) used a crossover design to test alternative methods of alleviating infant pain during heel-stick procedures. Infants were randomly assigned to a sequence of three treatments (nonnutritive sucking, facilitated tucking, and a control condition).

👉 **TIP:** Research reports do not always identify the specific experimental design that was used by name; this may have to be inferred from information about the data collection plan (in the case of posttest-only and pretest–posttest designs), or from such statements as: The subjects were used as their own controls (in the case of a crossover design).

## Experimental and Control Conditions

In designing experiments, researchers make many decisions about what the experimental and control conditions entail, and these decisions can affect the results. To give a new intervention a fair test, researchers need to design one that is of sufficient intensity and duration that effects on the outcome might reasonably be expected. Researchers describe the intervention in formal *protocols* that stipulate exactly what the treatment is for those in the experimental group.

The control group condition (the counterfactual) must also be carefully conceptualized. Researchers have choices about what to use as the control condition, and the decision affects the interpretation of the findings. Among the possibilities for the control condition are the following:

- No intervention—the control group gets no treatment at all
- "Usual care"—standard or normal procedures used to treat patients
- An alternative treatment (e.g., music versus massage)
- A **placebo** or pseudointervention presumed to have no therapeutic value, which is also called an *attention control condition* (the control group gets attention but not the intervention's active ingredients)
- A lower dose or intensity of treatment, or only parts of the treatment
- *Delayed treatment*, i.e., control group members are *wait-listed* and exposed to the experimental treatment at a later point

**Example of a wait-listed control group:**

White (2012) tested the effectiveness of an 8-week mindful yoga intervention for reducing stress and enhancing self-esteem in school-aged girls. Girls in the fourth and fifth grade were randomly assigned to the intervention group or a wait-listed control group.

From a methodologic standpoint, the best test is between two conditions that are as different as possible, as when the experimental group gets a strong intervention and the control group gets nothing. Ethically, however, the most appealing option is often the "delay of treatment" design, which is not always feasible. Testing two alternative interventions is also appealing ethically, but the risk is that the results will be inconclusive because it may be difficult to detect differential effects.

Researchers must also consider possibilities for *blinding*. Many nursing interventions do not lend themselves easily to blinding. For example, if the intervention were a smoking cessation program, participants would know whether they were receiving the intervention, and the intervener would know who was in the program. It is usually possible and desirable, however, to blind the participants' group status from the people collecting outcome data.

**Example of an experiment with blinding:**

Kassab and colleagues (2012) tested the efficacy of 25% oral glucose for pain relief in infants undergoing immunizations. Infants were randomized to receive either the glucose solution or sterile water. Researchers, nurses, parents, and infants were blinded with regard to which solution the infants received.

☞ **TIP:** The term *double blind* is widely used when more than one group is blinded (e.g., participants and interventionists). However, this term is falling into disfavor because of its ambiguity, in favor of clear specifications about exactly who was blinded and who was not.

## Advantages and Disadvantages of Experiments

RCTs are the most powerful designs for testing hypotheses of cause-and-effect relationships. RCTs are the "gold standard" for intervention studies (therapy questions) because they yield the highest-quality evidence about the effects of an intervention. Through randomization to groups, researchers come as close as possible to attaining an "ideal" counterfactual. Experiments offer greater corroboration than other designs that, *if* the independent variable (e.g., diet, drug dosage, counseling) is varied, *then* certain consequences in the outcome variable (e.g., weight loss, recovery of health, coping) may be expected to ensue.

The great strength of experiments, then, lies in the confidence with which causal relationships can be inferred. Through the controls imposed by intervening, comparing, and—especially—randomizing, alternative explanations to causal connections can often be ruled out. It is because of these strengths that meta-analyses of RCTs, which integrate evidence from multiple studies that used an experimental design, are at the pinnacle of evidence hierarchies for questions relating to causes (Figure 2.1, p. 23).

Despite the advantages of experiments, they have some limitations. First, a number of interesting variables simply are not amenable to intervention. A large number of human characteristics, such as disease or health habits, cannot be randomly conferred on people. That is why RCTs are not at the top of the hierarchy for prognosis questions (Table 9.2, p. 152), which concern the long-term consequences of health problems. For example, infants could not be randomly assigned to having cystic fibrosis to see if this disease causes poor psychosocial adjustment.

Second, there are many variables that could technically—but not ethically—be experimentally varied. For example, there have been no RCTs to study the effect of cigarette smoking on lung cancer. Such a study would require us to assign people randomly to a smoking group (people forced to smoke) or a nonsmoking group (people prohibited from smoking). Experimentation with humans will always be subject to such ethical constraints. Thus, although RCTs are technically at the top of the evidence hierarchy for etiology/harm questions (Table 9.2, p. 152), many etiology questions cannot be answered using an experimental design.

In many health care settings, RCTs may not be feasible even for therapy questions because of practical issues. It may, for instance, be impossible to secure the cooperation from administrators or other stakeholders to randomize people to groups.

Another potential problem is the *Hawthorne effect*, a term derived from experiments conducted at the Hawthorne plant of the Western Electric Corporation in which various environmental conditions (e.g., light, working hours) were varied to determine their effect on worker productivity. Regardless of what change was made (i.e., whether the light was made better or worse), productivity increased. Thus, knowledge of being in a study may cause people to change their behavior, thereby obscuring the effect of the research variables. In summary, experimental designs have some limitations that make them difficult to apply to real-world problems; nevertheless, RCTs have a clear superiority for testing causal hypotheses.

 **HOW-TO-TELL TIP:** How can you tell if a study is experimental? Researchers usually indicate in the method section of their reports that they have used an experimental or randomized design (RCT). If such terms are missing, you can conclude that a study is experimental if the article says that the study purpose was to *test or evaluate the effects of* an intervention or treatment, AND if individual participants were put into groups (or exposed to different conditions) at random.

## Quasi-Experiments

**Quasi-experiments** (called *trials without randomization* in the medical literature), also involve an intervention; however, quasi-experimental designs lack randomization, the signature of a true experiment. Some quasi-experiments even lack a control group. The signature of a quasi-experimental design, then, is an intervention in the absence of randomization.

### Quasi-Experimental Designs

A frequently used quasi-experimental design is the **nonequivalent control group pretest–posttest design**, which involves comparing two or more groups of people before and after implementing an intervention. As an example, suppose we were studying the effect of introducing a new hospital-wide model of care that involved having a patient care facilitator (PCF) be the primary point person for hospitalized patients (P) during their stay. Our main outcome is patient satisfaction (O). The new system is being implemented throughout the hospital, and so randomization to PCF (I) versus "usual care" (C) is not possible. We opt to collect data in a similar hospital that is not instituting the PCF model. Data on patient satisfaction is collected in both hospitals before the change is made (baseline) and again afterwards.

This quasi-experimental design is identical to the pretest–posttest experimental design discussed in the previous section, *except* participants were not randomized to groups. The quasi-experimental design is weaker because, without randomization, *it cannot be assumed that the experimental and comparison groups are equivalent at the outset.* Quasi-experimental comparisons are much farther from an ideal counterfactual than experimental comparisons. The design is, nevertheless, a strong one because the collection of baseline data allows us to see whether patients in the two hospitals had similar levels of satisfaction before the change was made. If the groups are comparable at baseline, we could be relatively confident inferring that posttest differences in satisfaction was the result of the new model of care. If patient satisfaction is different initially, however, it will be difficult to interpret postintervention differences. Note that in quasi-experiments, the term *comparison group* is sometimes used in lieu of *control group* to refer to the group against which outcomes in the treatment group are evaluated.

Now suppose we had been unable to collect baseline data. Such a design (*nonequivalent control group posttest-only*) has a flaw that is difficult to remedy. We no longer have information about the initial equivalence of the hospitals. If patient satisfaction in the experimental hospital is higher than that in the control hospital at the posttest, can we conclude that the new method of delivering care *caused* improved satisfaction? There could be other explanations for the differences. In particular, patient satisfaction in the two hospitals might have differed initially. Quasi-experiments lack some of the controlling properties of experiments, but the hallmark of strong quasi-experiments is the effort to introduce some controls, such as baseline measurements.

> ### Example of a nonequivalent control group design:
> Aitken, Burmeister, Clayton, Dalais, and Gardner (2011) used a nonequivalent control group pretest–posttest design to test the effect of launching clinical nursing rounds in intensive care units on nurses' satisfaction and perceived work environments. Nurses in the hospital that introduced nursing rounds were compared to nurses in a hospital that was similar in workload and staffing characteristics.

In the designs just described, a control group was used but randomization was not, but some quasi-experiments have neither. Suppose that a hospital implemented rapid response teams (RRTs) in its acute care units. We want to learn the effects on patient outcomes (e.g., mortality) and nurse outcomes (e.g., stress). For the purposes of this example, assume no other hospital would be a good comparison, and so the only comparison that can be made is a before–after contrast. If RRTs were implemented in January, we could compare the mortality rate, for example, during the 3 months before RRTs with the mortality rate in the subsequent 3-month period.

This **one-group pretest–posttest design** seems logical, but it has weaknesses. What if one of the 3-month periods is atypical, apart from the RRTs? What about the effect of other changes instituted during the same period? What about the effects of external factors, such as seasonal migration? The design in question offers no way of controlling these factors.

In this example, the design could be modified so that at least some alternative explanations for changes in mortality could be ruled out. For example, the **time-series design** involves collecting data over an extended time period, and introducing the treatment during that period. The present study could be designed with four observations before the RRTs are introduced (e.g., four quarters of mortality data for the prior year) and four observations after it (mortality for the next four quarters). Although a time-series design does not eliminate all the problems of interpreting changes in mortality, the extended time perspective strengthens the ability to attribute change to the intervention.

> ### Example of a time-series design:
> Polit and Chaboyer (2012) described a study that used a time-series design. Patient safety data were collected over a 33 month period, and a nursing practice improvement intervention was introduced in the 15th month. Patient harms decreased substantially after the introduction of the intervention.

## Advantages and Disadvantages of Quasi-Experiments

It is not always possible to conduct RCTs, and so a strength of quasi-experiments is that they may be practical. Nursing research often occurs in natural settings, where it is difficult to deliver an innovative treatment randomly to some people but not to others. Strong quasi-experimental designs introduce some research control when full experimental rigor is not possible.

Another issue is that people are not always willing to be randomized in clinical trials. Quasi-experimental designs, because they do not involve random assignment, are likely to be acceptable to a broader group of people. This, in turn, has implications for the generalizability of the results—but the problem is that the results are usually less conclusive.

The major disadvantage of quasi-experiments is that causal inferences cannot be made as readily as with RCTs. Alternative explanations for results abound with quasi-experiments. For example, suppose we administered a special diet to a group of frail nursing home residents to assess its impact on weight gain. If we use a nonequivalent control group and then observe a weight gain, we must ask: Is it *plausible* that some other factor caused the gain? Is it *plausible* that pretreatment differences between the intervention and comparison groups resulted in differential gain? Is it *plausible* that there was an average weight gain simply because the most frail died or were transferred to a hospital? If the answer to any of these *rival hypotheses* is yes, then the inferences about the causal effect of the intervention are weakened. With quasi-experiments, there is almost always at least one plausible rival explanation.

 **HOW-TO-TELL TIP:** How can you tell if a study is quasi-experimental? Researchers do not always identify their designs as quasi-experimental. If a study involves an intervention and if the report does not explicitly mention random assignment, it is probably safe to conclude that the design is quasi-experimental.

## Nonexperimental Studies

Many research questions—including cause-probing ones—cannot be addressed with an RCT or quasi-experimental design. For example, take this prognosis question: Do birth weights under 1,500 g *cause* developmental delays in children? Clearly, we cannot manipulate birth weight, the independent variable. Babies' weights are not subject to research control, nor are they random. When researchers do not intervene by controlling the independent variable, the study is **nonexperimental**, or, in the medical literature, **observational**.

There are various reasons for doing a nonexperimental study, including situations in which the independent variable inherently cannot be manipulated (prognosis questions) or in which it would be unethical to manipulate the independent variable (some etiology questions). Experimental designs are also not appropriate for descriptive questions.

### Types of Nonexperimental/Observational Studies

When researchers study the effect of a *cause* they cannot manipulate, they design **correlational studies** that examine relationships between variables. A **correlation** is an interrelationship or association between two variables, that is, a tendency for variation in one variable to be related to variation in another (e.g., people's height and weight). Correlations can be detected through statistical analyses.

As noted earlier, one criterion for causality is the existence of a relationship between variables, but it is risky to infer causal relationships in correlational research. In RCTs, investigators predict that deliberate variation of the independent variable will result in a change to the outcome variable. In correlational research, investigators do not control the independent variable, which often has already occurred. A famous research dictum is relevant: *correlation does not prove causation.* The mere existence of a relationship between variables is not enough to warrant the conclusion that one variable caused the other, even if the relationship is strong.

Correlational studies are weaker than RCTs for addressing cause-probing questions, but different designs offer varying degrees of supportive evidence. The strongest design for prognosis questions, and for etiology questions when randomization is impossible, is a cohort design (Table 9.2, p. 152). Observational studies with a **cohort design** (sometimes called a **prospective design**) start with a presumed cause and then go forward to the presumed effect. For example, in prospective lung cancer studies, researchers start with a cohort of adults (P) that includes smokers (I) and nonsmokers (C), and then later compare the two groups in terms of lung cancer incidence (O).

> **Example of a cohort (prospective) design:**
> Salamonson, Everett, Koch, Andrew, and Davidson (2012) studied the relationship between part-time employment among nursing students and their academic performance. Hours of paid work were measured in their first year of education, and academic performance was measured in their final year.

> ☞ **TIP:** All experimental studies are inherently prospective, because the researcher institutes the intervention (manipulates the independent variable) and subsequently examines its effect.

In **retrospective** correlational studies, an effect (outcome) observed in the present is linked to a potential cause occurring in the past. For example, in retrospective lung cancer research, researchers begin with some people who have lung cancer and others who do not, and then look for differences in antecedent behaviors or conditions, such as smoking habits. Such a retrospective study uses a **case–control design**—that is, *cases* with a certain condition, such as lung cancer, are compared to *controls* without it. In designing a case–control study, researchers try to identify controls who are as similar as possible to cases with regard to key confounding variables (e.g., age, gender). To the degree that researchers can demonstrate comparability between cases and controls with regard to confounding traits, causal inferences are enhanced. The difficulty, however, is that the two groups are almost never comparable with respect to *all* potential factors influencing the outcome.

> **Example of a case-control design:**
> Cora, Particino, Munafo, and Palomba (2012) conducted a pilot study of health risks among the family caregivers of terminally ill cancer patients. Their sample included 20 caregivers of terminally ill family members, and 20 noncaregivers who were matched to the cases by age and gender. The two groups were compared in terms of cardiovascular risk and emotional distress.

Prospective studies are more costly, but much stronger, than retrospective studies. For one thing, any ambiguity about the temporal sequence of phenomena is resolved in prospective research (i.e., smoking is known to precede the lung cancer). In addition, samples are more likely to be representative of smokers and nonsmokers.

A second broad class of nonexperimental studies is **descriptive research**. The purpose of descriptive studies is to observe, describe, and document aspects of a situation. For example, an investigator may wish to determine the percentage of teenagers who engage in risky behavior (e.g., drug use, unsafe sex)—i.e., the *prevalence* of such behaviors. Or sometimes a study design is **descriptive correlational**, meaning that researchers seek to describe relationships among variables, without attempting to infer causal connections. For example, researchers might be interested in describing the relationship between fatigue and psychological distress in patients with HIV. Because the intent in these situations is not to explain or to understand the underlying causes of the variables of interest, a descriptive nonexperimental design is appropriate.

**Example of a descriptive correlational study:**
Liou and colleagues (2012) conducted a descriptive correlational study with a sample of more than 15,000 Taiwanese adolescents to examine factors that correlated with self-induced vomiting as a weight-control strategy.

**TIP:** For descriptive questions, the strongest design is a nonexperimental study that relies on random sampling of participants. Sampling plans are discussed in the next chapter.

## Advantages and Disadvantages of Nonexperimental Research

The major disadvantage of nonexperimental studies is that they do not yield persuasive evidence for causal inferences. This is not a problem when the aim is description, but correlational studies are often undertaken with an underlying desire to discover causes. Yet correlational studies are susceptible to faulty interpretation because groups being compared have formed through **self-selection** (also called *selection bias*). A researcher doing a correlational study, unlike an RCT, cannot assume that the groups being compared were similar before the occurrence of the independent variable—the hypothesized cause or "I." Preexisting group differences may be a plausible alternative to the "I" as an explanation for any differences in "O" (outcomes).

As an example of such interpretive problems, suppose we studied differences in depression (O) of cancer patients (P) who do or do not have adequate social support (I). Suppose we found a correlation—that is, we found that patients without social support were more depressed than patients with adequate social support. We could interpret this to mean that people's emotional state is influenced by the adequacy of their social support, as diagrammed in Figure 9.1A. There are, however, alternative interpretations for the finding. Maybe a third variable influences *both* social support and depression, such as whether the patients are married. Having a spouse may affect how depressed the patients feel *and* the quality of their social support, as diagrammed in Figure 9.1B. A third possibility is reversed causality (Figure 9.1C). Depressed cancer patients may find it more difficult to elicit social support

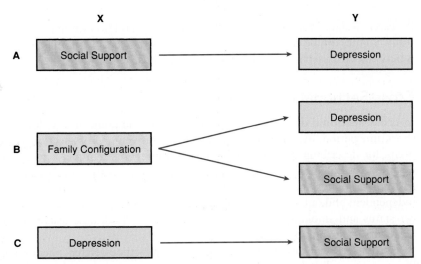

**FIGURE 9.1** ● Alternative explanations for correlation between depression and social support in cancer patients.

than patients who are more cheerful. In this interpretation, the person's depression causes the amount of received social support, and not the other way around. The point is that correlational results should be interpreted cautiously.

> ☞ **TIP:** Be prepared to think critically when a researcher claims to be studying the "effects" of one variable on another in a nonexperimental study. For example, if a report title were "The Effects of Eating Disorders on Depression," the study would be nonexperimental (i.e., participants were not randomly assigned to an eating disorder). In such a situation, you might ask, Did the eating disorder have an effect on depression—or did depression have an effect on eating patterns? Or, did a third variable (e.g., childhood abuse) have an effect on both?

Despite interpretive problems, nonexperimental studies play a crucial role in nursing because many interesting problems do not lend themselves to randomization or intervention. An example is whether smoking causes lung cancer. Despite the absence of any RCTs with humans, few people doubt that this causal connection exists. Thinking about the criteria for causality discussed earlier, there is ample evidence of a relationship between smoking and lung cancer and, through prospective studies, that smoking precedes lung cancer. Through numerous replications, researchers have been able to control for, and thus rule out, other possible "causes" of lung cancer. The findings have been consistent and coherent, and the criterion of biologic plausibility has been met through basic physiologic research.

Correlational research is often an efficient way to collect large amounts of data about a problem. For example, it would be possible to collect extensive information about people's health problems and eating habits. Researchers could then examine which problems correlate with which eating patterns. By doing this, many relationships could be discovered in a short time. By contrast, an experimenter looks at only a few variables at a time. For example, one RCT might manipulate cholesterol, whereas another might manipulate protein. Nonexperimental work is often necessary before interventions can be justified.

# THE TIME DIMENSION IN RESEARCH DESIGN

Research designs incorporate decisions about when and how often data will be collected in a study. Studies can be categorized in terms of how they deal with time. The major distinction is between cross-sectional and longitudinal designs.

## Cross-Sectional Designs

In **cross-sectional designs**, data are collected at one point in time (or multiple times in a short time period, such as 1 and 2 hours postoperatively). Cross-sectional designs are appropriate for describing phenomena at a fixed point. For example, a researcher might study whether psychological symptoms in menopausal women are correlated contemporaneously with physiologic symptoms. Retrospective studies are usually cross-sectional: data on the independent and outcome variables are collected concurrently (e.g., participants' lung cancer status and smoking habits), but the independent variable usually concerns events or behaviors occurring in the past.

Cross-sectional designs can be used to study time-related phenomena, but they are less persuasive than longitudinal designs. Suppose we were studying changes in children's health-promotion activities between ages 7 and 10. One way to investigate this would be to interview children at age 7 and then 3 years later at age 10—a longitudinal design. Or, we could question two groups of children, ages 7 and 10, at one point in time and then compare responses—a cross-sectional design. If 10-year-olds engaged in more health-promoting activities than 7-year-olds, it might be inferred that children made healthier choices as they aged. To make this inference, we have to assume that the older children would have responded as the younger ones did had they been questioned 3 years earlier, or, conversely, that 7-year-olds would report more health- promoting activities if they were questioned again 3 years later.

Cross-sectional designs are economical and easy to manage, but they pose problems for inferring changes over time. The amount of social and technological change that characterizes our society makes it questionable to assume that differences in the behaviors or characteristics of different age groups are the result of the passage through time rather than cohort differences. In the previous example, 7- and 10-year-old children may have different attitudes toward health and health promotion, independent of maturation. In such cross-sectional studies, there are often alternative explanations for observed group differences.

**Example of a cross-sectional study:**
Belanger, and colleagues (2012) examined the relationship between age on the one hand and physical activity preferences on the other in a cross-sectional study of 588 young adult cancer survivors, who were grouped into three age group clusters: 20 to 29, 30 to 39, and 40 to 44.

## Longitudinal Designs

**Longitudinal designs** involve collecting data multiple times over an extended period. Such designs are useful for studying changes over time and for establishing the sequencing of phenomena, which is a criterion for establishing causality. Multiple data collection points can also strengthen causal inferences, such as in a nonequivalent control group design in which collecting pretreatment data offers evidence about the initial comparability of groups.

Longitudinal studies can focus on general, nonclinical populations. For example, the well-known Harvard Nurses' Health Study has followed a sample of thousands of nurses for over 30 years. In nursing research, longitudinal studies are more likely to be *follow-up studies* of a clinical population, undertaken to assess the subsequent status of people with a specified condition or who received a specified intervention. For example, patients who received a smoking cessation intervention could be followed up to assess its long-term effectiveness. To take a nonexperimental example, samples of premature infants might be followed up to assess their subsequent motor development.

**Example of a follow-up study:**
McCullough and colleagues (2012) did a follow-up study of children with cerebral palsy 2½ years after an initial assessment to examine patterns of health and health behaviors.

In longitudinal studies, the number of data collection points and the time intervals between them depend on the nature of the study. When change or development is rapid, numerous data collection points at relatively short intervals may be required to understand trends. By convention, however, the term *longitudinal* implies multiple data collection points over an extended period of time.

A serious challenge in longitudinal studies is the loss of participants (**attrition**) over time. Attrition is problematic because those who drop out of the study usually differ in important respects from those who continue to participate, resulting in potential biases, the risk of faulty inferences, and concerns about the generalizability of the findings.

> ☞ **TIP:** Not all longitudinal studies are prospective, because sometimes the independent variable occurred even before the initial wave of data collection. And not all prospective studies are longitudinal in the classic sense. For example, an experimental study that collects data at 2, 4, and 6 hours after an intervention would be prospective but not longitudinal (i.e., data are not collected over a long time period.)

# TECHNIQUES OF RESEARCH CONTROL

A major goal of research design in quantitative studies is to maximize researchers' control over potentially confounding variables. There are two broad categories of confounders that need to be controlled—those that are intrinsic to study participants and those that are external, stemming from the research situation.

## Controlling the Study Context

Various external factors, such as the research environment, can affect outcomes. In carefully controlled quantitative research, steps are taken to minimize situational contaminants (i.e., to achieve *constancy of conditions*) so that researchers can be confident that outcomes reflect the influence of the independent variable and not the study context.

Researchers cannot totally control the context in natural settings, but many opportunities exist. For example, researchers can control *when* data are collected. If an investigator were studying fatigue, for example, all data should be collected at the same time of day. Blinding is another means of controlling external sources of bias. By keeping data collectors and others unaware of group allocation or study hypotheses, researchers minimize the risk that other people involved in the study will influence the results.

Most quantitative studies also standardize communications to participants. Formal scripts are often prepared to inform participants about the study purpose, the use that will be made of the data, and so forth. In research involving interventions, researchers develop formal intervention protocols that specify procedures. For example, in an experiment to test the effectiveness of a new medication, care would be needed to ensure that the participants in the intervention group received the same chemical substance and the same dosage, that the substance was administered in the same way, and so forth. Careful researchers pay attention to in *intervention fidelity*—that is, they take steps to monitor that an intervention is faithfully delivered in accordance with its plan and that the intended treatment was actually received. Intervention fidelity helps to avert biases and gives potential benefits a full opportunity to be realized.

> **Example of attention to intervention fidelity:**
> Robbins, Pfeiffer, Maier, Ladrig, and Berg-Smith (2012) described their efforts to monitor and enhance intervention fidelity in implementing a motivational interviewing intervention by school nurses to increase physical activity among middle school girls.

## Controlling Participant Factors

Control of study participants' characteristics is especially important and challenging. Outcomes in which nurse researchers are interested are affected by dozens of influences and attributes, and most are irrelevant to the research question. For example, suppose we were investigating the effects of a new physical fitness program on the cardiovascular functioning of nursing home residents. In this study, variables such as the participants' age, gender, and smoking history would be confounding variables; each is likely to be related to the outcome variable (cardiovascular functioning), independent of the physical fitness program. In other words, the effects that these variables have on the outcome are extraneous to the study. In this section, we review methods of controlling confounding subject characteristics.

## Randomization

Randomization is the most effective method of controlling participants' characteristics. Randomization yields a close approximation to an ideal counterfactual, that is, groups that are equal with respect to confounding variables. A critical advantage of randomization, compared with other methods of control, is that it controls *all* possible sources of extraneous variation, without any conscious decision about which variables need to be controlled. In our example of a physical fitness intervention, random assignment of elders to an intervention or control group would yield groups presumably comparable in terms of age, gender, smoking history, and hundreds of other characteristics that could affect the outcome. Randomization to different treatment orderings in a crossover design is especially powerful: participants serve as their own controls, thereby totally controlling all confounding characteristics.

## Homogeneity

When randomization is not feasible, other methods of controlling extraneous subject characteristics and achieving a counterfactual approximation can be used. One alternative is **homogeneity**, in which only people who are similar with respect to confounding variables are included in the study. Confounding variables, in this case, are not allowed to vary. In the physical fitness example, if gender were a confounding variable, we could recruit only men (or women) as participants. If age was considered a confounding influence, participation could be limited to those within a specified age range. Using a homogeneous sample is easy, but one problem is limited generalizability. Indeed, one problem with this approach is that researchers may exclude people who are extremely ill or incapacitated, which means that the findings cannot be generalized to the very people who perhaps are most in need of interventions.

> **Example of control through homogeneity:**
> Ngai, Chan, and Ip (2010) studied factors that predicted maternal role competence and satisfaction among mothers in Hong Kong. Several variables were controlled through homogeneity, including ethnicity (all were Chinese), parity (all primiparous), and marital status (all were married).

## Matching

A third method of controlling confounding variables is **matching**, which involves consciously forming comparable groups. For example, suppose we began with a group of nursing home residents who agreed to participate in the physical fitness program. A comparison group of nonparticipating residents could be created by matching participants, one by one, on the basis of important confounding variables (e.g., age and gender). This procedure results in groups known to be similar in terms of specific confounding variables. Matching is the technique often used to form comparable groups in case control designs.

Matching has some drawbacks, however. To match effectively, researchers must know in advance what the relevant confounders are. Also, after two or three variables, it becomes difficult to match. Suppose we wanted to control age, gender, race, and length of nursing home stay. In this situation, if a program participant were an African American woman, aged

80 years, whose length of stay was 5 years, we would have to seek another woman with these same characteristics as a comparison group counterpart. With more than three variables, matching becomes difficult. Thus, matching as a control method is usually used only when more powerful procedures are not feasible.

> **Example of control through matching:**
> Yin, Ma, Feng, and Wang (2012) compared levels of anxiety and depression among patients undergoing two types of surgery for congenital heart defects: thoracoscopic closure of defects versus conventional open heart surgery. The two groups were matched by age and sex.

### Statistical Control

Researchers can also control confounding variables statistically. You may be unfamiliar at this point with basic statistical procedures, let alone sophisticated techniques such as those referred to here. Therefore, a detailed description of powerful statistical control mechanisms, such as *analysis of covariance*, will not be attempted. You should recognize, however, that nurse researchers are increasingly using powerful statistical techniques to control confounding variables. A brief description of methods of statistical control is presented in Chapter 12.

> **Example of statistical control:**
> Grav, Hellzen, Romild, and Stordal (2012) studied the association between social support (both emotional and tangible) and depression in a general adult population in Norway. Both types of support were significantly correlated with depression, even after statistically controlling for age and gender—that is, the effect of support on depression was not because of male–female or age differences in support.

### Evaluation of Control Methods

Random assignment is the most effective approach to controlling confounding variables because randomization tends to control individual variation on all possible confounders. Crossover designs are especially powerful, but they cannot be used in many situations because of the possibility of carryover effects. The alternatives described here share two disadvantages. First, researchers must decide in advance which variables to control. To select homogeneous samples, match, or use statistical controls, researchers must identify which variables to control. Second, these methods control only identified characteristics, leaving others uncontrolled.

Although randomization is an excellent tool, it is not always feasible. If the independent variable cannot be manipulated, other techniques should be used. It is better to use matching or statistical control than to ignore the problem of confounding variables.

# CHARACTERISTICS OF GOOD DESIGN

A critical question in critiquing a quantitative study is whether the research design yielded valid evidence. Four key questions regarding research design, particularly in cause-probing studies, are as follows:

1. What is the strength of the evidence that a relationship between variables really exists?
2. If a relationship exists, what is the strength of the evidence that the independent variable of interest (e.g., an intervention), rather than other factors, *caused* the outcome?

3. What is the strength of evidence that observed relationships are generalizable across people, settings, and time?
4. What are the theoretical constructs underlying the related variables, and are those constructs adequately captured?

These questions, respectively, correspond to four aspects of a study's **validity**: (1) statistical conclusion validity; (2) internal validity; (3) external validity; and (4) construct validity (Shadish et al., 2002).

## Statistical Conclusion Validity

As noted previously, a criterion for establishing causality is showing that there is a relationship between the independent and dependent variable. Statistical tests are used to support inferences about whether such a relationship exists. Design decisions can influence whether statistical tests will actually be able to detect true relationships. Although we cannot discuss all aspects of **statistical conclusion validity**, we can describe a few design issues that can affect it.

One issue concerns **statistical power**, which refers to the capacity to detect true relationships. Statistical power can be achieved in various ways, the most straightforward of which is to use a large enough sample. With small samples, statistical power tends to be low, and the analyses may fail to show that the independent variable and the outcome are related—*even when they are*. Power and sample size are discussed in Chapter 10.

Another aspect of a powerful design concerns how the independent variable is defined. Results are clearer when differences between the groups (treatment conditions) being compared are large. Researchers should maximize group differences on the independent variables (i.e., make the *cause* powerful) so as to maximize differences on the outcome (the effect). If the groups or treatments are not very different, the statistical analysis might not be sufficiently sensitive to detect outcome effects that actually exist. Intervention fidelity can enhance the power of an intervention.

Thus, if you are critiquing a study in which outcomes for the groups being compared were not significantly different, one possibility is that the study had low statistical conclusion validity. The report might give clues about this possibility (e.g., too small a sample or substantial attrition) that should be taken into consideration in interpreting what the results mean.

## Internal Validity

**Internal validity** is the extent to which it can be inferred that the independent variable is truly causing the outcome. RCTs tend to have high internal validity because randomization enables researchers to rule out competing explanations for group differences. With quasi-experiments and correlational studies, there are competing explanations, which are sometimes called **threats to internal validity**. Evidence hierarchies rank study designs mainly in terms of internal validity.

### Threats to Internal Validity

#### Temporal Ambiguity

In a causal relationship, the cause must precede the effect. In RCTs, researchers create the independent variable and then observe performance on an outcome, so establishing a temporal sequence is never a problem. In correlational studies, however—especially ones using a cross-sectional design—it may be unclear whether the independent variable preceded the dependent variable, or vice versa, as illustrated in Figure 9.1 on page 161.

### Selection

The **selection threat** reflects biases stemming from preexisting differences between groups. When people are not assigned randomly to groups, the groups being compared may not be equivalent. In such a situation, group differences in the outcome may be caused by extraneous factors rather than by the independent variable. Selection bias is the most challenging threat to the internal validity of studies not using an experimental design (e.g., nonequivalent control group designs, case–control designs), but can be partially addressed using control mechanisms described in the previous section.

### History

The **history threat** is the occurrence of events concurrent with the independent variable that can affect the outcome. For example, suppose we were studying the effectiveness of a community-wide program to encourage flu shots among the elderly. Let us also suppose that a national media story about a flu epidemic occurred at about the same time. Our outcome variable, number of flu shots administered, is subject to the influence of at least two forces, and it would be hard to disentangle the two effects. In RCTs, history is not typically a threat because external events are as likely to affect one randomized group as another. The designs most likely to be affected by the history threat are one-group pretest–posttest designs and time-series designs.

### Maturation

The **maturation threat** arises from processes occurring as a result of time (e.g., growth, fatigue) rather than the independent variable. For example, if we were studying the effect of an intervention for developmentally delayed children, our design would have to deal with the fact that progress would occur without an intervention. *Maturation* does not refer only to developmental changes but to any change that occurs as a function of time. Phenomena such as wound healing or postoperative recovery occur with little intervention, and so maturation may be a rival explanation for favorable posttreatment outcomes in the absence of a nontreated group. One-group pretest–posttest designs are especially vulnerable to the maturation threat.

### Mortality/Attrition

**Mortality** is the threat that arises from attrition in groups being compared. If different kinds of people remain in the study in one group versus another, then these differences, rather than the independent variable, could account for group differences in outcomes. The most severely ill patients might drop out of an experimental condition because it is too demanding, for example. Attrition bias essentially is a selection bias that occurs after the study unfolds: groups initially equivalent can lose comparability because of subject loss, and differential group composition, rather than the independent variable, could be the "cause" of any group differences on outcomes.

> **TIP:** If attrition is random (i.e., those dropping out of a study are similar to those remaining in it), then there would not be bias. However, attrition is rarely random. In general, the higher the rate of attrition, the greater the risk of bias. Biases are usually of concern if the rate exceeds 10% to 15%.

## Internal Validity and Research Design

Quasi-experimental and correlational studies are especially susceptible to threats to internal validity. These threats compete with the independent variable as a cause of the dependent variable. *The aim of a good quantitative research design is to rule out these competing explanations*. The control mechanisms previously described are strategies for improving internal validity—and thus for strengthening the quality of evidence that studies yield.

An experimental design often, but not always, eliminates competing explanations. For example, if constancy of conditions is not maintained for experimental and control groups, history might be a rival explanation for obtained results. Experimental mortality is a particularly salient threat. Because researchers do different things with the groups, members may drop out of the study differentially. This is particularly likely to happen if the intervention is stressful or time-consuming or if the control condition is boring or disappointing. Participants remaining in a study may differ from those who left, nullifying the initial equivalence of the groups.

You should carefully consider possible rival explanations for study results, especially in non-RCT studies. When researchers do not have control over critical confounding variables, caution in drawing conclusions about the evidence is appropriate.

## External Validity

**External validity** concerns inferences about whether relationships found for study participants might hold true for different people, conditions, and settings. External validity has emerged as a major concern in an EBP world in which it is important to generalize evidence from controlled research settings to real-world practice settings.

External validity questions can take several different forms. For example, we may ask whether relationships observed with a study sample can be generalized to a larger population—for example, whether results about rates of postpartum depression in Boston can be generalized to mothers in the United States. Thus, one aspect of a study's external validity concerns its sampling plan. If the sample is representative of the population, the generalizability of results to the population is enhanced. Sampling is discussed in Chapter 10.

Other external validity questions are about generalizing to different types of people, settings, or situations. For example, can findings about a pain-reduction treatment in Canada be generalized to people in the United States? New studies are often needed to answer questions about generalizability, but sometimes external validity can be enhanced by design decisions.

An important concept relevant to external validity is *replication*. Multisite studies are powerful because more confidence in the generalizability of the results can be attained if the results have been replicated in several sites—particularly if the sites differ on important dimensions (e.g., size). Studies involving a diverse sample of participants can test whether study results are replicated for various subgroups—for example, whether an intervention benefits men *and* women. Systematic reviews represent a crucial aid to external validity precisely because they focus on replications across time, space, people, and settings to explore consistencies.

The demands for internal and external validity may conflict. If a researcher exercises tight control to maximize internal validity, the setting may become too artificial to generalize to more naturalistic environments. Compromises are often necessary.

## Construct Validity

Research cannot be undertaken without constructs. Researchers conduct a study with specific exemplars of treatments, outcomes, settings, and people, but these are all stand-ins for broad constructs. **Construct validity** involves inferences from the particulars of the study to the higher-order constructs they are intended to represent. If studies contain construct errors, there is a risk that the evidence will be misleading. One aspect of construct validity concerns the degree to which an intervention is a good representation of the underlying construct that was theorized as having the potential to cause beneficial outcomes. Lack of blinding also undermines construct validity: is it an intervention, or *awareness of* the intervention, that resulted in benefits? Another issue concerns whether the measures of the dependent variable are good operationalizations of the constructs for which they are intended. This aspect will be discussed more fully in Chapter 11.

# CRITIQUING QUANTITATIVE RESEARCH DESIGNS

A key evaluative question is whether the research design enabled researchers to get good answers to the research question. This question has both substantive and methodologic facets.

Substantively, the issue is whether the researcher selected a design that matches the aims of the research. If the research purpose is descriptive or exploratory, an experimental design is not appropriate. If the researcher is searching to understand the full nature of a phenomenon about which little is known, a structured design that allows little flexibility might block insights (flexible designs are discussed in Chapter 14). We have discussed research control as a bias-reducing strategy, but too much control can introduce bias—for example, when a researcher tightly controls how phenomena under study can be manifested and so obscures their true nature.

Methodologically, the main design issue in quantitative studies is whether the research design provides the most valid, unbiased, and interpretable evidence possible. Indeed, there usually is no other aspect of a quantitative study that affects the quality of evidence as much as research design. Box 9.1 provides questions to assist you in evaluating aspects of research designs; these questions are key to a meaningful critique of a quantitative study.

---

**BOX 9.1   Guidelines for Critiquing Research Design in a Quantitative Study**

1. Was the design experimental, quasi-experimental, or nonexperimental? What specific design was used? Was this a cause-probing study? Given the type of question (therapy, prognosis, etc.), was the most rigorous possible design used?
2. What type of comparison was called for in the research design? Was the comparison strategy effective in illuminating key relationships?
3. If the study involved an intervention, were the intervention and control conditions adequately described? Was blinding used, and if so, who was blinded? If not, is there a good rationale for failure to use blinding? Was attention paid to intervention fidelity?
4. If the study was nonexperimental, why did the researcher opt not to intervene? If the study was cause probing, which criteria for inferring causality were potentially compromised? Was a retrospective or prospective design used, and was such a design appropriate?
5. Was the study longitudinal or cross-sectional? Was the number and timing of data collection points appropriate?
6. What steps did the researcher take in designing the study to enhance statistical conclusion validity? Were these steps adequate?
7. What did the researcher do to control confounding external factors and intrinsic participant characteristics, and were the procedures effective? What are the threats to the study's internal validity? Does the design enable the researcher to draw causal inferences about the relationship between the independent variable and the outcome?
8. What are the major limitations of the design used? Are these limitations acknowledged by the researcher and taken into account in interpreting results? What can be said about the study's external validity?

## RESEARCH EXAMPLES WITH CRITICAL THINKING EXERCISES

This section presents examples of studies with different research designs. Read these summaries and then answer the critical thinking questions, referring to the full research reports if necessary.

Examples 1 and 2 below are also featured in our *Interactive Critical Thinking Activity* on thePoint website where you can easily record, print, and e-mail your responses to the related questions.

### EXAMPLE 1 ● A Randomized Controlled Trial

**Study:** "Investigation of standard care versus sham Reiki placebo versus actual Reiki therapy to enhance comfort and well-being in a chemotherapy infusion center" (Catlin & Taylor-Ford, 2011).

**Statement of Purpose:** The purpose of the study was to evaluate the efficacy of Reiki therapy in enhancing comfort and well-being among patients undergoing outpatient chemotherapy. Reiki is a form of energy work that involves laying of hands over a fully clothed person "for the purpose of unblocking energy centers" (p. E213).

**Treatment Groups:** Three groups of patients were compared: (1) an intervention group that received a Reiki intervention; (2) a placebo group that received a sham Reiki treatment; and (3) a control group that got usual care only.

**Method:** A sample of 189 participants was randomly assigned to one of the three groups, using a table of random numbers. The sample size was based on an analysis undertaken to ensure adequate statistical power. Patients in the intervention group received a 20-minute Reiki treatment during chemotherapy by an experienced Reiki therapist (an RN). For patients in the placebo group, the therapist pretended to perform a Reiki session. Patients in the control group received standard care. In terms of intervention fidelity, actual sessions were not monitored, but sessions held before the study allowed other Reiki instructors to see that the actual therapist and the sham therapist approached patients in identical ways. All patients completed scales that measured their comfort and well-being, both prior to the treatment and again after the chemotherapy session. Infusion center nurses and patients themselves were blinded as to whether the sham or actual Reiki therapy was being administered. There was no attrition from the study. A comparison of patients in the three study groups at baseline indicated that the three groups were comparable in terms of demographic characteristics (e.g., age, ethnicity) and treatment variables (e.g., round of chemotherapy).

**Key Findings:** Improvements in both comfort and well-being were observed from baseline to posttest for patients in both the Reiki group and the placebo group, but not for those in the standard care group. The standard care group had significantly lower comfort and well-being scores at the end of the trial than those in the Reiki and placebo groups.

**Conclusions:** The researchers concluded that the presence of an RN providing one-on-one support during a chemotherapy session helped to improve comfort and well-being, with or without an attempted healing energy field.

### CRITICAL THINKING EXERCISES

1. Answer the relevant questions from Box 9.1 on page 170 regarding this study.
2. Also consider the following targeted questions:
   a. Could a crossover design have been used in this study?
   b. Was randomization successful in creating comparable groups?
3. If the results of this study are valid, in what ways do you think the findings could be used in clinical practice?

### EXAMPLE 2 ● Quasi-Experimental Design

**Study:** "Efficacy of controlling nighttime noise and activities to improve patients' sleep quality in a surgical intensive care unit" (Li et al., 2011)

**Statement of Purpose:** The purpose of the study was to evaluate the effectiveness of implementing a set of sleep care guidelines for improving sleep quality of patients in a surgical intensive care unit (ICU) in a large medical center in Taiwan.

**Treatment Groups:** The control group of ICU patients received care as usual. Patients in the experimental group were cared for by nurses who followed special sleep care guidelines designed to reduce noise and light between the hours of 11:00 PM to 5:00 AM This entailed making several changes to nursing care, such as changing the time for chest X-rays from midnight to between 7:00 and 10:00 PM, and ensuring that the volume of IV fluid and tube feeding was adequate before 11:00 PM.

**Method:** A two-phase quasi-experimental design was used. In the first phase (December 2007 to February 2008), a control group of 30 patients got care as usual. In the second phase (March 2008 to May 2008), 30 patients were cared for under the new sleep care guidelines. Nurses received training in the use of the new guidelines, and fidelity to the new protocol was monitored during training. The sample size was based on an analysis designed to yield adequate statistical power. Blinding was not used in this study. Patients responded to a set of questions about sleep quality on the 3rd day after admittance to the ICU. A decibel meter was also used to continuously monitor environmental noise levels. The two groups of patients were similar in terms of such characteristics as age, sex, education, type of surgery, and disease severity. However, patients in the control group were more likely to have had a prior ICU experience that those in the experimental group. Out of the initial total sample of 60 patients, 5 were dropped from the study (2 in the intervention group, 3 in the control group).

**Key Findings:** Using data from the decibel meter, both the peak sound level and the average noise level were significantly lower after implementing the new guidelines. Patients in the experimental group also reported significantly better sleep quality and sleep efficiency than those in the control group.

**Conclusions:** The researchers concluded that the sleep care guidelines were effective and that nurses should make efforts to reduce environmental stimuli during nighttime hours.

## CRITICAL THINKING EXERCISES

1. Answer the relevant questions from Box 9.1 on page 170 regarding this study.
2. Also consider the following targeted questions:
   a. Is this study prospective or retrospective?
   b. What other quasi-experimental designs could have been used in this study?
3. If the results of this study are valid, in what ways do you think the findings could be used in clinical practice?

## EXAMPLE 3 ● Nonexperimental Study in Appendix A

• Read the method section from Howell and colleagues' (2007) study ("Anxiety, anger, and blood pressure in children") in Appendix A on page 395–402.

## CRITICAL THINKING EXERCISES

1. Answer the questions in Box 9.1 from page 170 regarding this study.
2. Also consider the following targeted questions:
   a. Could Howell and colleagues have used an experimental or quasi-experimental design to address the research questions?
   b. If the design was retrospective, how could the study have been done prospectively (or vice versa)?

**WANT TO KNOW MORE?** A wide variety of resources to enhance your learning and understanding of this chapter are available on the Point.

- Interactive Critical Thinking Activity
- Chapter Supplement on Selected Experimental and Quasi-Experimental Designs
- Answers to the Critical Thinking Exercises for Example 3
- Student Review Questions
- Full-text online
- Internet Resources with useful websites for Chapter 9

Additional study aids including eight journal articles and related questions are also available in *Study Guide for Essentials of Nursing Research, 8e.*

## SUMMARY POINTS

- The **research design** is the overall plan for answering research questions. In quantitative studies, the design designates whether there is an intervention, the nature of any comparisons, methods for controlling confounding variables, whether there will be blinding, and the timing and location of data collection.

- Therapy, prognosis, and etiology questions are cause probing, and there is a hierarchy of designs for yielding best evidence for these questions.

- Key criteria for inferring causality include the following: (1) a cause (independent variable) must precede an effect (outcome); (2) there must be a detectable relationship between a cause and an effect; and (3) the relationship between the two does not reflect the influence of a third (confounding) variable.

- A **counterfactual** is what would have happened to the same people simultaneously exposed *and* not exposed to a causal factor. The *effect* is the difference between the two. A good research design for cause-probing questions entails finding a good approximation to the idealized counterfactual.

- **Experiments** (or **randomized controlled trials [RCTs]**) involve an intervention (the researcher manipulates the independent variable by introducing an intervention; control (including the use of a **control group** that is not given the intervention and represents the comparative counterfactual); and **randomization** or **random assignment** (with participants allocated to experimental and control groups at random to make the groups comparable at the outset).

- RCTs are considered the gold standard because they come closer than any other design in meeting the criteria for inferring causal relationships.

- **Posttest-only designs** involve collecting data only once—after randomization and the introduction of the treatment; in **pretest–posttest designs**, data are collected both before the intervention (at **baseline**) and after it.

- In **crossover designs**, people are exposed to more than one experimental condition in random order and serve as their own controls. Crossover designs are not appropriate when there is a risk of *carryover effects*.

- The control group can undergo various conditions, including no treatment; an alternative treatment; a **placebo** or pseudointervention; standard treatment ("usual care"); different treatment doses; or a *wait-list* (*delayed treatment*) condition.

- **Quasi-experiments** (*trials without randomization*) involve an intervention but lack a comparison group or randomization. Strong quasi-experimental designs introduce controls to compensate for these missing components.

- **The nonequivalent control-group, pretest–posttest design** involves comparing an intervention group to a **comparison group** that was not created through randomization, and the collection of pretreatment data from both groups to assess initial group equivalence.

- In a **time-series design**, outcome data are collected over a period of time before and after the intervention, usually for a single group.

- **Nonexperimental** (*observational*) **research** includes **descriptive research**—studies that summarize the status of phenomena—and **correlational studies** that examine relationships among variables but involve no intervention.

- In **prospective cohort designs**, researchers begin with a possible cause, and then subsequently collect data about outcomes.

- **Retrospective designs** (**case–control designs**) involve collecting data about an outcome in the present and then looking back in time for possible causes.

- Making causal inferences in correlational studies is risky; a basic research dictum is that *correlation does not prove causation*.

- **Cross-sectional designs** involve the collection of data at one time period, whereas **longitudinal designs** involve data collection at two or more times over an extended period. In nursing, most longitudinal studies are **follow-up studies** of clinical populations.

- Longitudinal studies are typically expensive, time-consuming, and subject to the risk of **attrition** (loss of participants over time) but yield valuable information about time-related phenomena.

- Quantitative researchers strive to control external factors that could affect study outcomes and subject characteristics that are extraneous to the research question.

- Researchers delineate the intervention in formal *protocols* that stipulate exactly what the treatment is. Careful researchers attend to *intervention fidelity*—whether the intervention was properly implemented and actually received as intended.

- Techniques for controlling subject characteristics include **homogeneity** (restricting participants to reduce variability on confounding variables); **matching** (deliberately making groups comparable on some extraneous variables); statistical procedures; and randomization—the most effective method because it controls all possible confounding variables without researchers having to identify them.

- Study **validity** concerns the extent to which appropriate inferences can be made. **Threats to validity** are reasons that an inference could be wrong. A key function of quantitative research design is to rule out validity threats.

- **Statistical conclusion validity** concerns the strength of evidence that a relationship exists between two variables. Threats to statistical conclusion validity include low **statistical power** (the ability to detect true relationships among variables) and factors that undermine a strong treatment.

- **Internal validity** concerns inferences that the outcomes were caused by the independent variable, rather than by extraneous factors. Threats to internal validity include temporal ambiguity (uncertainty about whether the presumed cause preceded the outcome); **selection** (preexisting group differences); **history** (external events that could affect outcomes); **maturation** (changes due to the passage of time); and **mortality** (effects attributable to attrition).

- **External validity** concerns inferences about generalizability—whether findings hold true over variations in people, conditions, and settings.

# REFERENCES FOR CHAPTER 9

Aitken, L., Burmeister, E., Clayton, S., Dalais, C., & Gardner, G. (2011). The impact of Nursing Rounds on the practice environment and nursing satisfaction in intensive care. *International Journal of Nursing Studies, 48*, 918–925.

Belanger, L., Plotnikoff, R., Clark, A., & Courneya, K. (2012). A survey of physical activity programming and counseling preferences in young-adult cancer survivors. *Cancer Nursing, 35*, 48–54.

Carter, A., Deselms, J., Ruyle, S., Morrissey-Lucas, M., Kollar, S., Cannon, S., et al. (2012). Postanesthesia care unit visitation decreases family member anxiety. *Journal of Perisanesthesia Nursing, 27*, 3–9.

Catlin, A., & Taylor-Ford, R. (2011). Investigation of standard care versus sham Reiki placebo versus actual Reiki therapy to enhance comfort and well-being in a chemotherapy infusion center. *Oncology Nursing Forum, 38*, E212–E220.

Cora, A., Particino, M., Munafo, M., & Palomba, D. (2012). Health risk factors in caregivers of terminal cancer patients. *Cancer Nursing, 35*, 38–47.

Grav, S., Hellzen, O., Romild, U., & Stordal, E. (2012). Association between social support and depression in the general population. *Journal of Clinical Nursing, 21*, 111–120.

Kassab, M., Sheehy, A., King, M., Fowler, C., & Foureur, M. (2012). A double-blind randomized controlled trial of 25% oral glucose for pain relief in 2-month old infants undergoing immunization. *International Journal of Nursing Studies, 49*(3), 249–256.

Li, S., Wang, T., Wu, S., Liang, S., & Tung, H. (2011). Efficacy of controlling night-time noise and activities to improve patients' sleep quality in a surgical intensive care unit. *Journal of Clinical Nursing, 20*, 396–407.

Liaw, J. J., Yang, L., Katherine-Wang, K., Chen, C., Chang, Y., & Yin, T. (2012). Non-nutritive sucking and facilitated tucking relieve preterm infant pain during heel-stick procedures. *International Journal of Nursing Studies, 49*(3), 300–409.

Liou, Y. M., Hsu, Y., Ho, J., Lin, C., Hsu, W., & Liou, T. (2012). Prevalence and correlates of self-induced vomiting as weight control strategy among adolescents in Taiwan. *Journal of Clinical Nursing, 21*, 11–20.

McCullough, N., Parkes, J., Kerr, C., & McDowell. (2012). The health of children and young people with cerebral palsy. *International Journal of Nursing Studies*, PubMed ID 21329925.

Ngai, F., Chan, S., & Ip, W. (2010). Predictors and correlates of maternal role competence and satisfaction. *Nursing Research, 59*, 185–193.

Polit, D., & Chaboyer, W. (2012). Statistical process control in nursing research. *Research in Nursing & Health, 35*, 82–93.

Robbins, L., Pfeiffer, K., Maier, K., Ladrig, S., & Berg-Smith, S. (2012). Treatment fidelity of motivational interviewing delivered by a school nurse to increase girls' physical activity. *Journal of School Nursing, 28*, 70–78.

Salamonson, Y., Everett, B., Koch, J., Andrew, S., & Davidson, P. (2012). The impact of term-time paid work on academic performance in nursing students: A longitudinal study. *International Journal of Nursing Studies, 49*(5), 579–585.

Shadish, W. R., Cook, T. D., & Campbell, D. T. (2002). *Experimental and quasi-experimental designs for generalized causal inference.* Boston: Houghton Mifflin Co.

White, L. S. (2012). Reducing stress in school-age girls through mindful yoga. *Journal of Pediatric Health Care, 26*, 45–56.

Yin, Q., Ma, Z., Feng, F., & Wang, L. (2012). Postoperative anxiety and depression in patients undergoing thoracoscopic closure of congenital heart defects. *Journal of Cardiovascular Nursing*, PubMed ID 21926914.

# 10 Sampling and Data Collection in Quantitative Studies

## LEARNING OBJECTIVES

*On completing this chapter, you will be able to:*

● Distinguish between nonprobability and probability samples and compare their advantages and disadvantages

● Identify and describe several types of sampling designs in quantitative studies

● Evaluate the appropriateness of the sampling method and sample size used in a study

● Discuss the dimensions along which data collection approaches vary

● Identify phenomena that lend themselves to self-reports, observation, and biophysiologic measurement

● Describe various approaches to collecting self-report data (e.g., interviews vs. questionnaires, composite scales)

● Describe various methods of collecting, sampling, and recording observational data

● Describe the major features and advantages of biophysiologic measures

● Critique a researcher's decisions regarding the data collection plan and its implementation

● Define new terms in the chapter

## KEY TERMS

Accessible population
Category system
Checklist
Closed-ended question
Consecutive sampling
Convenience sampling
Eligibility criteria
Interview schedule
Questionnaire
Likert scale
Nonprobability sampling
Nonresponse bias

Observational methods
Open-ended question
Population
Power analysis
Probability sampling
Purposive sampling
Quota sampling
Random sampling
Rating scale
Representative sample
Response alternatives
Response rate

Response set bias
Sample size
Sampling
Sampling bias
Scale
Self-report
Simple random sampling
Strata
Stratified random sampling
Systematic sampling
Target population
Visual analog scale

This chapter covers two important research topics—how quantitative researchers select their study participants and how they collect data from them.

# SAMPLING IN QUANTITATIVE RESEARCH

Researchers answer their questions using a sample of participants. In testing the effects of an intervention for pregnant women, nurse researchers reach conclusions without testing it with all pregnant women. Quantitative researchers want samples that allow them to generalize their results to a broader population, and that have adequate power for statistical conculation validity. They develop a **sampling plan** that specifies in advance how participants will be selected and how many to include.

## Basic Sampling Concepts

Sampling is a critical part of the design of quantitative research. Let us first consider some terms associated with sampling—terms that are used primarily with quantitative studies.

### Populations

A **population** (the "P" in PICO questions) is the entire group of interest. For instance, if a researcher were studying American nurses with doctoral degrees, the population could be defined as all RNs in the United States who have acquired a doctoral-level degree. Other populations might be all patients who had cardiac surgery in St. Peter's Hospital in 2013 or all Australian children under age 10 with cystic fibrosis. Populations are not restricted to people. A population might consist of all hospital records in Memorial Hospital. Whatever the basic unit, the population is an entire aggregate of elements.

Researchers specify characteristics that delimit the population through **eligibility criteria**. For example, consider the population of American nursing students. Does the population include part-time students? Are RNs returning to school for a bachelor's degree included? Researchers establish criteria to determine whether a person qualifies as a member of the population (*inclusion* criteria) or should be excluded (*exclusion* criteria), for example, excluding patients who do not speak English or who are severely ill.

> **Example of inclusion and exclusion criteria:**
> Kvitvaer and colleagues (2012) sought to identify a group of symptoms that are highly correlated with unexplained infant crying commonly termed infant colic. Infants were eligible for the study if they were younger than 12 months and had been brought by their parents to a clinic because of excessive crying. Infants were excluded if they had a concurrent or systemic illness and if their parents could not speak English.

Quantitative researchers sample from an accessible population in the hope of generalizing to a target population. The **target population** is the entire population in which a researcher is interested. The **accessible population** is the portion of the target population that is accessible to the researcher. For example, the researcher's target population might be all diabetic patients in the United States, but, in reality, the population that is accessible might be diabetic patients in a particular hospital, from which a sample is selected.

### Samples and Sampling

**Sampling** involves selecting a portion of the population to represent the population. A **sample** is a subset of population elements. In nursing research, the *elements* (basic units) are usually humans. Researchers work with samples rather than populations because it is practical to do so.

Information from samples can, however, lead to erroneous conclusions. In quantitative studies, a key criterion for judging a sample is its representativeness. A **representative sample** is one whose characteristics closely approximate those of the population. Certain sampling plans are less likely to result in biased samples than others. **Sampling bias** is the systematic overrepresentation or underrepresentation of some segment of the population in terms of key characteristics.

### Strata

Populations consist of subpopulations, or **strata**. Strata are mutually exclusive segments of a population based on a specific characteristic. For instance, a population consisting of all RNs in the United Kingdom could be divided into two strata based on gender. Or, we could specify three strata based on years of experience (e.g., less than 10 years, 10 to 20 years, or more than 20 years). Strata are often used in sample selection to enhance the sample's representativeness.

> **TIP:** The sampling plan is usually discussed in a report's method section, sometimes in a subsection called "Sample" or "Study participants." Sample characteristics (e.g., average age) are often described at the beginning of the results section.

## Sampling Designs in Quantitative Studies

There are two broad classes of sampling designs in quantitative research: probability sampling and nonprobability sampling.

### Nonprobability Sampling

In **nonprobability sampling**, researchers select elements by nonrandom methods in which every element usually does not have a chance to be included. Nonprobability sampling is less likely than probability sampling to produce representative samples—and yet, *most* research samples in nursing and other disciplines are nonprobability samples.

**Convenience sampling** entails selecting the most conveniently available people as participants. A nurse who distributes questionnaires about vitamin use to 100 adults at a church picnic center is sampling by convenience, for example. The problem with convenience sampling is that people who are readily available might be atypical of the population, and so the price of convenience is the risk of bias. Convenience sampling is the weakest form of sampling, but it is also the most commonly used sampling method in many disciplines.

> **Example of a convenience sample:**
> Morrison and Ludington-Hoe (2012) studied interruptions to breast-feeding dyads in a community hospital birthing center. A convenience sample of 33 mothers who expressed the intent to breast-feed upon admission to the birth center yielded data on 1,596 interruptions over 360 hours of observation.

In **quota sampling**, researchers identify population strata and figure out how many people are needed from each stratum. By using information about the population, researchers can ensure that diverse segments are properly represented in the sample. As an example, suppose we were interested in studying nursing students' attitudes toward working on an AIDS unit. The accessible population is a nursing school with 500 undergraduates; a sample size of 100 students is desired. With a convenience sample, we could distribute questionnaires to 100 students as they entered classrooms. Suppose, though, that male and female students have

**TABLE 10.1　Numbers and Percentages of Students in Strata of a Population, Convenience Sample, and Quota Sample**

| Strata | Population | Convenience Sample | Quota Sample |
|--------|-----------|--------------------|--------------|
| Male | 100 (20%) | 5 (5%) | 20 (20%) |
| Female | 400 (80%) | 95 (95%) | 80 (80%) |
| **Total** | 500 (100%) | 100 (100%) | 100 (100%) |

different attitudes toward AIDS patients. A convenience sample might result in too many men, or too few. Table 10.1 presents some fictitious data showing the gender distribution for the population and for a convenience sample (columns 2 and 3). The convenience sample seriously underrepresents male students, which in turn means the results will be biased. We can use quota sampling to select participants so that the sample includes an appropriate number of men and women, as shown in the far-right column of Table 10.1.

Procedurally, quota sampling is similar to convenience sampling: participants are a convenience sample from each stratum. Because of this fact, quota sampling shares some of the weaknesses of convenience sampling. For instance, a trip to a dorm might be a convenient way to recruit the 20 needed male students. Yet this approach gives no representation to male students living off campus, who may feel differently about working with AIDS patients. Nevertheless, quota sampling is a big improvement over convenience sampling and does not require sophisticated skills or a lot of effort. Surprisingly, few researchers use this strategy.

**Example of a quota sample:**
Hung and colleagues (2011) used quota sampling to recruit 859 women from 18 Taiwanese hospitals or clinics into their study of factors predicting postpartum stress. The sample represented births from the 18 facilities proportionately.

**Consecutive sampling** is a nonprobability sampling method that involves recruiting *all* people from an accessible population over a specific time interval, or for a specified sample size. For example, in a study of ventilated-associated pneumonia in ICU patients, a consecutive sample might consist of all eligible patients who were admitted to an ICU over a 6-month period. Or it might be the first 250 eligible patients admitted to the ICU, if 250 were the targeted sample size. Consecutive sampling is a better approach than sampling by convenience, especially if the sampling period is sufficiently long to deal with potential biases that reflect seasonal fluctuations. Consecutive sampling is often the best possible choice when there is "rolling enrollment" into an accessible population.

**Example of a consecutive sample:**
Forni and colleagues (2011) conducted a study to evaluate the use of polyurethane foam inside plaster casts to prevent the onset of heel sores. Their intervention group was a consecutive sample of 71 patients requiring lower limb casts in an orthopedic hospital in Italy.

**Purposive sampling** is based on the belief that researchers' knowledge about the population can be used to hand-pick sample members. Researchers might decide purposely to select people who are judged to be particularly knowledgeable about the issues under study. This method can lead to bias, but can be a useful approach when researchers want a sample of experts.

> **Example of purposive sampling:**
> Castro and colleagues (2011) assessed the views of an expert panel of 22 nurses regarding the development of a taxonomy for the domain of clinical nursing research.

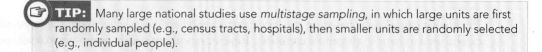 **HOW-TO-TELL TIP:** How can you tell what type of sampling design was used in a quantitative study? If the report does not explicitly mention or describe the sampling design, it is usually safe to assume that a convenience sample was used.

## Probability Sampling

**Probability sampling** involves random selection of elements from a population. Random selection should not be (although it often is) confused with random assignment, which is a signature of a randomized controlled trial (RCT) (Chapter 9). Random *assignment* to different treatment conditions has no bearing on how participants in the RCT were selected in the first place. With **random sampling**, each element in the population has an equal, independent chance of being selected.

**Simple random sampling** is the most basic probability sampling. In simple random sampling, researchers establish a *sampling frame*, the technical name for the list of population elements. If nursing students at the University of Connecticut were the accessible population, then a student roster would be the sampling frame. Elements in a sampling frame are numbered and then a table of random numbers or an online random sample generator is used to draw a random sample of the desired size. Samples selected in such a fashion are not subject to researcher biases. There is no *guarantee* of a representative sample, but random selection does guarantee that differences between the sample and the population are purely a function of chance. The probability of selecting a markedly atypical sample through random sampling is low, and this probability decreases as the sample size increases.

> **Example of a simple random sample:**
> Radzvin (2011) randomly sampled 800 certified registered nurse anesthetists (CRNAs) from the registry of the American Association of Nurse Anesthetists to study moral distress in CRNAs.

In **stratified random sampling**, the population is first divided into two or more strata, from which elements are randomly selected. As with quota sampling, the aim of stratified sampling is to enhance representativeness. Stratification is often based on demographic attributes, such as age or gender. Stratified sampling may not be possible if information on the stratifying variable is unavailable (e.g., student rosters may not include information on age).

> **Example of stratified random sampling:**
> Mattila and colleagues (2010) studied patients' perceived access to support from nursing staff. They sent questionnaires to a stratified random sample of patients in a Finnish hospital. The stratifying variable was type of hospital unit—surgical, internal medicine, and gynecologic.

**TIP:** Many large national studies use *multistage sampling*, in which large units are first randomly sampled (e.g., census tracts, hospitals), then smaller units are randomly selected (e.g., individual people).

**Systematic sampling** involves the selection of every *k*th case from a list, such as every 10th person on a patient list. Systematic sampling can be used in such a way that an essentially random sample is drawn. First, the size of the population is divided by the size of the desired sample to obtain the **sampling interval**, which is the standard distance between selected cases. For instance, if we needed a sample of 50 from a population of 5,000, our sampling interval would be 100 (5,000/50 = 100). Every 100th case on a sampling frame would be sampled, with the first case selected randomly. If our random number were 73, the people corresponding to numbers 73, 173, 273, and so on would be included in the sample. Systematic sampling done in this manner is essentially the same as simple random sampling, and is often more convenient.

> **Example of a systematic sample:**
> Gillespie and colleagues (2009) studied factors that predicted resilience in operating room (OR) nurses. The researchers sent a survey to 1,430 nurses—every other member of the professional association for OR nurses in Australia.

## Evaluation of Nonprobability and Probability Sampling

Probability sampling is the only viable method of obtaining representative samples. If all elements in a population have an equal probability of being selected, then the resulting sample is likely to do a good job of representing the population. A further advantage is that probability sampling allows researchers to estimate the magnitude of sampling error. *Sampling error* refers to differences between population values (e.g., the average age of the population) and sample values (e.g., the average age of the sample).

Nonprobability samples are rarely representative of the population. When every element in the population does not have a chance of being selected, it is likely that some segment of it will be underrepresented. When there is sampling bias, there is always a chance that the results could be misleading. Why, then, are nonprobability samples used in most nursing studies? Clearly, the advantages of these sampling designs lie in their ease and economy. Probability sampling, although highly respected, is often impractical. Quantitative researchers using nonprobability samples must be cautious about the inferences drawn from the data, and consumers should be alert to possible sampling biases.

☞ **TIP:** The quality of the sampling plan is of particular importance when the focus of the research is to obtain descriptive information about prevalence or average values for a population. All national surveys in the United States, such as the National Health Interview Survey, use probability samples. Probability samples are rarely used in randomized controlled trials. For studies whose purpose is primarily quantitative description, data from a probability sample is at the top of the evidence hierarchy for individual studies.

## Sample Size in Quantitative Studies

**Sample size**—the number of study participants—is a major concern in quantitative research. There is no simple formula to determine how large a sample should be, but larger is usually better than smaller. When researchers calculate a percentage or an average based on sample data, the purpose is to estimate a population value, and larger samples have less sampling error.

Researchers can estimate how large their samples should be for testing their research hypotheses through **power analysis**. A simple example can illustrate basic principles of power analysis. Suppose we were testing a new intervention to help people quit smoking;

smokers would be randomized to either an experimental or a control group. How many people should be in the sample? When using power analysis, researchers must estimate how large the group difference will be (e.g., group differences in average daily number of cigarettes smoked after the intervention). This estimate might be based on prior research or on a pilot test. When expected differences are large, a large sample is not needed to reveal group differences statistically but when small differences are predicted, large samples are necessary. For new areas of research, group differences are likely to be small or moderate. In our example, if a small group difference in postintervention smoking were expected, the sample size needed to test group differences in smoking, with standard statistical criteria, would be about 800 smokers (400 per group). If a small-to-moderate difference were expected, the total sample size would need to be about 250 smokers.

The risk of "getting it wrong" (statistical conclusion validity) increases when samples are too small: researchers risk gathering data that will not support their hypotheses *even when those hypotheses are correct*. Large samples are no assurance of accuracy, however. With nonprobability sampling, even a large sample can harbor bias. The famous example illustrating this point is the 1936 United States presidential poll conducted by the magazine *Literary Digest*, which predicted that Alfred M. Landon would defeat Franklin D. Roosevelt by a landslide. A sample of about 2.5 million people was polled, but biases arose because the sample was drawn from telephone directories and automobile registrations during a Depression year when only the well-to-do (who favored Landon) had a car or telephone.

A large sample cannot correct for a faulty sampling design; nevertheless, a large nonprobability sample is better than a small one. When critiquing quantitative studies, you must assess both the sample size and the sample selection method to judge how good the sample was.

> ☞ **TIP:** The sampling plan is often one of the weakest aspects of quantitative studies. Most nursing studies use samples of convenience, and many are based on samples that are too small to provide an adequate test of the research hypotheses. Small samples run a high risk of leading researchers to erroneously reject their research hypotheses. Therefore, you should give special scrutiny to the sampling plans of studies that fail to support research hypotheses.

## Critiquing Sampling Plans

In coming to conclusions about the quality of evidence that a study yields, the sampling plan merits special scrutiny. If the sample is seriously biased or too small, the findings may be misleading or just plain wrong.

In critiquing a description of a sampling plan, you should consider two issues. The first is whether the researcher has adequately described the sampling strategy. Ideally, research reports should describe the following:

- The type of sampling approach used (e.g., convenience, consecutive, random)
- The population under study and eligibility criteria for sample selection
- The sample size, with a rationale
- A description of the sample's main characteristics (e.g., age, gender, clinical status, and so on)
- The number and characteristics of potential subjects who declined to participate

If the description of the sample is inadequate, you may not be in a position to deal with the second and principal issue, which is whether the researcher made good sampling decisions.

**Box 10.1  Guidelines for Critiquing Quantitative Sampling Plans**

1. Is the population under study identified? Are eligibility criteria specified? Are the sample selection procedures clearly delineated?
2. What type of sampling design was used? Would an alternative sampling design have been preferable? Was the sampling design one that could be expected to yield a representative sample?
3. Did some factor other than the sampling design (e.g., a low response rate) affect the representativeness of the sample?
4. Are possible sample biases or weaknesses identified?
5. Are key characteristics of the sample described (e.g., mean age, percent female)?
6. Is the sample size sufficiently large to support statistical conclusion validity? Was the sample size justified on the basis of a power analysis or other rationale?
7. Does the sample support inferences about external validity? To whom can the study results reasonably be generalized?

And, if the description is incomplete, it will be difficult to draw conclusions about whether the evidence has relevance in your clinical practice.

We have stressed that a key criterion for assessing the quality of a sampling plan in quantitative research is whether the sample is representative of the population. You will never know for sure, of course, but if the sampling strategy is weak or if the sample size is small, there is reason to suspect some bias.

Even with a rigorous sampling plan, the sample may be biased if not all people invited to participate in a study agree to do so. If certain subgroups in the population refuse to participate, then a biased sample can result, even when probability sampling is used. The research report ideally should provide information about **response rates** (i.e., the number of people participating in a study relative to the number of people sampled), and about possible **nonresponse bias**—differences between participants and those who declined to participate (also sometimes referred to as *response bias)*. In a longitudinal study, attrition bias should be reported.

Your job as reviewer is to come to conclusions about the reasonableness of generalizing the findings from the researcher's sample to the accessible population and from the accessible population to a broader target population. If the sampling plan is seriously flawed, it may be risky to generalize the findings at all without replicating the study with another sample.

Box 10.1 presents some guiding questions for critiquing the sampling plan of a quantitative study.

# DATA COLLECTION IN QUANTITATIVE RESEARCH

Phenomena in which researchers are interested must be translated into data that can be analyzed. This section discusses the challenging task of collecting quantitative research data.

## Overview of Data Collection and Data Sources

Data collection methods vary along several dimensions. One issue is whether the researcher will collect original data or use existing data. Existing **records**, for example, are an important data source for nurse researchers. A wealth of data gathered for nonresearch purposes in clinical settings can be fruitfully analyzed to answer research questions.

> **Example of a study using records:**
> Garten and colleagues (2011) used data from the charts of 127 very low-birth-weight infants to study parental NICU visiting patterns during the first 28 days of life in a German hospital.

If existing data are unsuitable for a research question, researchers must collect new data. In developing their data collection plan, researchers make many important decisions, including the basic type of data to gather. Three types have been used most frequently by nurse researchers: self-reports, observations, and biophysiologic measures. **Self-report** data are participants' responses to questions posed by the researcher, such as in an interview. In nursing studies, self-reports are the most common data collection approach. Direct **observation** of people's behaviors, characteristics, and circumstances is an alternative to self-reports for certain questions. Nurses also use **biophysiologic measures** to assess important clinical variables. In quantitative studies, researchers decide upfront how to operationalize their variables and gather their data. Their data collection plans are almost always "cast in stone" before a single piece of data is collected.

Regardless of type of data collected in a study, data collection methods vary along several dimensions, including structure, quantifiability, and objectivity. Data for quantitative studies tend to be quantifiable and structured, with the same information gathered from all participants in a comparable, prespecified way. Quantitative researchers generally strive for methods that are as objective as possible.

> ☞ **TIP:** Most data that are analyzed quantitatively actually begin as qualitative data. If a researcher asked respondents if they have been severely depressed, moderately depressed, somewhat depressed, or not at all depressed in the past week, they answer in words, not numbers. The words are transformed, through *coding*, into quantitative categories.

## Self-Reports

A lot of information can be gathered by questioning people. If, for example, we wanted to learn about patients' eating habits, we would likely gather data by asking them relevant questions. The unique ability of humans to communicate verbally on a sophisticated level makes direct questioning an important part of nurse researchers' data collection repertoire.

Structured self-report methods are used when researchers know in advance exactly what they need to know and can frame appropriate questions to obtain the needed information. Structured self-report data are collected with a formal, written document—an *instrument*. The instrument is an **interview schedule** when the questions are asked orally face-to-face or by telephone or a **questionnaire** when respondents complete the instrument themselves.

### Question Form and Wording

In a totally structured instrument, respondents are asked to respond to the same questions in the same order. **Closed-ended** (or *fixed-alternative*) **questions** are ones in which the **response alternatives** are prespecified. The alternatives may range from a simple yes or no to complex expressions of opinion. The purpose of such questions is to ensure comparability of responses and to facilitate analysis. Some examples of closed-ended questions are presented in Table 10.2.

Some structured instruments, however, also include **open-ended questions**, which allow participants to respond to questions in their own words (e.g., What led to your decision to stop smoking?). When open-ended questions are included in questionnaires,

## TABLE 10.2  Examples of Closed-Ended Questions

| Question Type | Example |
|---|---|
| 1. Dichotomous question | Have you ever been pregnant?<br>1. Yes<br>2. No |
| 2. Multiple-choice question | How important is it to you to avoid a pregnancy at this time?<br>1. Extremely important<br>2. Very important<br>3. Somewhat important<br>4. Not important |
| 3. Rank-order question | People value different things in life. Below is a list of things that many people value. Please indicate their order of importance to you by placing a "1" beside the most important, "2" beside the second-most important, and so on.<br>_____ Career achievement/work<br>_____ Family relationships<br>_____ Friendships, social interactions<br>_____ Health<br>_____ Money<br>_____ Religion |
| 4. Forced-choice question | Which statement most closely represents your point of view?<br>1. What happens to me is my own doing.<br>2. Sometimes I feel I don't have enough control over my life. |
| 5. Rating question | On a scale from 0 to 10, where 0 means "extremely dissatisfied" and 10 means "extremely satisfied," how satisfied were you with the nursing care you received during your hospitalization?<br><br>0   1   2   3   4   5   6   7   8   9   10<br><br>Extremely dissatisfied                    Extremely satisfied |

respondents must write out their responses. In interviews, the interviewer writes down responses verbatim.

Good closed-ended questions are more difficult to construct than open-ended ones but easier to analyze. Closed-ended questions are also more efficient: people can complete more closed-ended questions than open-ended ones in a given amount of time. People may be unwilling to compose lengthy written responses to open-ended questions in questionnaires. A major drawback of closed-ended questions is that researchers might omit some potentially important responses. Closed-ended questions also can be superficial. Open-ended questions allow for richer information if the respondents are verbally expressive and cooperative. Finally, some respondents object to choosing from alternatives that do not reflect their opinions precisely.

In drafting (or borrowing) questions for a structured instrument, researchers must carefully monitor the wording of each question for clarity, sensitivity to respondents' psychological state, absence of bias, and (in questionnaires) reading level. Questions must be sequenced in a psychologically meaningful order that encourages cooperation and candor. Developing, pretesting, and refining a self-report instrument can take many months to complete.

### Interviews Versus Questionnaires

Researchers using structured self-reports must decide whether to use interviews or self-administered questionnaires. Questionnaires have the following advantages:

- Questionnaires are less costly and are advantageous for geographically dispersed samples. Internet questionnaires are especially economical and are an increasingly important means of gathering self-report data—although response rates to Internet questionnaires tend to be lower than for mailed questionnaires.
- Questionnaires offer the possibility of anonymity, which may be crucial in obtaining information about certain behavior, opinions, or traits.

**Example of mailed questionnaires:**

Krichbaum and colleagues (2011) developed and tested an instrument to measure *complexity compression* in nurses (being asked to assume new responsibilities in a compressed time frame). They sent questionnaires by mail to a random sample of 1,200 RNs in Minnesota.

The strengths of interviews outweigh those of questionnaires. Among the advantages are the following:

- Response rates tend to be high in face-to-face interviews. Respondents are less likely to refuse to talk to an interviewer than to ignore a questionnaire. Low response rates can lead to bias because respondents are rarely a random subset of the original sample. In the mailed questionnaire study of RNs described earlier (Krichbaum et al., 2011), the response rate was under 20%.
- Many people cannot fill out a questionnaire; examples include young children, the blind, and the very elderly. Interviews are feasible with most people.
- Interviewers can produce additional information through observation of respondents' behavior or living situation, which can be useful in interpreting responses.

Most advantages of face-to-face interviews also apply to telephone interviews. Complicated instruments are not well suited to telephone administration, but for relatively brief instruments, telephone interviews combine relatively low costs with high response rates.

**Example of personal interviews:**

Wu and co-researchers (2012) explored the relationship between fatigue and physical activity levels in patients with liver cirrhosis. Physical activity was assessed in interviews that involved a 7-day recall of all physical activities and their intensity and duration.

**TIP:** Even in interview situations, participants are sometimes asked some of their questions in a questionnaire format. Questions that are deeply personal (e.g., about sexuality) or that may require some reflection (e.g., about loneliness) are sometimes easier to answer privately on a form than to express out loud to an interviewer.

### Scales

Social-psychological scales are often incorporated into questionnaires or interview schedules. A **scale** is a device that assigns a numeric score to people along a continuum, like a scale for measuring weight. Social-psychological scales quantitatively discriminate among people with different attitudes, perceptions, and psychological traits.

One common scaling technique is the **Likert scale**, which consists of several declarative statements (*items*) that express a viewpoint on a topic. Respondents are asked to indicate

**TABLE 10.3 Example of a Likert Scale to Measure Attitudes Toward Condoms**

| Direction of Scoring* | Item | SA | A | ? | D | SD | Person 1 (✓) | Person 2 (X) |
|---|---|---|---|---|---|---|---|---|
| | | | **Responses†** | | | | **Score** | |
| + | 1. Using a condom shows you care about your partner. | | ✓ | | | X | 4 | 1 |
| − | 2. My partner would be angry if I talked about using condoms. | | | X | ✓ | | 5 | 3 |
| − | 3. I wouldn't enjoy sex as much if my partner and I used condoms. | | | X | ✓ | | 4 | 2 |
| + | 4. Condoms are a good protection against AIDS and other sexually transmitted diseases. | | | | ✓ | X | 3 | 2 |
| + | 5. My partner would respect me if I insisted on using condoms. | ✓ | | | | X | 5 | 1 |
| − | 6. I would be too embarrassed to ask my partner about using a condom. | | X | | ✓ | | 5 | 2 |
| | **Total score** | | | | | | 26 | 11 |

*Researchers would not indicate the direction of scoring on a Likert scale administered to participants. The scoring direction is indicated in this table for illustrative purposes only.
†SA, strongly agree; A, agree; ?, uncertain; D, disagree; SD, strongly disagree.

how much they agree or disagree with the statement. Table 10.3 presents an illustrative six-item Likert scale for measuring college students' attitudes toward condom use. In this example, agreement with positively worded statements is assigned a higher score. The first statement is positively worded; agreement indicates a favorable attitude toward condom use. Because there are five response alternatives, a score of 5 would be given for *strongly agree*, 4 for *agree*, and so on. Responses of two hypothetical participants are shown by a check or an X, and their item scores are shown in the right-hand columns. Person 1, who agreed with the first statement, has a score of 4, whereas person 2, who strongly disagreed, got a score of 1. The second statement is negatively worded, and so scoring is reversed—a 1 is assigned for *strongly agree*, and so forth. Item reversals ensure that a high score consistently reflects positive attitudes toward condom use.

A person's total score is the sum of item scores and so these scales are sometimes called *summated rating scales* or *composite scales*. In our example, person 1 has a more positive attitude toward condoms (total score = 26) than person 2 (total score = 11). Summing item scores makes it possible to finely discriminate among people with different opinions. A single Likert item puts people into only five categories. A six-item scale, such as the one in Table 10.3, permits finer gradation—from a minimum possible score of 6 (6 × 1) to a maximum possible score of 30 (6 × 5). Composite scales are often comprised of two or more *subscales* that measure different aspects of a construct. Developing high-quality scales requires a lot of skill and effort.

**Example of a Likert scale:**

Davidson and colleagues (2011) studied perceptions of cardiovascular risk in patients hospitalized for a percutaneous coronary intervention. They used several existing scales (e.g., the Perceived Stress Scale), and also developed a new Likert scale to measure perceived heart risk.

Another type of scale is the **visual analog scale** (VAS), which can be used to measure subjective experiences, such as pain, fatigue, and dyspnea. The VAS is a straight line, the end anchors of which are labeled as the extreme limits of the sensation or feeling being measured (Fig. 10.1). Participants mark a point on the line corresponding to the amount of sensation experienced. Traditionally, a VAS line is 100 mm in length, which makes it easy to derive a score from 0 to 100 by measuring the distance from one end of the scale to the mark on the line.

**Example of a visual analog scale:**

Taavoni and colleagues (2011) tested the effect of using birth balls on women's pain in the active phase of labor. Pain was measured using a visual analog scale.

Scales permit researchers to efficiently quantify subtle gradations in the intensity of individual characteristics. Scales can be administered either verbally or in writing and thus can be used with most people. Scales are susceptible to several common problems, however, many of which are referred to as **response set biases**. The most important biases include the following:

- *Social desirability response set bias*—a tendency to misrepresent attitudes or traits by giving answers that are consistent with prevailing social views
- *Extreme response set bias*—a tendency to consistently express extreme attitudes or feelings (e.g., strongly agree), leading to distortions because extreme responses may be unrelated to the trait being measured
- *Acquiescence response set bias*—a tendency to agree with statements regardless of their content by some people (*yea-sayers*). The opposite tendency for other people (*nay-sayers*) to disagree with statements independently of the question content is less common.

Researchers can reduce these biases by developing sensitively worded questions, creating a permissive, nonjudgmental atmosphere, and guaranteeing the confidentiality of responses.

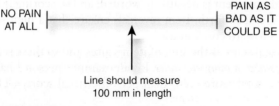

**FIGURE 10.1** ● Example of a visual analog scale.

> ☞ **TIP:** There are other special types of self-report approaches. *Vignettes*, for example, are brief descriptions of events or situations to which respondents are asked to react. *Q-sorts*, another example, present participants with a set of cards on which statements are written. Participants are asked to sort the cards along a specified dimension, such as most helpful/least helpful. Vignettes and Q-sorts are described in greater detail in the Chapter Supplement on thePoint website. ☀

### Evaluation of Self-Report Methods

If researchers want to know how people feel or what they believe, the most direct approach is to ask them. Self-reports frequently yield information that would be difficult or impossible to gather by other means. Behaviors can be *observed*, but only if people are willing to engage in them publicly—and engage in them at the time of data collection.

Despite these advantages, self-reports have some weaknesses. The most serious issue concerns the validity and accuracy of self-reports: How can we be sure that respondents feel or act the way they say they do? How can we trust the information that study participants provide, particularly if the questions ask them about potentially undesirable traits? Investigators usually have no choice but to assume that most respondents have been frank. Yet, we all have a tendency to present ourselves in the best light, and this may conflict with the truth. When reading research reports, you should be alert to potential biases in self-reported data.

## Observation

For some research questions, direct observation of people's behavior is an alternative to self-reports, especially in clinical settings. Observational methods can be used to gather such information as the conditions of individuals (e.g., the sleep–wake state of patients); verbal communication (e.g., exchange of information at change-of-shift report); nonverbal communication (e.g., body language); activities (e.g., geriatric patients' self-grooming activities); and environmental conditions (e.g., noise levels in nursing homes).

In observational studies, researchers have flexibility with regard to several important dimensions:

- *Focus of the observation*. The focus can be on broadly defined events (*e.g.*, patient mood swings), or on small, highly specific behaviors (e.g., facial expressions).
- *Concealment*. Researchers do not always tell people they are being observed, because awareness of being observed may cause people to behave atypically. Behavioral distortions due to the known presence of an observer is called *reactivity*.
- *Method of recording observations*. Observations can be made through the human senses and then recorded by paper-and-pencil methods, but they can also be done with sophisticated equipment (e.g., video equipment, audio recording equipment, computers).

Like self-report techniques, observational methods vary in terms of structure and quantifiability. Structured observation involves the use of formal instruments and protocols that dictate what to observe, how long to observe it, and how to record the data. Structured observation is not intended to capture a broad slice of ordinary life, but rather to document specific behaviors, actions, and events. Structured observation requires the formulation of a system for accurately categorizing, recording, and encoding the observations.

> ☞ **TIP:** Researchers often use structured observations when participants cannot be asked questions, or cannot be expected to provide reliable answers. Many observational instruments are designed to capture the behaviors of infants, children, or people whose communication skills are impaired.

## Categories and Checklists

The most common approach to making structured observations is to use a category system for classifying observed phenomena. A **category system** represents a method of recording in a systematic fashion the behaviors and events of interest that transpire within a setting.

Some category systems are constructed so that *all* observed behaviors within a specified domain (e.g., body positions and movements) can be classified into one and only one category. A contrasting technique is to develop a system in which only particular types of behavior (which may or may not be manifested) are categorized. For example, if we were studying children's aggressive behavior, we might develop such categories as "strikes another child" or "throws objects around the room." In this category system, many behaviors—all that are nonaggressive—would not be classified, and some children may exhibit *no* aggressive actions. Nonexhaustive systems are adequate for many purposes, but one risk is that resulting data might be difficult to interpret. When a large number of behaviors are not categorized, the investigator may have difficulty placing categorized behavior into perspective.

> **Example of nonexhaustive categories:**
> Happ and colleagues (2011) undertook a complex observational study of communication between nurses and patients in an intensive care unit. Among many different types of observations made, observers recorded instances of positive and negative nurse behaviors, according to carefully defined criteria. Nurse behaviors that were neutral were not categorized.

Category systems must be accompanied by, explicit operational definitions of the behaviors and characteristics to be observed. Each category must be carefully explained, giving observers clear-cut criteria for assessing the occurrence of the phenomenon. Even with detailed definitions of categories, observers often are faced with making numerous on-the-spot inferences. Virtually all category systems require observer inference, to greater or lesser degree.

> **Example of moderately low observer inference:**
> Tsai and colleagues (2011) examined factors that could predict osteoarthritic pain in elders, including nonverbal cues measured through observation. One predictor was motor patterns, which were videotaped in 10-minute sessions in which elders engaged in a set of activities. Observers coded for the presence of five behaviors (e.g., active rubbing of the knee or hip, joint flexion, rigidity) in 30-second intervals.

Category systems are the basis for constructing a **checklist**, which is the instrument observers use to record observations. The checklist is usually formatted with a list of behaviors from the category system on the left, and space for tallying the frequency or duration on the right. The task of the observer using an exhaustive category system is to place *all* observed behaviors in one category for each integral unit of behavior (e.g., a sentence in a conversation, a time interval). With nonexhaustive category systems, categories of behaviors that may or may not be manifested by participants are listed. The observer watches for instances of these behaviors and records their occurrence.

## Rating Scales

Another approach to structured observations is to use a **rating scale**, an instrument that requires observers to rate phenomena along a descriptive continuum. The observer may be required to make ratings of behavior at intervals throughout the observation or to summarize an entire event or transaction after observation is completed. Rating scales can be used as an extension of checklists, in which the observer records not only the occurrence of some behavior but also some qualitative aspect of it, such as its intensity. Although this approach yields a lot of information, the disadvantage is that it places an immense burden on observers.

> ### Example of observational ratings:
> The NEECHAM Confusion Scale, an observational instrument for recording the presence and severity of acute confusion, has subscales requiring behavioral ratings. For example, one rating in the Processing subscale concerns alertness/responsiveness; ratings are from 0 (responsiveness depressed) to 4 (full attentiveness). Ono and colleagues (2011) used NEECHAM scores as a measure of postoperative delirium in their study that tested the usefulness of bright light therapy after esophagectomy.

## Observational Sampling

Researchers must decide when to apply their structured observational systems. Observational sampling methods are a means of obtaining representative examples of the behaviors being observed. One system is **time sampling**, which involves the selection of time periods during which observations will occur. Time frames may be selected systematically (e.g., every 30 seconds at 2-minute intervals) or at random.

With **event sampling**, researchers select integral behaviors or events to observe. Event sampling requires researchers to either have knowledge about the occurrence of events (e.g., nursing shift changes) or be in a position to wait for their occurrence. Event sampling is preferable to time sampling when the events of interest are infrequent and may be missed if time sampling is used. When behaviors and events are relatively frequent, however, time sampling enhances the representativeness of the observed behaviors.

> ### Example of event and time sampling:
> In the previously mentioned observational study of nurse–patient communication in the ICU (Happ et al., 2011), events were first sampled (occasions of nurse–patient interaction), and then 3-minute segments of interaction on four separate occasions were videotaped and then coded for a range of outcomes (e.g., making eye contact, communication success).

## Evaluation of Observational Methods

Certain research questions are better suited to observation than to self-reports, such as when people cannot adequately describe their own behaviors. This may be the case when people are unaware of their own behavior (e.g., stress-induced behavior), when behaviors are emotionally laden (e.g., grieving), or when people are not capable of reporting their actions (e.g., young children). Observational methods have an intrinsic appeal for directly capturing behaviors. Often, nurses are in a position to watch people's behaviors and may, by training, be especially sensitive observers.

Shortcomings of observational methods include possible ethical problems and reactivity when the observer is conspicuous. One of the most pervasive problems, however, is the vulnerability of observations to bias. A number of factors interfere with objective observations, including the following:

- Emotions, prejudices, and values of the observer may lead to faulty inference.
- Personal views may color what observers see in the direction of what they want to see.
- Anticipation of what is to be observed may affect what is perceived.

Observational biases probably cannot be eliminated, but they can be minimized through careful observer training and assessment.

> ☞ **TIP:** As with self-report methods, structured observational methods require thorough pretesting and refinement.

## Biophysiologic Measures

Clinical nursing studies involve biophysiologic instruments both for creating independent variables (e.g., a biofeedback intervention) and for measuring dependent variables. Our discussion focuses on the use of biophysiologic measures as dependent (outcome) variables.

Nurse researchers have used biophysiologic measures for a wide variety of purposes. Examples include studies of basic biophysiologic processes, explorations of the ways in which nursing actions and interventions affect physiologic outcomes, product assessments, studies to evaluate the accuracy of biophysiologic information gathered by nurses, and studies of the correlates of physiologic functioning in patients with health problems.

Biophysiologic measures include both *in vivo* and *in vitro* measures. *In vivo* measures are those performed directly within or on living organisms, such as blood pressure, body temperature, and vital capacity measurement. Technological advances continue to improve the ability to measure biophysiologic phenomena more accurately and conveniently. With *in vitro* measures, data are gathered from participants by extracting biophysiologic material from them and subjecting it to analysis by specialized laboratory technicians. *In vitro* measures include chemical measures (e.g., the measurement of hormone levels); microbiologic measures (e.g., bacterial counts and identification); and cytologic or histologic measures (e.g., tissue biopsies).

> **Example of a study with *in vivo* and *in vitro* measures:**
> Yamamoto and Nagata (2011) examined the effects of a wrapped warm footbath to induce relaxation in patients with incurable cancer. The researchers measured heart rate variability to assess autonomic and sympathetic activities, and salivary cortisol to assess neuroimmunological parameters.

Biophysiologic measures offer a number of advantages to nurse researchers, including the following:

- ⊙ Biophysiologic measures are relatively accurate and precise, especially compared to psychological measures, such as self-report measures of anxiety or pain.
- ⊙ Biophysiologic measures are objective. Two nurses reading from the same spirometer output are likely to record identical tidal volume measurements, and two spirometers are likely to produce the same readouts.
- ⊙ Patients cannot easily distort measurements of biophysiologic functioning.
- ⊙ Biophysiologic instrumentation provides valid measures of targeted variables: thermometers can be relied on to measure temperature and not blood volume, and so forth. For nonbiophysiologic measures, there are typically concerns about whether an instrument is really measuring the target concept.

Biophysiologic measures are plentiful, tend to be accurate and valid, and are extremely useful in clinical nursing studies.

## Implementing the Data Collection Plan

Researchers must develop and implement a plan for gathering and recording the data. One important decision concerns who will collect the data. Researchers often hire assistants to collect data rather than collect it themselves, especially in large-scale quantitative studies.

From your perspective as a consumer, the critical issue is whether the people collecting data were able to produce valid and accurate data. Adequate training and monitoring of data collectors is essential. Also, blinding of data collectors (withholding information about study hypotheses or group assignments) is a good strategy in most quantitative studies.

Another issue concerns the circumstances under which data were gathered. For example, it may be critical to ensure privacy. In most cases, it is important for researchers to create a nonjudgmental atmosphere in which participants are encouraged to be candid or behave naturally. Again, you as a consumer must ask whether there is anything about the way in which the data were collected that could have created bias or otherwise affected data quality. In evaluating the data collection plan of a study, then, you should critically appraise not only the actual methods chosen but also the procedures used to collect and record the data.

## Critiquing Data Collection Methods

The goal of a data collection plan is to produce data that are of exceptional quality. Every decision researchers make about data collection methods and procedures can affect data quality, and hence the overall quality of the study.

It may, however, be difficult to critique data collection methods in studies reported in journals because researchers' descriptions are seldom detailed. Even though space constraints in journals make it impossible for researchers to fully elaborate their methods, however, researchers do have a responsibility to communicate basic information about their approach so that readers can assess the quality of evidence that the study yields.

Degree of structure is important in your assessment of a data collection plan. Researchers' decisions about structure are based on considerations that you can often evaluate, such as the status of knowledge on the topic (in a new area of inquiry, an unstructured approach may be preferred) and the nature of the research question. Another important issue is the *mix* of data collection approaches. Triangulation of methods (e.g., self-report and observation) is often extremely desirable. Finally, it is important to evaluate the actual procedures used to collect and record the data. This means giving consideration to who collected the data, how they were trained, whether formal instruments were adequately pretested, and whether efforts were made to reduce biases. Guidelines for critiquing data collection methods are presented in Box 10.2.

---

### Box 10.2 Guidelines for Critiquing Quantitative Data Collection Plans

1. Given the research question and characteristics of participants, did the researchers use the best method of capturing study phenomena (i.e., self-reports, observation, biophysiologic measures)? Was triangulation of methods used appropriately—that is, were multiple methods sensibly used?
2. Did the researchers make good data collection decisions with regard to structure, quantification, and objectivity?
3. If self-report methods were used, did the researchers make good decisions about the specific methods used to solicit information (e.g., in-person interviews, mailed questionnaires, and so on)? For structured self-reports, was there an appropriate mix of questions and composite scales?
4. Were efforts made to enhance data quality in collecting the self-report data (e.g., were efforts made to reduce or to evaluate response biases? Was the reading level of the instruments appropriate for self-administered questionnaires?)?

*(continued)*

> **Box 10.2   Guidelines for Critiquing Quantitative Data Collection Plans**
> **(Continued)**
>
> 5. If observational methods were used, did the report adequately describe what the observations entailed? Were risks of observational bias addressed? How much inference was required of the observers, and was this appropriate?
> 6. Were biophysiologic measures used in the study, and was this appropriate?
> 7. Did the report provide adequate information about data collection procedures? Were data collectors judiciously chosen and properly trained? Where and under what circumstances were data gathered? Were data gathered in a manner that promoted high-quality responses (e.g., in terms of privacy, efforts to put respondents at ease, etc.)?

## RESEARCH EXAMPLES WITH CRITICAL THINKING EXERCISES

In this section, we describe the sampling and data collection plan of a quantitative nursing study, followed by some questions to guide critical thinking.

Example 1 below is also featured in our *Interactive Critical Thinking Activity* on thePoint website where you can easily record, print, and e-mail your responses to the related questions.

### EXAMPLE 1 ● Sampling and Data Collection in a Quantitative Study

**Study:**  Family caregivers of hospitalized adults in Israel: A point-prevalence survey and exploration of tasks and motives (Auslander, 2011)

**Purpose:**  The purpose of this study was to examine the prevalence of family inpatient caregiving in acute care hospitals in Israel, to describe characteristics of caregivers and caregiving activities, and to examine the relationship between patient characteristics, caregiver characteristics, motivations for caregiving, and type and amount of caregiving activities.

**Design:**  The researchers collected data in a cross-sectional study of hospitalized patients and family caregivers. The design was descriptive correlational.

**Sampling:**  The sample consisted of adult family caregivers who provided care for patients during their hospitalization in six hospitals in central Israel. On a randomly selected week, a research coordinator gathered hospital record data about all eligible patients in three departments (internal medicine, surgery, and orthopedics) of the six hospitals. To be eligible for inclusion, patients had to be 18 years or older and hospitalized for at least 2 days. Tourists, foreign workers, and prisoners were excluded. A total of 1076 patients were identified in this manner. For each patient, a determination was made (via observations and patient questioning) regarding whether there was a family caregiver. A total of 744 patients had caregivers. All were invited to participate in the study, and 513 did so. Patients whose caregivers did or did not participate in the study were similar in terms of age, sex, ethnicity, residence, and length of stay. The total number in the sample exceeded the sample size that the researchers had estimated would be needed to yield sufficient statistical power.

**Data Collection:**  Background data and some clinical information (e.g., length of hospital stay) were obtained from the patients' charts. Information about the extent of in-hospital caregiving was obtained via observation. For each patient with a caregiver, observers recorded number of hours the caregiver and other family members spent in the hospital, frequency of visits, and whether the caregiver slept in the hospital. The researchers constructed a self-administered caregiver questionnaire that was developed on the basis of in-depth interviews with family caregivers and key informants, and pretested and refined in a pilot study with 200 families. The questionnaire included several composite scales, including one that measured various caregiving tasks and motivation for caregiving. The Motivation scale, for example, consisted of 29 items scored on 5 subscales. Respondents were asked the extent to which they agreed with each statement on a scale from 1 (not at all) to 5 (very much). Examples of items on this scale include: "I get satisfaction from being here" and "The staff expects family members to help."

**Key Findings:** Patients who lived further from the hospital were less likely to have family caregivers. Caregivers averaged 8 hours a day at the hospital. Their main motivation was the desire to help the patient. Factors that were related to the number of hours spent in caregiving were the patients' age, a caregiving motivation that involved the caregivers' peace of mind, and caregivers' own concerns about being separated from the patient.

## CRITICAL THINKING EXERCISES

1. Answer the relevant questions from Boxes 10.1 on page 183 and 10.2 on pages 193-94 regarding this study.
2. Also consider the following targeted questions:
    a. Are there variables in this study that could have been measured through observation, but were not?
    b. Where do you think this study belongs on an evidence hierarchy?
3. If the results of this study are valid and reliable, in what ways do you think the findings could be used in clinical practice?

## EXAMPLE 2 ● **Sampling and Data Collection in the Study in Appendix A**
● Read the method section from Howell and colleagues' (2007) study ("Anxiety, anger, and blood pressure in children") in Appendix A on page 395–402.

## CRITICAL THINKING EXERCISES

1. Answer the relevant questions from Boxes 10.1 on page 183 and 10.2 on pages 193-194 regarding this study.
2. Also consider the following targeted questions:
    a. What type of sampling plan might have improved the representativeness of the sample in this study?
    b. Identify some of the major potential sources of bias in the *sample*.
    c. Comment on factors that could have biased the *data* in this study.

**WANT TO KNOW MORE?** A wide variety of resources to enhance your learning and understanding of this chapter are available on thePoint.

- Interactive Critical Thinking Activity
- Chapter Supplement on Vignettes and Q-Sorts
- Answers to the Critical Thinking Exercises for Example 2
- Student Review Questions
- Full-text online
- Internet Resources with useful websites for Chapter 10

Additional study aids including eight journal articles and related questions are also available in *Study Guide for Essentials of Nursing Research, 8e.*

# SUMMARY POINTS

- **Sampling** is the process of selecting elements from a **population**, which is an entire aggregate of cases. An *element* is the basic unit of a population—usually humans in nursing research.

- **Eligibility criteria** (including both *inclusion criteria* and *exclusion criteria*) are used to define population characteristics.

- Researchers usually sample from an **accessible population**; a broader **target population** is the group to which they would like to generalize their results.

- A key criterion in assessing a sample in a quantitative study is its **representativeness**—the extent to which the sample is similar to the population and avoids bias. **Sampling bias** is the systematic overrepresentation or underrepresentation of some segment of the population.

- **Nonprobability sampling** (in which elements are selected by nonrandom methods) includes convenience, quota, consecutive, and purposive sampling. Nonprobability sampling is practical and economical; a major disadvantage is its potential for bias.

- **Convenience sampling** uses the most readily available or convenient group of people.

- **Quota sampling** divides the population into homogeneous **strata** (subpopulations) to ensure representation of the subgroups in the sample; within each stratum, people are sampled by convenience.

- **Consecutive sampling** involves taking *all* of the people from an accessible population who meet the eligibility criteria over a specific time interval, or for a specified sample size.

- In **purposive sampling**, participants are hand-picked to be included in the sample based on the researcher's knowledge about the population.

- **Probability sampling** designs, which involve the random selection of elements from the population, yield more representative samples than nonprobability designs and permit estimates of the magnitude of *sampling error*.

- **Simple random sampling** involves the random selection of elements from a **sampling frame** that enumerates all the elements; **stratified random sampling** divides the population into homogeneous subgroups from which elements are selected at random.

- **Systematic sampling** is the selection of every $k$th case from a list. By dividing the population size by the desired sample size, the researcher establishes the **sampling interval**, which is the standard distance between the selected elements.

- In quantitative studies, researchers can use a **power analysis** to estimate **sample size** needs. Large samples are preferable because they enhance statistical conclusion validity and tend to be more representative, but even large samples do not *guarantee* representativeness.

- Data collection methods vary in terms of structure, quantifiability, and objectivity. The three principal data collection methods for nurse researchers are self-reports, observations, and biophysiologic measures.

- **Self-reports**, which involve directly questioning study participants, are the most widely used method of collecting data for nursing studies.

- Structured self-reports for quantitative studies involve a formal *instrument*—a **questionnaire** or **interview schedule**—that may contain **open-ended questions** (which permit respondents to respond in their own words) and **closed-ended questions** (which offer respondents **response alternatives** from which to choose).

- Questionnaires are less costly than interviews and offer the possibility of anonymity, but interviews yield higher response rates, are suitable for a wider variety of people, and provide richer data than questionnaires.

- Social-psychological **scales** are self-report tools for quantitatively measuring such characteristics as attitudes, needs, and perceptions along a continuum.

- **Likert scales** (or **summated rating scales**) present respondents with a series of *items* worded favorably or unfavorably toward a phenomenon; responses indicating level of agreement or disagreement with each statement are scored and summed into a composite score.

- A **visual analog scale (VAS)** is used to measure subjective experiences (e.g., pain, fatigue) along a 100-mm line designating a bipolar continuum.

- Scales are versatile and powerful but are susceptible to **response set biases**—the tendency of some people to respond to items in characteristic ways, independently of item content.

- **Observational methods** are techniques for acquiring data through the direct observation of phenomena.

- Structured observations dictate what the observer should observe; they often involve **checklists**—tools based on **category systems** for recording the appearance, frequency, or duration of prespecified behaviors or events. Observers may also use **rating scales** to rate phenomena along a dimension of interest (e.g., intensity).

- Structured observations often use a sampling plan (such as **time sampling** or **event sampling**) for selecting the behaviors, events, and conditions to be observed.

- Observational techniques are a versatile and important alternative to self-reports, but observational biases can pose a threat to the validity and accuracy of observational data.

- Data may also be derived from **biophysiologic measures**, which include *in vivo* measurements (those performed within or on living organisms) and *in vitro* measurements (those performed outside the organism's body, such as blood tests). Biophysiologic measures have the advantage of being objective, accurate, and precise.

- In developing a data collection plan, the researcher must decide who will collect the data, how the data collectors will be trained, and what the circumstances for data collection will be.

# REFERENCES FOR CHAPTER 10

Auslander, G. K. (2011). Family caregivers of hospitalized adults in Israel: A point-prevalence survey and exploration of tasks and motives. *Research in Nursing & Health, 34*, 204–217.

Castro, K., Bevans, M., Miller-Davis, X., Cusack, G., Loscalzo, F., Matlock, A., et al. (2011). Validating the clinical research nursing domain of practice. *Oncology Nursing Forum, 38*, E72–E80.

Davidson, P., Salamonson, Y., Rolley, J., Everett, B., Fernandez, R., Andrew, S., et al. (2011). Perception of cardiovascular risk following a percutaneous coronary intervention. *International Journal of Nursing Studies, 48*, 973–978.

Forni, C., Loro, L., Tremosini, M., Mini, S., Pignotti, E., Bigoni, O., et al. (2011). Use of polyurethane foam inside plaster casts to prevent the onset of heel sores in the population at risk. *Journal of Clinical Nursing, 20*, 675–680.

Garten, L., Maass, E., Schmalisch, G., & Buhrer, C. (2011). O father, where art thou? Parental NICU visiting patterns during the first 28 days of life of very low-birth-weight infants. *Journal of Perinatal & Neonatal Nursing, 25*, 342–348.

Gillespie, B., Chaboyer, W., & Wallis, M. (2009). The influence of personal characteristics on the resilience of operating room nurses. *International Journal of Nursing Studies, 46*, 968–976.

Happ, M. B., Garrett, K., Thomas, D., Tate, J., George, E., Houze, M., et al. (2011). Nurse-patient communication interactions in the intensive care unit. *American Journal of Critical Care, 20*, e28–e40.

Hung, C., Lin, C., Stocker, J., & Yu, C. (2011). Predictors of postpartum stress. *Journal of Clinical Nursing, 20*, 666–674.

Krichbaum, K., Peden-McAlpine, C., Diemart, C., Koenig, P., Mueller, C., & Savik, K. (2011). Designing a measure of complexity compression in registered nurses. *Western Journal of Nursing Research, 33,* 7–25.

Kvitvaer, B., Miller, J., & Newell, D. (2012). Improving our understanding of the colicky infant. *Journal of Clinical Nursing, 21,* 63–69.

Matilla, E., Kaunonen, M., Aalto, P., Ollikainen, J., & Astedt-Kutki, P. (2010). Support for hospital patients and associated factors. *Scandinavian Journal of Caring Sciences, 24,* 734–745.

Morrison, B., & Ludington-Hoe, S. (2012). Interreuptions to breastfeeding dyads in an LDRP unit. *MCN:American Journal of Maternal/Child Nursing, 37,* 36–41.

Ono, H., Taguchi, T., Kido, Y., Fujino, Y., & Doki, Y. (2011). The usefulness of bright light therapy for patients after oesophagectomy. *Intensive and Critical Care Nursing, 27,* 158–166.

Radzvin, L. C. (2011). Moral distress in certified registered nurse anesthetists. *AANA Journal, 79,* 39–45.

Taavoni, S., Abdolahanian, S., Haghani, H., & Neysani, L. (2011). Effect of birth ball usage in the active phase of labor. *Journal of Midwifery & Women's Health, 56,* 137–140.

Tsai, P., Kuo, Y., Beck, C., Richards, K., Means, K., Pate, B., & Keefe, F. (2011). Nonverbal cues to osteoarthritis knee and/or hip pain in elders. *Research in Nursing & Health, 34,* 218–227.

Wu, L. J., Wu, M., Lien, G., Chen, F., & Tsai, J. (2012). Fatigue and physical activity levels in patients with liver cirrhosis. *Journal of Clinical Nursing, 21,* 129–138.

Yamamoto, K., & Nagata, S. (2011). Physiological and psychological evaluation of the wrapped warm footbath as a complementary nursing therapy to induce relaxation in hospitalized patients with incurable cancer. *Cancer Nursing, 34,* 185–192.

# 11 Measurement and Data Quality

## LEARNING OBJECTIVES

*On completing this chapter, you will be able to:*

- Describe the major characteristics of measurement and identify major sources of measurement error
- Describe aspects of reliability and validity, and specify how each aspect can be assessed
- Interpret the meaning of reliability and validity information
- Describe the function and meaning of sensitivity and specificity
- Evaluate the overall quality of a measuring tool used in a study
- Define new terms in the chapter

## KEY TERMS

| | | |
|---|---|---|
| Coefficient alpha | Interval measurement | Reliability |
| Construct validity | Interrater reliability | Reliability coefficient |
| Content validity | Level of measurement | Sensitivity |
| Content validity index (CVI) | Known-groups technique | Specificity |
| Criterion-related validity | Measurement | Test–retest reliability |
| Cronbach's alpha | Nominal measurement | True score |
| Error of measurement | Ordinal measurement | Validity |
| Factor analysis | Psychometric assessment | |
| Internal consistency | Ratio measurement | |

An ideal data collection procedure is one that captures a construct accurately, truthfully, and precisely. Few data collection procedures match this ideal perfectly. In this chapter, we discuss criteria for evaluating the quality of data obtained with structured instruments.

# MEASUREMENT

Quantitative studies derive data by measuring variables, and so we begin by discussing the concept of measurement.

## What is Measurement?

Early American psychologist L. L. Thurstone made a famous statement: "Whatever exists, exists in some amount and can be measured." **Measurement** involves rules for assigning numbers to objects or people to designate the *quantity* of an attribute. Attributes do not have inherent numeric values; humans invent rules to measure them. Attributes are not constant; they vary from day to day or from one person to another. This variability can be expressed numerically to signify *how much* of an attribute is present.

Measurement requires numbers to be assigned according to *rules*. Rules for measuring temperature and weight, for example, are familiar to us. Rules for measuring many variables for nursing studies, however, have to be created. Whether data are collected by observation, self-report, or any other method, researchers specify the criteria according to which numbers are to be assigned.

## Advantages of Measurement

Measurement removes guesswork and ambiguity in gathering and communicating information. Consider how handicapped health-care professionals would be without measures of body temperature, blood pressure, and so on. Because measurement has explicit rules, the resulting information tends to be objective; that is, it can be independently verified. Two people measuring the weight of a person using the same scale 5 minutes apart would get identical results. Not all measures are completely objective, but most have mechanisms for minimizing subjectivity.

Measurement also makes it possible to obtain reasonably precise information. Instead of describing Nathan as "tall," we can depict him as being 6 feet 3 inches tall. If necessary, we could achieve greater precision. Such precision allows researchers to make fine distinctions among people with different amounts of an attribute.

Measurement is a language of communication. Numbers are less vague than words and can communicate information clearly. If a researcher reported that the average temperature of a sample of patients was "somewhat high," different readers might have different interpretations, but if the researcher reported an average temperature of 99.6°F, there is no ambiguity.

## Levels of Measurement

In this chapter, we discuss how measurements can be evaluated. In the next chapter we consider what researchers *do* with measurements in their analyses. Statistical operations depend on a variable's **level of measurement**. There are four major classes, or levels, of measurement.

**Nominal measurement**, the lowest level, involves using numbers simply to categorize attributes. Gender and blood type are examples of nominally measured variables. The numbers used in nominal measurement do not have quantitative meaning. If we coded males as 1 and females as 2, the numbers have no quantitative implication—the number 2 does not mean "more than" 1. Nominal measurement provides information only about categorical equivalence and so the numbers cannot be treated mathematically. It makes no sense, for example, to compute a sample's average gender by adding all numeric values and dividing by the number of participants.

**Ordinal measurement** ranks people based on relative standing on an attribute. For example, consider this ordinal coding scheme for measuring ability to perform activities of daily living (ADL): 1 = completely dependent, 2 = needs another person's assistance, 3 = needs mechanical assistance, and 4 = completely independent. The numbers signify incremental ability to perform ADL independently. Ordinal measurement does not, however, tell us how much greater one level is than another. For example, we do not know if being completely independent is twice as good as needing mechanical assistance. As with nominal measures, the mathematic operations permissible with ordinal-level data are restricted.

Interval measurement occurs when researchers can rank people on an attribute *and* specify the distance between them. Most psychological tests yield interval-levels measures. For example, the Stanford-Binet intelligence test—a standardized IQ test—is an interval measure. A score of 140 on the test is higher than 120, which, in turn, is higher than 100. Moreover, the difference between 140 and 120 is equivalent to the difference between 120 and 100. Interval measures can be averaged, and many statistical procedures require interval data.

Ratio measurement is the highest level. Ratio scales, unlike interval scales, have a meaningful zero and thus provide information about the absolute magnitude of the attribute. The Fahrenheit scale for measuring temperature (interval measurement) has an arbitrary zero point. Zero on the thermometer does not signify the absence of heat; it would be inappropriate to say that 60°F is twice as hot as 30°F. Many physical measures, however, are ratio measures with a real zero. A person's weight, for example, is a ratio measure. It is meaningful to say that someone who weighs 200 pounds is twice as heavy as someone who weighs 100 pounds. Statistical procedures suitable for interval data are also appropriate for ratio-level data.

> **Example of different measurement levels:**
> Buck and colleagues (2012) examined the relationship between self-care and health-related quality of life in older adults with heart failure. The study included nominal-level variables (gender, ethnicity), ordinal-level variables (education, NY Heart Association classification), interval-level variables (scores on the Self-care of Heart Failure Index, quality-of-life scores), and ratio-level measures (age, body mass index).

Researchers usually strive to use the highest levels of measurement possible because higher levels yield more information and are amenable to more powerful analyses.

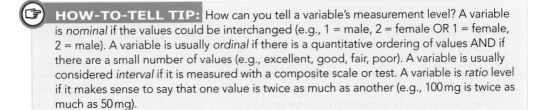

**HOW-TO-TELL TIP:** How can you tell a variable's measurement level? A variable is *nominal* if the values could be interchanged (e.g., 1 = male, 2 = female OR 1 = female, 2 = male). A variable is usually *ordinal* if there is a quantitative ordering of values AND if there are a small number of values (e.g., excellent, good, fair, poor). A variable is usually considered *interval* if it is measured with a composite scale or test. A variable is *ratio* level if it makes sense to say that one value is twice as much as another (e.g., 100 mg is twice as much as 50 mg).

## Errors of Measurement

Researchers work with fallible measures. The procedures used to take measurements and the people themselves are susceptible to influences that can alter the resulting data. We can think of every piece of quantitative data as consisting of two parts: a true component and an error component. This can be written as follows:

$$\text{Obtained score} = \text{True score} \pm \text{Error}$$

The *obtained* (or *observed*) *score* could be, for example, a patient's heart rate or score on an anxiety scale. The **true score** is the true value that would be obtained if it were possible to have an infallible measure. The true score is hypothetical—it cannot be known because measures are *not* infallible. The final term in the equation is the **error of measurement**. The difference between true and obtained scores is the result of distorting factors. Some errors are random, while others are systematic, representing a source of *bias*. Some common factors contributing to measurement error include

○ *Situational contaminants.* Scores can be affected by the conditions under which they are produced. For example, environmental factors (e.g., temperature, lighting, time of day) can introduce measurement error.

○ *Response-set biases.* Enduring characteristics of respondents can interfere with accurate measures (see Chapter 10).

○ *Transitory personal factors.* Temporary states such as fatigue, hunger, or mood can influence people's motivation or ability to cooperate, act naturally, or do their best.

○ *Item sampling.* Errors can reflect the sampling of items used to measure an attribute. For example, a student's score on a 100-item test of research methods will be influenced somewhat by *which* 100 questions are included.

This list is not exhaustive, but it illustrates that data are susceptible to measurement error from a variety of sources.

# RELIABILITY

The reliability of a quantitative measure is a major criterion for assessing its quality. **Reliability** is the consistency with which an instrument measures the attribute. If a scale weighed a person at 120 pounds 1 minute and 150 pounds the next, we would consider it unreliable. The less variation an instrument produces in repeated measurements, the higher its reliability.

Reliability also concerns accuracy. An instrument is reliable to the extent that it captures true scores. A reliable instrument maximizes the true score component and minimizes the error component of an obtained score.

Three aspects of reliability are of interest to quantitative researchers: stability, internal consistency, and equivalence.

## Stability

The *stability* of an instrument is the degree to which similar results are obtained on separate occasions. The reliability estimate focuses on the instrument's susceptibility to time-related influences, such as participant fatigue. Stability is assessed through **test–retest reliability** procedures. Researchers administer the measure to a sample twice and then compare the scores.

Suppose we were interested in the stability of a self-report self-esteem scale. Self-esteem is a fairly stable attribute, so we would expect a reliable measure of it to yield similar scores on two different days. To check the instrument's stability, we administer the scale 2 weeks apart to a sample of 10 people. Fictitious data for this example are presented in Table 11.1.

The scores on the two tests are not identical but most differences are small. Researchers compute a **reliability coefficient**, a numeric index that quantifies an instrument's reliability, to assess objectively how small the differences are. Reliability coefficients (designated as *r*) range from .00 to 1.00.* The higher the value, the more reliable (stable) is the measuring instrument. In the example shown in Table 11.1, the reliability coefficient is .95, which is high.

---

*Computation procedures for reliability coefficients are not presented in this textbook, but formulas can be found in Polit (2010). Although reliability coefficients can technically be less than .00 (i.e., a negative value), they are almost invariably a number between .00 and 1.00.

**TABLE 11.1　Fictitious Data for Test–Retest Reliability of Self-Esteem Scale**

| Subject Number | Time 1 | Time 2 | |
|:---:|:---:|:---:|:---:|
| 1 | 55 | 57 | |
| 2 | 49 | 46 | |
| 3 | 78 | 74 | |
| 4 | 37 | 35 | |
| 5 | 44 | 46 | |
| 6 | 50 | 56 | |
| 7 | 58 | 55 | |
| 8 | 62 | 66 | |
| 9 | 48 | 50 | |
| 10 | 67 | 63 | $r = .95$ |

**TIP:** Reliability coefficients higher than .70 are often considered adequate, but coefficients > .80 are far preferable.

Test–retest reliability is easy to compute, but one problem with this approach is that many traits do change over time, regardless of an instrument's stability. Attitudes, mood, and so forth can be changed by experiences between two measurements. Thus, stability indexes are most appropriate for fairly enduring characteristics, like temperament. Even with such traits, test–retest reliability tends to decline as the interval between the two administrations increases.

**Example of test–retest reliability:**
Hawthorne and colleagues (2011) assessed the stability of scores on the Spiritual Coping Strategies Scale. The 2-week test–retest reliability was .80 for the English version of the scale and .84 for the Spanish version.

## Internal Consistency

Composite scales and tests are usually evaluated for internal consistency. Most scales are composed of items that all measure one attribute and nothing else. On a scale to measure nurses' empathy, it would be inappropriate to include an item that measures resilience. An instrument is **internally consistent** to the extent that its items measure the same trait.

Internal consistency reliability is the most widely used reliability approach in nursing research. This approach is the best way to assess an important source of measurement error in scales, the sampling of items. Internal consistency is evaluated by calculating **coefficient alpha** (also called **Cronbach's alpha**). The normal range of values for this reliability index is from .00 to +1.00. The higher the coefficient, the more accurate (internally consistent) the measure.

> **Example of internal consistency reliability:**
> Abubakari and co-researchers (2012) evaluated the Illness Perception Questionnaire—Revised (IPQ-R), a scale that has been widely used with adults of European origin, but not evaluated with people from African cultures. In their study of 221 adults of African descent living in London, the internal consistency reliability on the seven subscales ranged from .61 to .90.

## Equivalence

*Equivalence*, in reliability assessment, primarily concerns the degree to which two or more independent observers or coders agree about scoring on an instrument. If there is a high level of agreement, then the assumption is that measurement errors have been minimized.

The degree of error can be assessed through **interrater** (or *interobserver*) **reliability** procedures, which involve having two or more observers or coders make independent observations. An index of agreement is then calculated with these data to evaluate the strength of the relationship between the ratings. When two independent observers score some phenomenon congruently, the scores are likely to be accurate and reliable.

> **Example of interrater reliability:**
> Kosits and Jones (2011) studied interruptions experienced by nurses in an emergency department. They developed an observational form to record nurses' tasks and types of interruption experiences. Interrater reliability was assessed and found to be very high (.825).

## Interpretation of Reliability Coefficients

Reliability coefficients are important indicators of data accuracy and quality. Unreliable measures reduce statistical power and hence lower statistical conclusion validity. If data fail to support a hypothesis, one possibility is that the instruments were unreliable—not necessarily that predicted relationships do not exist. Knowing an instrument's reliability is critical in interpreting research results, especially if research hypotheses are not supported.

Various things affect an instrument's reliability. For example, reliability is related to sample variability. The more homogeneous the sample (i.e., the more similar the scores), the lower the reliability coefficient will be. Scales are designed to measure differences, and if participants are similar to one another, it is more difficult for the scales to discriminate reliably among them. A depression scale is less reliable with a homeless group than with a general sample. Also, longer scales with more items tend to be more reliable than shorter ones.

Reliability estimates vary according to the procedure used to obtain them. Estimates of reliability computed by different procedures are not identical, and so it is important to consider which aspect of reliability is most important for the attribute being measured.

> **Example of different reliability estimates:**
> Pai and colleagues (2012) studied the relationship between sexual self-concept and sexual health behavior intentions among female adolescents in Taiwan. One scale they used was the Sexual Self-Concept Scale, which has three subscales: sexual arousability, sexual agency, and negative sexual affect. The internal consistency reliabilities of the three subscales were .92, .80, and .68, and the test–retest reliabilities were .74, .85, and .51, respectively.

☞ **TIP:** Many scales contain two or more subscales that tap distinct, but related, concepts (e.g., a measure of independent functioning might include subscales for motor activities, communication, and socializing). Subscale reliability typically is assessed and, if subscale scores are summed for an overall score, the scale's overall reliability would also be assessed.

# VALIDITY

The second major criterion for evaluating a quantitative instrument is its **validity**, the degree to which it measures what it is supposed to measure. When researchers develop a scale to measure hopelessness, how can they be sure that the scores validly reflect this construct and not something else, like depression?

Reliability and validity are not independent qualities of an instrument. *A measuring device that is unreliable cannot be valid.* An instrument cannot validly measure an attribute if it is erratic and inaccurate. An instrument can, however, be reliable without being valid. Suppose we had the idea to assess patients' anxiety by measuring the circumference of their wrists. We could obtain highly accurate measurements of wrist circumferences, but such measures would not be valid indicators of anxiety. Thus, an instrument's high reliability provides no evidence of its validity, but low reliability of a measure *is* evidence of low validity.

☞ **TIP:** Many studies are designed to evaluate the quality of instruments used by clinicians or researchers. In these **psychometric assessments**, information about the instrument's reliability and validity is carefully documented. As may be recalled from Chapter 2, an important evidence-based practice (EBP) question concerns diagnosis and assessment—whether tests yield accurate information for clinicians.

Like reliability, validity has several aspects, one of which is called face validity. *Face validity* refers to whether an instrument looks as though it is measuring the appropriate construct. Although it is good for an instrument to have face validity, three other aspects of validity are of greater importance: content validity, criterion-related validity, and construct validity.

## Content Validity

**Content validity** concerns the degree to which an instrument has an appropriate sample of items for the construct being measured. Researchers designing a new instrument should begin with a thorough conceptualization of the construct, so that the instrument can capture the full content domain. Such a conceptualization usually comes from a thorough literature review, a concept analysis, or findings from a qualitative inquiry.

An instrument's content validity is based on judgment. There are no totally objective methods for ensuring adequate content coverage, but often a panel of experts are asked to evaluate the content validity of new instruments. Researchers can calculate a **content validity index (CVI)** that indicates the extent of expert agreement. We suggest a CVI value of .90 or higher as the standard for establishing excellence in a scale's content validity.

> **Example of using a content validity index:**
> Mitchell and colleagues (2012) developed a scale to measure embarrassment as a barrier to colonoscopies. The content validity of their preliminary 26-item scale was assessed by three experts (two on colorectal screening and one on the concept of embarrassment). The scale's CVI was .93.

## Criterion-Related Validity

In **criterion-related validity** assessments, researchers examine the relationship between scores on an instrument and an external criterion. The instrument, whatever attribute it is measuring, is said to be valid if its scores correspond strongly with scores on the criterion. A **validity coefficient** is computed by using a mathematic formula that correlates the two scores. The magnitude of the coefficient is an estimate of the instrument's validity. These coefficients ($r$) range between .00 and 1.00, with higher values indicating greater criterion-related validity. Coefficients of .70 or higher are desirable.

Sometimes, a distinction is made between two types of criterion-related validity. *Predictive validity* is an instrument's ability to differentiate between people's performances on a *future* criterion. When a nursing school correlates students' high school grades with their subsequent grade-point averages, the predictive validity of high school grades for nursing school performance is being evaluated. *Concurrent validity* is an instrument's ability to distinguish among people who differ presently on a criterion. For example, a scale to differentiate between patients in a psychiatric hospital who could or could not be released could be correlated with nurses' contemporaneous behavioral ratings. The difference between predictive and concurrent validity is simply the timing of obtaining measurements on a criterion.

Validation via the criterion-related approach is most often used in applied situations. Criterion-related validity assists decision-makers by giving them some assurance that their decisions will be fair, appropriate, and, in short, valid.

> **Example of predictive validity:**
> Grossbach and Kuncel (2011) conducted a meta-analysis of 31 studies that examined the predictive validity of various nursing school admission variables for performance on the NCLEX-RN exam. Admissions tests (SAT and ACT) had good predictive validity, as did grades during baccalaureate degree nursing education.

## Construct Validity

As discussed in Chapter 9, **construct validity** is a key criterion for assessing research quality, and construct validity has most often been linked to measurement. Construct validity in measurement concerns these questions: What is this instrument *really* measuring? and Does it validly measure the abstract concept of interest? Construct validation is essentially a hypothesis-testing endeavor, typically linked to theoretical conceptualizations. In validating a measure of death anxiety, we would be less concerned with its relationship to a criterion than with its correspondence to a cogent conceptualization of death anxiety.

Construct validation can be approached in several ways, but it always involves logical analysis and testing relationships predicted on the basis of well-grounded conceptualizations. Constructs are explicated in terms of other abstract concepts; researchers make predictions about the manner in which the target construct will function in relation to other constructs.

One approach to construct validation is the **known-groups technique**. In this procedure, groups that are expected to differ on the target attribute are administered the instrument, and group scores are compared. For instance, in validating a measure of fear of the labor experience, the scores of primiparas and multiparas could be contrasted. On average, women who had never given birth would likely experience more anxiety than women who had already had children; one might question the validity of the instrument if such group differences did not emerge.

A similar method involves examining predicted relationships. Researchers might reason as follows: According to theory, construct X is related to construct Y; scales A and B are measures of constructs X and Y, respectively; scores on the two scales are related to each other, as predicted by the theory; therefore, it is inferred that A and B are valid measures of X and Y. This logical analysis is fallible, but offers supporting evidence.

Another approach to construct validation uses a statistical procedure called **factor analysis**, which is a method for identifying clusters of related items for a scale. Factor analysis identifies and groups together different measures into a unitary scale based on how participants reacted to the items, rather than based on the researcher's preconceptions.

In summary, construct validation employs logical and empirical procedures. Like content validity, construct validity requires judgments about what the instrument is measuring. Construct validity and criterion-related validity share an empirical component, but, in the latter case, there is a pragmatic, objective criterion with which to compare a measure rather than a second measure of an abstract theoretical construct.

**Example of construct validation:**

Gillespie, Polit and colleagues (2012) developed and tested the Perceived Perioperative Competence Scale. They used factor analysis to identify six distinct subscales, and tested hypotheses about the relationship between perceived competence and nurses' characteristics, such as years of experience.

## Interpretation of Validity

An instrument does not possess or lack validity; it is a question of degree. An instrument's validity is not proved or verified, but rather is supported to a greater or lesser extent by evidence.

Strictly speaking, researchers do not validate an instrument but rather an application of it. A measure of anxiety may be valid for presurgical patients but may not be valid for nursing students on the day of a test. Some instruments may be valid for a wide range of uses, but each use requires new supporting evidence. The more evidence that an instrument is measuring what it is supposed to be measuring, the more confidence people will have in its validity.

**TIP:** In quantitative studies, research reports usually provide validity and reliability information from an earlier study—often a study conducted by the researcher who developed the scale. If sample characteristics in the original study and the new study are similar, the citation provides valuable information about data quality in the new study. Ideally, researchers should also compute new reliability coefficients for the actual research sample.

# SENSITIVITY AND SPECIFICITY

Reliability and validity are key criteria for evaluating quantitative instruments, but for screening and diagnostic instruments—be they self-report, observational, or biophysiologic—sensitivity and specificity need to be evaluated.

**Sensitivity** is the ability of a measure to correctly identify a "case," that is, to correctly screen in or diagnosis a condition. A measure's sensitivity is its rate of yielding *true positives*. **Specificity** is the measure's ability to correctly identify noncases, that is, to screen *out* those without the condition. Specificity is an instrument's rate of yielding *true negatives*. To assess an instrument's sensitivity and specificity, researchers need a highly reliable and valid criterion of "caseness" against which scores on the instrument can be assessed.

To illustrate, suppose we wanted to test the accuracy of adolescents' self-reports about smoking, and we asked 100 teenagers whether they had smoked a cigarette in the previous 24 hours. The "gold standard" for nicotine consumption is cotinine levels in a body fluid, and so let us assume that we did a urinary cotinine assay. Some fictitious data are shown in Table 11.2.

Sensitivity, in this example, is calculated as the proportion of teenagers who said they smoked *and* who had high concentrations of cotinine, divided by all real smokers as indicated by the urine test. Put another way, it is the true positives divided by all *real* positives. In this case, there was underreporting of smoking and so the sensitivity of the self-report was only .50. Specificity is the proportion of teenagers who accurately reported they did not smoke, or the true negatives, divided by all *real* negatives. In our example, specificity is .83. There was much less overreporting of smoking ("faking bad") than underreporting ("faking good"). Sensitivity and specificity are sometimes reported as percentages rather than proportions, simply by multiplying the proportions by 100.

There is, unfortunately, a tradeoff between an instrument's sensitivity and specificity. When the sensitivity of a scale is increased to include more true positives, the number of false negatives increases. Thus, a critical task is to develop the appropriate *cutoff point*, that is, a score value to distinguish cases and noncases. Sophisticated procedures are used to make such a determination. It is difficult to set standards of acceptability for sensitivity and specificity. Both should be as high as possible, but the cutoff points may need to take into account the financial and emotional costs of having tests with false positive versus false negative results.

**TABLE 11.2  Fictitious Data to Illustrate Sensitivity and Specificity**

| Self-Reported Smoking | Urinary Cotinine Level | | Total |
| --- | --- | --- | --- |
| | Positive (Cotinine >200 ng/mL) | Negative (Cotinine 200 ng/mL) | |
| **Yes, smoked** | **A** (True positive) 20 | **B** (False positive) 10 | A+B 30 |
| **No, did not smoke** | **C** (False negative) 20 | **D** (True negative) 50 | C+D 70 |
| **TOTAL** | A+C ("Real" positives) 40 | B+D ("Real" negatives) 60 | A+B+C+D 100 |

Sensitivity = A/(A+C) = .50
Specificity = D/ (B+D) = .83

☞ **TIP:** In assessing evidence regarding the accuracy of diagnostic or assessment tests (Diagnosis questions, as shown in Table 1.3, p. 14), Level I evidence comes from systematic reviews of diagnostic studies with certain design features. Level II designs for Diagnosis questions are described in the Chapter Supplement on the**Point** website.

# CRITIQUING DATA QUALITY IN QUANTITATIVE STUDIES

If data are seriously flawed, the study cannot contribute useful evidence. In drawing conclusions about a study and its evidence, it is important to consider whether researchers have collected data that accurately reflect reality. Research consumers must ask: Can I trust the data? Do the data accurately and validly reflect the concepts under study?

Information about data quality should be provided in every quantitative research report. Reliability estimates are easy to communicate and are often reported. Ideally—especially for composite scales—the report should provide reliability coefficients based on data from the study itself, not just from previous research. Interrater or interobserver reliability is especially crucial for assessing data quality in observational studies. The values of the reliability coefficients should be sufficiently high to support confidence in the findings.

Validity is more difficult to document than reliability. At a minimum, researchers should defend their choice of existing measures based on validity information from the developers, and they should cite the relevant publication. If a study used a screening or diagnostic measure, information should also be provided about its sensitivity and specificity. Box 11.1 provides some guidelines for critiquing aspects of data quality of quantitative measures.

---

**BOX 11.1   Guidelines for Critiquing Data Quality in Quantitative Studies**

1. Does the report offer evidence of the reliability of measures? Does the evidence come from the research sample itself, or is it based on other studies? If the latter, is it reasonable to conclude that data quality would be similar for the research sample as for the reliability sample (e.g., are sample characteristics similar)?
2. If reliability is reported, which estimation method was used? Was this method appropriate? Should an alternative or additional method of reliability appraisal have been used? Is the reliability sufficiently high?
3. Does the report offer evidence of the validity of the measures? Does the evidence come from the research sample itself, or is it based on other studies? If the latter, is it reasonable to believe that data quality would be similar for the research sample as for the validity sample (e.g., are the sample characteristics similar)?
4. If validity information is reported, which validity approach was used? Was this method appropriate? Does the validity of the instrument appear to be adequate?
5. If there is no reliability or validity information, what conclusion can you reach about the quality of the data in the study?
6. If a diagnostic or screening tool was used, is information provided about its sensitivity and specificity, and were these qualities adequate?
7. Were the research hypotheses supported? If not, might data quality play a role in the failure to confirm the hypotheses?

## RESEARCH EXAMPLES WITH CRITICAL THINKING EXERCISES

In this section, we provide details about the development and testing of an instrument, followed by some questions to guide critical thinking.

☼ Example 1 below is also featured in our *Interactive Critical Thinking Activity* on thePoint website where you can easily record, print, and e-mail your responses to the related questions.

## EXAMPLE 1 ● Instrument Development and Psychometric Assessment

**Studies:** Postpartum Depression Screening Scale (PDSS): Development and psychometric testing (Beck & Gable, 2000); Further validation of the PDSS (Beck & Gable, 2001). ☼

**Background:** Beck had studied postpartum depression (PPD) in several qualitative studies. Based on her in-depth understanding of PPD, she created a scale to screen for PPD, the PDSS. Working with Gable, a psychometrician, Beck developed, refined, and validated the scale, and had it translated into Spanish.

**Scale Development:** The PDSS is a Likert scale tapping seven dimensions, such as sleeping/eating disturbances and mental confusion. A 56-item pilot form of the PDSS was initially developed. Beck's findings from her research on PPD and her knowledge of the literature were used to specify the domain and draft items.

**Content Validity:** Content validity was enhanced by using direct quotes from the qualitative studies as scale items (e.g., "I felt like I was losing my mind"). The pilot scale was subjected to content validation, and feedback from experts led to some revisions.

**Construct Validity:** The PDSS was administered to a sample of 525 new mothers in six states (Beck & Gable, 2000). The PDSS was finalized as a 35-item scale with seven subscales, each with five items. This version of the PDSS was subjected to factor analyses, which involved a validation of Beck's hypotheses about how individual items mapped onto underlying constructs. In a subsequent study, Beck and Gable (2001) administered the PDSS and other depression scales to 150 new mothers and tested hypotheses about how scores on the PDSS would correlate with scores on other scales, and these analyses suggested good construct validity.

**Criterion-Related Validity:** In the second study, Beck and Gable correlated scores on the PDSS with an expert clinician's diagnosis of PPD for each woman. The validity coefficient was .70.

**Internal Consistency:** In both studies, Beck and Gable found that the internal consistency reliability of the PDSS subscales was high, ranging from .83 to .94 in the first study and from .80 to .91 in the second study.

**Sensitivity and Specificity:** In the second validation study, Beck and Gable assessed the scale's sensitivity and specificity at different cutoff points, using the clinician's diagnosis to establish true positives and true negatives for PPD. The clinician diagnosed 46 of the 150 mothers as having major or minor depression. To illustrate tradeoffs in specificity and sensitivity, the researchers found that a cutoff score of 95 on the PDSS yielded a sensitivity of .41 (only 41% of the women actually diagnosed with PPD would be identified) but a specificity of 1.00 (all cases *without* an actual PPD diagnosis would be accurately screened out). At the other extreme, a cutoff score of 45 had a 1.00 sensitivity but only .28 specificity (i.e., 72% false positive), an unacceptable rate of overdiagnosis. Beck and Gable recommended a cutoff score of 60 for major or minor depression, which would accurately screen in 91% of PPD cases, and would mistakenly screen in 28% who do not have PPD. Using this cutoff point, 85% of their sample would have been correctly classified.

**Spanish Translation:** Beck (Beck & Gable, 2003, 2005) collaborated with translation experts to develop a Spanish version of the PDSS. The alpha reliability coefficient was .95 for the total Spanish scale, and ranged from .76 to .90 for the subscales. (Note: The PDSS has also been translated into Chinese (Li et al., 2011)).

## CRITICAL THINKING EXERCISES

1. Answer the relevant questions from Box 11.1 on page 209 regarding this study.
2. Also consider the following targeted questions:
   a. What is the level of measurement of scores on the PDSS?
   b. The researchers determined that there should be seven subscales to the PDSS. Why do you think this might be the case?
   c. Each item on the PDSS is scored on a 5-point scale from 1 to 5. What is the range of possible scores on the scale, and what is the range of possible scores on each subscale?
   d. Comment on the researchers' credentials for undertaking this study together, and on the appropriateness of their overall effort.
3. In what ways do you think the scale could be used in clinical practice?

## EXAMPLE 2 ● Measurement and Data Quality in the Study in Appendix A

Read the "Instruments" subsection from Howell and colleagues' (2007) study ("Anxiety, anger, and blood pressure in children") in Appendix A on page 395–402.

## CRITICAL THINKING EXERCISES

1. Answer the relevant questions from Box 11.1 on page 209 regarding this study.
2. Also consider the following targeted questions:
   a. What are some potential sources of measurement error in the measurement of trait anger, trait anxiety, and anger expression in this study?
   b. What is the level of measurement of the key variables in this study?

---

**WANT TO KNOW MORE?** A wide variety of resources to enhance your learning and understanding of this chapter are available on thePoint.

- Interactive Critical Thinking Activity
- Chapter Supplement on Level II Evidence for Diagnosis Questions
- Answers to the Critical Thinking Exercises for Example 2
- Student Review Questions
- Full-text online
- Internet Resources with useful websites for Chapter 11

Additional study aids including eight journal articles and related questions are also available in *Study Guide for Essentials of Nursing Research, 8e.*

# SUMMARY POINTS

- **Measurement** involves the assignment of numbers to objects or people to represent the amount of an attribute, using a set of rules.

- There are four **levels of measurement**: (1) **nominal measurement**—the classification of attributes into mutually exclusive categories; (2) **ordinal measurement**—the ranking of people based on their relative standing on an attribute; (3) **interval measurement**—indicating not only people's rank order but the distance between them; and (4) **ratio measurement**—distinguished from interval measurement by having a rational zero point.

- *Obtained scores* from an instrument consist of a **true score** component (the value that would be obtained for a hypothetical perfect measure of the attribute) and an error component, or **error of measurement**, that represents measurement inaccuracies.

- Sources of measurement error include situational contaminants, response-set biases, item sampling, and transitory personal factors, such as fatigue.

- **Reliability**, a primary criterion for assessing a quantitative instrument, is the degree of consistency or accuracy with which an instrument measures an attribute. The higher the reliability of an instrument, the lower the amount of error in obtained scores.

- There are different methods for assessing an instrument's reliability and for computing a **reliability coefficient**. Reliability coefficients typically range from .00 to 1.00, and should be at least .70 (but preferably > .80) to be considered satisfactory.

- The *stability* aspect of reliability, which concerns the extent to which an instrument yields similar results on two administrations, is evaluated by **test–retest procedures**.

- **Internal consistency** reliability, which refers to the extent to which all the instrument's items are measuring the same attribute, is usually assessed with **Cronbach's alpha**.

- When the reliability assessment focuses on *equivalence* between observers or coders assigning scores, estimates of **interrater** (or *interobserver*) **reliability** are obtained.

- **Validity** is the degree to which an instrument measures what it is supposed to measure.

- **Content validity** concerns the sampling adequacy of the content being measured. Expert ratings on the relevance of items can be used to compute a **content validity index** (**CVI**).

- **Criterion-related validity** (which includes both *predictive validity* and *concurrent validity*) focuses on the correlation between an instrument and an outside criterion.

- **Construct validity**, an instrument's adequacy in measuring the targeted construct, involves hypothesis-testing. One construct validation method, the **known-groups technique**, contrasts scores of groups hypothesized to differ on the attribute; another is **factor analysis**, a statistical procedure that identifies items that "go together."

- Sensitivity and specificity are important criteria for screening and diagnostic instruments. **Sensitivity** is the instrument's ability to identify a case correctly (i.e., its rate of yielding true positives). **Specificity** is the instrument's ability to identify noncases correctly (i.e., its rate of yielding true negatives).

- A **psychometric assessment** of a new instrument is undertaken with most scales to gather evidence about validity, reliability, and other assessment criteria.

# REFERENCES FOR CHAPTER 11

Abubakari, A., Jones, M., Lauder, W., Kirk, A., Devendra, D., & Anderson, J. (2012). Psychometric properties of the Revised Illness Perception Questionnaire: Factor structure and reliability among African-origin populations with type 2 diabetes. *International Journal of Nursing Studies, 49*(6), 672–681.

Beck, C. T., & Gable, R. K. (2000). Postpartum Depression Screening Scale: Development and psychometric testing. *Nursing Research, 49*, 272–282.

Beck, C. T., & Gable, R. K. (2001). Further validation of the Postpartum Depression Screening Scale. *Nursing Research, 50*, 155–164.

Beck, C. T., & Gable, R. K. (2003). Postpartum Depression Screening Scale: Spanish version. *Nursing Research, 52*, 296–306.

Beck, C. T., & Gable, R. K. (2005). Screening performance of the Postpartum Depression Screening Scale—Spanish version. *Journal of Transcultural Nursing, 16*(4), 331–338.

Buck, H., Lee, C., Moser, D., Albert, N., Lennie, T., Bentley, B., et al. (2012). Relationship between self-care and health-related quality of life in older adults with moderate to advanced heart failure. *Journal of Cardiovascular Nursing, 27*, 8–15.

Gillespie, B., Polit, D., Hamlin, L., & Chaboyer, W. (2012). Developing a model of competence in the operating theater: Psychometric validation of the perceived perioperative competence scale-revised. *International Journal of Nursing Studies, 49*, 90–101.

Grossbach, A., & Kuncel, N. (2011). The predictive validity of nursing admission measures for performance on the National Council Licensure Examination. *Journal of Professional Nursing, 27*, 124–128.

Hawthorne, D., Youngblut, J., & Brooten, D. (2011). Psychometric evaluation of the Spanish and English versions of the Spiritual Coping Strategies Scale. *Journal of Nursing Measurement, 19*, 46–54.

Kosits, L., & Jones, K. (2011). Interruptions experienced by registered nurses working in the emergency department. *Journal of Emergency Nursing, 37*, 3–8.

Li, L., Liu, F., Zhang, H., Wang, L., & Chen, X. (2011). Chinese version of the Postpartum Depression Screening Scale. *Nursing Research, 60*, 231–239.

Mitchell, K., Rawl, S., Champion, V., Jeffries, P., & Welch, J. (2012). Development and psychometric testing of the Colonoscopy Embarrassment Scale. *Western Journal of Nursing Research, 34*(4), 548–564.

Pai, H.C., Lee, S., & Yen, W. (2012). The effect of sexual self-concept on sexual health behaviour intentions. *Journal of Advanced Nursing, 68*, 47–55.

Polit, D. F. (2010). *Statistics and data analysis for nursing research* (2nd ed.). Upper Saddle River, NJ: Pearson.

## LEARNING OBJECTIVES

**On completing this chapter, you will be able to:**

- Describe characteristics of frequency distributions, and identify and interpret various descriptive statistics
- Describe the logic and purpose of parameter estimation, and interpret confidence intervals
- Describe the logic and purpose of statistical tests, and interpret *p* values
- Specify the appropriate applications for *t*-tests, analysis of variance, chi-squared tests, and correlation coefficients, and interpret the meaning of the calculated statistics
- Understand the results of simple statistical procedures described in a research report
- Define new terms in the chapter

## KEY TERMS

| | | |
|---|---|---|
| Absolute risk (AR) | Hypothesis testing | *r* |
| Absolute risk reduction (ARR) | Inferential statistics | *R²* |
| Alpha (α) | Level of significance | Range |
| Analysis of covariance (ANCOVA) | Logistic regression | Repeated measures ANOVA |
| | Mean | Risk ratio (RR) |
| Analysis of variance (ANOVA) | Median | Sampling distribution of the mean |
| Beta (β) | Mode | |
| Central tendency | Multiple regression | Skewed distribution |
| Chi-squared test | Multivariate statistics | Standard deviation |
| Confidence interval (CI) | *N* | Standard error of the mean (SEM) |
| Correlation | Negative relationship | |
| Correlation coefficient | Negative skew | Statistical test |
| Correlation matrix | Nonsignificant result (NS) | Statistically significant |
| Crosstabulation | Odds ratio (OR) | Symmetric distribution |
| *d* statistic | *p* value | Test statistic |
| Degrees of freedom | Pearson's *r* | *t*-test |
| Descriptive statistics | Positive relationship | Type I error |
| Effect size | Positive skew | Type II error |
| *F* ratio | Post hoc test | Variability |
| Frequency distribution | Predictor variable | |

Data collected in a study need to be systematically analyzed. This chapter describes procedures for using statistics to analyze quantitative data.

👉 **TIP:** Although the thought of learning about statistics may be anxiety provoking, consider Florence Nightingale's view of statistics: "To understand God's thoughts we must study statistics, for these are the measure of His purpose."

# DESCRIPTIVE STATISTICS

Statistical procedures enable researchers to organize and interpret numeric information. Statistics are either descriptive or inferential. **Descriptive statistics** are used to synthesize and describe data. When indexes such as averages and percentages are calculated with data from a population, they are **parameters**. A descriptive index from a sample is a **statistic**. Most research questions are about parameters; researchers calculate statistics to estimate parameters and use **inferential statistics** to make inferences about the population.

A set of data for a variable can be described in terms of three characteristics: the shape of the distribution of values, central tendency, and variability.

## Frequency Distributions

Data that are not organized are overwhelming. Without some structure, even broad trends are hard to discern. Consider the 60 numbers in Table 12.1. Let us assume that these numbers are the scores of 60 preoperative patients on a six-item scale of anxiety. Visual inspection of these numbers provides little insight on patients' anxiety.

Frequency distributions impose order on numeric data. A **frequency distribution** is a systematic arrangement of values from lowest to highest, together with a count or percentage of how many times each value occurred. A frequency distribution for the 60 anxiety scores (Table 12.2, p. 128) makes it easy to see the highest and lowest scores, the most common score, where the scores clustered, and how many patients were in the sample (total sample size is designated as *N* in research reports). None of this was apparent before the data were organized.

**TABLE 12.1  Patients' Anxiety Scores**

| | | | | | | | | | |
|----|----|----|----|----|----|----|----|----|----|
| 22 | 27 | 25 | 19 | 24 | 25 | 23 | 29 | 24 | 20 |
| 26 | 16 | 20 | 26 | 17 | 22 | 24 | 18 | 26 | 28 |
| 15 | 24 | 23 | 22 | 21 | 24 | 20 | 25 | 18 | 27 |
| 24 | 23 | 16 | 25 | 30 | 29 | 27 | 21 | 23 | 24 |
| 26 | 18 | 30 | 21 | 17 | 25 | 22 | 24 | 29 | 28 |
| 20 | 25 | 26 | 24 | 23 | 19 | 27 | 28 | 25 | 26 |

**TABLE 12.2  Frequency Distribution of Patients' Anxiety Scores**

| Score | Frequency | Percentage (%) |
|---|---|---|
| 15 | 1 | 1.7 |
| 16 | 2 | 3.3 |
| 17 | 2 | 3.3 |
| 18 | 3 | 5.0 |
| 19 | 2 | 3.3 |
| 20 | 4 | 6.7 |
| 21 | 3 | 5.0 |
| 22 | 4 | 6.7 |
| 23 | 5 | 8.3 |
| 24 | 9 | 15.0 |
| 25 | 7 | 11.7 |
| 26 | 6 | 10.0 |
| 27 | 4 | 6.7 |
| 28 | 3 | 5.0 |
| 29 | 3 | 5.0 |
| 30 | 2 | 3.3 |
| | N = 60 | 100.0% |

Frequency data can be displayed graphically in a *frequency polygon* (Fig. 12.1). In such graphs, scores typically are on the horizontal line, with the lowest value on the left, and frequency counts or percentages are on the vertical line. Data distributions can be described by their shapes. **Symmetric distribution** occurs if, when folded over, the two halves of a frequency polygon would be superimposed (Fig. 12.2). In an asymmetric or **skewed distribution**, the peak is off center, and one tail is longer than the other. When the longer tail points to the right, the distribution has a **positive skew**, as in the first graph of Figure 12.3. Personal income is a positively skewed attribute. Most people have moderate incomes, with only a few people with very high incomes at the right end of the distribution. If the longer tail points to the left, the distribution has a **negative skew**, as in the second graph in Figure 12.3. Age at death is negatively skewed: the bulk of people are at the far right end of the distribution, with relatively few people dying at an early age.

Another aspect of a distribution's shape concerns how many peaks it has. A *unimodal distribution* has one peak (graph A of Figure 12.2), whereas a *multimodal distribution* has two or more peaks—that is, two or more values of high frequency. A multimodal distribution with two peaks is *bimodal* (graph B of Figure 12.2).

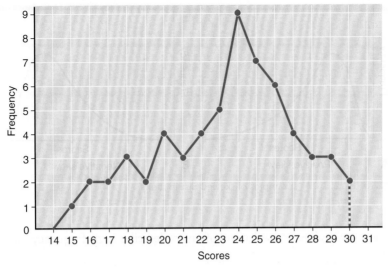

**FIGURE 12.1** ● Frequency polygon of patients' anxiety scores.

A special distribution called the **normal distribution** (*a bell-shaped curve*) is symmetric, unimodal, and not very peaked (graph A of Figure 12.2). Many human attributes (e.g., height, intelligence) approximate a normal distribution.

## Central Tendency

Frequency distributions help to clarify patterns, but often a pattern is less useful than an overall summary. Researchers usually ask a question such as, "What is the *average* oxygen consumption of myocardial infarction patients during bathing?" Such a question seeks a single number to represent a distribution of values. Indexes of "typicalness" are called measures of **central tendency**. Researchers avoid using the term *average* because there are three indexes of central tendency: the mode, the median, and the mean.

● **Mode:** The mode is the number that occurs most frequently in a distribution. In the following distribution, the mode is 53:

50 51 51 52 53 53 53 53 54 55 56

The value of 53 occurred four times, a higher frequency than for other numbers. The mode of the patients' anxiety scores in Table 12.2 was 24. The mode, which identifies the

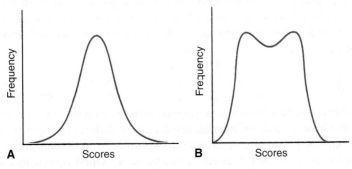

**FIGURE 12.2** ● Examples of symmetric distributions.

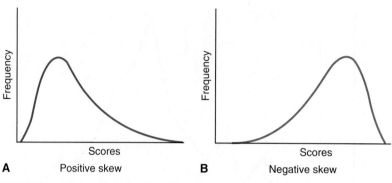

**FIGURE 12.3** ● Examples of skewed distributions.

most "popular" value, is used most often to describe high-frequency values for nominal measures.

● **Median**: The median is the point in a distribution that divides scores in half. Consider the following set of values:

2 2 3 3 4 5 6 7 8 9

The value that divides the cases in half is midway between 4 and 5, and thus 4.5 is the median. The median for the anxiety scores in Table 12.2 is 24, the same as the mode. The median does not take into account individual values and so is insensitive to extremes. In the above set of numbers, if the value of 9 were changed to 99, the median would remain 4.5. Because of this property, the median is the preferred index to describe a highly skewed distribution. In research articles, the median may be abbreviated as *Md* or *Mdn*.

● **Mean**: The mean equals the sum of all values divided by the number of participants—what people refer to as the average. The mean of the patients' anxiety scores is 23.4 (1,405 ÷ 60). As another example, here are the weights of eight people:

85 109 120 135 158 177 181 195

In this example, the mean is 145. Unlike the median, the mean is affected by the value of every score. If we exchanged the 195-lb person for one weighing 275 lb, the mean would increase from 145 to 155 lb. In research articles, the mean is often symbolized as $M$ or $\bar{X}$ (e.g., $\bar{X} = 145$).

For interval-level or ratio-level measurements, the mean is usually the statistic reported. Of the three indexes, the mean is the most stable: if repeated samples were drawn from a population, the means would fluctuate less than the modes or medians. Because of its stability, the mean usually is the best estimate of a population's central tendency. When a distribution is highly skewed, however, the median is preferred. For example, the median is a better central tendency measure of family income than the mean because income is positively skewed.

## Variability

Two distributions with identical means could differ with respect to shape (e.g., how skewed they are) and how spread out the data are (i.e., how different people are from one another on an attribute). This section describes the **variability** of distributions.

Consider the two distributions in Figure 12.4, which represent hypothetical scores for students from two schools on an IQ test. Both distributions have a mean of 100, but

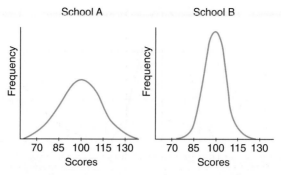

**FIGURE 12.4** ● Two distributions of different variability.

the patterns are different. School A has a wide range of scores, with some below 70 and some above 130. In school B, by contrast, there are few low or high scores. School A is more *heterogeneous* (i.e., more varied) than school B, and school B is more *homogeneous* than school A. Researchers compute an index of variability to express the extent to which scores in a distribution differ from one another. Two common indexes are the range and standard deviation.

○ **Range**: The range is the highest score minus the lowest score in a distribution. In our anxiety score example, the range is 15 (30–15). In the distributions in Figure 12.4, the range for school A is about 80 (140–60), whereas the range for school B is about 50 (125–75). The chief virtue of the range is ease of computation. Because it is based on only two scores, however, the range is unstable: from sample to sample drawn from a population, the range can fluctuate greatly. The range is used largely as a gross descriptive index.

○ **Standard deviation**: The most widely used variability index is the standard deviation. Like the mean, the standard deviation is calculated based on every value in a distribution. The standard deviation summarizes the *average* amount of deviation of values from the mean.[*] In the anxiety scale example, the standard deviation is 3.725.[**] In research reports, the standard deviation may be abbreviated as *s* or *SD*.

👉 **TIP:** Occasionally, *SD*s are shown in relation to the mean without a formal label. For example, the anxiety scores might be shown as *M* = 23.4 (3.7) or *M* = 23.4 ± 3.7, where 23.4 is the mean and 3.7 is the standard deviation.

A standard deviation (*SD*) is more difficult to interpret than the range. For the *SD* of anxiety scores, you might ask, 3.725 *what?* What does the number mean? We can answer these questions from several angles. First, the *SD* is an index of how variable scores in a distribution are and so if (for example) male and female patients had means of 23 on the anxiety scale, but their *SD*s were 7 and 3, respectively, we would know that females were more homogeneous (i.e., their scores were more similar to one another).

---

[*]Formulas for computing the standard deviation, as well as other statistics discussed in this chapter, are not shown in this textbook. The emphasis here is on helping you to understand statistical applications. Polit (2010) can be consulted for computation formulas.
[**]Another index of variability is the variance which is simply the value of the standard deviation squared. In the example of patients' anxiety scores, the variance is $3.725^2$, or 13.88.

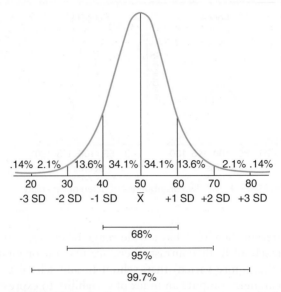

**FIGURE 12.5** ● Standard deviations in a normal distribution.

The *SD* represents the *average* of deviations from the mean. The mean tells us the best value for summarizing an entire distribution, and an *SD* tells us how much, on average, the scores deviate from the mean. In the anxiety scale example, scores deviated by an average of just under 4 points. A standard deviation can be interpreted as our degree of error when we use a mean to describe an entire sample.

In normal and near-normal distributions, there are roughly three *SD*s above and below the mean. For a normal distribution with a mean of 50 and an *SD* of 10 (Fig. 12.5), a fixed percentage of cases fall within certain distances from the mean. Sixty-eight percent of all cases fall within 1 *SD* above and below the mean. Thus, nearly 7 of 10 scores are between 40 and 60. In a normal distribution, 95% of the scores fall within 2 *SD*s of the mean. Only a handful of cases—about 2% at each extreme—lie more than 2 *SD*s from the mean. Using this figure, we can see that a person with a score of 70 achieved a higher score than about 98% of the sample.

☞ **TIP:** Descriptive statistics (percentages, means, standard deviations, and so on) are used for various purposes, but they are most often used to summarize sample characteristics, describe key research variables, and document methodological features (e.g., response rates). They are seldom used to answer research questions—inferential statistics usually are used for this purpose.

**Example of descriptive statistics:**
Table 12.3 presents descriptive statistics from Padden and colleagues' (2011) study of stress, coping, and well-being in military spouses during deployment separation. The table shows, for three self-report scale scores, the theoretical and actual range of scores, means, and *SD*s. We can see that the scale scores were heterogeneous, with wide ranges. Scores on the Health Survey appear skewed: the mean (69.6) was much higher than the midpoint between the lowest and highest value (42.5), suggesting a negative skew.

**TABLE 12.3 Example of Descriptive Statistics: Scores on Selected Scales of Stress, Coping, and Well-Being in Military Spouses During Deployment Separation ($N = 105$)[a]**

| | Scale Range | Range of Actual Scores | M (SD) |
|---|---|---|---|
| Perceived Stress Scale scores | 0–40 | 1–34 | 17.5 (6.6) |
| Jalowiec Coping Scale scores | 0–180 | 48–150 | 101.1 (19.1) |
| Rand Health Survey, total scores | 0–100 | 14–99 | 69.9 (17.9) |

[a]Adapted from Padden, D., Connors, R., & Agazia, J. (2011). Stress, coping, and well-being in military spouses during deployment separation. *Western Journal of Nursing Research, 33*, 247–267.

## Bivariate Descriptive Statistics

So far, our discussion has focused on *univariate* (one-variable) *descriptive statistics*. A mean or *SD* describe one variable at a time. *Bivariate* (two-variable) *descriptive statistics* describe relationships between two variables.

### Crosstabulations

A **crosstabs table** (or *contingency table*) is a two-dimensional frequency distribution in which the frequencies of two variables are **crosstabulated.** Suppose we had data on patients' sex and whether they were nonsmokers, light smokers (less than one pack of cigarettes a day), or heavy smokers (one or more packs a day). The question is whether men smoke more heavily than women, or vice versa (i.e., whether there is a *relationship* between smoking and sex). Fictitious data for this example are shown in Table 12.4. Six **cells** are created by placing one variable (sex) along one dimension and the other variable (smoking status) along the other dimension. After subjects' data are allocated to the appropriate cells, percentages are computed. The crosstab allows us to see at a glance that women were more likely than men

**TABLE 12.4 Crosstabs Table for Relationship Between Sex and Smoking Status**

| | Sex | | | | | |
|---|---|---|---|---|---|---|
| | Women | | Men | | Total | |
| **Smoking Status** | *n* | % | *n* | % | *n* | % |
| Nonsmoker | 10 | 45.4 | 6 | 27.3 | 16 | 36.4 |
| Light smoker | 8 | 36.4 | 8 | 36.4 | 16 | 36.4 |
| Heavy smoker | 4 | 18.2 | 8 | 36.4 | 12 | 27.3 |
| TOTAL | 22 | 100.0 | 22 | 100.0 | 44 | 100.0 |

to be nonsmokers (45.4% vs. 27.3%) and less likely to be heavy smokers (18.2% vs. 36.4%). Crosstabs are used with nominal data or ordinal data with few values. In this example, sex is nominal, and smoking, as defined, is ordinal.

## Correlation

Relationships between two variables can be described by **correlation** methods. The correlation question is: To what extent are two variables related to each other? For example, to what degree are anxiety scores and blood pressure values related? This question can be answered by calculating a **correlation coefficient**, which describes *intensity* and *direction* of a relationship.

Two variables that are related are height and weight: tall people tend to weigh more than short people. The relationship between height and weight would be a *perfect relationship* if the tallest person in a population was the heaviest, the second tallest person was the second heaviest, and so on. A correlation coefficient indicates how "perfect" a relationship is. Possible values for a correlation coefficient range from –1.00 through .00 to +1.00. If height and weight were perfectly correlated, the correlation coefficient would be 1.00 (the actual correlation coefficient is in the vicinity of .50 to .60 for a general population). Height and weight have a **positive relationship** because greater height tends to be associated with greater weight.

When two variables are unrelated, the correlation coefficient is zero. One might anticipate that women's shoe size is unrelated to their intelligence. Women with large feet are as likely to perform well on IQ tests as those with small feet. The correlation coefficient summarizing such a relationship would be in the vicinity of .00.

Correlation coefficients between .00 and –1.00 express a **negative** (*inverse*) **relationship**. When two variables are inversely related, increments in one variable are associated with decrements in the second. For example, there is a negative correlation between depression and self-esteem. This means that, on average, people with *high* self-esteem tend to be *low* on depression. If the relationship were perfect (i.e., if the person with the highest self-esteem score had the lowest depression score and so on), then the correlation coefficient would be –1.00. In actuality, the relationship between depression and self-esteem is moderate—usually in the vicinity of –.40 or –.50. Note that the higher the *absolute value* of the coefficient (i.e., the value disregarding the sign), the stronger the relationship. A correlation of –.80, for instance, is much stronger than a correlation of +.20.

The most commonly used correlation index is **Pearson's *r*** (the *product–moment correlation coefficient*), which is computed with interval or ratio measures. There are no fixed guidelines on what should be interpreted as strong or weak relationships, because it depends on the variables. If we measured patients' body temperature orally and rectally, an *r* of .70 between the two measurements would be low. For most psychosocial variables (e.g., stress and depression), however, an *r* of .70 would be high. Perfect correlations (+1.00 and –1.00) are rare.

> **TIP:** Validity coefficients, such as those described in Chapter 11, are usually calculated using Pearson's correlation coefficients.

In research articles, correlation coefficients are sometimes shown in a two-dimensional **correlation matrix**, in which variables are displayed in both rows and columns. To read a correlation matrix, one finds the row for one variable and reads across until the row intersects with the column for another variable, as described in the following example.

**Example of a correlation matrix:**

Greenslade and Jimmieson (2011) studied the relationship between organizational factors and patient satisfaction. They hypothesized that patient satisfaction is influenced by the setting in which they are treated. Table 12.5, adapted from their report, shows a correlation matrix for some of the variables. This table lists, on the left, four variables: Variable 1: the service climate of the nursing unit in which the patient was cared for, Variable 2: effectiveness of nurses' task performance (e.g., administering medications), Variable 3: effectiveness of nurses' contextual performance (e.g., making special arrangements for patients), and Variable 4: patient satisfaction. The numbers in the top row, from 1 to 4, correspond to the four variables: 1 is service climate, and so on. The correlation matrix shows, in column 1, the correlation coefficient between service climate and all variables. At the intersection of row 1-column 1, we find 1.00, which indicates that service climate scores are perfectly correlated with themselves. The next entry in column 1 is the value of $r$ between service climate and task performance. The value of .31 (which can be read as +.31) indicates a modest, positive relationship between these two variables: effective performance tends to be higher in units with a positive service climate. The bottom entry in column 1 shows a positive correlation between service climate and patient satisfaction (.42), indicating greater satisfaction in units with a positive service climate.

## Describing Risk

The evidence-based practice (EBP) movement has made decision-making based on research findings an important issue. Several descriptive indexes can be used to facilitate such decision-making. Many of these indexes involve calculating changes in risk—for example, a change in risk after exposure to a potentially beneficial intervention.

In this section, we focus on describing dichotomous outcomes (e.g., had a fall/did not have a fall) in relation to exposure or nonexposure to a beneficial treatment or protective factor. This situation results in a $2 \times 2$ crosstabs table with four cells. The four cells in the crosstabs table in Table 12.6 are labeled so that various indexes can be explained. *Cell a* is the number with an undesirable outcome (e.g., a fall) in an intervention/protected group; *cell b* is the number with a desirable outcome (e.g., no fall) in an intervention/protected group; and *cells c* and *d* are the two outcome possibilities for a nontreated or unprotected group. We can now explain the meaning and calculation of some indexes of interest to clinicians.

### Absolute Risk

Absolute risk can be computed for those exposed to an intervention or protective factor, and for those not exposed. **Absolute risk (AR)** is simply the proportion of people who

**TABLE 12.5  Example of a Correlation Matrix: Study of Organizational Factors Affecting Patient Satisfaction ($N = 172$)**

| Variable | 1 | 2 | 3 | 4 |
|---|---|---|---|---|
| 1. Service climate in nursing unit | 1.00 | | | |
| 2. Effectiveness of nurses' task performance | .31 | 1.00 | | |
| 3. Effectiveness of nurses' contextual performance | .22 | .52 | 1.00 | |
| 4. Global patient satisfaction | .42 | .49 | .26 | 1.00 |

Adapted from Table 1 of Greenslade, J., & Jimmieson, N. (2011). Organizational factors impacting on patient satisfaction. *International Journal of Nursing Studies, 48*, 1188–1198.

## TABLE 12.6   Indexes of Risk and Association in a 2 × 2 Table

| Exposure to an Intervention or Protective Factor | Outcome | | Total |
|---|---|---|---|
| | **Undesirable Outcome** | **Desirable Outcome** | |
| **Yes** (Exposed) | a | b | a + b |
| **No** (Not Exposed) | c | d | c + d |
| **TOTAL** | a + c | b + d | a + b + c + d |

Absolute Risk, exposed group ($AR_E$)   $= a / (a + b)$

Absolute Risk, non - exposed group ($AR_{NE}$)   $= c / (c + d)$

Absolute Risk Reduction (ARR)   $= (c / (c + d)) - (a / (a + b))$   Or $AR_{NE} - AR_E$

Odds Ratio (OR)   $= \dfrac{ad}{bc}$   Or $\dfrac{a/b}{c/d}$

experienced an undesirable outcome in each group. To illustrate, suppose 200 smokers were randomly assigned to a smoking cessation intervention or to a control group (Table 12.7). The outcome is smoking status 3 months after the intervention. In this example, the absolute risk of continued smoking is .50 in the intervention group and .80 in the control group. Without the intervention, 20% of those in the experimental group would presumably have stopped smoking anyway, but the intervention boosted the rate to 50%.

## TABLE 12.7   Hypothetical Data for Smoking Cessation Intervention Example

| Exposure to Intervention | Outcome | | Total |
|---|---|---|---|
| | **Continued Smoking** | **Stopped Smoking** | |
| **Yes** (Experimental Group) | 50 | 50 | 100 |
| **No** (Control Group) | 80 | 20 | 100 |
| **TOTAL** | 130 | 70 | 200 |

Absolute Risk, exposed group ($AR_E$)   $= 50 / 100 = .50$

Absolute Risk, non - exposed group ($AR_{NE}$)   $= 80 / 100 = .80$

Absolute Risk Reduction (ARR)   $= .80 - .50 = .30$

Odds Ratio (OR)   $= \dfrac{(50 / 50)}{(80 / 20)} = .25$

## Absolute Risk Reduction

The **absolute risk reduction (ARR)** index, a comparison of the two risks, is computed by subtracting the absolute risk for the exposed group from the absolute risk for the unexposed group. This index is the estimated proportion of people who would be spared the undesirable outcome through exposure to an intervention or protective factor. In our example, the value of ARR is .30: 30% of the control group subjects would presumably have stopped smoking if they had received the intervention, over and above the 20% who stopped without it.

## Odds Ratio

The odds ratio is a widely reported risk index. The *odds*, in this context, is the proportion of subjects *with* the adverse outcome relative to those *without* it. In our example, the odds of continued smoking for the intervention group is 1.0: 50 (the number who continued smoking) divided by 50 (the number who stopped). The odds for the control group is 80 divided by 20, or 4.0. The **odds ratio (OR)** is the ratio of these two odds—.25 in our example. The estimated odds of continuing to smoke are one-fourth as high for those in the intervention group as for those in the control group. Turned around, we could say that the estimated odds of continued smoking is four times higher among smokers who do not get the intervention as among those who do.

> **Example of odds ratios:**
> Matthews and colleagues (2011) examined factors associated with smoking risk among sexual minority women (lesbian, bisexual, transgender). The OR for smoking was, for example, 2.21 among those with any recreational drug use in the prior 6 months. The risk of smoking was also higher among those who frequented lesbian/gay clubs once a week or more (OR = 2.60).

> ☞ **TIP:** An index known as the **risk ratio** (RR) is another risk index. The RR (also known as *relative risk*) is the estimated proportion of the original risk of an adverse outcome (in our example, continued smoking) that persists when people are exposed to the intervention. In our example, RR is .625 (.50/.80): the risk of continued smoking is estimated as 62.5% of what it would have been without the intervention.

# INTRODUCTION TO INFERENTIAL STATISTICS

Descriptive statistics are useful for summarizing data, but researchers usually do more than describe. **Inferential statistics**, based on the *laws of probability*, provide a means for drawing conclusions about a population, given data from a sample.

## Sampling Distributions

When estimating population attributes from a sample, the sample should be representative, and random sampling is the best means to secure such a sample. Inferential statistics are based on the assumption of random sampling from populations—although this assumption is widely violated.

Even with random sampling, however, sample characteristics are seldom identical to those of the population. Suppose we had a population of 50,000 nursing school applicants whose mean score on an entrance exam was 500 with a standard deviation of 100. Assume we do not know these parameters, but must estimate them based on scores from a random sample of 25 applicants. Should we expect a mean of exactly 500 and an *SD* of 100 for the sample? It would be improbable to obtain identical values. Our sample mean might be, for example, 505. If we drew a completely new random sample of 25 applicants and computed the mean, we might obtain a value of 497. Sample statistics fluctuate and are unequal to the parameter because of sampling error. Researchers need a way to assess whether sample statistics are good estimates of population parameters.

To understand the logic of inferential statistics, we must perform a mental exercise. Consider drawing a sample of 25 students from the population of applicants, calculating a mean score, replacing the students, and drawing a new sample. If we drew 5,000 samples, we would have 5,000 means (data points) that we could use to construct a frequency polygon (Fig. 12.6). This distribution is called a ***sampling distribution of the mean***. A sampling distribution is theoretical: in practice no one *actually* draws consecutive samples from a population and plots their means. Statisticians have shown that (1) sampling distributions of means are normally distributed and (2) the mean of a sampling distribution equals the population mean. In our example, the mean of the sampling distribution is 500, the same as the population mean.

Remember that when scores are normally distributed, 68% of the cases fall between +1 *SD* and –1 *SD* from the mean. For a sampling distribution of means, the probability is 68 out of 100 that a randomly drawn sample mean lies between +1 *SD* and –1 *SD* of the population mean. The problem is to determine the *SD* of the sampling distribution—called the **standard error of the mean** (or **SEM**). The word *error* signifies that the sample means contain some error as estimates of the population mean. The smaller the standard error (i.e., the less variable the sample means), the more accurate are the means as estimates of the population value.

Because no one actually constructs a sampling distribution, how can its standard deviation be computed? Statisticians have a formula for estimating the SEM from data from a single sample, using two pieces of information: the *SD* for the sample and sample size. In the present example, the SEM is 20 (Fig. 12.6), which is an estimate of how much sampling error there would be from one sample mean to another in an infinite number of samples of 25 applicants.

We can now estimate the probability of drawing a sample with a certain mean. With a sample size of 25 and a population mean of 500, the chances are 95 out of 100 that a sample mean would fall between 460 and 540—2 *SD*s above and below the mean. Only 5 times

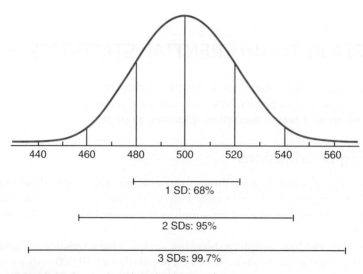

**FIGURE 12.6** ● Sampling distribution of a mean.

out of 100 would the mean of a random sample of 25 applicants be greater than 540 or less than 460. In other words, only 5 times out of 100 would we be likely to draw a sample whose mean deviates from the population mean by more than 40 points.

Because the SEM is partly a function of sample size, we need only increase sample size to increase the estimate's accuracy. Suppose we used a sample of 100 applicants to estimate the population mean. With this many students, the SEM would be 10, not 20. The probability would be 95 in 100 that a sample mean would be between 480 and 520. The chances of drawing a sample with a mean very different from that of the population are reduced as sample size increases—large numbers promote the likelihood that extreme values will cancel each other out.

You may wonder why you need to learn about these abstract statistical notions. Consider, though, that we are talking about how likely it is that a researcher's results are accurate. As an intelligent consumer, you need to evaluate critically how believable research evidence is so that you can decide whether to incorporate it into your nursing practice. The concepts underlying the standard error are important in such an evaluation and are related to an issue we stressed in Chapter 10 on sampling: the larger the sample size, the greater is the degree of accuracy.

## Parameter Estimation

Statistical inference consists of two techniques: parameter estimation and hypothesis testing. *Parameter estimation* is used to estimate a population parameter—for example, a mean, a proportion, or a mean difference between two groups (e.g., men vs. women). *Point estimation* involves calculating a single statistic to estimate the parameter. To continue with the earlier example, if we calculated the mean entrance exam score for a sample of 25 applicants and found that it was 510, then this would be the point estimate of the population mean.

Point estimates convey no information about the estimate's margin of error. *Interval estimation* of a parameter is useful because it indicates a range of values within which the parameter has a specified probability of lying. With interval estimation, researchers construct a **confidence interval (CI)** around the estimate; the upper and lower limits are called *confidence limits*. The confidence interval around a sample mean establishes a range of values for the population value and the probability of being right—the estimate is made with a certain degree of confidence. By convention, researchers use either a 95% or a 99% confidence interval.

👉 **TIP:** Confidence intervals (CIs) address a key EBP question for appraising evidence, as presented in Box 2.1 (p. 32): How *precise* is the estimate of effects?

Calculating confidence limits around a mean involves the SEM. As shown in Figure 12.6, 95% of the scores in a normal distribution lie within about 2 *SD*s (more precisely, 1.96 *SD*s) from the mean. In our example, if the point estimate for mean scores is 510 and the *SD* is 100, the SEM for a sample of 25 would be 20. We can build a 95% confidence interval using this formula: $95\% \text{ CI} = (\bar{X} \pm 1.96 \times \text{SEM})$. That is, the confidence is 95% that the population mean lies between the values equal to 1.96 times the SEM, above and below the sample mean. In our example, we would obtain the following:

$$95\% \text{ CI} = (510 \pm [1.96 \times 20.0])$$

$$95\% \text{ CI} = (510 \pm [39.2])$$

$$95\% \text{ CI} = (470.8 \text{ to } 549.2)$$

The final statement indicates that the confidence is 95% that the population mean is between 470.8 and 549.2.

CIs reflect how much risk researchers are willing to take of being wrong. With a 95% CI, researchers accept the risk that they will be wrong 5 times out of 100. A 99% CI sets the risk at only 1% by allowing a wider range of possible values. The formula is: CI 99% ($\bar{X} \pm 2.58 \times SEM$). The 2.58 reflects the fact that 99% of all cases in a normal distribution lie within ±2.58 *SD* units from the mean. In our example, the 99% CI is 458.4 to 561.6. The price of having lower risk of being wrong is reduced precision. For a 95% interval, the CI range is about 80 points; for a 99% interval, the range is more than 100 points.

The acceptable risk of error depends on the nature of the problem, but for most studies, a 95% confidence interval is sufficient. CIs are often constructed around risk indexes, such as the OR or RR, and around descriptive indexes like means and percentages.

> **Example of confidence intervals:**
> Kottner and colleagues (2011) studied pressure ulcer occurrence in a sample of more than 50,000 German hospital patients. The overall proportion of patients with a pressure ulcer at the trunk was 2.0% (99% CI = 1.8%–2.2%) for staging category 2 and 0.9% (99% CI = 0.8%–1.0%) for staging categories 3 or 4. The narrow CI range resulted from the huge sample size.

## Hypothesis Testing

Statistical **hypothesis testing** uses objective criteria for deciding whether research hypotheses should be accepted as true or rejected as false. Suppose we hypothesized that maternity patients exposed to a film on breastfeeding would breastfeed longer than mothers who did not see the film. We find that the mean number of days of breastfeeding is 131.5 for 25 experimental subjects and 125.1 for 25 control subjects. Should we conclude that the hypothesis has been supported? True, group differences are in the predicted direction, but perhaps in another sample, the group means would be nearly identical. Two explanations for the observed outcome are possible: (1) the film is truly effective in encouraging breastfeeding or (2) the difference in this sample was due to chance factors (e.g., differences in the characteristics of the two groups even before the film was shown, reflecting a bias).

The first explanation is the *research hypothesis*, and the second is the *null hypothesis*. The null hypothesis, it may be recalled, states that there is no relationship between the independent and dependent variables. Statistical hypothesis testing is a process of disproof. It cannot be demonstrated directly that the research hypothesis is correct. But it is possible to show, using sampling distributions, that the null hypothesis has a high probability of being incorrect, and such evidence lends support to the research hypothesis. Hypothesis testing helps researchers to make objective decisions about whether results are likely to reflect chance differences or hypothesized effects. The rejection of the null hypothesis is what researchers seek to accomplish through **statistical tests**.

Null hypotheses are accepted or rejected based on sample data, but hypotheses are about population values. The real interest in testing hypotheses, as in all statistical inference, is to use a sample to make inferences about a population.

### Type I and Type II Errors

Researchers decide whether to accept or reject the null hypothesis by estimating how probable it is that observed group differences are due to chance. Because information about the population is not available, it cannot be asserted that the null hypothesis is or is not true. Researchers must be content to say that hypotheses are either *probably* true or *probably* false.

The actual situation is that the null hypothesis is:

|  | True | False |
|---|---|---|
| **True**<br>(Null accepted) | Correct decision | Type II error |
| **False**<br>(Null rejected) | Type I error | Correct decision |

The researcher calculates
a test statistic and decides
that the null hypothesis is:

**FIGURE 12.7** ● Outcomes of statistical decision-making.

Researchers can make two types of error: rejecting a true null hypothesis or accepting a false null hypothesis. Figure 12.7 summarizes possible outcomes of researchers' decisions. Researchers make a **Type I error** by rejecting a null hypothesis that is, in fact, true. For instance, if we concluded that the film was effective in promoting breastfeeding when, in fact, group differences were merely due to sampling error, we would be making a Type I error—a false positive conclusion. Or, we might conclude that observed differences in breastfeeding were due to sampling fluctuations, when the film actually *did* have an effect. Acceptance of a false null hypothesis is a **Type II error**—a false negative conclusion.

### Level of Significance

Researchers do not know when they have made an error in statistical decision-making. The validity of a null hypothesis could only be known by collecting data from the population, in which case there would be no need for statistical inference.

Researchers control the risk for a Type I error by selecting a **level of significance**, which is the probability of making a Type I error. The two most frequently used levels of significance (referred to as **alpha ($\alpha$)**) are .05 and .01. With a .05 significance level, we accept the risk that out of 100 samples from a population, a true null hypothesis would be wrongly rejected 5 times. In 95 out of 100 cases, however, a true null hypothesis would be correctly accepted. With a .01 significance level, the risk of a Type I error is lower: In only 1 sample out of 100 would we wrongly reject the null. By convention, the minimal acceptable alpha level is .05.

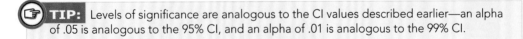 **TIP:** Levels of significance are analogous to the CI values described earlier—an alpha of .05 is analogous to the 95% CI, and an alpha of .01 is analogous to the 99% CI.

Researchers would like to reduce the risk of committing both types of error, but unfortunately, lowering the risk of a Type I error increases the risk of a Type II error. The stricter the criterion for rejecting a null hypothesis, the greater the probability of accepting a false null. However, researchers can reduce the risk of a Type II error by increasing their sample size.

The probability of committing a Type II error, called **beta ($\beta$)**, can be estimated through *power analysis*, the procedure we mentioned in Chapter 10 with regard to sample size. *Power* is the ability of a statistical test to detect true relationships, and is the complement of beta (that is, power equals 1-$\beta$). The standard criterion for an acceptable risk for a Type II error is .20, and thus researchers ideally use a sample size that gives them a minimum power of .80.

👉 **TIP:** Quantitative researchers should do a power analysis before starting their study, but many do not. If a report indicates that a research hypothesis was not supported by the data, consider whether a Type II error might have occurred because of inadequate sample size.

## Tests of Statistical Significance

In hypothesis testing, researchers use study data to compute a **test statistic**. For every test statistic, there is a theoretical sampling distribution, similar to the sampling distribution of means. Hypothesis testing uses theoretical distributions to establish *probable* and *improbable* values for the test statistics, which are used to accept or reject the null hypothesis.

An example from our study of gender bias in nursing research (Polit & Beck, 2009) illustrates the process. We tested the hypothesis that females are over-represented as participants in nursing studies—that is, the average percentage of females in published studies is greater than 50%. We found, using a consecutive sample of 843 studies from eight nursing research journals published over a 2-year period, that the mean percentage of females was 71.0. Using statistical procedures, we tested the hypothesis that the mean of 71.0 is not merely a chance fluctuation from the true population mean of 50.0.

In hypothesis testing, researchers assume that the null hypothesis is true—and then gather evidence to disprove it. Assuming a mean percentage of 50.0 for the entire population of recently published nursing studies, a theoretical sampling distribution can be constructed. For simplicity, let us say that the SEM is 2.0 (in our study, the SEM was actually less than 2.0). This is shown in Figure 12.8. Using a normal distribution, we can determine probable and improbable values of sample means from the population of nursing studies. If, as is assumed in the null hypothesis, the population mean is 50.0 percent, 95% of all sample means would fall between 46.0% and 54.0%, that is, within 2 *SD*s above and below the mean of 50.0%. The obtained sample mean of 71.0% is in the region considered *improbable* if the null hypothesis were correct—in fact, any value greater than 54.0% would be improbable if the true population mean were 50.0%, when alpha = .05. The *improbable* range beyond 2 *SD*s corresponds to only 5% (100% – 95%) of the sampling distribution. In our study, the probability of obtaining a value of 71.0% female by chance alone was less than 1 in 10,000. We rejected the null

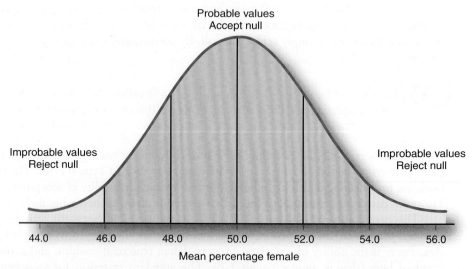

**FIGURE 12.8** ● Sampling distribution for hypothesis test example: Percentage female among participants in nursing studies. Based on Polit, D., & Beck, C. (2009). International gender bias in nursing research. *International Journal of Nursing Studies, 46,* 1102–1110.

hypothesis that the mean percentage of female participants in nursing studies was 50.0. We would not be justified in saying that we had *proved* the research hypothesis because the possibility of having made a Type I error remains—but the possibility is, in this case, remote.

Researchers reporting the results of hypothesis tests state whether their findings are **statistically significant**. The word *significant* does not mean important or meaningful. In statistics, the term *significant* means that results are not likely to have been due to chance, at some specified level of probability. A **nonsignificant result (NS)** means that any observed difference or relationship could have been the result of a chance fluctuation.

 **TIP:** It may help to keep in mind that inferential statistics are just a tool to help us evaluate whether study results are likely to be *real* and replicable, or simply spurious.

## Overview of Hypothesis Testing Procedures

In the next section, a few statistical tests are discussed. We emphasize applications and interpretations of statistical tests, not computations. Each statistical test can be used with specific kinds of data, but the overall hypothesis-testing process is similar for all tests:

1. *Selecting a test statistic.* Researchers select a test based on such factors as whether certain assumptions are justified, which levels of measurement were used, and, if relevant, how many groups are being compared.
2. *Specifying the level of significance.* An $\alpha$ level of .05 is usually chosen.
3. *Computing a test statistic.* A test statistic is calculated based on the collected data.
4. *Determining degrees of freedom.* The term *degrees of freedom (df)* refers to the number of observations free to vary about a parameter. The concept is too complex for elaboration, but computing degrees of freedom is easy.
5. *Comparing the test statistic to a theoretical value.* Theoretical distributions have been developed for all test statistics, and values for these distributions are available for specified degrees of freedom. The computed value of the test statistic is compared to a theoretical value to establish significance or nonsignificance.

When a computer is used for the analysis, as is almost always the case, researchers follow only the first step and then give commands to the computer. The computer calculates the test statistic, degrees of freedom, and the actual probability that the relationship being tested is due to chance. For example, the computer may print that the probability ($p$) of an experimental group doing better on a measure of postoperative recovery than the control group on the basis of chance alone is .025. This means that fewer than 3 times out of 100 (only 25 times out of 1,000) would a group difference of the size observed occur by chance. The computed $p$ level (probability) is then compared with the desired alpha. In the present example, if the significance level were .05, the results would be significant because .025 is more stringent than .05. Any computed probability greater than .05 (e.g., .15) indicates a nonsignificant relationship (sometimes abbreviated *NS*), that is, one that could have occurred on the basis of chance in more than 5 out of 100 samples.

 **TIP:** Most tests discussed in this chapter are *parametric tests*, which are ones that focus on population parameters and involve certain assumptions about variables in the analysis, notably the assumption that they are normally distributed in the population. *Nonparametric tests*, by contrast, do not estimate parameters and involve less restrictive assumptions about the distribution's shape.

# BIVARIATE STATISTICAL TESTS

Researchers use a variety of statistical tests to make inferences about their hypotheses. Several frequently used bivariate tests are briefly described and illustrated.

## t-Tests

Researchers frequently compare two groups of people on an outcome. A parametric test for testing the significance of differences in two group means is called a *t*-test.

Suppose we wanted to test the effect of early discharge of maternity patients on perceived maternal competence. We administer a scale of perceived maternal competence at discharge to 20 primiparas who had a vaginal delivery: 10 who remained in the hospital 25 to 48 hours (regular discharge group) and 10 who were discharged 24 hours or less after delivery (early discharge group). Data for this example are presented in Table 12.8. Mean scores for these two groups are 25.0 and 19.0, respectively. Are these differences *real* (i.e., would they exist in the population of early-discharge and later-discharge mothers?), or do group differences reflect chance fluctuations? The 20 scores vary from one mother to another. Some variation reflects individual differences in perceived maternal competence. Some variation might reflect the scale's low reliability, some could result from participants' moods on a particular day, and so forth. The research question is:

**TABLE 12.8 Fictitious Data for *t*-Test Example: Scores on a Perceived Maternal Competence Scale**

| Early-Discharge Mothers | Regular-Discharge Mothers |
|:---:|:---:|
| 30 | 23 |
| 27 | 17 |
| 25 | 22 |
| 20 | 18 |
| 24 | 20 |
| 32 | 26 |
| 17 | 16 |
| 18 | 13 |
| 28 | 21 |
| 29 | 14 |
| Mean = 19.0 | Mean = 25.0 |

$t = 2.86$, $df = 18$, $p = .011$

Can a significant portion of the variation be attributed to the independent variable—time of hospital discharge? The *t*-test allows us to make inferences about this question objectively.

The formula for calculating the *t* statistic uses group means, variability, and sample size. The computed value of *t* for the data in Table 12.8 is 2.86. Degrees of freedom in this example are equal to the total sample size minus 2 ($df = 20 - 2 = 18$). For an $\alpha$ level of .05, the theoretical cutoff value for *t* with 18 degrees of freedom is 2.10. *This value establishes an upper limit to what is probable if the null hypothesis is true.* Thus, the calculated *t* of 2.86, which is larger than the theoretical value of *t*, is improbable (i.e., statistically significant). We can say that the primiparas discharged early had significantly lower perceived maternal competence than those who were not discharged early. The group difference was sufficiently large that it is unlikely to reflect chance fluctuations. In fewer than 5 out of 100 samples would a difference in means this great be found by chance alone. In fact, the actual *p* value is .011: only in about 1 sample out of 100 would this difference be found by chance.

The situation we just described calls for an *independent groups t-test*: mothers in the two groups were different people, independent of each other. There are situations for which this type of *t*-test is not appropriate. For example, if means for a single group of people measured before and after an intervention were being compared, researchers would use a *paired t-test* (also called a *dependent groups t-test*), which involves a different formula.

> **Example of *t*-tests:**
> Karatay and Akkus (2012) tested the effectiveness of a multistimulant home-based program on cognitive function in older adults in Turkey. They used independent group *t*-tests to compare cognitive functioning scores of those in the experimental and control groups, and also used paired *t*-tests to assess differences before and after the program within each group.

As an alternative to *t*-tests, CIs can be constructed around the difference between two means. The results provide information about both statistical significance (i.e., whether the null hypothesis should be rejected) and precision of the estimated difference. In the example in Table 12.8, we can construct CIs around the mean difference of 6.0 in maternal competence scores ($25.0 - 19.0 = 6.0$). For a 95% CI, the confidence limits are 1.6 and 10.4: we can be 95% confident that the true difference between population means for early- and regular-discharge mothers lies between these values.

With CI information, we learn the range in which the mean difference probably lies and we can also see that it is significant at $p < .05$ *because the range does not include 0.* There is a 95% probability that the mean difference is not lower than 1.6, so this means that there is less than a 5% probability that there is no difference at all—thus, the null hypothesis can be rejected.

## Analysis of Variance

**Analysis of variance (ANOVA)** is used to test mean group differences of three or more groups. ANOVA sorts out the variability of an outcome variable into two components: variability due to the independent variable (e.g., experimental group status) and variability due to all other sources (e.g., individual differences, measurement error). Variation *between* groups is contrasted with variation *within* groups to yield an *F* ratio statistic.

Suppose we were comparing the effectiveness of interventions to help people stop smoking. One group of smokers receives nurse counseling (group A), a second group is treated by a nicotine patch (group B), and a control group gets no special treatment (group C). The outcome is 1-day cigarette consumption measured 1 month after the intervention.

**TABLE 12.9  Fictitious Data for ANOVA Example: Number Of Cigarettes Smoked In 1 Day, Post-Treatment**

| Group A Nurse Counseling | | Group B Nicotine Patch | | Group C Untreated Controls | |
|---|---|---|---|---|---|
| 28 | 19 | 0 | 27 | 33 | 35 |
| 0 | 24 | 31 | 0 | 54 | 0 |
| 17 | 0 | 26 | 3 | 19 | 43 |
| 20 | 21 | 30 | 24 | 40 | 39 |
| 35 | 2 | 24 | 27 | 41 | 36 |
| $Mean_A$ = 16.6 | | $Mean_B$ = 19.2 | | $Mean_C$ = 34.0 | |

$F = 4.98$, $df = 2, 27$, $p = .01$

Thirty smokers who wish to quit smoking are randomly assigned to one of the three groups. The null hypothesis is that the population means for post-treatment cigarette smoking is the same for all three groups, and the research hypothesis is inequality of means. Table 12.9 presents fictitious data for the 30 participants. The mean numbers of post-treatment cigarettes consumed are 16.6, 19.2, and 34.0 for groups A, B, and C, respectively. These means are different, but are they significantly different—or do differences reflect random fluctuations?

An ANOVA applied to these data yields an $F$ ratio of 4.98. For $\alpha$ = .05 and $df$ = 2 and 27 (2 $df$ between groups and 27 $df$ within groups), the theoretical $F$ value is 3.35. Because our obtained $F$-value of 4.98 exceeds 3.35, we reject the null hypothesis that the population means are equal. The *actual* probability, as calculated by a computer, is .014. In only 14 samples out of 1,000 would differences this great be obtained by chance alone.

ANOVA results support the hypothesis that different treatments were associated with different cigarette smoking, but we cannot tell from these results whether treatment A was significantly more effective than treatment B. Statistical analyses known as **post hoc tests** (or *multiple comparison procedures*) are used to isolate the differences between group means that are responsible for rejecting the overall ANOVA null hypothesis. Note that it is *not* appropriate to use a series of $t$-tests (group A vs. B, A vs. C, and B vs. C) because this increases the risk of a Type I error.

ANOVA also can be used to test the effect of two independent variables on an outcome variable. Suppose we wanted to assess whether the two smoking cessation interventions (nurse counseling and nicotine patch) were equally effective for men and women. We randomly assign men and women, separately, to the two treatment conditions, without a control condition. Suppose the analysis revealed the following about two *main effects*: On average, people in the nurse-counseling group smoked less than those in the nicotine-patch group (19.0 vs. 25.0), and, overall, women smoked less than men (21.0 vs. 23.0). In addition, there is an *interaction effect*: Female smoking was especially low in the counseling condition (mean = 16.0), whereas male smoking was especially high in that condition (mean = 30.0). By performing a *two-way ANOVA* on these data, it would be possible to test the statistical significance of these differences.

A type of ANOVA known as **repeated measures ANOVA (RM-ANOVA)** can be used when the means being compared are means at different points in time (e.g., mean blood pressure at 2, 4, and 6 hours after surgery). This is analogous to a paired *t*-test, extended to three or more points of data collection. When two or more groups are measured several times, a repeated measures ANOVA provides information about a main effect for time (do the measures change significantly over time, irrespective of group?), a main effect for groups (do the group means differ significantly, irrespective of time?), and an interaction effect (do the groups differ more at certain times?).

**Example of an ANOVA:**

Lee, Chao, Yiin, Chiang, and Chao (2011) conducted a randomized trial to test the effects of music on preoperative anxiety. Patients were assigned to a headphone music group, a broadcast music group, or a control group with no music. Analysis of variance revealed significant group differences on anxiety ($F = 13.0$, $p < .001$). Post hoc tests revealed that both music groups had significantly lower anxiety than the control group, but anxiety in the two music groups did not differ significantly.

## Chi-Squared Test

The **chi-squared** ($\chi^2$) **test** is used to test hypotheses about the proportion of cases in different categories, as in a crosstabulation. For example, suppose we were studying the effect of nursing instruction on patients' compliance with self-medication. Nurses implement a new instructional strategy with 50 patients, while 50 control group patients get usual care. The research hypothesis is that a higher proportion of people in the treatment than in the control condition will be compliant. Some fictitious data for this example are presented in Table 12.10, which shows that 60% of those in the experimental group were compliant, compared to 40% in the control group. But is this 20 percentage point difference statistically significant—that is, likely to be "real"?

The chi-squared statistic is computed by summing differences between the *observed frequencies* in each cell (such as those in Table 12.10) and the *expected frequencies*—those that would be expected if there were *no* relationship between the variables. The value of the chi-squared statistic here is 4.00, which we can compare with the value from a theoretical chi-squared distribution. In this example, the theoretical value that must be exceeded to establish significance at the .05 level is 3.84. The obtained value of 4.00 is larger than would be expected by chance (the actual $p = .046$). We can conclude that a significantly larger proportion of experimental patients than control patients were compliant.

**TABLE 12.10  Observed Frequencies for Chi-Squared Example: Rates of Compliance with Medications**

| Patient Compliance | Group | | | | | Total |
|---|---|---|---|---|---|---|
| | Experimental | | Control | | | |
| | *n* | % | *n* | % | | *n* |
| Compliant | 30 | 60.0 | 20 | 40.0 | | 50 |
| Noncompliant | 20 | 40.0 | 30 | 60.0 | | 50 |
| TOTAL | 50 | 100.0 | 50 | 100.0 | | 100 |

$\chi^2 = 4.0$, *df* = 1, $p = .046$

**Example of chi-squared test:**

Fukui, Fujita, Tsujimura, and Hayashi (2011) studied factors associated with a home death, versus a hospital death, in home palliative cancer care patients in Japan. They used chi-squared tests to study differences between the two groups on a wide range of variables. For example, a significantly higher proportion of patients who died at home (37%) than who died in the hospital (23%) had a daughter or daughter-in-law as a primary caretaker ($\chi^2$ = 12.6, $df$ =1, $p$ < .001).

As with means, it is possible to construct CIs around the difference between two proportions. In our example, the group difference in proportion compliant was .20. The 95% CI in this example is .06 to .34. We can be 95% confident that the true population difference in compliance rates between those exposed to the intervention and those not exposed is between 6% and 34%. This interval does not include 0%, so we can be 95% confident that group differences are "real" in the population.

## Correlation Coefficients

Pearson's $r$ is both descriptive and inferential. As a descriptive statistic, $r$ summarizes the magnitude and direction of a relationship between two variables. As an inferential statistic, $r$ tests hypotheses about population correlations; the null hypothesis is that there is no relationship between two variables, that is, that the population $r$ = .00.

Suppose we were studying the relationship between patients' self-reported level of stress (higher scores indicate more stress) and the pH level of their saliva. With a sample of 50 patients, we find that $r$ = –.29. This value indicates a tendency for people with high stress to have lower pH levels than those with low stress. But we need to ask whether this finding can be generalized to the population. Does the $r$ of –.29 reflect a random fluctuation, observed only in this sample, or is the relationship significant? Degrees of freedom for correlation coefficients equal $N$ minus 2, which is 48 in this example. The theoretical value for $r$ with $df$ = 48 and $\alpha$ = .05 is .28. Because the absolute value of the calculated $r$ is .29, the null hypothesis is rejected. There is a modest but significant relationship between patients' stress level and the acidity of their saliva.

CIs can be constructed around Pearson $r$s. In our example, the 95% CI around the $r$ of .29 for stress levels and saliva pH, with a sample of 50 subjects, is .01 and .53. Because the upper confidence limit is less than .00, the correlation in this example was statistically significant at the .05 level (but note that the range of possible values for the population $r$ is very large because of the small sample size).

**Example of Pearson's r:**

Suhonen et al. (2012) studied the correlation between patient satisfaction and perceptions of individualized care in a sample of 1,315 surgical patients from five European countries. Pearson correlation coefficients were moderately strong and significant. For example, the $r$ between satisfaction and a subscale called "Decisional control over care" was .63, $p$ < .001.

**TIP:** Most tests discussed in this chapter (e.g., $t$-tests, ANOVA, Pearson's $r$) are *parametric tests*, which focus on population parameters. The chi-squared test is nonparametric.

## Effect Size Indexes

Effect size indexes are estimates of the magnitude of effects of an "I" component on an "O" component in PICO questions, as described in Chapter 2—an important issue in EBP (see Box 2.1, p. 32). Effect size information can be crucial because, with large samples, even miniscule effects can be statistically significant. *P* values tell you whether results are likely to be *real*, but effect sizes suggest whether they are important. Effect size plays an important role in meta-analyses.

It is beyond our scope to explain effect sizes in detail, but we offer an illustration. A frequently used effect size index is the *d* statistic, which summarizes the magnitude of differences in two means, such as the difference between experimental and control group means on an outcome. Thus, *d* can be calculated to estimate effect size when *t*-tests are used. When *d* is zero, it means that there is no effect of the independent variable—the means of the two groups being compared are the same. By convention, a *d* of .20 or less is considered *small*, a *d* of .50 is considered *moderate*, and a *d* of .80 or greater is considered *large*.

Different effect size indexes and interpretive conventions are associated with different situations. For example, the *r* statistic can be interpreted directly as an effect size index, as can the OR. The key point is that they encapsulate information about how powerful the effect of an independent variable is on an outcome.

> **TIP:** Researchers who conduct a power analysis to estimate how big a sample size they need to adequately test their hypotheses (i.e., to avoid a Type II error) must estimate in advance how large the effect size will be—usually based on prior research or a pilot study.

**Example of calculated effect size:**
Krampe (2012) conducted a pilot study to test the effectiveness of a dance-therapy intervention on balance and mobility in older adults. Although differences between the intervention and control groups were not significant due to the small sample size (*N* = 27), effect size calculations suggested several positive moderate effects. For example, the effect size for backward reach was *d* = .48.

## Guide to Bivariate Statistical Tests

The selection of a statistical test depends on several factors, such as number of groups and the levels of measurement of the research variables. To aid you in evaluating the appropriateness of statistical tests used by nurse researchers, Table 12.11 summarizes key features of the bivariate tests mentioned in this chapter.

> **TIP:** Every time a report presents information about statistical tests, such as those described in this section, it means that the researcher was testing hypotheses—whether or not those hypotheses were formally stated in the introduction.

# MULTIVARIATE STATISTICAL ANALYSIS

Many nurse researchers now use complex **multivariate statistics** to analyze their data. We use the term *multivariate* to refer to analyses dealing with at least three—but usually

## TABLE 12.11   Guide to Major Bivariate Statistical Tests

| Name | Test Statistic | Purpose | Measurement Level Independent Variable | Dependent Variable |
|------|----------------|---------|----------------------------------------|--------------------|
| *t*-test for independent groups | *t* | To test the difference between the means of two independent groups (e.g., experimental vs. control, men vs. women) | Nominal | Interval, Ratio |
| *t*-test for paired groups | *t* | To test the difference between the means of a paired group (e.g., pretest vs. posttest for same people) | Nominal | Interval, Ratio |
| Analysis of variance (ANOVA) | *F* | To test the difference among means of 3+ independent groups or means for 2+ independent variables | Nominal | Interval, Ratio |
| Repeated measures ANOVA | *F* | To test the difference among means of 3+ related groups, e.g., the same group over time, or to compare 2+ groups over time | Nominal | Interval, Ratio |
| Pearson's correlation coefficient | *r* | To test the existence of a relationship between two variables | Interval, Ratio | Interval, Ratio |
| Chi-squared test | $\chi^2$ | To test the difference in proportions in 2+ independent groups | Nominal (or ordinal, few categories) | Nominal (or ordinal, few categories) |

more—variables simultaneously. The evolution to more sophisticated methods of analysis has resulted in increased rigor in nursing studies, but one unfortunate side effect is that it has become more challenging for those without statistical training to understand research reports.

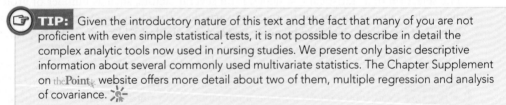 **TIP:** Given the introductory nature of this text and the fact that many of you are not proficient with even simple statistical tests, it is not possible to describe in detail the complex analytic tools now used in nursing studies. We present only basic descriptive information about several commonly used multivariate statistics. The Chapter Supplement on thePoint website offers more detail about two of them, multiple regression and analysis of covariance.

## Multiple Regression

Correlations enable researchers to make predictions. For example, if the correlation between secondary school grades and nursing school grades were .60, nursing school administrators could make predictions—albeit imperfect ones—about applicants' future performance. Researchers can improve their prediction of an outcome by performing a **multiple regression** in which multiple independent variables are included in the analysis. As an example, we might predict infant birth weight (the outcome) from such variables as mothers' smoking, amount of prenatal care, and gestational period. In multiple regression, outcome variables are interval- or ratio-level variables. Independent variables (also called **predictor variables** in regression) are either interval- or ratio-level variables or dichotomous nominal-level variables, such as male/female.

The coefficient in multiple regression is the **multiple correlation coefficient**, symbolized as $R$. Unlike the bivariate correlation coefficient $r$, $R$ does not have negative values. $R$ varies from .00 to 1.00, showing the *strength* of the relationship between several independent variables and an outcome, but not *direction*. Researchers can test whether $R$ is statistically significant (i.e., different from .00). An interesting feature of $R$ is that, when squared, it can be interpreted as the proportion of the variability in the outcome variable that is explained by the predictors. In predicting birth weight, if we achieved an $R$ of .60 ($R^2 = .36$), we could say that the predictors accounted for just over one third (36%) of the variation in birth weights. Two thirds of the variation, however, resulted from factors not identified or measured. Researchers usually report multiple correlation results in terms of $R^2$ rather than $R$.

> **Example of multiple regression analysis:**
> Buck and colleagues (2012), in their study of older adults with moderate to advanced heart failure, studied the relationship between several demographic, clinical, and psychosocial predictors on the one hand and health-related quality of life (HRQL) on the other. Using multiple regression, they found that the patient's self-care management and their self-care confidence were significant predictors of HRQL ($R^2 = .10$, $p = .008$). ⚘

## Analysis of Covariance

**Analysis of covariance (ANCOVA)**, which combines features of ANOVA and multiple regression, is used to control confounding variables statistically—that is to "equalize" groups being compared. This approach is valuable in certain situations, for example, when a nonequivalent control group design is used. When control through randomization is lacking, ANCOVA offers the possibility of statistical control.

In ANCOVA, the confounding variables being controlled are called *covariates*. Analysis of covariance tests the significance of differences between group means on an outcome after eliminating the effect of covariates. ANCOVA produces $F$ statistics to test the significance of group differences. ANCOVA is a powerful and useful analytic technique for controlling confounding influences on outcomes.

> **Example of ANCOVA:**
> Keough and colleagues (2011) studied differences in self-management behaviors in managing diabetes among youth in early, middle, and late adolescence. The three age groups were compared with regard to problem solving and collaboration with parents, using gender and type of regimen (flexible or conventional) as covariates.

## Multivariate Analysis of Variance

*Multivariance analysis of variance (MANOVA)* is the extension of ANOVA to more than one outcome. MANOVA is used to test the significance of differences between the means of two or more groups on two or more outcome variables, considered simultaneously. For instance, if we wanted to compare the effect of two exercise regimens on both blood pressure and heart rate, then a MANOVA would be appropriate. Covariates can also be included to control confounding variables, in which case, the analysis is a *multivariate analysis of covariance (MANCOVA)*.

> **Example of MANOVA:**
> Leiter and colleagues (2011) investigated the anxiolytic effects of myristicin (a major compound found in nutmeg) in male Sprague-Dawley rats. Rats were divided into five groups (two control groups, a myristicin group, and two groups with myristicin plus other compounds). MANOVA was used to test differences in the five groups with respect to a behavioral measure of anxiety and two other outcomes.

### Logistic Regression

**Logistic regression** analyzes the relationships between multiple independent variables and a nominal-level outcome (e.g., compliant vs. noncompliant). It is similar to multiple regression, although it employs a different statistical estimation procedure. Logistic regression transforms the probability of an event occurring (e.g., that a woman will practice breast self-examination or not) into its *odds*. After further transformations, the analysis examines the relationship of the predictor variables to the transformed outcome variable. For each predictor, the logistic regression yields an *odds ratio*, which is the factor by which the odds change for a unit change in the predictors after controlling other predictors. Logistic regression also yields CIs around the ORs.

> **Example of logistic regression:**
> Kim and colleagues (2012) used logistic regression to identify various risk factors (e.g., parental education, children's use of computers) for childhood obesity (obese vs. not obese) in a sample of 1,644 Korean children.

### Guide to Multivariate Statistical Analyses

In selecting a multivariate analysis, researchers attend to such issues as the number of independent variables, the number of outcome variables, the measurement level of all variables, and the desirability of controlling confounding variables. Table 12.12 is an aid to help you evaluate the appropriateness of multivariate statistics used in many nursing studies.

# READING AND UNDERSTANDING STATISTICAL INFORMATION

Statistical findings are communicated in the results section of research reports and are described in the text and in tables (or, less frequently, figures). This section offers assistance in reading and interpreting statistical information.

## Tips on Reading Text with Statistical Information

Several types of information are reported in results sections. First, descriptive statistics typically summarize sample characteristics. Information about the participants' background helps readers to draw conclusions about the people to whom the findings can be applied. Second, researchers may provide statistical information for evaluating biases. For example, when a quasi-experimental or case-control design has been used, researchers often test the equivalence of the groups being compared on baseline or background variables, using tests such as *t*-tests.

## TABLE 12.12   Guide to Selected Multivariate Analyses

| Test Name | Purpose | Measurement Level of Variables[a,b] | | | Number of Variables[a] | | |
| --- | --- | --- | --- | --- | --- | --- | --- |
| | | IV | DV | Covar | IVs | DVs | Covar |
| Multiple regression | To test relationship between 2+ IVs and 1 DV; to predict a DV from 2+ IVs | N, I, R | I, R | | 2+ | 1 | |
| Analysis of covariance (ANCOVA) | To test the difference between the means of 2+ groups, while controlling for 1+ covariate | N | I, R | N, I, R | 1+ | 1 | 1+ |
| Multivariate analysis of variance (MANOVA) | To test the difference between the means of 2+ groups for 2+ DVs simultaneously | N | I, R | | 1+ | 2+ | |
| Multivariate analysis of covariance (MANCOVA) | To test the difference between the means of 2+ groups for 2+ DVs simultaneously, while controlling for 1+ covariate | N | I, R | N, I, R | 1+ | 2+ | 1+ |
| Logistic regression | To test the relationship between 2+ IVs and 1 DV; to predict the probability of an event; to estimate relative risk | N, I, R | N | | 2+ | 1 | |

[a]Variables: IV, independent variables; DV, dependent variable; Covar, covariate.
[b]Measurement levels: N, nominal; I, interval; R, ratio.

The text of research articles usually provides certain information about statistical tests, including (1) which test was used, (2) the value of the calculated statistic, (3) degrees of freedom, and (4) level of statistical significance. Examples of how the results of various statistical tests might be reported in the text are shown below.

1. $t$-test: $t = 1.68$; $df = 160$; $p = .09$
2. Chi-squared: $\chi^2 = 16.65$; $df = 2$; $p < .001$
3. Pearson's $r$: $r = .36$; $df = 100$; $p < .01$
4. ANOVA: $F = 0.18$; $df = 1, 69$, $ns$

Note that the significance level is sometimes reported as the *actual* computed probability that the null hypothesis is correct (example 1), which is the preferred approach. In this case, the observed group mean differences could be found by chance in 9 out of 100 samples. This result is not statistically significant, because the mean difference had an unacceptably high chance of being spurious. The probability level is sometimes reported simply as falling below or above certain thresholds (examples 2 and 3). These results are significant because the probability of obtaining such results by chance is <1 in 100. You must be careful to read the symbol following the $p$ value correctly: The symbol < means *less than*—i.e., the results are statistically significant. The symbol > means *greater than*—i.e., the results are not significant. When results do not achieve statistical significance at the desired level, researchers may simply indicate that the results were not significant (*ns*), as in example 4.

Statistical information usually is noted parenthetically in a sentence describing the findings, as in the following example: Patients in the intervention group had a significantly lower rate of infection than those in the control group ($\chi^2$ = 5.41, $df$ = 1, $p$ = .02). In reading research reports, it is not important to absorb numeric information for the test statistics. For example, the actual value of $\chi^2$ has no inherent interest. What is important is to grasp whether the statistical tests indicate that the research hypotheses were accepted as probably true (as demonstrated by significant results) or rejected as probably false (as demonstrated by nonsignificant results).

## Tips on Reading Statistical Tables

The use of tables allows researchers to condense a lot of statistical information, and minimizes redundancy. Consider, for example, putting information from a correlation matrix (Table 12.5, p.22) into the text: "The correlation between service climate and nurses' task performance was .31; the correlation between task performance and patient satisfaction was .49..."

Tables are efficient but they may be daunting, partly because of the absence of standardization. There is no universally accepted method of presenting $t$-test results, for example. Thus, each table may present a new deciphering challenge. Another problem is that some researchers try to include too much information in their tables; we deliberately used tables of relative simplicity as examples in this chapter.

We have a few suggestions for helping you to comprehend statistical tables. First, read the text and the tables simultaneously—the text may help you figure out what the table is communicating. Second, before trying to understand the numbers in a table, try to glean information from the accompanying words. Table titles and footnotes often present critical pieces of information. Table headings should be carefully scrutinized because they indicate what the variables in the analysis are (often listed as row labels in the first column, as in Table 12.3, p. 221) and what statistical information is included (often specified in the top

**TABLE 12.13 Effects of Parenting Intervention on Selected Maternal and Infant Outcomes at the 4-Week Follow-Up[a]**

| Outcome | Intervention Group (N = 93) M | SD | Community Group (N = 85) M | SD | P | Mean Difference | 95% CI, Mean Difference |
|---------|------|------|------|------|------|------|------|
| Maternal Confidence | 61.4 | 4.7 | 60.0 | 4.2 | .046 | 1.4 | .03, 2.75 |
| Parenting Sense of Competence | 56.3 | 8.2 | 53.9 | 7.0 | .045 | 2.4 | .06, 4.73 |
| Postnatal Depression | 5.6 | 4.2 | 6.1 | 3.4 | .38 | −0.5 | −.63. 1.66 |
| Maternal Anxiety | 2.7 | 1.7 | 2.9 | 1.5 | .27 | −0.2 | −.22,.78 |

[a]The p values are for intervention group versus community group comparisons on each outcome using analysis of covariance (ANCOVA), controlling for the baseline measure of the respective outcome, baby's age, and parity; F statistic values were not reported.

Adapted from Hauck, Y., Hall, W., Dhaliwal, S., Bennett, E., & Wells, G. (2012). The effectiveness of an early parenting intervention for mothers with infants with sleep and settling concerns. *Journal of Clinical Nursing, 21*, 52–62.

row as the column headings). Third, you may find it helpful to consult the glossary of symbols on the inside back cover of this book to check the meaning of a statistical symbol. Not all symbols in this glossary were described in this chapter, so it may be necessary to refer to a statistics textbook, such as that of Polit (2010), for further information.

> 👉 **TIP:** In tables, probability levels associated with the significance tests are sometimes presented directly (e.g., $p < .05$), as in Table 12.13. Here, the significance of each test is indicated in the third-to-last column, headed "$p$". However, researchers often indicate significance levels in tables through asterisks placed next to the value of the test statistic. One asterisk usually signifies $p < .05$, two asterisks signify $p < .01$, and three asterisks signify $p < .001$ (but there should be a key at the bottom of the table indicating what the asterisks mean). Thus, a table might show: $t = 3.00$, $p < .01$ or $t = 3.00^{**}$. When asterisks are used, the absence of an asterisk would signify a nonsignificant result.

# CRITIQUING QUANTITATIVE ANALYSES

It is often difficult to critique statistical analyses. We hope this chapter has helped to demystify statistics, but we also recognize the limited scope of our coverage. It would be unreasonable to expect you to be adept at evaluating statistical analyses, but you can be on the lookout for certain things in reviewing research articles. Some specific guidelines are presented in Box 12.1.

---

**BOX 12.1  Guidelines for Critiquing Statistical Analyses**

1. Did the descriptive statistics in the report sufficiently describe the major key variables and background characteristics of the sample? Were appropriate descriptive statistics used—for example, was a mean presented when percentages would have been more informative?
2. Were statistical analyses undertaken to assess threats to the study's validity (e.g., to test for selection bias or attrition bias)?
3. Does the report include any inferential statistics? If inferential statistics were not used, should they have been?
4. Was information provided about both hypothesis testing and parameter estimation (i.e., confidence intervals)? Were effect sizes (or risk indexes) reported? Overall, did the reported statistics provide readers with sufficient information about the evidence the study yielded?
5. Were any multivariate procedures used? If not, should they have been used—for example, would the internal validity of the study be strengthened by statistically controlling confounding variables?
6. Were the selected statistical tests appropriate, given the level of measurement of the variables and the nature of the hypotheses?
7. Were the results of any statistical tests significant? What do the tests tell you about the plausibility of the research hypotheses? Were effects sizeable?
8. Were the results of any statistical tests nonsignificant? Is it plausible that these reflect Type II errors? What factors might have undermined the study's statistical conclusion validity?
9. Was there an appropriate amount of statistical information? Were findings clearly and logically organized? Were tables or figures used judiciously to summarize large amounts of statistical information? Are the tables clearly presented, with good titles and carefully labeled column headings? Is the information presented in the text and the tables redundant?

One aspect of the critique should focus on which analyses were reported in the article. You should assess whether the statistical information adequately describes the sample and reports the results of statistical tests for all hypotheses. Another presentational issue concerns the researcher's judicious use of tables to summarize statistical information.

A thorough critique also addresses whether researchers used the appropriate statistics. Tables 12.11 on page 238 and 12.12 on page 241 provide guidelines for some frequently used statistical tests. The major issues to consider are the number of independent and dependent variables, the levels of measurement of the research variables, and the number of groups (if any) being compared.

If researchers did not use a multivariate technique, you should consider whether the bivariate analysis adequately tests the relationship between the independent and dependent variables. For example, if a *t*-test or ANOVA was used, could the internal validity of the study have been enhanced through the statistical control of confounding variables using ANCOVA? The answer will often be "yes."

Finally, you can be alert to possible exaggerations or subjectivity in the reported results. Researchers should never claim that the data proved, verified, confirmed, or demonstrated that the hypotheses were correct or incorrect. Hypotheses should be described as being *supported* or *not supported*, *accepted* or *rejected*.

The main task for beginning consumers in reading a results section of a research report is to understand the meaning of the statistical tests. What do the quantitative results indicate about the researcher's hypothesis? How believable are the findings? The answer to such questions form the basis for interpreting the research results, a topic discussed in Chapter 13.

## RESEARCH EXAMPLES WITH CRITICAL THINKING EXERCISES

In this section, we provide details about analytic portion of a study, followed by some questions to guide critical thinking.

☀ Example 1 below is also featured in our *Interactive Critical Thinking Activity* on thePoint website where you can easily record, print, and e-mail your responses to the related questions.

### EXAMPLE 1 ● Descriptive and Bivariate Inferential Statistics

**Study:** The effectiveness of an early parenting intervention for mothers with infants with sleep and settling concerns (Hauck et al., 2012)

**Statement of Purpose:** The purpose of this study was to test the effects of a parenting intervention offered at an early parenting center in Australia on maternal well-being and children's sleep and settling behavior.

**Methods:** A nonequivalent control group before–after design was used. Parents whose 4- to 6-month-old infants exhibited sleep behavior problems were recruited to participate in a Day Stay intervention that emphasized the development of parental confidence and competence relating to infants' sleep patterns. The intervention group (n = 93) was compared to a similar community comparison group (n = 85) in terms of maternal confidence, competence, depression, and anxiety, and in terms of infants' sleep and settling behaviors. Outcomes were measured for both groups at baseline and again 4 weeks later. Mothers completed self-administered questionnaires about their emotional state, bedtime practices with their infants, and the infants' night waking and settling behavior.

**Descriptive Statistics:** The researchers presented descriptive statistics (means, *SDs*, and percentages) to describe the characteristics of sample members prior to the intervention. For example, the mean age of the participants was 32.8 (± 4.3) for the intervention group and 32.9 (± 4.0) for the community group. The typical participant was married (94.9%) and had a college degree (63.5%).

**Analysis of Bias:** Recognizing that the groups might not be equivalent, the researchers assessed their baseline comparability. Using chi-squared tests and *t*-tests, they found the two groups comparable in terms of maternal age, marital status, and educational level. However, mothers in the intervention groups were significantly less likely than those in the community group to be primiparas (54% vs. 79%, respectively), and babies in the intervention group were significantly older (21.5 weeks vs. 20.1 weeks, respectively), both $p < .05$.

**Hypothesis Tests:** The researchers used paired *t*-tests to test changes over time on all major outcomes for both groups. They found, for example, that maternal confidence increased in both groups from baseline to follow-up, but the change was significant only in the intervention group (from $M = 57.6$ at baseline to $M = 60.5$ four weeks later, $p < .001$). The 95% CI around the mean improvement of 2.9 was 1.9 to 4.1. The researchers also used ANCOVA to test whether posttest scores were significantly different in the two groups. For each outcome, the group means at follow-up were compared after statistically controlling the baseline measure of the outcome, plus the baby's age and mother's parity. The two groups were significantly different on some of the outcomes, but there were no differences on others (see Table 12.13). For example, the two groups differed significantly on maternal confidence and perceived competence, but not on depression or anxiety. Finally, a logistic regression analysis was undertaken to explore factors that might predict whether an infant had a long settling time (>20 minutes). The predictors in the analysis included the baby's age, maternal parity, whether the mother had received the intervention, and whether the infant had needed a long or short time to settle at baseline. The only significant predictor of a long postintervention settling time was a long settling time at baseline. The OR for infants who had a settling time >20 minutes at baseline for predicting a long subsequent settling time was 3.35 (95% CI = 1.47 to 7.62).

## CRITICAL THINKING EXERCISES

1. Answer the relevant questions from Box 12.1 on page 243 regarding this study.
2. Also consider the following targeted questions:
   a. Table 12.13 on page 242 shows that the group difference in maternal depression was not statistically significant. State the findings for this outcome in words, including information about the means and *p* value.
   b. Explain what the OR and CI information means regarding the prediction of postintervention settling time.
3. In what ways do you think the findings could be used in clinical practice?

## EXAMPLE 2 ● Statistical Analysis in the Study in Appendix A

- Read the "Results" section of Howell and colleagues' (2007) study ("Anxiety, anger, and blood pressure in children") in Appendix A on pages 395–402.

## CRITICAL THINKING EXERCISES

1. Answer the relevant questions in Box 12.1 on page 243 regarding this study.
2. Also consider the following targeted questions:
   a. In reporting information about scale scores for boys and girls (Table 1, Appendix A), the researchers stated that "Boys had higher mean anger scores but lower mean anxiety scores than girls." Did the researchers test whether the sex differences were statistically significant? What test was used or would have been used?
   b. Looking at Table 1 of Appendix A, write one or two sentences about the results for diastolic blood pressure, making sure to mention *SD* values.
   c. In Table 2 of Appendix A, which variable was most highly correlated with Systolic blood pressure (SBP) and Diastolic blood pressure (DBP)?

**WANT TO KNOW MORE?** A wide variety of resources to enhance your learning and understanding of this chapter are available on thePoint.

• Interactive Critical Thinking Activity
• Chapter Supplement on Multiple Regression and Analysis of Covariance
• Answers to the Critical Thinking Exercises for Example 2
• Student Review Questions
• Full-text online
• Internet Resources with useful websites for Chapter 12

Additional study aids including eight journal articles and related questions are also available in *Study Guide for Essentials of Nursing Research, 8e.*

## SUMMARY POINTS

- **Descriptive statistics** are used to summarize and describe quantitative data.

- In **frequency distributions**, numeric values are ordered from lowest to highest, together with a count of the number (or percentage) of times each value was obtained.

- Data for a variable can be completely described in terms of the shape of the distribution, central tendency, and variability.

- The shape of a distribution can be **symmetric** or **skewed**, with one tail longer than the other; it can also be unimodal with one peak (i.e., one value of high frequency) or multimodal with more than one peak. A **normal distribution** (bell-shaped curve) is symmetric, unimodal, and not too peaked.

- Measures of **central tendency** represent the average or typical value of a set of scores. The **mode** is the value that occurs most frequently; the **median** is the point above which and below which 50% of the cases fall; and the mean is the arithmetic average of all scores. The **mean** is the most stable measure of central tendency.

- Measures of **variability**—how spread out the data are—include the range and standard deviation. The **range** is the distance between the highest and lowest scores. The **standard** deviation (*SD*) indicates how much, on average, scores deviate from the mean.

- In a normal distribution, 95% of values lie within 2 *SD*s above and below the mean.

- A **crosstabs table** is a two-dimensional frequency distribution in which the frequencies of two nominal- or ordinal-level variables are **cross tabulated**.

- **Correlation coefficients** describe the direction and magnitude of a relationship between two variables, and range from –1.00 (perfect *negative correlation*) through .00 to +1.00 (perfect *positive correlation*). The most frequently used correlation coefficient is **Pearson's *r***, used with interval- or ratio-level variables.

- Statistical indexes that describe the effects of exposure to risk factors or interventions provide useful information for clinical decisions. A widely reported risk index is the **odds ratio (OR)**, which is the ratio of the odds for an exposed vs unexposed group, with the *odds* reflecting the proportion of people with an adverse outcome relative to those without it.

- **Inferential statistics**, based on laws of probability, allow researchers to make inferences about a population based on data from a sample.

- The *sampling distribution of the mean* is a theoretical distribution of the means of an infinite number of same-sized samples drawn from a population. Sampling distributions are the basis for inferential statistics.

- The **standard error of the mean (SEM)**—the standard deviation of this theoretical distribution—indicates the degree of average error of a sample mean; the smaller the SEM, the more accurate are estimates of the population value.

- Statistical inference consists of two types of approach: estimating parameters and testing hypotheses. *Parameter estimation* is used to estimate a population parameter.

- *Point estimation* provides a single value of a population estimate (e.g., a mean). *Interval estimation* provides limits of a range of values—the **confidence interval (CI)**—between which the population value is expected to fall, at a specified probability. Most often the 95% CI is reported, which indicates that there is a 95% probability that the true population value lies between the upper and lower confidence limit.

- **Hypothesis testing** through statistical tests enables researchers to make objective decisions about relationships between variables.

- The *null hypothesis* states that no relationship exists between variables; rejection of the null hypothesis lends support to the research hypothesis. In testing hypotheses, researchers compute a test statistic and then determine whether the statistic falls beyond a critical region on the relevant theoretical distribution. The value of the test statistic indicates whether the null hypothesis is "improbable."

- A **Type I error** occurs if a null hypothesis is wrongly rejected (false positives). A **Type II error** occurs when a null hypothesis is wrongly accepted (false negatives).

- Researchers control the risk of making a Type I error by selecting a **level of significance** (or **alpha** level), which is the probability that such an error will occur. The .05 level (the conventional standard) means that in only 5 out of 100 samples would the null hypothesis be rejected when it should have been accepted.

- The probability of committing a Type II error is **beta** ($\beta$). *Power*, the ability of a statistical test to detect true relationships, is the complement of beta (i.e., power equals $1 - \beta$). The standard criterion for an acceptable level of power is .80.

- Results from hypothesis tests are either significant or nonsignificant; **statistically significant** means that the obtained results are not likely to be due to chance fluctuations at a given probability level (*p* **value**).

- Two common statistical tests are the *t*-**test** and **analysis of variance (ANOVA)**, both of which can be used to test the significance of the difference between group means; ANOVA is used when there are three or more groups or when there is more than one independent variable. **Repeated measures ANOVA (RM-ANOVA)** is used when data are collected over multiple time periods.

- The **chi-squared test** is used to test hypotheses about differences in proportions.

- Pearson's r can be used to test whether a correlation is significantly different from zero.

- **Effect size** indexes (such as the *d* **statistic**) summarize the strength of the effect of an independent variable (e.g., an intervention) on an outcome variable.

- **Multivariate statistics** are used in nursing research to untangle complex relationships among three or more variables.

- **Multiple regression analysis** is a method for understanding the effect of two or more **predictor** (independent) **variables** on a continuous dependent variable. The square multiple correlation coefficient ($R^2$) is an estimate of the proportion of variability in the outcome variable accounted for by the predictors.

- **Analysis of covariance (ANCOVA)** controls confounding variables (called *covariates*) before testing whether group mean differences are statistically significant.

- Other multivariate procedures used by nurse researchers include **logistic regression** and *multivariate analysis of variance (MANOVA)*.

# REFERENCES FOR CHAPTER 12

Buck, H., Lee, C., Moser, D., Albert, N., Lennie, T., Bentley, B., et al. (2012). Relationship between self-care and health-related quality of life in older adults with moderate to advanced heart failure. *Journal of Cardiovascular Nursing, 27,* 8–15.

Fukui, S., Fujita, J., Tsujimura, Y., & Hayashi, Y. (2011). Predictors of home death of home palliative cancer care patients. *International Journal of Nursing Studies, 48,* 1393–1400.

Greenslade, J., & Jimmieson, N. (2011). Organizational factors impacting on patient satisfaction. *International Journal of Nursing Studies, 48,* 1188–1198.

Hauck, Y., Hall, W., Dhaliwal, S., Bennett, E., & Wells, G. (2012). The effectiveness of an early parenting intervention for mothers with infants with sleep and settling concerns. *Journal of Clinical Nursing, 21,* 52–62.

Karatay, G., & Akkus, Y. (2012). Effectiveness of a multistimulant home-based program on cognitive function of older adults. *Western Journal of Nursing Research,* PubMed ID 21685369.

Keough, L., Sullivan-Bolyai, S., Crawford, S., Schilling, L., & Dixon, J. (2011). Self-management of type 1 diabetes across adolescence. *The Diabetes Educator, 37,* 486–500.

Kim, B., Lee, C., Kim, H., Ko, I., Park, C., & Kim, G. (2012). Ecological risk factors of childhood obesity in Korean elementary school children. *Western Journal of Nursing Research,* PubMed ID 22045783.

Kottner, J., Gefen, A., & Lahman, N. (2011). Weight and pressure ulcer occurrence. *International Journal of Nursing Studies, 48,* 1339–1148.

Krampe, J. (2012). Exploring the effects of dance-based therapy on balance and mobility in older adults. *Western Journal of Nursing Research,* PubMed ID 22045782.

Lee, K., Chao, Y., Yiin, J., Chiang, P., & Chao, Y. (2011). Effectiveness of different music-playing devices for reducing pre-operative anxiety. *International Journal of Nursing Studies, 48,* 1180–1187.

Leiter, E., Hitchcock, G., Godwin, S., Johnson, M., Sedgwick, W., Jones, W., et al. (2011). Evaluation of the anxiolytic properties of myristicin, a component of nutmeg, in the male Sprague-Dawley rat. *AANA Journal, 79,* 109–114.

Matthews, A., Hotton, A., DuBois, S., Fingerhut, D., & Kuhns, L. (2011). Demographic, psychosocial, and contextual correlates of tobacco use in sexual minority women. *Research in Nursing and Health, 34,* 141–152.

Padden, D., Connors, R., & Agazia, J. (2011). Stress, coping, and well-being in military spouses during deployment separation. *Western Journal of Nursing Research, 33,* 247–267.

Polit, D. F. (2010). *Statistics and data analysis for nursing research* (2nd ed.). Upper Saddle River, NJ: Pearson Education.

Polit, D., & Beck, C. (2009). International gender bias in nursing research. *International Journal of Nursing Studies, 46,* 1102–1110.

Suhonen, R., Papastavrou, E., Efstanthiou, G., Tsangari, H., Leino-Kilpi, H., Patiraki E., et al. (2012). Patient satisfaction as an outcome of individualized nursing care. *Scandinavian Journal of Caring Sciences, 26*(2), 372–380.

# 13 Rigor and Interpretation in Quantitative Research

## LEARNING OBJECTIVES

*On completing this chapter, you will be able to:*

● Describe dimensions key aspects for interpreting quantitative research results

● Describe the mindset conducive to a critical interpretation of research results

● Identify approaches to an assessment of the credibility of quantitative results, and undertake such an assessment

● Critique researchers' interpretation of their results in a discussion section of a report

● Define new terms in the chapter

## KEY TERMS

CONSORT guidelines
Results

In this chapter, we consider approaches to interpreting researchers' statistical results, which requires consideration of the various theoretical, methodological, and practical decisions that researchers have made in designing and implementing their studies.

# INTERPRETATION OF QUANTITATIVE RESULTS

Study **results** from statistical analyses are summarized in the Results section of a research article. Researchers present their *interpretations* of the results in Discussion sections—but researchers are seldom totally objective, and so you should develop your own interpretations.

This chapter offers guidance to help you in interpreting quantitative results and in critiquing Discussion sections of research articles. Another aim of this chapter is to encourage you to think critically about all aspects of a quantitative study. At this point, you are better able to apply the critiquing guidelines in Table 4.1 on page 69 than you were earlier. Results need to be understood and then evaluated within the context of the study aims, its theoretical basis, related research evidence, and the strengths and limitations of the research methods.

## Aspects of Interpretation

Interpreting study results involves attending to six different but overlapping considerations, which intersect with the "Questions for Appraising the Evidence" presented in Box 2.1 on page 32:

- The credibility and accuracy of the results
- The precision of the parameter estimates
- The magnitude of effects and importance of the results
- The meaning of the results, especially with regard to causality
- The generalizability of the results
- The implications of the results for nursing practice, theory development, or further research

Before discussing these considerations, we want to remind you about the role of inference in research thinking and interpretation.

## Inference and Interpretation

An *inference* is the act of drawing conclusions based on limited information, using logical reasoning. Interpreting research findings involves making a series of inferences. In research, virtually everything is a "stand-in" for something else: A sample is a stand-in for a population, a scale yields scores that are proxies for the magnitude of abstract attributes, and so on.

Figure 13.1 shows that research findings are meant to reflect "truth in the real world"—the findings themselves are "stand-ins" for the true state of affairs. Inferences about the real world are valid, however, to the extent that the researchers have made rigorous methodologic decisions in selecting proxies and have controlled sources of bias. This chapter offers several vantage points for assessing whether study findings really do reflect "truth in the real world."

## The Interpretive Mindset

Evidence-based practice (EBP) involves integrating best research evidence into clinical decision-making. EBP encourages clinicians to think critically about clinical practice and to challenge the status quo when it conflicts with "best evidence." Thinking critically and demanding evidence are also part of a research interpreter's job. Just as clinicians should ask, "What *evidence* is there that this intervention or strategy will be beneficial?" so must interpreters ask, "What *evidence* is there that the results are real and true?"

To be a good interpreter of research results, you can profit by starting with a skeptical attitude and a null hypothesis. *The "null hypothesis" in interpretation is that the results are wrong and the evidence is flawed.* The "research hypothesis" is that the evidence reflects the truth. Interpreters decide whether the null hypothesis has merit by critically examining methodologic evidence. The greater the evidence that the researcher's design and methods were sound, the less plausible is the null hypothesis that the evidence is inaccurate.

> **TIP:** In doing a critical interpretation of study results, it is appropriate to adopt a "show me" attitude. You should expect researchers to "show you" that their design is strong, their measurements are reliable and valid, their sample is adequately large and representative, and that their statistical decision-making is sound.

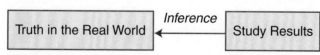

**FIGURE 13.1** ● Inferences in interpreting research results.

# CREDIBILITY OF QUANTITATIVE RESULTS

One of the most important interpretive tasks is to assess whether the results are *right*. This corresponds to the first question we posed in Box 2.1 on page 32: "What is the quality of the evidence—i.e., how rigorous and reliable is it?" If the results are not judged to be credible, the remaining interpretive issues (the meaning, magnitude, precision, or generalizability, and implications of results) are not likely to be relevant.

A credibility assessment requires a careful analysis of the study's methodologic and conceptual limitations and strengths. To come to a conclusion about whether the results closely approximate "truth in the real world," each aspect of the study—its research design, sampling plan, data collection plan, and analytic approach—must be subjected to critical scrutiny.

There are various ways to approach the issue of credibility, including the use of the critiquing guidelines we have offered throughout this book, and the overall critiquing protocol presented in Table 4.1 on page 69. We share some additional perspectives in this section.

## Proxies and Interpretation

Researchers begin with ideas and constructs, and then devise ways to operationalize them. The constructs are linked to the actual strategies and outcomes in a series of approximations, each step of which can be evaluated. The better the proxies, the more credible the results are likely to be. In this section, we illustrate successive proxies using sampling concepts, to highlight the potential for inferential challenges.

When researchers formulate research questions, the population of interest is often abstract. For example, suppose we wanted to test the effectiveness of an intervention to increase physical activity in low-income women. Figure 13.2 shows the series of steps between the abstract population construct (low-income women) and the actual participants. Using data from the actual sample on the far right, the researcher would like to make inferences about the effectiveness of the intervention for a broader group, but each proxy along the way represents a potential problem for achieving the desired inference. In interpreting a study, readers must consider how *plausible* it is that the actual sample reflects the recruited sample, the accessible population, the target population, and the population construct.

Table 13.1 presents a description of a hypothetical scenario in which the researchers moved from the population construct of low-income women to an actual sample of 161 participants. The table identifies some questions that might be asked in drawing inferences about the study results. Answers to these questions would affect the interpretation of whether the intervention *really* is effective with low-income women—or only with cooperative welfare recipients from two neighborhoods of Los Angeles who were recently approved for public assistance.

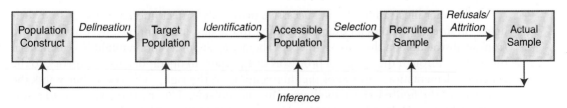

**FIGURE 13.2**  ● Inferences about populations: from final sample to the population.

## TABLE 13.1  Example of Successive Series of Proxies in Sampling

| Element | Description | Possible Inferential Challenges |
|---|---|---|
| Population construct | Low-income women | |
| Target population | All women who receive public assistance (cash welfare) in California | * Why only welfare recipients—why not the working poor?<br>* Why not those on disability?<br>* Why California? |
| Accessible population | All women who receive public assistance in Los Angeles and who speak English or Spanish | * Why Los Angeles?<br>* What about non-English/non-Spanish speakers? |
| Recruited sample | A consecutive sample of 300 female welfare recipients (English or Spanish speaking) who applied for benefits in January, 2013 at two randomly selected welfare offices in Los Angeles | * Why only new applicants—what about women with long-term receipt?<br>* Why only two offices? Are these representative?<br>* Is January a typical month? |
| Actual sample | 161 women from the recruited sample who fully participated in the study | * Who refused to participate (or was too ill, etc.)?<br>* Who dropped out of the study? |

As Figure 13.2 suggests, researchers make methodologic decisions that affect inferences, and these decisions must be carefully scrutinized. However, participant behavior and external circumstances also need to be considered in the interpretation. In our example, 300 women were recruited for the study, but only 161 provided data. The final sample of 161 almost surely would differ in important ways from the 139 who were not in the study, and these differences affect inferences about the study evidence.

Fortunately, researchers are increasingly documenting participant flow in their studies—especially in intervention studies. Guidelines called the Consolidated Standards of Reporting Trials or **CONSORT guidelines** have been adopted by major medical and nursing journals to help readers track study participants. CONSORT flow charts, when available, should be scrutinized in interpreting study results.

### Example of a CONSORT flow chart:

Qi and colleagues (2011) tested the effectiveness of a self-efficacy program aimed at preventing osteoporosis among Chinese immigrants. Figure 13.3 shows the progression of study participants through the study, from 111 originally assessed for eligibility to 72 who provided final data. As this figure shows, one person did not meet the inclusion criteria, and another 26 were eliminated because they were a member of a dyad and only one from each dyad was chosen (at random). All of those who enrolled ($N = 83$) did receive the allocated intervention, but 11 participants were lost to follow-up, leaving 72 for the final analysis.

As another illustration of how successive proxies can affect inferences about study evidence, Figure 13.4 shows an example relating to nursing interventions. Researchers move from an abstraction on the left—a "theory" about why an intervention might have beneficial outcomes—through the design of protocols that purport to operationalize the theory, to the actual implementation and use of the intervention on the right. The researcher wants the right side of the figure to be a good proxy for the left side. The interpreter's job is to assess the plausibility that the researcher was successful in the transformation.

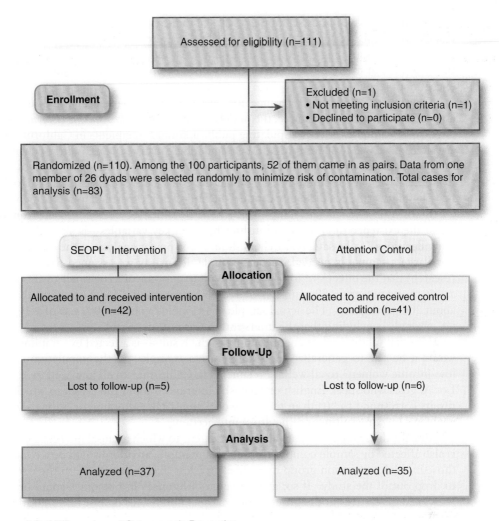

* Self Efficacy-based Osteoporosis Prevention

**FIGURE 13.3** ● Consort flow diagram of participant recruitment. (Adapted from Figure 1, Qi, B., Resnick, B., Smeltzer, S., & Bausell, B. (2011). Self-efficacy program to prevent osteoporosis among Chinese immigrants. *Nursing Research, 60,* 393–404.

## Credibility and Validity

Inference and validity are inextricably linked. As the research methodology experts Shadish and colleagues (2002) have stated, "We use the term *validity* to refer to the approximate truth of an inference" (p. 34). To be careful interpreters, readers must search for evidence that the desired inferences are, in fact, valid. Part of this process involves considering alternative competing hypotheses about the credibility and meaning of the results.

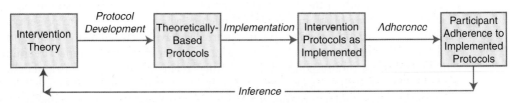

**FIGURE 13.4** ● Inferences about interventions: from actual operations to the theory.

In Chapter 9, we discussed four key types of validity that relate to the credibility of study results: statistical conclusion validity, internal validity, external validity, and construct validity. We use our sampling example (Fig. 13.2, p. 251 and Table 13.1, p. 252) to demonstrate the relevance of methodologic decisions to all four types of validity—and hence to inferences about study results.

Construct validity has relevance for measurement (Chapter 11), and also for many aspects of a study. In our example, the population construct is *low-income women*, which led to population eligibility criteria stipulating public assistance recipients in California. Yet, there are alternative operationalizations of the population construct (e.g., California women living below the official poverty level). Construct validity, it may be recalled, involves inferences from the particulars of the study to higher-order constructs. So it is fair to ask, Do the specified eligibility criteria adequately capture the population construct, low-income women?

Statistical conclusion validity—the extent to which correct inferences can be made about the existence of "real" relationships between key variables—is also affected by sampling decisions. To be safe, researchers should do a power analysis at the outset to estimate how large a sample is needed. In our example, let us say we assumed (based on previous research) that the effect size for the exercise intervention would be small-to-moderate, with $d = .40$. For a power of .80, with risk of a Type I error set at .05, we would need a sample of about 200 participants. The actual sample of 161 yields a nearly 30% risk of a Type II error, i.e., wrongly concluding that the intervention was not successful.

External validity—the generalizability of the results—is affected by sampling. To whom would it be safe to generalize the results in this example—to the population construct of low-income women? to all welfare recipients in California? to all new welfare recipients in Los Angeles who speak English or Spanish? Inferences about the extent to which the study results correspond to "truth in the real world" must take sampling decisions and sampling problems (e.g., recruitment difficulties) into account.

Finally, the study's internal validity (the extent to which a causal inference can be made) is also affected by sample composition. In this example, attrition would be a concern. Were those in the intervention group more likely (or less likely) than those in the control group to drop out of the study? If so, any observed differences in outcomes could be caused by individual differences in the groups (for example, differences in motivation), rather than by the intervention itself.

Methodological decisions and the careful implementation of those decisions—whether they be about sampling, intervention design, measurement, research design, or analysis—inevitably affect the rigor of a study. And all of them can affect the four types of validity and hence, the interpretation of the results.

## Credibility and Bias

A researcher's job is to translate abstract constructs into plausible and meaningful proxies. Another major job concerns efforts to eliminate, reduce, or control biases—or, as a last resort, to detect and understand them. As a reader of research reports, your job is to be on the lookout for biases, and to consider them in your assessment about the credibility of the results.

Biases are factors that create distortions and that undermine researchers' efforts to capture and reveal "truth in the real world." Biases are pervasive. It is not so much a question of whether there *are* biases in a study, so much as what types of bias are present, and how extensive, sizeable, and systematic the biases are. We have discussed many types of bias in this book—some reflect design inadequacies (e.g., selection bias), others reflect recruitment or sampling problems (nonresponse bias), and others relate to measurement (social desirability). Table 13.2 presents a list of some of the biases and errors mentioned in this book. This table is meant to serve as a reminder of some of the problems to consider in interpreting study results.

**TABLE 13.2  Selected List of Major Biases or Errors in Quantitative Studies in Four Research Domains**

| Research Design | Sampling | Measurement | Analysis |
|---|---|---|---|
| Expectation bias | Sampling error | Social desirability bias | Type I error |
| Hawthorne effect | Volunteer bias | Acquiescence bias | Type II error |
| Contamination of treatments | Nonresponse bias | Nay-sayers bias | |
| Carryover effects | | Extreme response set bias | |
| Noncompliance bias | | Recall/memory bias | |
| Selection bias | | Reactivity | |
| Attrition bias | | Observer biases | |
| History bias | | | |

**TIP:** The supplement to this chapter on thePoint website includes a longer list of biases, including many that were not described in this book. We offer definitions and notes for all biases listed. Different disciplines, and different writers, may use different names for the same or similar biases. The actual names are not important—what is important is to reflect on how different forces can distort the results and affect inferences.

## Credibility and Corroboration

Earlier, we noted that research interpreters should seek evidence to disconfirm the "null hypothesis" that the research results of a study are wrong. Some evidence to discredit the null hypothesis comes from the plausibility that proxies were good stand-ins for abstractions. Other evidence involves ruling out biases. Yet another strategy is to seek corroboration for the results.

Corroboration can come from internal and external sources, and the concept of *replication* is an important one in both cases. Interpretations are aided by considering prior research on the topic, for example. Interpreters can examine whether the study results replicate (are congruent with) those of other studies. Consistency across studies tends to discredit the "null hypothesis" of erroneous results.

Researchers may have opportunities for replication themselves. For example, in multisite studies, if the results are similar across sites, this suggests that something "real" is occurring with some regularity. Triangulation can be another form of replication. For example, if the results are similar across different measures of a key outcome, then there can perhaps be greater confidence that the results are "real" and do not reflect some peculiarity of an instrument.

Finally, we are strong advocates of mixed methods studies, a special type of triangulation (see Chapter 18). When findings from the analysis of qualitative data are consistent with the results of statistical analyses, internal corroboration can be especially powerful and persuasive.

# OTHER ASPECTS OF INTERPRETATION

If an assessment of the study leads you to accept that the results are probably "real," you have gone a long way in interpreting the study findings. Other interpretive tasks depend on a conclusion that the results appear to be credible.

## Precision of the Results

Results from statistical hypothesis tests indicate whether a relationship or group difference is probably real and replicable. A $p$ value in hypothesis testing indicates how strong the evidence is that the study's null hypothesis is false—it is not an estimate of any quantity of direct relevance to practicing nurses. A $p$ value offers information that is important, but incomplete.

Confidence intervals (CIs), by contrast, communicate information about how precise (or imprecise) the study results are. Dr. David Sackett, a founding father of the EBP movement, had this to say about CIs: "*P* values on their own are…not informative…. By contrast, CIs indicate the strength of evidence about quantities of direct interest, such as treatment benefit. Thus they are of particular relevance to practitioners of evidence-based medicine" (2000, p. 232). It seems likely that nurse researchers will increasingly report CI information in the years ahead because of the value of this information for interpreting study results and assessing their potential utility for nursing practice.

## Magnitude of Effects and Importance

Attaining statistical significance does not necessarily mean that the results are meaningful to nurses and clients. Statistical significance indicates that the results are unlikely to be due to chance—not that they are necessarily important. With large samples, even modest relationships are statistically significant. For instance, with a sample of 500, a correlation coefficient of .10 is significant at $p < .05$ level, but a relationship this weak may have little practical value. When assessing the importance of findings, interpreters must attend to actual numeric values and also, if available, to effect sizes. Effect size information is important in addressing the important EBP question (Box 2.1, p. 32): "What *is* the evidence—what is the magnitude of effects?"

The absence of statistically significant results, conversely, does not always mean that the results are unimportant—although because nonsignificant results could reflect a Type II error, the case is more complex. Suppose we compared two procedures for making a clinical assessment (e.g., body temperature) and that we found no statistically significant differences between the two methods. If an effect size analysis suggested a small effect size for the differences *despite a large sample size*, we might be justified in concluding that the two procedures yield equally accurate assessments. If one procedure is more efficient or less painful than the other, nonsignificant findings could be clinically important. Nevertheless, corroboration in replication studies would be needed before firm conclusions could be reached.

> **Example of contrasting statistical and clinical significance:**
> Nitz and Josephson (2011) studied whether a balance strategy training program for elders was effective in improving functional mobility and reducing falls. They found statistically significant improvements on several outcomes, but concluded that the improvement was clinically significant for only one of them, 5 sit-to-stands (timed). As the investigators noted, "Statistically significant improvement does not necessarily equate to a meaningful clinical effect" (p. 108).

## The Meaning of Quantitative Results

In quantitative studies, statistical results are in the form of test statistic values, $p$ levels, effect sizes, and CIs, to which researchers and consumers must attach meaning. Many questions about the meaning of statistical results reflect a desire to interpret causal connections.

Interpreting what results mean is not typically a challenge in descriptive studies. For example, suppose we found that, among patients undergoing electroconvulsive therapy (ECT), the percentage who experience an ECT-induced headache is 59.4% (95% CI = 56.3, 63.1). This result is directly interpretable. But if we found that headache prevalence is significantly lower in a cryotherapy intervention group than among patients given acetaminophen, we would need to interpret what the results mean. In particular, we need to interpret whether it is plausible that cryotherapy *caused* the reduced prevalence of headaches. Clearly, internal validity is a key issue in interpreting the meaning of results with a potential for causal inference—even if the results have previously been deemed to be "real," i.e., statistically significant.

In this section, we discuss the interpretation of various research outcomes within a hypothesis testing context. The emphasis in on the issue of causal interpretations.

### Interpreting Hypothesized Results

Interpreting the meaning of statistical results is easiest when hypotheses are supported. Researchers have already considered prior findings, a theoretical framework, and logical reasoning in developing hypotheses. Nevertheless, a few caveats should be kept in mind.

First, it is important to be conservative in drawing conclusions from the results and to avoid the temptation of going beyond the data to explain what results mean. For example, suppose we hypothesized that pregnant women's anxiety level about childbearing is correlated with the number of children they have. The data reveal a significant negative relationship between anxiety levels and parity ($r = -.40$). We interpret this to mean that increased experience with childbirth results in decreased anxiety. Is this conclusion supported by the data? The conclusion appears logical, but in fact, there is nothing in the data that leads directly to this interpretation. An important, indeed critical, research precept is: *correlation does not prove causation*. The finding that two variables are related offers no evidence suggesting which of the two variables—if either—caused the other. In our example, perhaps causality runs in the opposite direction—perhaps a woman's anxiety level influences how many children she bears. Or maybe a third variable, such as the woman's relationship with her husband, influences both anxiety and number of children. As discussed in Chapter 9, inferring causality is especially difficult in studies that have used a nonexperimental design.

Empirical evidence supporting research hypotheses never constitutes *proof* of their veracity. Hypothesis testing is probabilistic. There is always a possibility that observed relationships resulted from chance—that is, a Type I error has occurred. Researchers must be tentative about their results and about interpretations of them. Thus, even when the results are in line with expectations, researchers should draw conclusions with restraint and should give due consideration to limitations identified in assessing the accuracy of the results.

**Example of corroboration of a hypothesis:**
Houck and colleagues (2011) studied factors associated with self-concept in 145 children with attention deficit hyperactivity disorder (ADHD). They hypothesized that behavior problems in these children would be associated with less favorable self-concept, and they found that internalizing behavior problems were significantly predictive of lower self-concept scores. In their discussion, they stated that "age and internalizing behaviors were found to negatively influence the child's self-concept" (p. 245).

This study is a good example of the challenges of interpreting findings in correlational studies. The researchers' interpretation was that behavior problems were a factor that *influenced* ("caused") low self-concept. This is a conclusion supported by earlier research, yet there is nothing in the data that would rule out the possibility that a child's self-concept *influenced* the child's behavior, or that some other factor influenced both behavior and self-concept. The researchers' interpretation is certainly plausible, but their cross-sectional design makes it difficult to rule out other explanations. A major threat to the internal validity of the inference in this study is temporal ambiguity.

## Interpreting Nonsignificant Results

Nonsignificant results pose interpretative challenges because statistical tests are geared toward disconfirmation of the null hypothesis. Failure to reject a null hypothesis can occur for many reasons, and the real reason is usually difficult to discern. The null hypothesis *could* actually be true, for example, accurately reflecting the absence of a relationship among research variables.

On the other hand, the null hypothesis could be false. Retention of a false null hypothesis (a Type II error) can result from a variety of methodologic problems, such as poor internal validity, an anomalous sample, a weak statistical procedure, or unreliable measures. In particular, failure to reject null hypotheses is often a consequence of insufficient power, usually reflecting too small a sample size.

In any event, a retained null hypothesis should not be considered as proof of the *absence* of relationships among variables. *Nonsignificant results provide no evidence of the truth or the falsity of the hypothesis.* Interpreting the meaning of nonsignificant results can, however, be aided by considering such factors as sample size and effect size estimates.

> **Example of nonsignificant results:**
> Griffin, Polit, and Byrnes (2007) hypothesized that stereotypes about children (based on children's gender, race, and attractiveness) would influence pediatric nurses' perceptions of children's pain and their pain treatment recommendations. None of the hypotheses was supported—i.e., there was no evidence of stereotyping. The conclusion that stereotyping was absent was bolstered by the fact that the sample was randomly selected and rather large ($N = 334$) and nurses were blinded to the manipulation, i.e., child characteristics. Very small effect sizes offered additional support for the conclusion that stereotyping was absent.

Because statistical procedures are designed to provide support for rejecting null hypotheses, they are not well-suited for testing *actual* research hypotheses about the absence of relationships between variables or about equivalence between groups. Yet sometimes, this is exactly what researchers want to do, especially in clinical situations in which the goal is to test whether one practice is as effective as another. When the actual research hypothesis is null (i.e., a prediction of no group difference or no relationship), stringent additional strategies must be used to provide supporting evidence. In particular, it is imperative to compute effect sizes and CIs as a means of illustrating that the risk of a Type II error was small.

> **Example of support for a hypothesized nonsignificant result:**
> Rickard and colleagues (2010) conducted a clinical trial to test whether resite of peripheral intravenous devices (IVDs) based on clinical indications was equivalent to the recommended routine resite every 3 days in terms of IVD complications. Complication rates were 68 per 1,000 IVD days for clinically indicated replacement and 66 per 1,000 IVD days for routine replacement. The large sample ($N = 362$ patients), high $p$ value (.86), and negligible effect size (OR = 1.03) led the researchers to conclude that the evidence supported "the extended use of peripheral IVDs with removal only on clinical indication" (p. 53).

## Interpreting Unhypothesized Significant Results

Unhypothesized significant results can occur in two situations. The first involves exploring relationships that were not considered during the design of the study. For example, in examining correlations among research variables, a researcher might notice that two variables that were not central to the research questions were nevertheless significantly correlated—and interesting.

**Example of a serendipitous significant finding:**
Latendress and Ruiz (2011) studied the relationship between chronic maternal stress and preterm birth. They observed an unexpected finding that maternal use of selective serotonin reuptake inhibitors (SSRIs) was associated with a 12-fold increase in preterm births.

The second situation is more perplexing, and it does not happen often: obtaining results *opposite* to those hypothesized. For instance, a researcher might hypothesize that individualized teaching about AIDS risks is more effective than group instruction, but the results might indicate that the group method was significantly better. Although this might seem embarrassing, research should not be undertaken to corroborate predictions, but rather to arrive at truth. There is no such thing as a study whose results "came out wrong" if they reflect the truth.

When significant findings are opposite to what was hypothesized, it is less likely that the methods are flawed than that the reasoning or theory is problematic. The interpretation of such findings should involve comparisons with other research, a consideration of alternate theories, and a critical scrutiny of the research methods.

**Example of significant results contrary to hypothesis:**
Strom and colleagues (2011), who studied diabetes self-care in a national sample of more than 50,000 people with type 2 diabetes, hypothesized that rural dwellers would have poorer diabetes self-care than urban dwellers. However, they found the opposite: foot self-checks and daily blood glucose testing were significantly higher among those in rural areas.

## Interpreting Mixed Results

Interpretation is often complicated by *mixed results*: some hypotheses are supported, but others are not. Or a hypothesis may be accepted with one measure of the dependent variable, but rejected with a different measure. When only some results run counter to a theory or conceptual scheme, the research methods deserve critical scrutiny. Differences in the validity or reliability of the measures may account for such discrepancies, for example. On the other hand, mixed results may suggest that a theory needs to be qualified. Mixed results sometimes present opportunities to make conceptual advances because efforts to make sense of conflicting evidence may lead to a breakthrough.

**Example of mixed results:**
Dhruva and colleagues (2012) hypothesized that objective sleep/wake circadian rhythm parameters would be correlated with subjective ratings of sleep disturbance and fatigue in family caregivers of oncology patients. They found significant correlations for some variables (e.g., fatigue and subjective indicators of sleep disturbance), but not for others (e.g., fatigue and objective measures of sleep disturbance). The modest sample ($N = 103$) might have resulted from a Type II error for some of the relationships examined.

In summary, interpreting the meaning of research results is a demanding task, but it offers the possibility of intellectual rewards. Interpreters must play the role of scientific detectives, trying to make pieces of the puzzle fit together so that a coherent picture emerges.

### Generalizability of the Results

Researchers typically seek evidence that can be used by others. If a new nursing intervention is found to be successful, perhaps others will want to adopt it. Therefore, an important interpretive question is whether the intervention will "work" or whether the relationships will "hold" in other settings, with other people. Part of the interpretive process involves asking the question, "To what groups, environments, and conditions can the results reasonably be applied?"

In interpreting a study's generalizability, it is useful to consider our earlier discussion about proxies. For which higher-order constructs, which populations, which settings, or which versions of an intervention were the study operations good "stand-ins"?

### Implications of the Results

Once you have reached conclusions about the credibility, precision, importance, meaning, and generalizability of the results, you are ready to draw inferences about their implications. You might consider the implications of the findings with respect to future research: What should other researchers in this area do—what is the right "next step"? You are most likely to consider the implications for nursing practice: How should the results be used by nurses in their practice?

Clearly, all of the dimensions of interpretation that we have discussed are critical in evidence-based nursing practice. With regard to generalizability, it may not be enough to ask a broad question about to whom the results could apply—you need to ask, Are these results relevant to *my* particular clinical situation? Of course, if you have reached the conclusion that the results have limited credibility or importance, they may be of little utility to your practice.

# CRITIQUING INTERPRETATIONS

Researchers offer an interpretation of their findings and discuss what the findings might imply for nursing in the discussion section of research articles. When critiquing a study, your own interpretation can be contrasted against those of the researchers.

A good discussion section should point out study limitations. Researchers are in the best position to detect and assess sampling deficiencies, practical constraints, data quality problems, and so on, and it is a professional responsibility to alert readers to these difficulties. Also, when researchers acknowledge methodologic shortcomings, readers know that these limitations were considered in interpreting the results. Of course, researchers are unlikely to note all relevant limitations. Your task as reviewer is to develop your own interpretation and assessment of methodologic problems, to challenge conclusions that do not appear to be warranted, and to consider how the study's evidence could have been enhanced.

You should also carefully scrutinize causal interpretations, especially in nonexperimental studies. Sometimes, even the titles of reports suggest a potentially inappropriate causal inference. If the title of a nonexperimental study includes terms like "the effect of...," or "the impact of...," this may signal the need for critical scrutiny of the researcher's inferences.

In addition to comparing your interpretation with that of the researchers, your critique should also draw conclusions about the stated implications of the study. Some researchers make grandiose claims or offer unfounded recommendations on the basis of modest results. Some guidelines for evaluating researchers' interpretation are offered in Box 13.1.

**Box 13.1 Guidelines for Critiquing Interpretations/Discussions in Quantitative Research Reports**

**Interpretation of the Findings**

1. Did the researchers discuss any study limitations and their possible effects on the credibility of the results? In discussing limitations, were key threats to the study's validity and biases mentioned? Did the interpretations take limitations into account?
2. What types of evidence were offered in support of the interpretation, and was that evidence persuasive? If results were "mixed," were possible explanations offered? Were results interpreted in light of findings from other studies?
3. Did the researchers make any unjustifiable causal inferences? Were alternative explanations for the findings considered? Were the rationales for rejecting these alternatives convincing?
4. Did the interpretation take into account the precision of the results and/or the magnitude of effects? Did the researchers distinguish between practical and statistical significance?
5. Did the researchers draw any unwarranted conclusions about the generalizability of the results?

**Implications of the Findings and Recommendations**

6. Did the researchers discuss the study's implications for clinical practice or future nursing research? Did they make specific recommendations?
7. If yes, are the stated implications appropriate, given the study's limitations and the magnitude of the effects—as well as consistent with evidence from other studies? Are there important implications that the report neglected to include?

## RESEARCH EXAMPLES WITH CRITICAL THINKING EXERCISES

In this section, we provide details about the interpretive portion of a study, followed by some questions to guide critical thinking.

Example 1 below is also featured in our *Interactive Critical Thinking Activity* on thePoint website where you can easily record, print, and e-mail your responses to the related questions.

### EXAMPLE 1 ● Interpretation in a Quantitative Study

**Study:** An office-based health promotion intervention for overweight and obese uninsured adults: A feasibility study (Buchholz et al., 2012)

**Statement of Purpose:** The purpose of this study was to assess the feasibility and initial efficacy of a nurse-delivered tailored physical activity intervention for uninsured overweight or obese adults seen at a free clinic.

**Method:** The researchers used a one-group pretest–posttest design with a convenience sample of 123 adults recruited from two free clinics in a midsized county in Indiana. The health intervention promotion (HIP) was designed as a 30-minute nutrition and physical activity intervention to be incorporated into monthly clinic visits for 6 months. Outcomes, measured at baseline and 6 months later, included body mass index values, physical activity, and self-reported nutrition measures. Adherence, the primary feasibility outcome, was measured by recording attendance at the HIP visits.

**Analyses:** The researchers used a number of descriptive statistics (means, standard deviations, percentages) to describe their sample and examine rates of adherence. Paired t-tests or chi-squared tests were used to examine changes over time for those who fully adhered to the program (attended all six sessions). The researchers also examined differences between those who fully adhered, and those who only partially adhered to HIP (i.e., attended fewer than six sessions).

**Results:** A total of 123 people (89% female) agreed to participate, but only 23 (19%) completed all 6 months of the program. About half of the enrollees (49%) completed three or more visits. The body mass index (BMI) of the full adherers declined significantly between baseline and follow-up, from 37.3 to 36.7. The BMI of partial adherers also declined, but the change was not significant. Partial and full adherers were not significantly different in terms of gender, ethnicity, or baseline BMI classification, but full adherers were older ($M = 53.4$) than partial adherers ($M = 45.1$).

**Discussion:** Here are a few excerpts from the Discussion section of this report:

"The strategies used in this study to recruit uninsured people from two free clinics proved effective. The participants were receptive to a nurse-delivered moderate-intensity counseling program to decrease or maintain weight through nutrition and physical activity…The challenge was to retain people in the study through and beyond 3 months. Once a participant missed an appointment (nonadherence), he/she did not return. Repeated attempts were made to find out why these participants did not adhere to the nurse visits. From those we reached, we learned that time and health issues were among the primary reasons for nonadherence. Furthermore, anecdotal staff notes show that conflicting responsibilities because of care of a family member, of other family-related responsibilities, and scheduling difficulties interfered with the ability of some participants to keep appointments with the nurse." (p. 72).

"A program such as this one, with appointments 1 month apart and no intervening contacts, can be problematic when participants miss an appointment…Telephone contacts with patients between visits may provide the additional intervention intensity needed. However, multiple calls often have to be made to make contact, increasing the effort and cost of this strategy…Mobile phone text messaging may offer a nonintrusive, cost-effective way to maintain contact.." (p. 73).

"Throughout this 6-month intervention, participants' step counts remained in the range of 5,000 to 7,500, which has been classified as 'low active.' Likewise, there was little change in fruit and vegetable intake…These findings suggest that additional attention may need to be given to the availability of recreational facilities and grocery stores with adequate produce" (p. 73).

"The main limitation of this pilot study was the lack of a control group with random assignment to group, thereby decreasing the ability to attribute the weight loss to the intervention. Also, the small number of participants who completed all six intervention sessions made it difficult to evaluate the impact of the full intervention on BMI" (p.73).

"This feasibility study demonstrates that a moderate-intensity nurse counseling intervention was modestly effective in decreasing BMI in those participants who were able to fully adhere to the visits…Although this study demonstrates that, for a small percentage of the sample, this intervention was successful in reducing BMI, study results also showed that a large number of participants did not adhere after the 3-month mark, suggesting this time frame needs to be more closely examined in regard to frequency of nurse contact as well as participant loss of interest" (pp. 73–74).

## CRITICAL THINKING EXERCISES

1. Answer the relevant questions from Box 13.1 on page 261 regarding this study. (We encourage you to read the report in its entirety, especially the Discussion, to answer these questions).
2. Also consider the following targeted questions:
   a. Comment on the statistical conclusion validity of this study.
   b. Was a CONSORT-type flow-chart included in this report? Should one have been included?
3. What might be some of the uses to which the findings could be put in clinical practice?

## EXAMPLE 2 ● Discussion Section in the Study in Appendix A

- Read the "Discussion" section of Howell and colleagues' (2007) study ("Anxiety, anger, and blood pressure in children") in Appendix A on pages 395–402.

## CRITICAL THINKING EXERCISES

1. Answer the relevant questions in Box 13.1 on page 261 regarding this study.
2. Also consider the following targeted questions:
   a. Were there any statistically significant correlations that were unanticipated or unhypothesized in this study? Did the researchers discuss them? If yes, do you agree with their interpretation?
   b. Comment on the researchers' recommendations about gender-specific research in the discussion section.

## EXAMPLE 3 ● Quantitative Study in Appendix C

- Read McGillion and colleagues' (2008) study (Randomized controlled trial of a psychoeducational program for the self-management of chronic cardiac pain) in Appendix C on pages 413–428 and then address the following suggested activities or questions.

## CRITICAL THINKING EXERCISES

1. Before reading our critique, which accompanies the full report, write your own critique or prepare a list of what you think are the study's major strengths and weaknesses. Pay particular attention to validity threats and bias. Then contrast your critique with ours. Remember that you (or your instructor) do not necessarily have to agree with all of the points made in our critique, and you may identify strengths and weaknesses that we overlooked. You may find the broad critiquing guidelines in Table 4.1 on page 69 helpful.
2. Write a short summary of how credible, important, and generalizable you find the study results to be. Your summary should conclude with your interpretation of what the results mean, and what their implications are for nursing practice. Contrast your summary with the discussion section in the report itself.
3. In selecting studies to include in this textbook, we avoided choosing a poor-quality study because we did not wish to embarrass any researchers. In the questions below, we offer some "pretend" scenarios in which the researchers for the study in Appendix C made different methodologic decisions than the ones they in fact did make. Write a paragraph or two critiquing these "pretend" decisions, pointing out how these alternatives would have affected the rigor of the study and the inferences that could be made.
   a. Pretend that the researchers had been unable to randomize subjects to treatments. The design, in other words, would be a nonequivalent control-group quasi-experiment.
   b. Pretend that 130 participants were randomized (this is actually what did happen), but that only 80 participants remained in the study 3 months after randomization.
   c. Pretend that the health-related quality of life measure (the SF-36 scale) and the Seattle Angina Questionnaire (SAQ) were of lower quality—for example, that they had internal consistency reliabilities of .60.

**WANT TO KNOW MORE?** A wide variety of resources to enhance your learning and understanding of this chapter are available on thePoint.

- Interactive Critical Thinking Activity
- Chapter Supplement on Research Biases
- Answers to the Critical Thinking Exercises for Examples 2 and 3
- Student Review Questions
- Full-text online
- Internet Resources with useful websites for Chapter 13

Additional study aids including eight journal articles and related questions are also available in *Study Guide for Essentials of Nursing Research, 8e.*

# SUMMARY POINTS

- The interpretation of quantitative research **results** (the outcomes of the statistical analyses) typically involves consideration of: (1) the credibility of the results, (2) precision of estimates of effects, (3) magnitude of effects, (4) underlying meaning, (5) generalizability, and (6) implications for future research and nursing practice.

- The particulars of the study—especially the methodologic decisions made by researchers—affect the inferences that can be made about the correspondence between study results and "truth in the real world."

- A cautious and even skeptical outlook is appropriate in drawing conclusions about the credibility and meaning of study results.

- An assessment of a study's credibility can involve various approaches, one of which involves an evaluation of the degree of congruence between abstract constructs or idealized methods on the one hand and the proxies actually used on the other.

- Credibility assessments also involve an assessment of study rigor through an analysis of validity threats and biases that could undermine the accuracy of the results.

- Corroboration (replication) of results, through either internal or external sources, is another approach in a credibility assessment.

- Researchers can facilitate interpretations by carefully documenting methodologic decisions and the outcomes of those decisions (e.g., by using the **CONSORT guidelines** to document participant flow).

- In their discussions of study results, researchers should themselves always point out known study limitations, but readers should draw their own conclusions about the rigor of the study and about the plausibility of alternative explanations for the results.

# REFERENCES FOR CHAPTER 13

Buchholz, S. W., Wilbur, J., Miskovich, L., & Gerard, P. (2012). An office-based health promotion intervention for overweight and obese uninsured adults: A feasibility study. *Journal of Cardiovascular Nursing, 27,* 68–75.

Dhruva, A., Lee, K., Paul, S., West, C., Dunn, L., Dodd, M., et al. (2012). Sleep-wake circadian activity rhythms and fatigue in family caregivers of oncology patients. *Cancer Nursing, 35,* 70–81.

Griffin, R., Polit, D., & Byrnes, M. (2007). Stereotyping and nurses' treatment of children's pain. *Research in Nursing & Health, 30,* 655–666.

Houck, G., Kendall, J., Miller, A., Morrell, P., & Wiebe, G. (2011). Self-concept in children and adolescents with attention deficit hyperactivity disorder. *Journal of Pediatric Nursing, 26,* 239–247.

Latendresse, G., & Ruiz, R. (2011). Maternal corticotrophin-releasing hormone and the use of selective serotonin reuptake inhibitors independently predict the occurrence of preterm birth. *Journal of Midwifery & Women's Health, 56,* 118–126.

Nitz, J., & Josephson, D. (2011). Enhancing functional balance and mobility among older people living in long-term care facilities. *Geriatric Nursing, 32,* 106–113.

Qi, B., Resnick, B., Smeltzer, S., & Bausell, B. (2011). Self-efficacy program to prevent osteoporosis among Chinese immigrants. *Nursing Research, 60,* 393–404.

Rickard, C., McCann, D., Munnings, J., & McGrail, M. (2010). Routine resite of peripheral intravenous devices every 3 days did not reduce complication compared with clinically indicated resite. *BMC Medicine, 8,* 53–65.

Sackett, D. L., Straus, S.E., Richardson, W.S., Rosenberg, W., & Haynes, R. B. (2000). *Evidence-based medicine: How to practice and teach EBM* (2nd ed.), Edinburgh, UK: Churchill Livingstone.

Shadish, W. R., Cook, T. D., & Campbell, D. T. (2002). *Experimental and quasi-experimental designs for generalized causal inference.* Boston, MA: Houghton Mifflin.

Strom, J., Lynch, C., & Egede, L. (2011). Rural/urban variations in diabetes self-care and quality of care in a national sample of U. S. adults with diabetes. *The Diabetes Educator, 37,* 254–262.

# Qualitative Research

# 14 Qualitative Designs and Approaches

## LEARNING OBJECTIVES

*On completing this chapter, you will be able to:*

- Discuss the rationale for an emergent design in qualitative research, and describe qualitative design features
- Identify the major research traditions for qualitative research and describe the domain of inquiry of each
- Describe the main features of ethnographic, phenomenologic, and grounded theory studies
- Discuss the goals and methods of various types of research with an ideological perspective
- Define new terms in the chapter

## KEY TERMS

Basic social process (BSP)
Bracketing
Case study
Constant comparison
Constructivist grounded theory
Core variable
Critical ethnography

Critical theory
Descriptive phenomenology
Descriptive qualitative study
Emergent design
Ethnonursing research
Feminist research
Field work
Hermeneutics

Interpretive phenomenology
Narrative analysis
Participant observation
Participatory action research (PAR)
Reflexive journal

Quantitative researchers specify a research design before collecting even one piece of data, and rarely depart from that design once the study is underway: they design and *then* they do. In qualitative research, by contrast, the study design typically evolves during the project: qualitative researchers design *as* they do. Decisions about how best to obtain data, from whom to obtain data, and how long a data collection session should last are made as the study unfolds.

# THE DESIGN OF QUALITATIVE STUDIES

Qualitative studies use an **emergent design** that evolves as researchers make ongoing decisions based on what they have already learned. An emergent design in qualitative studies is a reflection of the researchers' desire to have the inquiry based on the realities and viewpoints of those under study—realities and viewpoints that are not known at the outset.

## Characteristics of Qualitative Research Design

Qualitative inquiry has been guided by different disciplines, and each has developed methods for addressing questions of interest. Some characteristics of qualitative research design tend to apply across disciplines, however. In general, qualitative design:

- Is flexible and elastic, capable of adjusting to what is being learned during data collection
- Often involves merging together various data collection strategies (i.e., triangulation)
- Tends to be holistic, striving for an understanding of the whole
- Requires researchers to become intensely involved and can necessitate a lengthy period of time
- Benefits from ongoing data analysis to guide subsequent strategies and decisions about when data collection is done.

Although design decisions are not finalized in advance, qualitative researchers typically do advance planning that supports their flexibility. That is, they plan for broad contingencies that may pose decision opportunities once the study has begun. For example, qualitative researchers make advance decisions with regard to their research tradition, the study site, the maximum amount of time available for the study, a broad data collection strategy, and the equipment they will need in the field. Qualitative researchers plan for a variety of circumstances, but decisions about how to deal with them must be resolved when the social context of time, place, and human interactions are better understood.

## Qualitative Design Features

Some of the design features discussed in Chapter 9 apply to qualitative studies. However, qualitative design features are often posthoc characterizations of what happened in the field rather than features specifically planned in advance. To contrast qualitative and quantitative research design, we consider the design elements identified in Table 9.1 on page 150.

### Intervention, Control, and Blinding

Qualitative research is almost always nonexperimental—although a qualitative substudy may be embedded in an experiment (see Chapter 18). Qualitative researchers do not conceptualize their studies as having independent and dependent variables, and they rarely control any aspect of the people or environment under study. Blinding is rarely used by qualitative researchers. The goal is to develop a rich understanding of a phenomenon as it exists and as it is constructed by individuals within their own context.

### Comparisons

Qualitative researchers typically do not plan to make group comparisons because the intent is to thoroughly describe or explain a phenomenon. Yet, patterns emerging in the data sometimes suggest illuminating comparisons. Indeed, as Morse (2004) noted in an editorial in *Qualitative Health Research*, "All description requires comparisons" (p. 1323). In analyzing qualitative data and in determining whether categories are saturated, there is a need to compare "this" to "that."

> **Example of qualitative comparisons:**
> Baum and colleagues (2012) explored the experiences of 30 Israeli mothers of very-low-birth-weight babies when the babies were still in neonatal hospitalization. The researchers discovered that there were three patterns with regard to attribution of blame for not carrying to full term: those who blamed themselves, those who blamed others, and those who believed that premature delivery was fortunate because it saved their baby's life.

## Research Settings

Qualitative researchers usually collect their data in real-world, naturalistic settings. And, whereas a quantitative researcher usually strives to collect data in one type of setting to maintain constancy of conditions (e.g., conducting all interviews in participants' homes), qualitative researchers may deliberately strive to study phenomena in a variety of natural contexts, especially in ethnographic research.

> **Example of variation in settings and sites:**
> Bohman and colleagues (2011) studied the experience of being old and in care-related relationships in a changing South African context. Interviews with elders were supplemented with observations in a variety of community contexts where the care of elders takes place and in participants' homes.

## Timeframes

Qualitative research, like quantitative research, can be either cross-sectional, with one data collection point, or longitudinal, with multiple data collection points designed to observe the evolution of a phenomenon. In terms of the retrospective/prospective distinction, most qualitative research is retrospective: an "outcome" or situation occurring in the present may give rise to inquiries into previously occurring factors that led up to or contributed to it.

> **Examples of a longitudinal qualitative study:**
> Taylor and colleagues (2011) conducted a longitudinal study over a 12-month period of the experience of surviving colorectal cancer treatment and dealing with fears about recurrence.

## Causality and Qualitative Research

In evidence hierarchies that rank evidence in terms of its support of causal inferences (e.g., the one in Figure 2.1 on page 23), qualitative inquiry is often near the base, which has led some to criticize evidence-based practice initiatives. The issue of causality, which has been controversial throughout the history of science, is especially contentious in qualitative research.

Some qualitative researchers think that causality is not an appropriate concept within the constructivist paradigm. For example, Lincoln and Guba (1985) devoted an entire chapter of their book to a critique of causality and argued that it should be replaced with a concept that they called *mutual shaping*. According to their view, "Everything influences everything else, in the here and now" (p. 151).

Others, however, believe that qualitative methods are particularly well suited to understanding causal relationships. For example, Huberman and Miles (1994) argued that qualitative studies "can look directly and longitudinally at the local processes underlying a temporal series of events and states, showing how these led to specific outcomes, and ruling out rival hypotheses" (p. 434).

In attempting to not only describe but also to explain phenomena, qualitative researchers who undertake in-depth studies will inevitably reveal patterns and processes suggesting causal interpretations. These interpretations can be (and often are) subjected to more systematic testing using more controlled methods of inquiry.

# QUALITATIVE RESEARCH TRADITIONS

Although some features are shared by many qualitative research designs, there is a wide variety of approaches. One useful taxonomic system is to describe qualitative research according to disciplinary traditions. These traditions vary in their conceptualization of what types of questions are important to ask and in the methods considered appropriate for answering them. Table 14.1 provides an overview of several such traditions, some of which we have previously introduced. This section describes traditions that have been especially prominent in nursing research.

## Ethnography

Ethnography is a type of qualitative inquiry that involves the description and interpretation of a culture and cultural behavior. *Culture* refers to the way a group of people live—the patterns of human activity and the symbolic structures (for example, the values and norms) that give such activity significance. Ethnographies typically involve extensive **field work**, which is the process by which the ethnographer comes to understand a culture. Because culture is, in itself, not visible or tangible, it must be inferred from the words, actions, and products of members of a group and then constructed through ethnographic writing.

Ethnographic research sometimes concerns broadly defined cultures (e.g., the Maori culture of New Zealand), in what is sometimes referred to as a *macroethnography*. However, ethnographies sometimes focus on more narrowly defined cultures in a *microethnography* or focused ethnography. Focused ethnographies are fine-grained studies of small units in a group or culture (e.g., the culture of an intensive care unit). An underlying assumption

## TABLE 14.1 Overview of Qualitative Research Traditions

| Discipline | Domain | Research Tradition | Area of Inquiry |
| --- | --- | --- | --- |
| Anthropology | Culture | Ethnography | Holistic view of a culture |
| Psychology/ Philosophy | Lived experience | Phenomenology | Experiences and meanings of individuals within their lifeworld |
| | | Hermeneutics | Interpretations and meanings of individuals' experiences |
| Sociology | Social settings | Grounded theory | Social psychological and structural processes within a social setting |
| History | Past behavior, events, conditions | Historical analysis | Description/interpretation of historical events |

of the ethnographer is that every human group eventually evolves a culture that guides the members' view of the world and the way they structure their experiences.

> **Example of a focused ethnography:**
> MacKinnon (2011) used an ethnographic approach to explore the work of rural nurses, with specific focus on their safeguarding work to maintain patient safety.

Ethnographers seek to learn from (rather than to study) members of a cultural group—to understand their world view. Ethnographic researchers refer to "emic" and "etic" perspectives. An **emic perspective** refers to the way the members of the culture regard their world—the insiders' view. The emic is the local language, concepts, or means of expression that are used by the members of the group under study to name and characterize their experiences. The **etic perspective**, by contrast, is the outsiders' interpretation of the experiences of that culture—the words and concepts they use to refer to the same phenomena. Ethnographers strive to acquire an emic perspective of a culture and to reveal *tacit knowledge*—information about the culture that is so deeply embedded in cultural experiences that members do not talk about it or may not even be consciously aware of it.

Three broad types of information are usually sought by ethnographers: cultural behavior (what members of the culture do), cultural artifacts (what members make and use), and cultural speech (what they say). Ethnographers rely on a wide variety of data sources, including observations, in-depth interviews, records, and other types of physical evidence (e.g., photographs, diaries). Ethnographers typically use a strategy called **participant observation** in which they make observations of the culture under study while participating in its activities. Ethnographers observe people day after day in their natural environments to observe behavior in a wide array of circumstances. Ethnographers also enlist the help of **key informants** to help them understand and interpret the events and activities being observed.

Ethnographic research is labor-intensive and time-consuming—months and even years of fieldwork may be required to learn about a culture. Ethnography requires a certain level of intimacy with members of the cultural group, and such intimacy can be developed only over time and by working directly with those members as active participants.

The product of ethnographies is a rich and holistic description of the culture under study. Ethnographers also interpret the culture, describing normative behavioral and social patterns. Among health care researchers, ethnography provides access to the health beliefs and health practices of a culture. Ethnographic inquiry can thus help to foster understanding of behaviors affecting health and illness. Leininger coined the phrase **ethnonursing research**, which she defined as "the study and analysis of the local or indigenous people's viewpoints, beliefs, and practices about nursing care behavior and processes of designated cultures" (1985, p. 38).

> **Example of an ethnonursing study:**
> Schumacher (2010) explored the meanings, beliefs, and practices of care for rural people in the Dominican Republic. Leininger's theory of culture-care diversity and universality was the conceptual basis for the study, and her four-phase ethnonursing methods were adopted. Interviews were conducted with 29 informants.

Ethnographers are often, but not always, "outsiders" to the culture under study. A type of ethnography that involves self-scrutiny (including scrutiny of groups or cultures to which researchers themselves belong) is called *autoethnography* or *insider research*.

Autoethnography has several advantages, including ease of access and recruitment and the ability to get candid data based on pre-established trust. The drawback is that an "insider" may have biases about certain issues or may be so entrenched in the culture that valuable data are overlooked.

## Phenomenology

Phenomenology, rooted in a philosophical tradition developed by Husserl and Heidegger, is an approach to exploring and understanding people's everyday life experiences.

Phenomenologic researchers ask: What is the *essence* of this phenomenon as experienced by these people and what does it *mean?* Phenomenologists assume there is an *essence*—an essential structure—that can be understood, in much the same way that ethnographers assume that cultures exist. Essence is what makes a phenomenon what it is, and without which it would not be what it is. Phenomenologists investigate subjective phenomena in the belief that critical truths about reality are grounded in people's lived experiences. The topics appropriate to phenomenology are ones that are fundamental to the life experiences of humans, such as the meaning of suffering or the quality of life with chronic pain.

Phenomenologists believe that lived experience gives meaning to each person's perception of a particular phenomenon. The goal of phenomenologic inquiry is to understand fully lived experience and the perceptions to which it gives rise. Four aspects of lived experience that are of interest to phenomenologists are *lived space*, or spatiality; *lived body*, or corporeality; *lived time*, or temporality; and *lived human relation*, or relationality.

Phenomenologists view human existence as meaningful and interesting because of people's consciousness of that existence. The phrase *being-in-the-world* (or *embodiment*) is a concept that acknowledges people's physical ties to their world—they think, see, hear, feel, and are conscious through their bodies' interaction with the world.

In phenomenologic studies, the main data source is in-depth conversations. Through these conversations, researchers strive to gain entrance into the informants' world, and to have access to their experiences as lived. Phenomenologic studies usually involve a small number of participants—often 10 or fewer. For some phenomenologic researchers, the inquiry includes not only gathering information from informants but also efforts to experience the phenomenon, through participation, observation, and reflection. Phenomenologists share their insights in rich, vivid reports that describe key *themes*. The results section in a phenomenological report should help readers "see" something in a different way that enriches their understanding of experiences.

Phenomenology has several variants and interpretations. The two main schools of thought are descriptive phenomenology and interpretive phenomenology (hermeneutics).

### Descriptive Phenomenology

**Descriptive phenomenology** was developed first by Husserl, who was primarily interested in the question: *What do we know as persons?* His philosophy emphasized descriptions of human experience. Descriptive phenomenologists insist on the careful portrayal of ordinary conscious experience of everyday life—a depiction of "things" as people experience them. These "things" include hearing, seeing, believing, feeling, remembering, deciding, and evaluating.

Descriptive phenomenologic studies often involve the following four steps: bracketing, intuiting, analyzing, and describing. **Bracketing** refers to the process of identifying and holding in abeyance preconceived beliefs and opinions about the phenomenon under study. Researchers strive to bracket out presuppositions in an effort to confront their data in pure form. Phenomenological researchers (as well as other qualitative researchers) often maintain a **reflexive journal** in their efforts to bracket.

*Intuiting*, the second step in descriptive phenomenology, occurs when researchers remain open to the meanings attributed to the phenomenon by those who have experienced it. Phenomenologic researchers then proceed to an analysis (i.e., extracting significant statements, categorizing, and making sense of the essential meanings of the phenomenon). Finally, the descriptive phase occurs when researchers come to understand and define the phenomenon.

**Example of a descriptive phenomenological study:**

Porter and colleagues (2012) used a descriptive phenomenological approach in their longitudinal study of the intentions of elderly homebound women with regard to reaching help quickly.

## Interpretive Phenomenology

Heidegger, a student of Husserl, is the founder of **interpretive phenomenology** or hermeneutics. Heidegger's critical question is: *What is being?* He stressed interpreting and understanding—not just describing—human experience. He believed that lived experience is inherently an interpretive process and argued that **hermeneutics** ("understanding") is a basic characteristic of human existence. (The term *hermeneutics* refers to the art and philosophy of interpreting the meaning of an object, such as a *text* or work of art). The goals of interpretive phenomenological research are to enter another's world and to discover the wisdom and understandings found there.

Gadamer, another influential interpretive phenomenologist, described the interpretive process as a circular relationship known as the *hermeneutic circle* where one understands the whole of a text (for example, a transcribed interview) in terms of its parts and the parts in terms of the whole. Researchers continually question the meanings of the text.

In an interpretive phenomenologic study, bracketing does not occur. For Heidegger, it was not possible to bracket one's being-in-the-world. Hermeneutics presupposes prior understanding on the part of the researcher. Interpretive phenomenologists ideally approach each interview text with openness—they must be open to hearing what it is the text is saying.

Interpretive phenomenologists, like descriptive phenomenologists, rely primarily on in-depth interviews with individuals who have experienced the phenomenon of interest, but they may go beyond a traditional approach to gathering and analyzing data. For example, interpretive phenomenologists sometimes augment their understandings of the phenomenon through an analysis of supplementary texts, such as novels, poetry, or other artistic expressions—or they use such materials in their conversations with study participants.

**Example of an interpretive phenomenological study:**

Vatne and Nåden (2012) used a hermeneutic approach to explore the experiences and reflections of 10 people after suicidal crisis or recently completed suicide attempts.

👉 **HOW-TO-TELL TIP:** How can you tell if a phenomenological study is descriptive or interpretive? Phenomenologists often use terms that can help you make this determination. In a descriptive phenomenological study such terms may be bracketing, description, essence, and Husserl. The names of Colaizzi, Van Kaam, or Giorgi may appear in the methods section. In an interpretive phenomenological study, key terms can include being-in-the-world, hermeneutics, understanding, and Heidegger. The names van Manen, Benner, or Diekelmann may appear in the method section. These names are discussed in Chapter 16 on qualitative data analysis.

## Grounded Theory

Grounded theory has contributed to the development of many middle-range theories of phenomena relevant to nurses. Grounded theory was developed in the 1960s by two sociologists, Glaser and Strauss (1967), whose theoretical roots were in *symbolic interaction*, which focuses on the manner in which people make sense of social interactions.

Grounded theory tries to account for people's actions from the perspective of those involved. Grounded theory researchers seek to understand the actions by first discovering the main concern or problem, and then the behavior that is designed to address it. The manner in which people resolve this main concern is called the **core variable**. One type of core variable is a **basic social process (BSP)**. The goal of grounded theory is to discover the main concern and the basic social process that explains how people resolve it. Grounded theory researchers generate conceptual categories and integrate them into a substantive theory grounded in the data.

### Grounded Theory Methods

Grounded theory methods constitute an entire approach to the conduct of field research. A study that truly follows Glaser and Strauss's precepts does not begin with a focused research problem. The problem, and the process used to solve it, emerge from the data and are discovered during the study. In grounded theory research, data collection, data analysis, and sampling of participants occur simultaneously. The grounded theory process is recursive: researchers collect data, categorize them, describe the emerging central phenomenon, and then recycle earlier steps.

A procedure called **constant comparison** is used to develop and refine theoretically relevant concepts and categories. Categories elicited from the data are constantly compared with data obtained earlier so that commonalities and variations can be detected. As data collection proceeds, the inquiry becomes increasingly focused on emerging theoretical concerns.

In-depth interviews and participant observation are common data sources in grounded theory studies, but existing documents and other data may also be used. Typically, a grounded theory study involves interviews with a sample of about 20 to 30 people.

> **Example of a grounded theory study:**
> Lundh and colleagues (2012) used grounded theory methods to understand the process of trying to quit smoking from the perspective of patients with COPD. Analysis of data from interviews with 18 patients led to a theoretical model that illuminated factors related to the decision to try to quit smoking, including constructive and destructive strategies.

### Alternate Views of Grounded Theory

In 1990, Strauss and Corbin published the first edition of a controversial book, *Basics of qualitative research: Grounded theory procedures and techniques*. The stated purpose of the book was to provide beginning grounded theory researchers with basic procedures involved in building theory at a substantive level.

Glaser, however, disagreed with some procedures advocated by Strauss (his original coauthor) and Corbin (a nurse researcher). Glaser (1992) believed that Strauss and Corbin developed a method that is not grounded theory but rather what he called "full conceptual description." According to Glaser, the purpose of grounded theory is to generate concepts and theories about their relationships that explain, account for, and interpret variation in behavior in the substantive area under study. *Conceptual description*, in contrast, is aimed at describing the full range of behavior of what is occurring in the substantive area.

Nurse researchers have conducted grounded theory studies using both the original Glaser and Strauss and the Strauss and Corbin approaches. They are also using an approach called **constructivist grounded theory** (Charmaz, 2006). Charmaz viewed Glaser and Strauss' grounded theory as being based in the positivist tradition. In Charmaz's approach, the developed grounded theory is viewed as an interpretation. The data collected and analyzed are acknowledged to be constructed from shared experiences and relationships between the researcher and the participants. Data and analyses are viewed as social constructions.

## Historical Research

One other qualitative tradition springs from the discipline of history. **Historical research** is the systematic collection and critical evaluation of data relating to past occurrences. Historical research relies primarily on qualitative (narrative) data but can sometimes involve statistical analysis of quantitative data. Nurses use historical research methods to examine a wide range of phenomena in both the recent and more distant past.

Historical research should not be confused with a review of the literature about historical events. Like other types of research, historical inquiry has as its goal discovering *new* knowledge, not summarizing existing knowledge.

Data for historical research are usually in the form of written records: diaries, letters, newspapers, medical or legal documents, and so forth. Nonwritten materials may also be of interest. For example, visual materials, such as photographs and films, are forms of data. In some cases, it is possible to conduct interviews with people who participated in historical events (e.g., nurses who served in recent wars).

Historical research is usually interpretive. Historical researchers try to describe what happened, and also how and why it happened. Relationships between events and ideas, between people and organizations, are explored and interpreted within their historical context and within the context of new viewpoints about what is historically significant.

> **Example of historical research:**
> Connolly and Gibson (2011) conducted a historical study of the role nurses played in pediatric tuberculosis care in Virginia from 1900 to 1935. They concluded that although nurses were leaders in designing a template for children's care, they also helped to forge "a system funded by a complicated, poorly coordinated, race- and class-based mix of public and private support" (p. 230). Yet, the researchers also found that these nurses took courageous action and helped invent pediatric nursing.

# OTHER TYPES OF QUALITATIVE RESEARCH

Qualitative studies often can be characterized and described in terms of the disciplinary research traditions discussed in the previous section. However, several other important types of qualitative research not associated with a particular discipline also deserve mention.

## Case Studies

**Case studies** are in-depth investigations of a single entity or small number of entities. The entity may be an individual, family, institution, community, or other social unit. Case study researchers attempt to analyze and understand issues that are important to the history, development, or circumstances of the entity under study.

One way to think of a case study is to consider what is at center stage. In most studies, whether qualitative or quantitative, certain phenomena or variables are the core of the inquiry. In a case study, the *case* itself is central. The focus of case studies is typically on understanding *why* an individual thinks, behaves, or develops in a particular manner rather than on *what* his or her status or actions are. Probing research of this type often requires detailed study over a considerable period. Data are often collected that relate not only to the person's present state but also to past experiences and situations relevant to the problem being examined.

The greatest strength of case studies is the depth that is possible when a small number of entities is being investigated. Case study researchers have opportunities to gain an intimate knowledge of a person's feelings, actions (past and present), intentions, and environment. Yet, this same strength is a potential weakness: researchers' familiarity with the person or group may make objectivity more difficult—especially if the data are collected by observational techniques for which the researchers are the main (or only) observers. Another criticism of case studies concerns generalizability: If researchers discover important relationships, it is difficult to know whether the same relationships would occur with others. However, case studies can often play a critical role in challenging generalizations based on other types of research.

**Example of a case study:**
Moro and colleagues (2011) conducted in-depth case studies of parents' decision-making for life support for extremely premature infants, based on multiple in-depth interviews and data from medical records.

## Narrative Analyses

**Narrative analysis** focuses on *story* as the object of inquiry, to understand how individuals make sense of events in their lives. The underlying premise of narrative research is that people most effectively make sense of their world—and communicate these meanings—by constructing and narrating stories. Individuals construct stories when they wish to understand specific events and situations that require linking an inner world of desire to an external world of observable actions. Analyzing stories opens up *forms* of telling about experience, and is more than just content. Narrative analysts ask, *Why did the story get told that way?*

A number of structural approaches can be used to analyze stories, including ones based on literary analysis and linguistics. Burke's (1969) *pentadic dramatism* is one approach for narrative analysis. For Burke there are five key elements of a story: act, scene, agent, agency, and purpose. The five terms of Burke's pentad are meant to be understood paired together as ratios such as, act: agent, agent: agency, and purpose: agent. The analysis focuses on the internal relationships and tensions of these five terms to each other. Each pairing of terms in the pentad provides a different way of directing the researcher's attention. What drives the narrative analysis is not just the interaction of the pentadic terms but an imbalance between two or more of these terms.

**Example of a narrative analysis using Burke's approach:**
Beck (2006), one of this book's authors, did a narrative analysis on birth trauma. Eleven mothers sent their stories of traumatic childbirth to Beck. Burke's pentad of terms was used to analyze these narratives. The most problematic ratio imbalance was between act and agency. Frequently, in the mothers' narratives it was the "how" an act was carried out by the labor and delivery staff that led to the women perceiving their childbirth as traumatic.

## Descriptive Qualitative Studies

Many qualitative studies claim no particular disciplinary or methodologic roots. The researchers may simply indicate that they have conducted a qualitative study, a naturalistic inquiry, or a *content analysis* of qualitative data (i.e., an analysis of themes and patterns that emerge in the narrative content). Thus, some qualitative studies do not have a formal name or do not fit into the typology we have presented in this chapter. We refer to these as **descriptive qualitative studies**.

Descriptive qualitative studies tend to be eclectic in their designs and methods and are based on the general premises of constructivist inquiry. These studies, which are actually more common in nursing than studies based on a disciplinary tradition, are infrequently discussed in research methods textbooks.

☞ **TIP:** The Chapter Supplement on the**Point**₭ website for this chapter presents additional material relating to descriptive qualitative studies and to studies that nurse researcher Sally Thorne (2008) called interpretive description. ☀

**Example of a descriptive qualitative study:**
Stewart and colleagues (2012) did a descriptive qualitative study to explore the biopsychosocial burden of chronic hepatitis C and patients' coping and help-seeking. In-depth interviews were conducted with 13 patients, 5 hepatologists, and 2 counselors.

# RESEARCH WITH IDEOLOGICAL PERSPECTIVES

Some qualitative researchers conduct inquiries within an ideological framework, typically to draw attention to certain social problems or the needs of certain groups and to bring about change. These approaches represent important investigative avenues.

## Critical Theory

**Critical theory** originated with a group of Marxist-oriented German scholars in the 1920s. Variants of critical theory abound in the social sciences. Essentially, a critical researcher is concerned with a critique of society and with envisioning new possibilities.

Critical social science is typically action oriented. Its aim is to make people aware of contradictions and disparities in their beliefs and social practices, and become inspired to change them. Critical researchers, who reject the idea of an objective, disinterested inquirer, are oriented toward a transformation process. Critical theory calls for inquiries that foster enlightened self-knowledge and social or political change.

The design of research in critical theory often begins with an analysis of certain aspects of the problem. For example, critical researchers might analyze and critique taken-for-granted assumptions that underlie the problem, the language used to depict the situation, and the biases of prior researchers investigating the problem. Critical researchers often triangulate methods, and emphasize multiple perspectives (e.g., alternative racial or social class perspectives) on problems. Critical researchers typically interact with participants in ways that emphasize participants' expertise. Some features that distinguish more traditional qualitative research and critical research are summarized in Table 14.2.

Critical theory has been applied in several disciplines, but has played an especially important role in ethnography. **Critical ethnography** focuses on raising consciousness in the hope of effecting social change. Critical ethnographers address the historical, social, political, and economic dimensions of cultures and their value-laden agendas. Critical ethnographers

**TABLE 14.2  Comparison of Traditional Qualitative Research and Critical Research**

| Issue | Traditional Qualitative Research | Critical Research |
|---|---|---|
| Research aims | Understanding, reconstruction of multiple constructions | Critique, transformation, consciousness raising, advocacy |
| View of knowledge | Transactional/subjective: knowledge is created in interactions between investigator and participants | Transactional/subjective: value-mediated and value-dependent |
| Methods | Dialectic: truth is arrived at logically through conversations | Dialectic and didactic: dialogue designed to transform naivety and misinformation |
| Evaluative criteria for inquiry quality | Authenticity, trustworthiness | Historical situatedness of the inquiry, erosion of ignorance, stimulus for change |
| Researcher's role | Facilitator of multivoice reconstruction | Transformative agent, advocate, activist |

attempt to increase the political dimensions of cultural research and undermine oppressive systems. Critical ethnography has been viewed as especially well suited to health promotion research because both are concerned with enabling people to take control over their own situation.

> **Example of a critical ethnography:**
> Baumbusch (2011) used a critical ethnographic approach to explore disenfranchised groups in the context of long-term residential care in British Columbia, Canada.

## Feminist Research

**Feminist research** is similar to critical theory research, but the focus is on gender domination and discrimination within patriarchal societies. Similar to critical researchers, feminist researchers seek to establish collaborative and nonexploitative relationships with their informants and to conduct research that is transformative. Feminist investigators seek to understand how gender and a gendered social order have shaped women's lives and their consciousness. The aim is to facilitate change in ways relevant to ending women's unequal social position.

The scope of feminist research ranges from studies of the subjective views of individual women to studies of social movements, structures, and broad policies that affect (and often exclude) women. Feminist research methods typically include in-depth, interactive, and collaborative individual interviews or group interviews that offer the possibility of reciprocally educational encounters. Feminists usually seek to negotiate the meanings of the results with those participating in the study, and to be self-reflective about what they themselves are learning.

> **Example of feminist research:**
> Van Daalen-Smith (2011) used feminist theory to explore women's experiences of electroshock, which the women—but not their nurses—believed resulted in damage and devastating loss.

## Participatory Action Research

A type of research known as participatory action research is closely allied to both critical research and feminist research. **Participatory action research (PAR)** is based on a recognition that the production of knowledge can be political and used to exert power. Researchers in this approach typically work with groups or communities that are vulnerable to the control or oppression of a dominant group.

PAR is, as the name implies, participatory. Researchers and study participants collaborate in the definition of the problem, the selection of research methods, the analysis of the data, and the use to which findings are put. The aim of PAR is to produce not only knowledge, but also action, empowerment, and consciousness-raising as well. The PAR tradition has as its starting point a concern for the powerlessness of the group under study. Thus, a key objective is to produce an impetus that is directly used to make improvements through education and sociopolitical action.

In PAR, the research methods are designed to facilitate processes of collaboration and dialogue that can motivate, increase self-esteem, and generate community solidarity. Thus, "data-gathering" strategies used are not only the traditional methods of interview and observation (including both qualitative and quantitative approaches), but may also include storytelling, sociodrama, photography, drawing, skits, and other activities designed to encourage people to find creative ways to explore their lives, tell their stories, and recognize their own strengths.

> **Example of PAR:**
> Kneipp and colleagues (2011) designed and tested a public health nursing case-management intervention for women with chronic health problems who received public assistance. The community-based intervention had been developed on the basis of PAR.

# CRITIQUING QUALITATIVE DESIGNS

Evaluating a qualitative design is often difficult. Qualitative researchers do not always document design decisions and are even less likely to describe the process by which such decisions were made. Researchers often do, however, indicate whether the study was conducted within a specific qualitative tradition. This information can be used to come to some conclusions about the study design. For example, if a report indicated that the researcher conducted 2 months of field work for an ethnographic study, you might well suspect that insufficient time had been spent in the field to obtain a true emic perspective of the culture under study. Ethnographic studies may also be critiqued if their only source of information was from interviews, rather than from a broader range of data sources, particularly participant observations.

In a grounded theory study, you might also be concerned if the researcher relied exclusively on data from interviews; a stronger design might have been obtained by including participant observations. Also, look for evidence about when the data were collected and analyzed. If the researcher collected all the data before analyzing any of it, you might question whether the constant comparative method was used correctly.

In critiquing a phenomenological study, you should first determine if the study is descriptive or interpretive. This will help you to assess how closely the researcher kept to the basic tenets of that qualitative research tradition. For example, in a descriptive phenomenological study, did the researcher bracket? When critiquing a phenomenological study, in

## BOX 14.1   Guidelines for Critiquing Qualitative Designs

1. Is the research tradition for the qualitative study identified? If none was identified, can one be inferred? If more than one was identified, is this justifiable or does it suggest "method slurring"?
2. Is the research question congruent with a qualitative approach and with the specific research tradition (i.e., is the domain of inquiry for the study congruent with the domain encompassed by the tradition)? Are the data sources, research methods, and analytic approach congruent with the research tradition?
3. How well is the research design described? Are design decisions explained and justified? Does it appear that the researcher made all design decisions up-front, or did the design emerge during data collection, allowing researchers to capitalize on early information?
4. Is the design appropriate, given the research question? Does the design lend itself to a thorough, in-depth, intensive examination of the phenomenon of interest? What design elements might have strengthened the study (e.g., a longitudinal perspective rather than a cross-sectional one)?
5. Was there evidence of reflexivity in the design?
6. Was the study undertaken with an ideological perspective? If so, is there evidence that ideological methods and goals were achieved? (e.g., was there evidence of full collaboration between researchers and participants? Did the research have the power to be transformative, or is there evidence that a transformative process occurred?)

addition to critiquing the methodology, you should also look at its power in capturing the meaning of the phenomena being studied.

No matter what qualitative design is identified in a study, look to see if the researchers stayed true to a single qualitative tradition throughout the study or if they mixed qualitative traditions ("method slurring"). For example, did the researcher state that grounded theory was used, but then presents results that described *themes* instead of generating a substantive theory?

The guidelines in Box 14.1 are designed to assist you in critiquing the designs of qualitative studies.

## RESEARCH EXAMPLES WITH CRITICAL THINKING EXERCISES

This section presents examples of different types of qualitative studies. Read these summaries and then answer the critical thinking questions, referring to the full research report if necessary.

⚡ Example 1 below is also featured in our *Interactive Critical Thinking Activity* on thePoint website where you can easily record, print, and e-mail your responses to the related questions.

### EXAMPLE 1  ●  A Grounded Theory Study

**Study:** Preserving the self: The process of decision-making about hereditary breast cancer and ovarian cancer risk reduction (Howard et al., 2011).

**Statement of Purpose:** The purpose of the study was to understand how women make decisions about strategies to reduce the risk of hereditary breast and ovarian cancer (HBOC), such as cancer screening and risk-reducing surgeries.

**Method:** The researchers used a constructivist grounded theory approach to understanding women's decision-making processes. Participants were recruited through a hereditary cancer program. Women were eligible for the study if they were older than 18 and tested positive for BRCA1/2 mutations in genetic testing. The researchers initially invited all eligible women to participate, but as the study progressed, they used preliminary findings to recruit women who might best refine conceptualizations. Data saturation was achieved with a total of 22 participants. In-depth interviews, lasting 45 to 90 minutes, were audiotaped and subsequently transcribed for analysis. Early interviews covered broad questions about decision-making and changes in decisions over time. Later in the study, the questions became more focused, to explore certain issues in greater depth and to verify emerging findings. Four women, whose decision experiences varied, were interviewed a second time to obtain clarification and feedback about preliminary findings. The analysis of the data was guided by theories of relational autonomy and gender: "Using gender as an analytic tool helped us explore the role of femininity in decision-making in the context of HBOC.... It also enabled us to examine the influence of gendered roles in relation to family, friends, and health professionals on HBOC decision-making" (p. 505).

**Key Findings:** The women's main concern was making a decision about risk-reducing strategies, and the analysis suggested that the overarching decision-making process entailed *preserving the self*. The process was shaped by various contextual conditions, including characteristics of health services, gendered roles, the nature of the risk-reducing strategies to be considered, and the women's perceptions of their proximity to cancer. These contextual conditions contributed to different decision-making approaches and five distinct decision-making styles: "snap" decision-making, intuitive decision-making, deliberate decision-making, deferred decision-making, and "if-then" decision-making. The researchers concluded that the findings provide insights that could inform the provision of decisional support to BRCA1/2 carriers.

## CRITICAL THINKING EXERCISES

1. Answer the relevant questions from Box 14.1 on page 278 regarding this study.
2. Also consider the following targeted questions:
   a. Was this study cross-sectional or longitudinal?
   b. Could this study have been undertaken as an ethnography? A phenomenological inquiry?
3. If the results of this study are trustworthy, in what ways do you think the findings could be used in clinical practice?

## EXAMPLE 2 ● Phenomenological Study in Appendix B

- Read the method section from Beck and Watson's (2010) study ("Subsequent childbirth after a previous traumatic birth") in Appendix B on pages 403–412.

## CRITICAL THINKING EXERCISES

1. Answer the relevant questions from Box 14.1 on page 278 regarding this study.
2. Also consider the following targeted questions:
   a. Was this study a descriptive or interpretive phenomenology?
   b. Could this study have been conducted as a grounded theory study? As an ethnographic study? Why or why not?
   c. Could this study have been conducted as a feminist inquiry? If yes, what might Beck have done differently?

**WANT TO KNOW MORE?** A wide variety of resources to enhance your learning and understanding of this chapter are available on thePoint.

- Interactive Critical Thinking Activity
- Chapter Supplement on Qualitative Descriptive Studies
- Answers to the Critical Thinking Exercises for Example 2
- Student Review Questions
- Full-text online
- Internet Resources with useful websites for Chapter 14

Additional study aids including eight journal articles and related questions are also available in *Study Guide for Essentials of Nursing Research, 8e.*

## SUMMARY POINTS

- Qualitative research involves an **emergent design**—a design that emerges in the field as the study unfolds.

- Although qualitative design is elastic and flexible, qualitative researchers plan for broad contingencies that can pose decision opportunities for study design in the field.

- Ethnography focuses on the culture of a group of people and relies on extensive **field work** that usually includes **participant observation** and in-depth interviews with **key informants**. Ethnographers strive to acquire an **emic** (insider's) perspective of a culture rather than an **etic** (outsider's) perspective.

- Nurses sometimes refer to their ethnographic studies as **ethnonursing research**. Most ethnographers study cultures other than their own; *autoethnographies* are ethnographies of a group or culture to which the researcher belongs.

- Phenomenologists seek to discover the *essence* and *meaning* of a phenomenon as it is experienced by people, mainly through in-depth interviews with people who have had the relevant experience.

- In **descriptive phenomenology**, which seeks to describe lived experiences, researchers strive to **bracket** out preconceived views and to *intuit* the essence of the phenomenon by remaining open to meanings attributed to it by those who have experienced it.

- **Interpretive phenomenology (hermeneutics)** focuses on interpreting the meaning of experiences, rather than just describing them.

- **Grounded theory** researchers try to account for people's actions by focusing on the main concern that their behavior is designed to resolve. The manner in which people resolve this main concern is the **core variable**. The goal of grounded theory is to discover this main concern and the **basic social process (BSP)** that explains how people resolve it.

- Grounded theory uses **constant comparison**: categories elicited from the data are constantly compared with data obtained earlier.

- A controversy in grounded theory concerns whether to follow the original Glaser and Strauss procedures or to use procedures adapted by Strauss and Corbin; Glaser has argued that the latter approach does not result in *grounded theories* but rather in *conceptual descriptions*. More recently, Charmaz's **constructivist grounded theory** has emerged, emphasizing interpretive aspects in which the grounded theory is constructed from shared experiences and relationships between the researcher and participants.

- **Case studies** are intensive investigations of a single entity or a small number of entities, such as individuals, groups, families, or communities.

- **Narrative analysis** focuses on *story* in studies in which the purpose is to determine how individuals make sense of events in their lives. Several different structural approaches can be used to analyze narrative data (e.g., Burke's *pentadic dramatism*).

- **Descriptive qualitative studies** are not embedded in a disciplinary tradition. Such studies may be referred to as qualitative studies, naturalistic inquiries, or as qualitative content analyses.

- Research is sometimes conducted within an ideological perspective, and such research tends to rely primarily on qualitative research.

- **Critical theory** is concerned with a critique of existing social structures. Critical researchers conduct studies that involve collaboration with participants and that foster enlightened self-knowledge and transformation. **Critical ethnography** uses the principles of critical theory in the study of cultures.

- **Feminist research**, like critical research, aims at being transformative, but the focus is on how gender domination and discrimination shape women's lives and their consciousness.

- **Participatory action research (PAR)** produces knowledge through close collaboration with groups that are vulnerable to control or oppression by a dominant culture; in PAR research, methods take second place to emergent processes that can motivate people and generate community solidarity.

# REFERENCES FOR CHAPTER 14

Baum, N., Weidberg, Z., Osher, Y., & Kohelet, D. (2012). No longer pregnant, not yet a mother: Giving birth prematurely to a very-low-birth-weight baby. *Qualitative Health Research, 22*, 595–606.

Baumbusch, J. (2011). Conducting critical ethnography in long-term residential care. *Journal of Advanced Nursing, 67*, 184–192.

Beck, C. T. (2006). Pentadic cartography: Mapping birth trauma narratives. *Qualitative Health Research,16*, 453–466.

Bohman, D., van Wyck, N., & Ekman, S. (2011). South Africans' experiences of being old and of care and caring in a transitional period. *International Journal of Older People Nursing, 6*, 187–195.

Burke, K. (1969). *A grammer of motives.* Berkley, CA: University of California Press.

Charmaz, K. (2006). *Constructing grounded theory: A practical guide through qualitative analysis.* Thousand Oaks, CA: Sage Publications.

Connolly, C., & Gibson, M. (2011). The "white plague" and color: Children, race, and tuberculosis in Virginia 1900–1935. *Journal of Pediatric Nursing, 26*, 230–238.

Glaser, B. G. (1992). *Emergence versus forcing: Basics of grounded theory analysis.* Mill Valley, CA: Sociology Press.

Glaser, B. G., & Strauss, A. L. (1967). *The discovery of grounded theory: Strategies for qualitative research.* Chicago, IL Aldine.

Howard, A. F., Balneaves, L., Bottorff, J., & Rodney, P. (2011). Preserving the self: The process of decision making about hereditary breast cancer and ovarian cancer risk reduction. *Qualitative Health Research, 21*, 502–519.

Huberman, A. M., & Miles, M. (1994). Data management and analysis methods. In Denzin, N. K., & Lincoln, Y. S. (Eds.), *Handbook of qualitative research.* (1st ed.). Thousand Oaks, CA: Sage.

Kneipp, S., Kairalla, J., Lutz, B., Pereira, D., Hall, A., Flocks, J., et al. (2011). Public health nursing case management for women receiving Temporary Assistance for Needy Families: A randomized controlled trial using community-based participatory research. *American Journal of Public Health, 101*, 1759–68.

Leininger, M. M. (Ed.). (1985). *Qualitative research methods in nursing.* New York: Grune and Stratton.

Lincoln, Y. S., & Guba, E. G. (1985). *Naturalistic inquiry.* Newbury Park, CA: Sage.

Lundh, L., Hylander, I., & Tornkvist, L. (2012). The process of trying to quit smoking from the perspective of patients with chronic obstructive pulmonary disease. *Scandinavian Journal of Caring Sciences,* PubMed ID 22117588

MacKinnon, K. (2011). Rural nurses' safeguarding work: Reembodying patient safety. *Advances in Nursing Science, 34*, 119–129.

Moro, T., Kavanagh, K., Savage, T., Reyes, M., Kimura, R., & Bhat, R. (2011). Parent decision making for life support for extremely premature infants. *The Journal of Perinatal & Neonatal Nursing, 25*, 52–60.

Morse, J. M. (2004). Qualitative comparison: Appropriateness, equivalence, and fit. *Qualitative Health Research, 14*(10), 1323–1325.

Porter, E., Ganong, L., & Matsuda, S. (2012). Intentions of older homebound women with regard to reaching help quickly. *Western Journal of Nursing Research,* PubMed ID 22146885.

Schumacher, G. (2010). Culture care meanings, beliefs, and practices in rural Dominican Republic. *Journal of Transcultural Nursing, 21,* 93–103.

Stewart, B., Mikocka-Walus, A., Harley, H., & Andrews, J. (2012). Help-seeking and coping with the psychosocial burden of chronic hepatitis C. *International Journal of Nursing Studies, 49*(5), 560–569.

Strauss, A., & Corbin, J. (1998). *Basics of qualitative research: Grounded theory procedures and techniques* (2nd ed.). Thousand Oaks, CA: Sage.

Taylor, C., Richardson, A., & Cowley, B. (2011). Surviving cancer treatment. *European Journal of Oncology Nursing, 15,* 243–249.

Thorne, S. (2008). *Interpretive description.* Walnut Creek, CA: Left Coast Press.

Van Daalen-Smith, C. (2011). Waiting for oblivion: women's experiences with electroshock. *Issues in Mental Health Nursing, 32,* 457–472.

Vatne, M., & Nåden, D. (2012). Finally, it became too much—experiences and reflections in the aftermath of attempted suicide. *Scandinavian Journal of Caring Sciences, 26*(2), 304–312.

# 15 Sampling and Data Collection in Qualitative Studies

## LEARNING OBJECTIVES

*On completing this chapter, you will be able to:*

- Describe the logic of sampling for qualitative studies
- Identify and describe several types of sampling in qualitative studies
- Evaluate the appropriateness of the sampling method and sample size used in a qualitative study
- Identify and describe methods of collecting unstructured self-report data
- Identify and describe methods of collecting and recording unstructured observational data
- Critique a qualitative researcher's decisions regarding the data collection plan (general method, informational adequacy, mode of administration)
- Define new terms in the chapter

## KEY TERMS

| | | |
|---|---|---|
| Critical incidents technique | Log | Semistructured interview |
| Data saturation | Maximum variation sampling | Snowball sampling |
| Field notes | Photo-elicitation interview | Theoretical sampling |
| Focus group interview | Photovoice | Topic guide |
| Grand tour question | Purposive (purposeful) | Unstructured interview |
| Key informant |    sampling | |

This chapter covers two important aspects of qualitative studies—sampling (selecting good study participants) and data collection (gathering the right types and amount of information to address the research question).

# SAMPLING IN QUALITATIVE RESEARCH

Qualitative studies almost always use small, nonprobability samples. This does not mean that qualitative researchers are unconcerned with the quality of their samples; rather, they use different considerations in selecting study participants.

## The Logic of Qualitative Sampling

Quantitative research is concerned with measuring attributes and identifying relationships in a population, and therefore a representative sample is desirable so that the findings can be generalized. The aim of most qualitative studies is to discover *meaning* and to uncover multiple realities, not to generalize to a target population.

Qualitative researchers ask such sampling questions as: Who would be an *information-rich* data source for my study? Whom should I talk to, or what should I observe, to maximize my understanding of the phenomenon? A first step in qualitative sampling is selecting settings with high potential for information richness.

As the study progresses, new sampling questions emerge, such as the following: Whom can I talk to or observe who would confirm my understandings? Challenge or modify my understandings? Enrich my understandings? As with the overall design, sampling design in qualitative studies is an emergent one that capitalizes on early information to guide subsequent action.

> 👉 **TIP:** Like quantitative researchers, qualitative researchers often identify eligibility criteria for their studies. Although they do not specify an explicit population to whom results could be generalized, they do establish the kinds of people who are eligible to participate in their research.

## Types of Qualitative Sampling

Qualitative researchers avoid random samples because they are not the best methods for selecting people who will make good informants, that is, people who meet the conceptual needs of the study and are knowledgeable, articulate, reflective, and willing to talk at length with researchers. Qualitative researchers use various nonprobability sampling designs.

### Convenience and Snowball Sampling

Qualitative researchers often begin with a convenience sample (also called a *volunteer sample*). Often, volunteer samples are used when researchers want participants to come forward and identify themselves. For example, if we wanted to study the experiences of people with frequent nightmares, we might recruit them by placing a notice on a bulletin board, in a newspaper, or on the Internet. We would be less interested in obtaining a representative sample of people with nightmares, than in recruiting a diverse group with various nightmare experiences.

Sampling by convenience is efficient, but is not a preferred approach, even in qualitative studies. The aim in qualitative studies is to extract the greatest possible information from a small number of people, and a convenience sample may not provide the most information-rich sources. However, convenience sampling may be an economical way to launch the sampling process.

> **Example of a convenience sample:**
> Beal and colleagues (2012) did a narrative analysis of women's early symptom experience of ischemic stroke. The convenience sample of nine women was recruited through fliers distributed at community stroke groups and at hospitals, and an advertisement was placed in a local newspaper.

Qualitative researchers also use **snowball sampling** (or *network sampling*), asking early informants to make referrals for other participants. A weakness of this approach is that the eventual sample might be restricted to a small network of acquaintances. Also, the quality of the referrals may be affected by whether the referring sample member trusted the researcher and truly wanted to cooperate.

> **Example of a snowball sample:**
> Cooke and colleagues (2012) studied factors influencing women's decisions to delay childbearing
> beyond the age of 35. The initial participant referred a further potential participant, and snowball
> sampling continued until the full sample of 18 women was obtained.

## Purposive Sampling

Qualitative sampling may begin with volunteer informants and may be supplemented with new participants through snowballing. Many qualitative studies, however, evolve to a purposive (or *purposeful*) sampling strategy in which researchers deliberately choose the cases or types of cases that will best contribute to the study. Regardless of how initial participants are selected, qualitative researchers often strive to select sample members purposefully based on the information needs that emerge from the early findings.

Within purposive sampling, dozens of strategies have been identified (Patton, 2002), only some of which are mentioned here. Researchers do not necessarily refer to their sampling plans with Patton's labels; his classification shows the kind of diverse strategies qualitative researchers have adopted to meet the conceptual needs of their research:

- **Maximum variation sampling** involves deliberately selecting cases with wide variation on dimensions of interest.
- *Extreme (deviant) case sampling* provides opportunities for learning from the most unusual and extreme informants (e.g., outstanding successes and notable failures).
- *Typical case sampling* involves the selection of participants who illustrate or highlight what is typical or average.
- *Criterion sampling* involves studying cases that meet a predetermined criterion of importance.

Maximum variation sampling is often the sampling mode of choice in qualitative research because it is useful in illuminating the scope of a phenomenon and in identifying important patterns that cut across variations. Other strategies can also be used advantageously, however, depending on the nature of the research question.

> **Example of maximum variation sampling:**
> Tierney and colleagues (2011) did an in-depth study of factors that influence physical activity in people
> with heart failure. Their sample included 22 patients aged between 53 and 82 who were purposively
> selected to provide variation in gender, age, heart failure duration and severity, and activity levels.

A strategy of sampling confirming and disconfirming cases is another purposive strategy that is used toward the end of data collection. As researchers note trends and patterns in the data, emerging conceptualizations may need to be checked. **Confirming cases** are additional cases that fit researchers' conceptualizations and strengthen credibility. **Disconfirming cases** are new cases that do not fit and serve to challenge researchers' interpretations. These "negative" cases may offer new insights into how the original conceptualization needs to be revised.

> **TIP:** Some qualitative researchers call their sample *purposive* simply because they "purposely" selected people who experienced the phenomenon of interest. Exposure to the phenomenon is, however, an eligibility criterion. If the researcher then recruits *any* person with the desired experience, the sample is selected by convenience, not purposively. Purposive sampling implies an intent to choose *particular* exemplars or *types* of people who can best enhance the researcher's understanding of the phenomenon.

## Theoretical Sampling

**Theoretical sampling** is a method used in grounded theory studies. Theoretical sampling involves decisions about what data to collect next and where to find those data to develop an emerging theory optimally. The basic question in theoretical sampling is: What groups or subgroups should the researcher turn to next? Groups are chosen for their relevance in furthering the emerging conceptualization. These groups are not chosen before the research begins but only as they are needed for their theoretical relevance in developing and refining emerging categories.

Theoretical sampling is not the same as purposeful sampling. The objective of theoretical sampling is to discover categories and their properties and to offer new insights into interrelationships that occur in the substantive theory.

**Example of a theoretical sampling:**
Porr and colleagues (2012) used theoretical sampling in their grounded theory study that elucidated how public health nurses develop therapeutic relationships with vulnerable, low-income single mothers. After identifying a fundamental pattern of interactional behaviors by interviewing and observing nurses and mothers, the researchers saw that theory construction could be enhanced by interviewing a family physician, two social workers, and other service providers so that they could compare other relationship experiences with the mothers.

## Sample Size in Qualitative Research

Sample size in qualitative research is usually determined based on informational needs. A guiding principle is **data saturation**—that is, sampling to the point at which no new information is obtained and redundancy is achieved. The number of participants needed to reach saturation depends on various factors. For example, the broader the scope of the research question, the more participants will likely be needed. Data quality can also affect sample size. If participants are able to reflect on their experiences and communicate effectively, saturation can be achieved with a relatively small sample. Type of sampling strategy may also be relevant: a larger sample is likely to be needed with maximum variation sampling than with typical case sampling.

**Example of saturation:**
Bertrand (2012) studied nurses' integration of traditional Chinese medicine into their triage process. She thought she had achieved saturation after 15 interviews, but when she conducted the 16th interview, "an operating nurse told me a story I had not heard before" (p. 266). Interviewing continued and saturation was reached at 20 interviews.

☞ **TIP:** Sample size adequacy in a qualitative study is difficult to evaluate because the main criterion is redundancy of information, which consumers have insufficient information to judge. Some qualitative reports explicitly mention that data saturation was achieved.

## Sampling in the Three Main Qualitative Traditions

There are similarities among the main qualitative traditions with regard to sampling: samples are usually small, nonrandom methods are used, and final sampling decisions usually take place during data collection. However, there are some differences as well.

## Sampling in Ethnography

Ethnographers may begin with a "big net" approach—that is, they mingle and converse with as many members of the culture as possible. Although they may talk to many group members (usually 25 to 50), ethnographers often rely heavily on a smaller number of **key informants**, who are highly knowledgeable about the culture and who develop special, ongoing relationships with the researcher. Key informants are the researcher's main link to the "inside."

Key informants are chosen purposively, guided by the ethnographer's informed judgments. Developing a pool of potential key informants often depends on ethnographers' ability to construct a relevant framework. For example, an ethnographer might decide to seek out different types of key informants based on their *roles* (e.g., health care practitioners, advocates). Once a pool of potential key informants is identified, key considerations for final selection are their level of knowledge about the culture and how willing they are to collaborate with the ethnographer in revealing and interpreting the culture.

Sampling in ethnography typically involves sampling *things* as well as people. For example, ethnographers make decisions about observing *events* and *activities*, about examining *records* and *artifacts*, and about exploring *places* that provide clues about the culture. Key informants can play an important role in helping ethnographers decide what to sample.

**Example of an ethnographic sample:**
Lori and Boyle (2011) conducted an ethnographic study exploring cultural childbirth practices, beliefs, and traditions in postconflict Liberia. The researchers engaged in participant observation, which involved participation "in many community activities around the hospital and at out-patient clinics" (p. 457). They also conducted interviews with 56 key informants: 10 postpartum women who had experienced a childbirth complication, 18 family members of women who had died or suffered severe morbidity, and 26 health care workers, indigenous healers, and tribal chiefs in a rural county of Liberia.

## Sampling in Phenomenological Studies

Phenomenologists tend to rely on very small samples of participants—typically 10 or fewer. Two principles guide the selection of a sample for a phenomenological study: (1) all participants must have experienced the phenomenon and (2) they must be able to articulate what it is like to have lived that experience. Phenomenological researchers often want to explore diversity of individual experiences and so they may specifically look for people with demographic or other differences who have shared a common experience.

**Example of a sample in a phenomenological study:**
Roscigno and Swanson (2011) recruited a larger-than-typical purposive sample in their phenomenological study of the experiences of parents from across the United States whose child had a traumatic brain injury. Their sample included 42 parents from 37 families. The goal was to recruit a diverse group of parents and children with varied sociodemographic characteristics.

Interpretive phenomenologists may, in addition to sampling people, sample artistic or literary sources. Experiential descriptions of a phenomenon may be selected from literature, such as poetry, novels, biographies, autobiographies, or diaries. These sources can help increase phenomenologists' understanding of the phenomena under study. Art—including paintings, sculpture, film, photographs, and music—can offer additional insights into lived experience.

## Sampling in Grounded Theory Studies

Grounded theory research is typically done with samples of about 20 to 30 people, using theoretical sampling. The goal in a grounded theory study is to select informants who can best contribute to the evolving theory. Sampling, data collection, data analysis, and theory construction occur concurrently, and so study participants are selected serially and contingently (i.e., contingent on the emerging conceptualization). Sampling might evolve as follows:

1. The researcher begins with a general notion of where and with whom to start. The first few cases may be solicited by convenience or through snowballing.
2. In the early part of the study, a strategy such as maximum variation sampling might be used, to gain insights into the range and complexity of the phenomenon.
3. The sample is adjusted in an ongoing fashion. Emerging conceptualizations help to inform the theoretical sampling process.
4. Sampling continues until saturation is achieved.
5. Final sampling may include a search for confirming and disconfirming cases to test, refine, and strengthen the theory.

**Example of sampling in a grounded theory study:**
Hall and colleagues (2012) conducted a grounded theory study of Canadian health care providers' and pregnant women's approaches to managing birth. They began with purposeful sampling and then used theoretical sampling to further develop categories. The sample included 9 pregnant women, and 56 health care providers including physicians, nurses, midwives, and doulas.

## Critiquing Qualitative Sampling Plans

In a qualitative study, the sampling plan can be evaluated in terms of its adequacy and appropriateness (Morse, 1991). *Adequacy* refers to the sufficiency and quality of the data the sample yielded. An adequate sample provides data without "thin" spots. When researchers have truly obtained saturation, informational adequacy has been achieved, and the resulting description or theory is richly textured and complete.

*Appropriateness* concerns the methods used to select a sample. An appropriate sample results from the selection of participants who can best supply information that meets the study's conceptual requirements. The sampling strategy must yield the fullest possible understanding of the phenomenon of interest. A sampling approach that excludes negative cases or that fails to include people with unusual experiences may not fully address the study's information needs.

Another important issue concerns the potential for transferability of the findings. The transferability of study findings is a direct function of the similarity between the sample of the original study and other people to whom the findings might be applied. Thus, in critiquing a report you should assess whether the researcher provided an adequately *thick description* of the sample and the study context so that someone interested in transferring the findings could make an informed decision. Further guidance in critiquing qualitative sampling decisions is presented in Box 15.1.

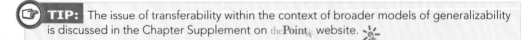

**TIP:** The issue of transferability within the context of broader models of generalizability is discussed in the Chapter Supplement on thePoint website.

# DATA COLLECTION IN QUALITATIVE STUDIES

Qualitative researchers typically go into the field knowing the most likely data sources, while not ruling out other possibilities that might come to light as data collection progresses. In-depth interviews are the most common method of collecting qualitative data.

---

**BOX 15.1   Guidelines for Critiquing Qualitative Sampling Plans**

1. Is the setting appropriate for addressing the research question, and is it adequately described?
2. What type of sampling strategy was used? Are sampling procedures clearly delineated?
3. Were the eligibility criteria for the study specified? How were participants recruited into the study? Did the recruitment strategy yield information-rich participants?
4. Given the information needs of the study—and, if applicable, its qualitative tradition—was the sampling approach appropriate? Are dimensions of the phenomenon under study adequately represented?
5. Is the sample size adequate and appropriate? Did the researcher indicate that saturation had been achieved? Do the findings suggest a richly textured and comprehensive set of data without any apparent "holes" or thin areas?
6. Are key characteristics of the sample described (e.g., age, gender)? Is a rich description of participants and context provided, allowing for an assessment of the transferability of the findings?

---

Observation is used in some qualitative studies as well. Physiologic data are rarely collected in a constructivist inquiry.

Table 15.1 compares the types of data and aspects of the data collection process used by researchers in the three main qualitative traditions. Ethnographers typically collect a wide array of data, with observation and interviews being the primary methods. Ethnographers also gather or examine products of the culture under study, such as documents, records, artifacts, photographs, and so on. Phenomenologists and grounded theory researchers rely primarily on in-depth interviews, although participant observation can also play a role in grounded theory studies.

**TABLE 15.1   Comparison of Data Collection in Three Qualitative Traditions**

| Issue | Ethnography | Phenomenology | Grounded Theory |
|---|---|---|---|
| Types of data | Primarily observation and interviews, plus artifacts, documents, photographs, social network diagrams | Primarily in-depth interviews, sometimes diaries or other written or artistic materials | Primarily individual interviews, sometimes group interviews, observation, diaries, documents |
| Unit of data collection | Cultural system | Individuals | Individuals |
| Data collection points | Mainly longitudinal | Mainly cross-sectional | Cross-sectional or longitudinal |
| Length of time for data collection | Typically long, many months or years | Typically moderate | Typically moderate |
| Salient field issues | Gaining entrée, determining a role, learning how to participate, reactivity, encouraging candor, loss of objectivity, premature exit, reflexivity | Bracketing one's views, building rapport, encouraging candor, listening while preparing what to ask next, keeping "on track," handling emotionality | Building rapport, encouraging candor, listening while preparing what to ask next, keeping "on track," handling emotionality |

## Qualitative Self-Report Techniques

Qualitative researchers do not have a set of questions that must be asked in a specific order and worded in a given way. Instead, they start with general questions and allow respondents to tell their stories in a naturalistic fashion. Qualitative self-reports, usually obtained through interviews, tend to be conversational. Interviewers encourage respondents to define the important dimensions of a phenomenon and to elaborate on what is relevant to them, rather than relying on investigators' *a priori* notions of relevance.

### Types of Qualitative Self-Reports

Several approaches can be used to collect qualitative self-report data. Researchers use completely **unstructured interviews** when they have no preconceived view of the information to be gathered. They aim to learn about respondents' perceptions and experiences without imposing their own views. Researchers begin by asking a **grand tour question** such as, "What happened when you first learned that you had AIDS?" Subsequent questions are guided by initial responses. Ethnographic and phenomenologic studies often rely on unstructured interviews.

**Semistructured** (or *focused*) **interviews** are used when researchers have a list of topics or broad questions that must be covered in an interview. Interviewers use a written **topic guide** to ensure that all question areas are addressed. The interviewer's function is to encourage participants to talk freely about all the topics on the guide.

> **Example of a semistructured interview:**
> Coombs and colleagues (2012) explored how nurses and doctors make the transition from active intervention to palliative and end-of-life care. They collected their data via semistructured interviews with 13 nurses and 13 medical staff. Interviews began with the question, "Could you tell me about what happened around the time of (patient's name) death?" Then a series of probes elicited additional information about end-of-life decisions and the process of care withdrawal.

**Focus group interviews** involve groups of about 5 to 10 people whose opinions and experiences are solicited simultaneously. The interviewer (or *moderator*) guides the discussion using a topic guide. A group format is efficient and can generate a lot of dialogue, but one problem is that not everyone is comfortable sharing their views or experiences in front of a group. Focus groups have been used by researchers in many qualitative traditions and in qualitative descriptive research.

> **Example of focus group interviews:**
> Beck and colleagues (2012) studied nurse assistants' experiences of palliative care in residential care settings in Sweden. Six focus group interviews were conducted with two to six nurse assistants from different residential care units. Examples of questions from the interview guide are: What does palliative care mean to you? What are the major difficulties when providing palliative care?

Personal **diaries** are a standard data source in historical research. It is also possible to generate new data for a study by asking participants to maintain a diary over a specified period. Diaries can be useful in providing an intimate description of a person's everyday life. The diaries may be completely unstructured; for example, individuals who have had an organ transplantation could be asked to spend 15 minutes a day jotting down or audiotaping their thoughts. Frequently, however, people are asked to make diary entries regarding some specific aspect of their lives.

**Example of diaries:**
Buchwald and colleagues (2012) studied how children aged 11 to 17 handle life when their mother or father was seriously ill and dying. The researchers asked the children to maintain video diaries in daily sessions for 1 month, in which the children were asked to share their feelings, reflections, and the day's events with the camera.

The **critical incidents technique** is a method of gathering information about people's behaviors in specific circumstances. The method focuses on a factual *incident*—an integral episode of human behavior; *critical* means that the incident must have had a discernible impact on some outcome. The technique focuses on incidents about which respondents can testify as expert witnesses. Generally, data on 50 to 100 critical incidents are collected, but this typically involves interviews with a smaller number of people, because each person can often describe multiple incidents.

**Example of a critical incident study:**
Pavlish and colleagues (2011) used the critical incident technique in a study of nurses' experiences with ethically difficult situations and risk factors for such situations.

**Photo elicitation** involves an interview stimulated and guided by photographic images. This procedure, most often used in ethnographies and participatory action research (PAR), can help to promote a collaborative discussion. The photographs sometimes are ones that researchers have made of the participants' world, through which researchers can gain insights into a new culture. Photo elicitation can also be used with photos that participants have in their homes. Researchers have also used the technique of asking participants to take photographs themselves and then interpret them, a method sometimes called **photovoice**.

**Example of a photovoice study:**
Findholt and colleagues (2011), in their PAR study of childhood obesity prevention, used photovoice to engage rural youth in discussions about community assets and barriers that influenced children's physical activity and diets.

## Gathering Qualitative Self-Report Data

Researchers gather narrative self-report data to develop a construction of a phenomenon that is consistent with that of participants. This goal requires researchers to overcome communication barriers and to enhance the flow of information. Although qualitative interviews are conversational, the conversations are purposeful ones that require preparation. For example, the wording of questions should reflect the participants' world view and language. In addition to being good questioners, researchers must be good listeners. Only by attending carefully to what respondents are saying can in-depth interviewers develop appropriate follow-up questions.

Unstructured interviews are typically long, sometimes lasting several hours, and so an important issue is how best to record such abundant information. Some researchers take notes during the interview, filling in the details after the interview is completed. This method is, however, risky in terms of data accuracy. Most prefer tape recording the interviews for later transcription. Although some respondents are self-conscious when their conversation is recorded, they typically forget about the presence of recording equipment after a few minutes.

> ☞ **TIP:** Although qualitative self-report data are often gathered in face-to-face interviews, they can also be collected in writing. Internet "interviews" are increasingly common.

## Evaluation of Qualitative Self-Report Methods

In-depth interviews are an extremely flexible approach to gathering data and, in many research contexts, offer distinct advantages. In clinical situations, for example, it is often appropriate to let people talk freely about their problems and concerns, allowing them to take much of the initiative in directing the flow of conversation. Unstructured self-reports may allow investigators to ascertain what the basic issues or problems are, how sensitive or controversial the topic is, how individuals conceptualize and talk about the problems, and what range of opinions or behaviors exist relevant to the topic. In-depth interviews may also help to elucidate the underlying meaning of a pattern or relationship repeatedly observed in more structured research. On the other hand, qualitative methods are extremely time-consuming and demanding of researchers' skills in gathering, analyzing, and interpreting the resulting data.

## Qualitative Observational Methods

Qualitative researchers sometimes collect loosely structured observational data, often as an important supplement to self-report data. The aim of qualitative observation is to understand the behaviors and experiences of people as they occur in naturalistic settings. Skillful unstructured observation permits researchers to see the world as the study participants see it, to develop a rich understanding of the phenomena of interest, and to grasp subtleties of cultural variation.

Unstructured observational data are often gathered in field settings through **participant observation**. Participant observers take part in the functioning of the group under study and strive to observe, ask questions, and record information within the contexts and structures that are relevant to group members. Participant observation is characterized by prolonged periods of social interaction between researchers and participants, in the participants' sociopolitical and cultural milieu. By assuming a participating role, observers often have insights that would have eluded more passive or concealed observers.

> ☞ **TIP:** Not all qualitative observational research is *participant* observation (i.e., with observations occurring from *within* the group under study). Some unstructured observations involve watching and recording behaviors without the observers' active participation in activities. Be on the alert for the misuse of the term "participant observation." Some researchers use the term inappropriately to refer to all unstructured observations conducted in the field. A description of what participation actually entailed should be included in reports of participant observational studies.

### The Observer-Participant Role in Participant Observation

In participant observation, the role that observers play in the group is important because their social position determines what they are likely to see. The extent of the observers' actual participation in a group is best thought of as a continuum. At one extreme is complete immersion in the setting, with researchers assuming full participant status; at the other extreme is complete separation, with researchers as onlookers. Researchers may in some cases assume a fixed position on this continuum throughout the study, but often researchers' role as participants evolves over the course of the field work. Leininger and McFarland (2006) describe a participant observer's role as evolving through a four-phase sequence:

1. Primarily observation and active listening
2. Primarily observation with limited participation
3. Primarily participation with continued observation
4. Primarily reflection and reconfirmation of findings with informants

In the initial phase, researchers observe and listen to people, allowing everyone to get more comfortable in their interactions. In phase 2, observation is enhanced by a modest degree of participation in the social group. In phase 3, researchers strive to become more active participants, learning by the experience of doing rather than just watching and listening. In phase 4, researchers reflect on the total process of what transpired.

Observers must overcome at least two major hurdles in assuming a satisfactory role vis-à-vis participants. The first is to gain entrée into the social group under study; the second is to establish rapport and trust within that group. Without gaining entrée, the study cannot proceed; but without the trust of the group, the researcher will be restricted to "front stage" knowledge—that is, information distorted by the group's protective facades. The goal of participant observers is to "get backstage"—to learn about the true realities of the group's experiences and behaviors. On the other hand, being a fully participating member does not *necessarily* offer the best perspective for studying a phenomenon—just as being an actor in a play does not offer the most advantageous view of the performance.

**Example of participant-observer roles:**
Michaelson (2012) conducted a study that focused on nurses' relationships with patients they regard as being difficult. Data were collected by means of participant observation and in-depth interviews over an 18-month period. Michaelson conducted 18 observation sessions, lasting between 3 and 4 hours, of the nurses interacting with patients during home visits. She kept "a balance between being an 'insider' and an 'outsider,' between participation and observation." (p. 92).

## Gathering Participant Observation Data

Participant observers typically place few restrictions on the nature of the data collected, but they often have a broad plan for the types of information to be gathered. Among the aspects of an observed activity likely to be considered relevant are the following:

1. *The physical setting—"where" questions.* Where is the activity happening? What are the main features of the setting?
2. *The participants—"who" questions.* Who is present? What are their characteristics and roles? Who is given access to the event? Who is denied access?
3. *Activities—"what" questions.* What is going on? What are participants doing? What methods do they use to communicate?
4. *Frequency and duration—"when" questions.* When did the activity begin and end? Is the activity a recurring one and, if so, how regularly does it recur?
5. *Process—"how" questions.* How is the activity organized? How does it unfold?
6. *Outcomes—"why" questions.* Why is the activity happening, or why is it happening in this manner? What did not happen (especially if it ought to have happened) and why?

Participant observers must decide how to sample events and to select observational locations. They often use a combination of positioning approaches. *Single positioning* means staying in a single location for a period to observe transactions in that location. *Multiple positioning* involves moving around the site to observe behaviors from different locations. *Mobile positioning* involves following a person throughout a given activity or period.

Because participant observers cannot be in more than one place at a time, observation is usually supplemented with information from unstructured interviews. For example, informants may be asked to describe what went on in a meeting the observer was unable to attend, or to describe an event that occurred before the observer entered the field. In such cases, the informant functions as the observer's observer.

### Recording Observations

The most common forms of record keeping for participant observation are logs and field notes, but photographs and videotapes may also be used. A **log** (or *field diary)* is a daily record of events and conversations. **Field notes** are broader and more interpretive. Field notes represent the observer's efforts to record information and to synthesize and understand the data.

Field notes can be categorized according to their purpose. *Descriptive notes* (or *observational notes)* are objective descriptions of events and conversations, and the contexts in which they occurred. The goal of participant observers' descriptive notes is thick description.

*Reflective notes* document researchers' personal experiences, reflections, and progress in the field, and can serve different purposes. *Theoretical notes* document interpretive efforts to attach meaning to observations. *Methodologic notes* are reminders about how subsequent observations should be made. *Personal notes* are comments about the researcher's own feelings during the research process. Box 15.2 presents examples of various types of field notes from Beck's (2002) grounded theory study of mothering twins.

The success of any participant observation study depends on the quality of the logs and field notes. It is clearly essential to record observations as quickly as possible, but participant observers cannot usually record information by openly carrying a clipboard or a tape recorder because this would undermine their role as ordinary participants. Observers must develop skills in making detailed mental notes that can later be written or tape recorded.

### Evaluation of Unstructured Observational Methods

Qualitative observational methods, and especially participant observation, can provide a deeper and richer understanding of human behaviors and social situations than is possible with structured methods. Participant observation is valuable for its ability to "get inside" a situation and provide understanding of its complexities. This approach is inherently flexible and thus gives observers the freedom to reconceptualize problems once they are in the field. Participant observation is a good method for answering questions about phenomena that are difficult for insiders themselves to explain because these phenomena are taken for granted.

Like all research methods, however, participant observation faces potential problems. Observer bias is a prominent risk. Observers may lose objectivity in sampling, viewing, and recording observations. Once they begin to participate in a group's activities, the possibility of emotional involvement becomes a concern. Researchers in their member role may fail to attend to scientifically relevant aspects of the situation or may develop a myopic view on issues of importance to the group. Finally, the success of participant observation depends on the observer's observational and interpersonal skills—skills that may be difficult to cultivate.

### Critiquing the Collection of Unstructured Data

It is often difficult to critique the decisions that researchers made in collecting qualitative data because details about those decisions are seldom spelled out in research articles. In

---

**BOX 15.2    Example of Field Notes for Unstructured Observations (From a Grounded Theory Study)**

**Observational Notes**: O.L. attended the Mothers of Multiples Support Group again this month, but she looked worn-out today. She wasn't as bubbly as she had been at the March meeting. She explained why she wasn't doing as well this month. She and her husband had just found out that their house has lead-based paint in it. Both twins do have increased lead levels. She and her husband are in the process of buying a new house.

**Theoretical Notes**: So far, all the mothers have stressed the need for routine in order to survive the first year of caring for twins. Mothers, however, have varying definitions of routine. I.R. had the firmest routine with her twins. B.L. is more flexible with her routine, i.e., the twins are always fed at the same time but aren't put down for naps or bed at night at the same time. Whenever one of the twins wants to go to sleep it is fine with her. B.L. does have a daily routine with regard to housework. For example, when the twins are down in the morning for a nap, she makes their bottles up for the day (14 bottles total).

**Methodologic Notes**: The first sign-up sheet I passed around at the Mothers of Multiples Support Group for women to sign up to participate in interviews for my grounded theory study only consisted of two columns: one for the mother's name and one for her telephone number. I need to revise this sign-up sheet to include extra columns for the age of the multiples, the town where the mother lives, and older siblings and their ages. My plan is to start interviewing mothers with multiples around 1 year of age so that the moms can reflect back over the process of mothering their infants for the first 12 months of their lives. Right now I have no idea of the ages of the infants of the mothers who signed up to be interviewed.

I will need to call the nurse in charge of this support group to find out the ages.

**Personal Notes**: Today was an especially challenging interview. The mom had picked the early afternoon for me to come to her home to interview her because that is the time her 2-year-old son would be napping. When I arrived at her house, her 2-year-old ran up to me and said hi. The mom explained that he had taken an earlier nap that day and that he would be up during the interview. Also in the living room with us during our interview were her two twin daughters (3 months old) swinging in the swings and her 2-year-old son. One of the twins was quite cranky for the first half hour of the interview. During the interview, the 2-year-old sat on my lap and looked at the two books I had brought as a little present. If I didn't keep him occupied with the books, he would keep trying to reach for the microphone of the tape recorder.

From Beck, C. T. (2002). Releasing the pause button: Mothering twins during the first year of life. *Qualitative Health Research, 12,* 593–608.

---

particular, there is often scant information about participant observation. It is not uncommon for a report to simply say that the researcher undertook participant observation, without descriptions of how much time was spent in the field, what exactly was observed, how observations were recorded, and what level of participation was involved. Thus, one aspect of a critique is likely to involve an appraisal of how much information the article provided about the data collection methods used. Even though space constraints in journals make it impossible for researchers to fully elaborate their methods, researchers have a responsibility to communicate basic information about their approach so that readers can assess the quality of evidence that the study yields. Researchers should provide examples of questions asked and types of observations made.

> **BOX 15.3 Guidelines for Critiquing Data Collection Methods in Qualitative Studies**
>
> 1. Given the research question and the characteristics of study participants, did the researcher use the best method of capturing study phenomena (i.e., self-reports, observation)? Should supplementary data collection methods have been used to enrich the data available for analysis?
> 2. If self-report methods were used, did the researcher make good decisions about the specific method used to solicit information (e.g., focus group interviews, critical incident interviews, and so on)? Was the modality of obtaining the data appropriate (e.g., in-person interviews, Internet questioning, etc.)?
> 3. If a topic guide was used, did the report present examples of specific questions? Were the questions appropriate and comprehensive? Did the wording encourage full and rich responses?
> 4. Were interviews tape recorded and transcribed? If interviews were not tape recorded, what steps were taken to ensure the accuracy of the data?
> 5. Were self-report data gathered in a manner that promoted high-quality responses (e.g., in terms of privacy, efforts to put respondents at ease, etc.)? Who collected the data, and were they adequately prepared for the task?
> 6. If observational methods were used, did the report adequately describe what the observations entailed? What did the researcher actually observe, in what types of setting did the observations occur, and how often and over how long a period were observations made? Were decisions about positioning described? Were risks of observational bias addressed?
> 7. What role did the researcher assume in terms of being an observer and a participant? Was this role appropriate?
> 8. How were observational data recorded? Did the recording method maximize data quality?

As we discuss more fully in Chapter 17, triangulation of methods provides important opportunities for qualitative researchers to enhance the integrity of their data. Thus, an important issue to consider in evaluating unstructured data is whether the types and amount of data collected are sufficiently rich to support an in-depth, holistic understanding of the phenomena under study. Box 15.3 provides guidelines for critiquing the collection of unstructured data.

## RESEARCH EXAMPLES WITH CRITICAL THINKING EXERCISES

In the following section, we describe the sampling plans and data collection strategies used in a nursing study, followed by some questions to guide critical thinking.

Example 1 below is also featured in our *Interactive Critical Thinking Activity* on thePoint website where you can easily record, print, and e-mail your responses to the related questions.

### EXAMPLE 1 ● Sampling and Data Collection in a Qualitative Study

**Study:** Everyday nursing practice values in the NICU and their reflection on breastfeeding promotion. (Cricco-Lizza, 2011) (A related article by Cricco-Lizza appears in its entirety in the appendix to the accompanying the *Study Guide*).

**Method:** Cricco-Lizza used ethnographic methods to collect contextually rich and detailed information about NICU nurses, with a particular focus on infant feeding. The research was undertaken over a 14-month period in a level IV NICU in a pediatric hospital in northeastern United States. Data were collected primarily through observations and interviews.

**Sampling Strategy:** Approximately 250 nurses worked in the NICU; 114 of them participated as general informants. These nurses were observed or informally interviewed during routine NICU activities, and they provided a broad overview of infant feeding on the unit. From these 114 nurses, 18 nurses with a variety of professional experiences and educational backgrounds were purposefully sampled to be key informants. These key informants, who were followed more intensively during the fieldwork, were chosen from different expertise levels (novice to clinical expert) to obtain varied views of the NICU culture with regard to infant feeding.

**Data Collection:** The researcher observed nurses during the usual course of their activities in the NICU. The researcher focused on the nurses' interactions with babies, families, nurses, and other staff throughout the course of diverse activities. The observational sessions, which lasted for an hour or two, involved sampling of activities on varying days, work shifts, and times of the week. Cricco-Lizza noted that her "role evolved from observation to informal interviewing over the course of 128 participant-observation session" (p. 401). General informants were observed and informally interviewed an average of 3.5 times each over the study period. Cricco-Lizza documented all observational data in detailed field notes immediately after each session. Key informants agreed to formal interviews that lasted about 1 hour each. The researcher asked open-ended questions about breastfeeding and formula feeding, the nature of the nurses' work, and their roles in the NICU. During the formal interviews, the researcher followed up in greater depth on questions that arose during participant observation. Key informants were also observed and informally interviewed a total of 3 to 43 times each, with an average of 13.1 interactions over the study. The repeated contacts during the course of the study "allowed for deeper exploration about everyday practices, values, and breastfeeding in the NICU" (p. 401).

**Key Findings:** Cricco-Lizza's analysis revealed that uncertainty was a central concern underlying everyday practice values. Three themes described these values: (1) maximizing babies' potentials in the midst of uncertainty, (2) relying on the sisterhood of NICU nurses to deal with uncertainty, and (3) confronting uncertainty through tight control of actions, reliance on technology, and maximal efficiency in use of time.

## CRITICAL THINKING EXERCISES

1. Answer the relevant questions from Box 15.1 on page 289 and Box 15.3 on page 296 regarding this study.
2. Also consider the following targeted questions:
    a. Comment on the variation the researcher achieved in type of study participants.
    b. How likely is it that the researcher's presence in the NICU affected the nurses' behaviors?
    c. Comment on the researchers' overall data collection plan in terms of the amount of information gathered and the timing of the data collection.
3. If the results of this study are valid and trustworthy, in what ways do you think the findings could be used in clinical practice?

## EXAMPLE 2 ● Sampling and Data Collection in the Study in Appendix B

- Read the method section from Beck and Watson's (2010) study ("Subsequent childbirth after a previous traumatic birth") in Appendix B on pages 403–412.

## CRITICAL THINKING EXERCISES

1. Answer the relevant questions from Boxes 15.1 on page 289 and 15.3 on page 296 regarding this study.
2. Also consider the following targeted questions:
    a. Comment on the characteristics of the participants, given the purpose of the study.
    b. Do you think that Beck and Watson should have limited their sample to women from one country only? Provide a rationale for your answer.
    c. Could any of the variables in this study have been captured by observation? Should they have been?
    d. Did Beck and Watson's study involve a "grand tour" question?

**WANT TO KNOW MORE?** A wide variety of resources to enhance your learning and understanding of this chapter are available on thePoint.

• Interactive Critical Thinking Activity
• Chapter Supplement on Transferability and Generalizability
• Answers to the Critical Thinking Exercises for Example 2
• Student Review Questions
• Full-text online
• Internet Resources with useful websites for Chapter 11

Additional study aids including eight journal articles and related questions are also available in *Study Guide for Essentials of Nursing Research, 8e.*

## SUMMARY POINTS

- Qualitative researchers use the conceptual demands of the study to select articulate and reflective informants with certain types of experience in an emergent way, capitalizing on early learning to guide subsequent sampling decisions.

- Qualitative researchers may start with convenience or **snowball** sampling, but usually rely eventually on **purposive sampling** to guide them in selecting data sources that maximize information richness.

- One purposive strategy is **maximum variation sampling**, which entails purposely selecting cases with a wide range of variation. Another important strategy is sampling **confirming cases** and **disconfirming cases**—i.e., selecting cases that enrich and challenge the researchers' conceptualizations. Other types of purposive sampling include *extreme case sampling* (selecting the most unusual or extreme cases), *typical case sampling* (selecting cases that illustrate what is typical), and *criterion sampling* (studying cases that meet a predetermined criterion of importance).

- Samples in qualitative studies are typically small and based on information needs. A guiding principle is **data saturation**, which involves sampling to the point at which no new information is obtained and redundancy is achieved.

- Ethnographers make numerous sampling decisions, including not only *whom* to sample but *what* to sample (e.g., activities, events, documents, artifacts); decision making is often aided by their **key informants** who serve as guides and interpreters of the culture.

- Phenomenologists typically work with a small sample of people (often 10 or fewer) who meet the criterion of having lived the experience under study.

- Grounded theory researchers typically use **theoretical sampling** in which sampling decisions are guided in an ongoing fashion by the emerging theory. Samples of about 20 to 40 people are typical in grounded theory studies.

- In-depth interviews are the most widely used method of collecting data for qualitative studies. Self-reports in qualitative studies include completely **unstructured interviews**, which are conversational discussions on the topic of interest; **semi-structured** (or *focused*) **interviews**, using a broad **topic guide**; **focus group interviews**, which involve discussions with small groups; **diaries**, in which respondents are asked to maintain daily records about some aspects of their lives; the **critical incidents technique**, which involve probes about the circumstances surrounding an incident that is critical to an outcome of interest; and **photo elicitation** interviews, which are guided and stimulated by photographic images, sometimes using photos that participants themselves take (**photovoice**).

● In qualitative research, self-reports are often supplemented by direct observation in naturalistic settings. One type of unstructured observation is **participant observation**, in which the researcher gains entrée into a social group and participates to varying degrees in its functioning while making in-depth observations of activities and events. Maintaining **logs** of daily events and **field notes** of the observer's experiences and interpretations constitute the major data collection strategies.

# REFERENCES FOR CHAPTER 15

Beal, C., Stuifbergen, A., & Volker, D. (2012). A narrative study of women's early symptom experience of ischemic stroke. *Journal of Cardiovascular Nursing, 27*(3), 240–252.

Beck, C. T. (2002). Releasing the pause button: Mothering twins during the first year of life. *Qualitative Health Research, 12*, 593–608.

Beck, I., Tornquist, A., Brostrom, L., & Edberg, A. (2012). Having to focus on doing rather than being: Nurse assistants' experiences of palliative care in municipal residential care settings. *International Journal of Nursing Studies, 49, 455–464.*

Bertrand, S. (2012). Registered nurses integrate traditional Chinese medicine into the triage process. *Qualitative Health Research, 22*, 263–273.

Buchwald, D., Delmar, C., & Schantz-Laursen, B. (2012). How children handle life when their mother or father is seriously ill and dying. *Scandinavian Journal of Caring Sciences, 26*(2), 228–235.

Cooke, A., Mills, T., & Lavender, T. (2012). Advanced maternal age: Delayed childbearing is rarely a conscious choice. *International Journal of Nursing Studies, 49*, 30–39.

Coombs, M., Addington-Hall, J., & Long-Sutehall, T. (2012). Challenges in transition from intervention to end of life care in intensive care. *International Journal of Nursing Studies, 49*(5), 519–527.

Cricco-Lizza, R. (2011). Everyday nursing practice values in the NICU and their reflection on breastfeeding promotion. *Qualitative Health Research, 21*, 399–409.

Findholt, N., Michael, Y., & Davis, M. (2011). Photovoice engages rural youth in childhood obesity prevention. *Public Health Nursing, 28*, 186–192.

Hall, W., Tomkinson, J., & Klein, M. (2012). Canadian care providers' and pregnant women's approaches to managing birth: Minimizing risk while maximizing integrity. *Qualitative Health Research, 22*, 575–586.

Leininger, M. M., & McFarland, M. R. (2006). *Culture care diversity and universality: A worldwide nursing theory.* Boston, MA Jones & Bartlett.

Lori, J., & Boyle, J. (2011). Cultural childbirth practices, beliefs, and traditions in postconflict Liberia. *Health Care for Women International, 32*, 454–473.

Michaelson, J. J. (2012). Emotional distance to so-called difficult patients. *Scandinavian Journal of Caring Sciences, 26*(1), 90–97.

Morse, J. M. (1991). Strategies for sampling. In J. M. Morse (Ed.), *Qualitative nursing research: A contemporary dialogue.* Newbury Park, CA: Sage.

Patton, M. Q. (2002). *Qualitative evaluation and research methods* (3rd ed.). Thousand Oaks, CA: Sage.

Pavlish, C., Brown-Saltzman, K., Hersh, M., Shirk, M., & Nudelman, O. (2011). Early indicators and risk factors for ethical issues in clinical practice. *Journal of Nursing Scholarship, 43*, 13–21.

Porr, C., Drummond, J., & Olson, K. (2012). Establishing therapeutic relationships with vulnerable and potentially stigmatized clients. *Qualitative Health Research, 22*, 384–396.

Roscigno, C., & Swanson, K. (2011). Parents' experiences following children's moderate to severe traumatic brain injury. *Qualitative Health Research, 21*, 1413–1426.

Tierney, S., Elwers, H., Sange, C., Mams, M., Rutter, M., Gibson, M., et al. (2011). What influences physical activity in people with heart failure? *International Journal of Nursing Studies, 48*, 1234–1243.

# 16 Analysis of Qualitative Data

## LEARNING OBJECTIVES

*On completing this chapter, you will be able to:*

● Describe activities that qualitative researchers perform to manage and organize their data

● Discuss the procedures used to analyze qualitative data, including both general procedures and those used in ethnographic, phenomenologic, and grounded theory research

● Assess the adequacy of researchers' descriptions of their analytic procedures, and evaluate the suitability of those procedures

● Define new terms in the chapter

## KEY TERMS

| | | |
|---|---|---|
| Axial coding | Content analysis | Open coding |
| Basic social process (BSP) | Core category | Paradigm case |
| Category scheme | Domain | Selective coding |
| Central category | Emergent fit | Substantive coding |
| Conceptual file | Focused coding | Taxonomy |
| Constant comparison | Hermeneutic circle | Theme |
| Constitutive pattern | Level I, II, and III codes | Theoretical coding |

Qualitative data are derived from narrative materials, such as transcripts from audio-taped interviews or participant observers' field notes. This chapter describes methods for analyzing such qualitative data.

# INTRODUCTION TO QUALITATIVE ANALYSIS

Qualitative data analysis is challenging, for several reasons. First, there are no universal rules for analyzing qualitative data. The absence of standard procedures makes it difficult to explain how to do such analyses.

A second challenge of qualitative analysis is the enormous amount of work required. Qualitative analysts must organize and make sense of hundreds or even thousands of pages of narrative materials. Qualitative researchers typically scrutinize their data carefully and deliberatively, often reading the data over and over in a search for meaning and understanding. Insights and theories cannot emerge until researchers become completely familiar with their data.

A third challenge is that doing qualitative analysis well requires creativity, sensitivity, and strong inductive skills (inducing universals from particulars). A good qualitative analyst must be skillful in discerning patterns and weaving them together into an integrated whole.

Another challenge comes in reducing data for reporting purposes. Quantitative results can often be summarized in a few tables. Qualitative researchers, by contrast, must balance the need to be concise with the need to maintain the richness and evidentiary value of their data.

> ☞ **TIP:** Qualitative analyses are more difficult to *do* than quantitative ones, but qualitative findings are easier to understand than quantitative ones because the stories are told in everyday language. Qualitative analyses are often harder to critique than quantitative analyses, however, because readers cannot know firsthand if researchers adequately captured thematic patterns in the data.

# QUALITATIVE DATA MANAGEMENT AND ORGANIZATION

Qualitative analysis is supported by several tasks that help to organize and manage the mass of narrative data. A key first step is checking the accuracy of transcribed data. Researchers should begin data analysis with the best-possible quality data, which requires careful training of transcribers, ongoing feedback, and continuous efforts to verify accuracy.

## Developing a Category Scheme

Qualitative researchers begin their analysis by developing a method to classify and index their data. Researchers must be able to gain access to parts of the data, without having repeatedly to reread the data set in its entirety. This phase of data analysis is essentially reductionist—data must be converted to smaller, more manageable units that can be retrieved and reviewed.

A widely used procedure is to develop a **category scheme** and then to code data according to the categories. A preliminary category system is sometimes drafted before data collection, but more typically qualitative analysts develop categories based on a scrutiny of actual data. Developing a high-quality category scheme involves a careful reading of the data, with an eye to identifying underlying concepts and clusters of concepts. The nature of the categories may vary in level of detail or specificity, as well as in level of abstraction.

Researchers whose aims are primarily descriptive tend to use categories that are fairly concrete. For example, the category scheme may focus on differentiating various types of actions or events, or different phases in a chronologic unfolding of an experience. In developing a category scheme, related concepts are often grouped together to facilitate the coding process.

> **Example of a descriptive category scheme:**
> Elfström and colleagues (2012) explored situations that affect support of a partner's use of continuous positive airway pressure (CPAP) for sleep apnea, using data gathered through the critical incidents technique. The category system of situations negatively affecting partner support included such descriptive categories as *problems with the mask, complicated routines, being fatigued,* and *poor knowledge.*

Studies designed to develop a theory are more likely to involve abstract, conceptual categories. In creating conceptual categories, researchers break the data into segments, closely examine them, and compare them to other segments for similarities and dissimilarities to uncover what the meaning of those phenomena are. This is part of the process referred to as *constant comparison* by grounded theory researchers. The researcher asks questions such as the following about discrete events, incidents, or statements: What is this? What is going on? What else is like this? What is this distinct from?

Important concepts that emerge from examination of the data are then given a label. These names are necessarily abstractions, but the labels are usually sufficiently graphic that the nature of the material to which they refer is clear—and often provocative.

---

**Example of a conceptual category scheme:**
Box 16.1 shows the category scheme developed by Beck and Watson (2010) to code data from their interviews on childbirth after a previous traumatic birth (the full study is in Appendix B). The coding scheme includes major thematic categories with subcodes. For example, an excerpt that described a mother interviewing various obstetrical clinicians to determine who would be the best match to care for her would be coded 2J, for "interviewing perspective obstetricians and midwives." (Note that the original coding scheme, as shown in Box 16.1, was refined and made more parsimonious during the analysis. For example, codes 2F, 2J, and 2N, were collapsed into a larger category called "Interactions with obstetrical care providers.")

---

☞ **TIP:** A good category scheme is crucial to the analysis of qualitative data. Unfortunately, research reports rarely present the category scheme for readers to critique, but they may provide information that may help you evaluate its adequacy (e.g., researchers may say that the scheme was reviewed by peers or developed and independently verified by other researchers).

---

## Coding Qualitative Data

After a category scheme has been developed, the data are read in their entirety and coded for correspondence to the categories—a task that is seldom straightforward. Researchers may have difficulty deciding the most appropriate code, for example. It sometimes takes several readings of the material to grasp its nuances.

Also, researchers often discover during coding that the initial category system was incomplete. It is common for categories to emerge that were not initially identified. When this happens, it is risky to assume that the category was absent in materials that have already been coded. A concept might not be identified as salient until it has emerged three or four times. In such a case, it would be necessary to reread all previously coded material to check if the new code should be applied.

Another issue is that narrative materials usually are not linear. For example, paragraphs from transcribed interviews may contain elements relating to three or four different categories, embedded in a complex fashion.

---

**Example of a multitopic segment:**
Figure 16.1 shows an example of a multitopic segment of an interview from Beck and Watson's (2010) subsequent childbirth after a previous traumatic birth study. The codes in the margin represent codes from the category scheme presented in Box 16.1.

---

## Methods of Organizing Qualitative Data

Before the advent of computer programs for qualitative data management, analysts often developed **conceptual files** for organizing their data. This approach involves creating a physical file for each category, and then cutting out and inserting all of the materials relating

**Box 16.1 Beck and Watson's (2010) Coding Scheme for Subsequent Childbirth after a Previous Traumatic Birth**

**Theme 1. Riding the turbulent wave of panic during pregnancy**

A. Fear
B. Panic
C. Anxiety
D. Terror
E. Dread
F. Denial

**Theme 2. Strategizing: Attempts to reclaim their body and complete the journey to motherhood**

A. Keeping a journal
B. Nurturing self
C. Reading about childbirth process
D. Hiring a doula
E. Hypnobirthing
F. Discussing previous traumatic birth with obstetric health care providers
G. Sharing their fears with partners
H. Writing detailed birth plan
I. Birth art
J. Interviewing prospective obstetricians and midwives
K. Homeopathic remedies
L. Using Internet support group
M. Regaining control
N. Building trust with obstetrical clinicians

**Theme 3. Bringing reverence to the birthing process and empowering women**

A. Treated with respect during labor and delivery
B. Pain relief taken seriously
C. Mother's wishes listened to
D. Not rushed during labor and delivery
E. Good communication with labor and delivery staff
F. Regaining sense of control
G. Caring health care providers during labor and delivery
H. Mother's body allowed to birth without medical interventions
I. Birth plan honored by labor and delivery staff
J. Feeling empowered

**Theme 4. Still elusive: The longed-for healing birth experience**

A. Unsuccessful home birth
B. Contrast in way woman was treated emphasized how badly her prior birth was
C. No sense of healing
D. Failed again as a woman

| | |
|---|---|
| The 9 months of pregnancy after my traumatic delivery in 2003 were 9 of the longest months of my life! I can honestly say I have never felt so anxious about anything. I had only been diagnosed as suffering with postpartum PTSD 2 months prior to falling pregnant (accidentally) with my 2nd child and was only just coming to terms with the fact that the emotions and physical reactions I was feeling were normal reactions to such an abnormal situation. | 1C |
| The emotions I experienced ranged from sheer terror about the thought of another birth to a conscious effort to regain my composure and take control of the situation. On a "good day" I would consider my birth plan and attempt to put various instructions into it that would put me into the driving seat–control being such an important issue to me following the total lack of control during my previous birth. | 1D 2H 2M |
| Working in a hospital I was incredibly lucky in that I could speak to my obstetrician on a daily basis. He recognized that all was not well when I told him about my first birth and he recommended that I speak with the head of midwifery for a debriefing session. When I did this, she suggested that for this subsequent pregnancy she would put herself "on call" for my delivery and would attend all my prenatal appointments. She was true to her word and this made me feel incredibly safe. | 2F 2N |
| I also read Heidi Gordon's book, *Birth and Beyond*, and referred to it like a bible. It helped to feel I was in full understanding of the birth process. I also spoke with other women to find out if birth second time around would be easier! My husband and I spoke at length about the birth and my fears. | 2C 2L 2G |

**FIGURE 16.1** ● Coded excerpt from Beck and Watson's (2010) study.

to that category into the file. Researchers can then retrieve all of the content on a particular topic by reviewing the applicable file folder.

Creating conceptual files is a cumbersome, labor-intensive task. This is particularly true when segments of the narrative materials have multiple codes, such as the excerpt shown in Figure 16.1. In this situation, there would need to be three copies of the second paragraph—one for each file corresponding to the three codes that were used (1D, 2H, 2M). Researchers must also be sensitive to the need to provide enough context that the cut-up material can be understood. Thus, it is often necessary to include material preceding or following the directly relevant materials.

*Computer-assisted qualitative data analysis software (CAQDAS)* can help to remove some of the work of cutting and pasting pages of narrative material. Dozens of CAQDAS have been developed. These programs permit an entire data set to be entered onto the computer, each portion of an interview or observational record coded, and then portions of the text corresponding to specified codes retrieved for analysis. The software can also be used to examine relationships between codes. Software cannot, however, *do* the coding, and it cannot tell the researcher how to analyze the data.

Computer programs offer many advantages for managing qualitative data, but some people prefer manual methods because they allow researchers to get closer to the data. Others object to having a cognitive process turned into an activity that is technical. Despite concerns, many researchers have switched to computerized data management. Proponents insist that it frees up their time and permits them to pay greater attention to important conceptual issues.

# ANALYTIC PROCEDURES

Data *management* in qualitative research is reductionist in nature: It involves converting large masses of data into smaller, more manageable segments. By contrast, qualitative data *analysis* is constructionist: It is an inductive process that involves putting segments together into meaningful conceptual patterns. There are various approaches to qualitative data analysis, but some elements are common to several of them.

## A General Analytic Overview

The analysis of qualitative materials usually begins with a search for broad categories or themes. In their review of how the term *theme* is used among qualitative researchers, DeSantis and Ugarriza (2000) offered this definition: "A **theme** is an abstract entity that brings meaning and identity to a current experience and its variant manifestations. As such, a theme captures and unifies the nature or basis of the experience into a meaningful whole" (p. 362).

Themes emerge from the data. They often develop within categories of data (i.e., within categories of the coding scheme used for indexing materials), but may also cut across them. For example, in Beck and Watson's (2010) study (Box 16.1), one theme that emerged was bringing reverence to the birthing process and empowering women; this theme included categories 3A (treated with respect by labor and delivery staff), 3C (mother's wishes listened to), 3E (good communication with labor and delivery staff), and 3I (birth plan honored by labor and delivery staff).

The search for themes involves not only discovering commonalities across participants but also seeking variation. Themes are never universal. Researchers must attend not only to what themes arise but also to how they are patterned. Does the theme apply only to certain types of people or in certain contexts? At certain periods? What are the conditions that precede the observed phenomenon, and what are the apparent consequences of it? In other words, the qualitative analyst must be sensitive to *relationships* within the data.

> **TIP:** Qualitative researchers often use major themes as the subheadings in the results section of their reports. For example, in their analysis of interviews with older Korean women about health behavior, Yang and Yang (2011) identified seven themes that were used to organize their results, including "Being modest and free from greed" and "Staying in harmony with nature."

Researchers' search for themes, regularities, and patterns in the data can sometimes be facilitated by charting devices that enable them to summarize the evolution of behaviors, events, and processes. For example, for qualitative studies that focus on dynamic experiences—such as decision making—it is often useful to develop flow charts or timelines that highlight time sequences, major decision points, and events.

The identification of key themes and categories is seldom a tidy, linear process—iteration is usually necessary. That is, researchers derive themes, go back to the narrative materials with the themes in mind to see if there is a true fit, and then refine the themes. Sometimes apparent insights early in the process have to be abandoned.

Some qualitative researchers use metaphors as an analytic strategy. A **metaphor** is a symbolic comparison, using figurative language to evoke a visual analogy. A metaphor can be a powerfully expressive tool for qualitative analysts, although they can run the risk of "supplanting creative insight with hackneyed cliché masquerading as profundity" (Thorne & Darbyshire, 2005, p. 1111).

> **Example of a metaphor:**
> Sun and colleagues (2011) conducted a study of Taiwanese women's journey from a prior pregnancy loss to motherhood. They used the nautical metaphor "sailing against the tide" to capture the essence of the women's journey because "the sea has deep cultural meaning of uncertainty in life for the Taiwanese people" (p. 127).

A further step involves validation. In this phase, the concern is whether the themes accurately represent the perspectives of the participants. Several validation procedures can be used, as we discuss in Chapter 17. If more than one researcher is working on the study, sessions in which the themes are reviewed and specific cases discussed can be productive. Such review cannot ensure thematic validity, but it can minimize idiosyncratic biases.

In validating and refining themes, some researchers introduce **quasi-statistics**—a tabulation of the frequency with which certain themes or insights are supported by the data. The frequencies cannot be interpreted in the same way as frequencies in quantitative studies because of imprecision in enumerating the themes, but, as Becker (1970) pointed out, "Quasi-statistics may allow the investigator to dispose of certain troublesome null hypotheses. A simple frequency count of the number of times a given phenomenon appears may make untenable the null hypothesis that the phenomenon is infrequent" (p. 81).

> **Example of tabulating data:**
> Crowe and colleagues (2012) examined how women describe their decisions relating to the use of menopausal hormone therapy following surgical menopause. In their interviews with 30 women, the researchers found three themes that distinguished how the women managed risks associated with hormone therapy: *Waiting for someone to tell me* (13 women), *Life has to go on* (14 women), and *Relying on my body to get me through* (3 women).

> ☞ **TIP:** Although relatively few qualitative researchers make formal efforts to quantify features of their data, be alert to quantitative implications when you read a qualitative report. Qualitative researchers routinely use words like "some," "most," or "many" in characterizing participants' experiences and actions, which implies some level of quantification.

In the final analysis stage, researchers strive to weave the thematic pieces together into a cohesive whole. The various themes are integrated to provide an overall structure (such as a theory or full description) to the data. The integration task demands creativity and intellectual rigor if it is to be successful.

## Qualitative Content Analysis

In the remainder of this section, we discuss analytic procedures used by ethnographers, phenomenologists, and grounded theory researchers. Qualitative researchers who conduct descriptive qualitative studies may, however, simply say that they performed a content analysis. Qualitative **content analysis** involves analyzing the content of narrative data to identify prominent themes and patterns among the themes. Qualitative content analysis involves breaking down data into smaller *units*, coding and naming the units according to the content they represent, and grouping coded material based on shared concepts.

There are different types of units that can be identified in a text (Krippendorff, 2013). For example, physical units are defined by time, length, or size (not by type of information). Syntactical units are based on grammatical divisions within the data—i.e., words, sentences, paragraphs. Categorical distinctions define units by identifying something they have in common i.e., membership in a category. Thematic distinctions delineate units according to themes. Krippendorff suggested *clustering* as a way to represent the results of content analyses. Clustering is based on similarities among units of analysis and hierarchies that conceptualize the text on different levels of abstraction.

> **Example of a content analysis:**
> Ackerson (2012) undertook a content analysis of semistructured interviews with 15 low-income African American women who had a history of sexual trauma to understand their experiences in undergoing gynecological examinations and Pap smear testing. Coding of content was guided by the Interaction Model of Client Health Behavior.

## Ethnographic Analysis

Analysis typically begins the moment ethnographers set foot in the field. Ethnographers are continually looking for *patterns* in the behavior and thoughts of participants, comparing one pattern against another, and analyzing many patterns simultaneously. As they analyze the organization and rhythms of everyday life, ethnographers acquire a deeper understanding of the culture being studied. Maps, flowcharts, and organizational charts are also useful tools that help to crystallize and illustrate the data being collected. Matrices (two-dimensional displays) can also help to highlight a comparison graphically, to cross-reference categories, and to discover emerging relationships.

Spradley's (1979) research sequence is often used for ethnographic data analyses. His method assumes that language is the primary means that relates cultural meaning in a culture. The task of ethnographers is to describe cultural symbols and to identify their coding rules. His sequence of 12 steps, which includes both data collection and data analysis, follows:

1. Locating an informant
2. Interviewing an informant
3. Making an ethnographic record
4. Asking descriptive questions
5. Analyzing ethnographic interviews
6. Making a domain analysis
7. Asking structural questions
8. Making a taxonomic analysis
9. Asking contrast questions
10. Making a componential analysis
11. Discovering cultural themes
12. Writing the ethnography

Thus, in Spradley's method there are four levels of data analysis, the first of which is *domain analysis*. **Domains**, which are units of cultural knowledge, are broad categories that encompass smaller categories. During this first level of data analysis, ethnographers identify relational patterns among terms in the domains that are used by members of the culture. The ethnographer focuses on the cultural meaning of terms and symbols (objects and events) used in a culture, and their interrelationships.

In *taxonomic analysis*, the second level of data analysis, ethnographers decide how many domains the data analysis will encompass. Will only one or two domains be analyzed in depth, or will a number of domains be studied less intensively? After making this decision, a **taxonomy**—a system of classifying and organizing terms—is developed to illustrate the internal organization of a domain and the relationship among the subcategories of the domain.

In *componential analysis*, multiple relationships among terms in the domains are examined. The ethnographer analyzes data for similarities and differences among cultural terms in a domain. Finally, in *theme analysis*, cultural themes are uncovered. Domains are connected in cultural themes, which help to provide a holistic view of the culture being studied. The discovery of cultural meaning is the outcome.

> **Example using Spradley's method:**
>
> Bourbonnais and Ducharme (2010) conducted an ethnographic study in a nursing home. They used Spradley's method of ethnographic analysis to explore *screaming* among elders in the nursing home environment as a unique language of communication.

Other approaches to ethnographic analysis have also been developed. For example, in their ethnonursing research method, Leininger and McFarland (2006) provided ethnographers with a four-phase ethnonursing data analysis guide. In the first phase ethnographers collect, describe, and record data. The second phase involves identifying and categorizing descriptors. In phase 3, data are analyzed to discover repetitive patterns in their context. The fourth and final phase involves abstracting major themes and presenting findings.

> **Example using Leininger's method:**
>
> Schumacher (2010) studied culture care meanings, beliefs, and practices in rural areas of the Dominican Republic. Interviews were conducted with 19 general and 10 key informants. Using Leininger's four-phase analytic method, three major cultural themes were identified.

## Phenomenological Analysis

Schools of phenomenology have developed different approaches to data analysis. Three frequently used methods for descriptive phenomenology are the methods of Colaizzi (1978), Giorgi (1985), and Van Kaam (1966), all of whom are from the *Duquesne School* of phenomenology, based on Husserl's philosophy. Table 16.1 presents a comparison of these three analytic methods. The basic outcome of all three methods is the description of the essential nature of an experience, often through the identification of essential themes.

Phenomenologists search for common themes emerging from particular instances. There are, however, some important differences among these three approaches. Colaizzi's method, for example, is the only one that calls for a validation of results by querying study participants. Giorgi's view is that it is inappropriate either to return to participants to validate findings or to use external judges to review the analysis. Van Kaam's method requires that intersubjective agreement be reached with other expert judges.

> **Example of a study using Colaizzi's method:**
>
> Doyle and colleagues (2012) explored dietary decision making among patients attending a secondary prevention clinic following myocardial infarction. Transcribed interviews with nine people were analyzed using Colaizzi's method. The analysis identified six recurrent themes, three that facilitated change (fear, determination, and self-control) and three that impeded change (lack of willpower, poor recall of information, and need for support).

Phenomenologists from the *Utrecht School*, such as Van Manen (1997), combine characteristics of descriptive and interpretive phenomenology. Van Manen's approach involves six activities: (1) turning to the nature of the lived experience; (2) exploring the experience as we live it; (3) reflecting on essential themes; (4) describing the phenomenon through the art of writing and rewriting; (5) maintaining a strong relation to the phenomenon; and (6) balancing the research context by considering parts and whole. According to Van Manen,

## TABLE 16.1 Comparison of Three Descriptive Phenomenologic Methods

| Colaizzi (1978) | Giorgi (1985) | Van Kaam (1966) |
|---|---|---|
| 1. Read all protocols to acquire a feeling for them. | 1. Read the entire set of protocols to get a sense of the whole. | 1. List and group preliminarily the descriptive expressions which must be agreed upon by expert judges. Final listing presents percentages of these categories in that particular sample. |
| 2. Review each protocol, and extract significant statements. | 2. Discriminate units from participants' description of phenomenon being studied. | 2. Reduce the concrete, vague, and overlapping expressions of the participants to more descriptive terms. (Intersubjective agreement among judges needed.) |
| 3. Spell out the meaning of each significant statement (i.e., formulate meanings). | 3. Articulate the psychological insight in each of the *meaning units.* | 3. Eliminate elements not inherent in the phenomenon being studied or that represent blending of two related phenomena. |
| 4. Organize the formulated meanings into clusters of themes.<br>a. Refer these clusters back to the original protocols to validate them.<br>b. Note discrepancies among or between the various clusters, avoiding the temptation of ignoring data or themes that do not fit. | 4. Synthesize all of the transformed meaning units into a consistent statement regarding participants' experiences (referred to as the "structure of the experience"); can be expressed on a specific or general level. | 4. Write a hypothetical identification and description of the phenomenon being studied. |
| 5. Integrate results into an exhaustive description of the phenomenon under study. | | 5. Apply hypothetical description to randomly selected cases from the sample. If necessary, revise the hypothesized description, which must then be tested again on a new sample. |
| 6. Formulate an exhaustive description of the phenomenon under study in as unequivocal a statement of identification as possible. | | 6. Consider the hypothesized identification as a valid identification and description once preceding operations have been carried out successfully. |
| 7. Ask participants about the findings thus far as a final validating step. | | |

thematic aspects of experience can be uncovered or isolated from participants' descriptions of the experience by three methods: the holistic, selective, or detailed approach. In the *holistic approach*, researchers view the text as a whole and try to capture its meanings. In the *selective* (or highlighting) *approach*, researchers highlight or pull out statements that seem essential to the experience under study. In the *detailed* (or line-by-line) *approach*, researchers analyze every sentence. Once themes have been identified, they become the objects of reflection and interpretation through follow-up interviews with participants. Through this process, essential themes are discovered.

> **Example of a study using Van Manen's method:**
> Haahr and colleagues (2011) studied the experience of living with advanced Parkinson's disease using van Manen's approach. They illustrated with interview excerpts how holistic, selective, and detailed approaches were used to reveal how participants lived with unpredictability.

In addition to identifying themes from participants' descriptions, Van Manen also called for gleaning thematic descriptions from artistic sources. Van Manen urged qualitative researchers to keep in mind that literature, painting, and other art forms can provide rich experiential data that can increase insights into the essential meaning of the experience being studied.

A third school of phenomenology is an interpretive approach called Heideggerian hermeneutics. Central to analyzing data in a hermeneutic study is the notion of the **hermeneutic circle**. The circle signifies a methodological process in which, to reach understanding, there is continual movement between the parts and the whole of the text being analyzed. Gadamer (1975) stressed that, to interpret a text, researchers cannot separate themselves from the meanings of the text and must strive to understand possibilities that the text can reveal.

Diekelmann, Allen, and Tanner (1989) proposed a seven-stage process of data analysis in hermeneutics that involves collaborative effort by a *team* of researchers. The goal of this process is to describe common meanings. Diekelmann and colleagues' stages include the following:

1. All the interviews or texts are read for an overall understanding.
2. Interpretive summaries of each interview are written.
3. A team of researchers analyzes selected transcribed interviews or texts.
4. Any disagreements on interpretation are resolved by going back to the text.
5. Common meanings and shared practices are identified by comparing and contrasting the text.
6. Relationships among themes emerge.
7. A draft of the themes along with exemplars from texts are presented to the team. Responses or suggestions are incorporated into the final draft.

According to Diekelmann and colleagues, the discovery in step 6 of a **constitutive pattern**— a pattern that expresses the relationships among relational themes and is present in all the interviews or texts—is the highest level of hermeneutical analysis. A situation is constitutive when it gives content to a person's self-understanding or to a person's way of being in the world.

> **Example of a Diekelmann's hermeneutical analysis:**
> Crotser and Dickerson (2011) described the experiences of women with at-risk relatives who learned of a family potential for cancer through genetic testing. Using team interpretation and Diekelman's seven-step analytic method, they discovered several themes, including *Redefining future possibilities* and *Navigating a twist in the road.*

Benner (1994) offered another analytic approach for hermeneutic phenomenology. Her interpretive analysis consists of three interrelated processes: the search for paradigm cases, thematic analysis, and analysis of exemplars. **Paradigm cases** are "strong instances of concerns or ways of being in the world" (Benner, 1994, p.113). Paradigm cases are used early in the analytic process as a strategy for gaining understanding. Thematic analysis is done to compare and contrast similarities across cases. Lastly, paradigm cases and thematic analysis can be enhanced by *exemplars* that illuminate aspects of a paradigm case or theme. The presentation of paradigm cases and exemplars in research reports allows readers to play a role in consensual validation of the results by deciding whether the cases support the researchers' conclusions.

> **Example using Benner's hermeneutical analysis:**
> Tzeng and colleagues (2010) conducted an interpretive phenomenological study of suicide survivors in Taiwan. They used Benner's approach in their analysis. A paradigm case was developed, and the researchers used it to compare and contrast other cases to identify commonalities and differences.

## Grounded Theory Analysis

The grounded theory method emerged in the 1960s in connection with research that focused on dying in hospitals by two sociologists, Glaser and Strauss. The two co-originators eventually split and developed divergent schools of thought, which have been called the "Glaserian" and "Straussian" versions of grounded theory. A third analytic approach by Charmaz, constructivist grounded theory, has also emerged.

### Glaser and Strauss' Grounded Theory Method

Grounded theory in all three analytic systems uses **constant comparison**, a method that involves comparing elements present in one data source (e.g., in one interview) with those in another. The process continues until the content of all sources has been compared so that commonalities are identified. The concept of fit is an important element in Glaserian grounded theory analysis. **Fit** has to do with how closely the emerging concepts fit with the incidents they are representing—which depends on how thoroughly constant comparison was done.

Coding in the Glaserian approach is used to conceptualize data into categories. Coding helps the researcher to discover the basic problem with which participants must contend. The substance of the topic under study is conceptualized through **substantive codes**, of which there are two types: open and selective. **Open coding**, used in the first stage of constant comparison, captures what is going on in the data. Open codes may be the actual words participants used. Through open coding, data are broken down and their similarities and differences are examined.

There are three levels of open coding that vary in degree of abstraction. **Level I codes** (or *in vivo codes*) are derived directly from the language of the substantive area. They have vivid imagery and "grab." Table 16.2 presents five level I codes and illustrative interview excerpts from Beck's (2002) grounded theory study on mothering twins.

As researchers constantly compare new level I codes with previously identified ones, they condense them into broader **level II codes**. For example, in Table 16.2, Beck's five level I codes were collapsed into a single level II code, "Reaping the Blessings." **Level III codes** (or theoretical constructs) are the most abstract. Collapsing level II codes aids in identifying constructs.

> ☞ **TIP:** Additional material relating to Beck's twin study is presented in the Chapter Supplement on the Point website. ☀

Open coding ends when the core category is discovered, and then selective coding begins. The **core category** (or *core variable*) is a pattern of behavior that is relevant and/or problematic for study participants. In **selective coding**, researchers code only those data that are related to the core category. One kind of core category is a **basic social process**

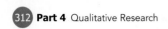

**TABLE 16.2** Collapsing Level I Codes into the Level II Code of
*"REAPING THE BLESSINGS"* (Beck, 2002)

| Excerpt | Level I Code |
| --- | --- |
| I enjoy just watching the twins interact so much. Especially now that they are mobile. They are not walking yet but they are crawling. I will tell you they are already playing. Like one will go around the corner and kind of peek around and they play hide and seek. They crawl after each other. | Enjoying Twins |
| With twins it's amazing. She was sick and she had a fever. He was the one acting sick. She didn't seem like she was sick at all. He was. We watched him for like 6 to 8 hours. We gave her the medicine and he started calming down. Like WOW! That is so weird. 'Cause you read about it but it's like, Oh come on! It's really neat to see. | Amazing |
| These days it's really neat 'cause you go to the store or you go out and people are like, "Oh, they are twins, how nice." And I say, "Yeah they are. Look, look at my kids." | Getting Attention |
| I just feel blessed to have two. I just feel like I am twice as lucky as a mom who has one baby. I mean that's the best part. It's just that instead of having one baby to watch grow and change and develop and become a toddler and school-age child, you have two. | Feeling Blessed |
| It's very exciting. It's interesting and it's fun to see them and how the twin bond really is. There really is a twin bond. You read about it and you hear about it, but until you experience it, you just don't understand. One time they were both crying and they were fed. They were changed and burped. There was nothing wrong. I couldn't figure out what was wrong. So I said to myself, "I am just going to put them together and close the door." I put them in my bed together, and they patty-caked their hands and put their noses together and just looked at each other and went right to sleep. | Twin Bonding |

**(BSP)** that evolves over time in two or more phases. All BSPs are core categories, but not all core categories have to be BSPs.

Glaser (1978) provided nine criteria to help researchers decide on a core category. Here are a few examples: It must be central, meaning that it is related to many categories; it must recur frequently in the data; it relates meaningfully and easily to other categories; and it has clear and grabbing implications for formal theory.

**Theoretical codes** provide insights into how substantive codes relate to each other. Theoretical codes help grounded theorists to weave the broken pieces of data back together again. Glaser (1978) proposed 18 families of theoretical codes that researchers can use to conceptualize how substantive codes relate to each other (although he subsequently expanded possibilities in 2005). Four examples of his families of theoretical codes include the following:

- Process: stages, phases, passages, transitions
- Strategy: tactics, techniques, maneuverings
- Cutting point: boundaries, critical junctures, turning points
- The six Cs: causes, contexts, contingencies, consequences, covariances, and conditions

Throughout coding and analysis, grounded theory analysts document their ideas about the data and emerging conceptual scheme in *memos*. Memos encourage researchers to reflect on and describe patterns in the data, relationships between categories, and emergent conceptualizations.

Glaser's grounded theory method is concerned with the *generation* of categories and hypotheses rather than testing them. The product of the typical grounded theory analysis is a theoretical model that endeavors to explain a pattern of behavior that is relevant for study participants. Once the basic problem emerges, the grounded theorist goes on to discover the process these participants experience in coping with or resolving this problem.

> **Example of Glaser and Strauss grounded theory analysis:**
> Figure 16.2 presents Beck's (2002) model from a study in which "Releasing the Pause Button" was conceptualized as the core category and process through which mothers of twins progressed as they tried to resume their lives after giving birth. The process involves four phases: Draining Power, Pausing Own Life, Striving to Reset, and Resuming Own Life. Beck used 10 coding families in her theoretical coding for the study. The family *cutting point* offers an illustration. Three months seemed to be a turning point for mothers, when life started to be more manageable. Here is an excerpt from an interview that Beck coded as a cutting point: "Three months came around and the twins sort of slept through the night and it made a huge, huge difference."

Glaser and Strauss cautioned against consulting the literature before a framework is stabilized, but they also saw the benefit of scrutinizing other work. Glaser discussed the evolution of grounded theories through the process of **emergent fit**, to prevent individual substantive theories from being "respected little islands of knowledge" (Glaser, 1978, p. 148). As he noted, generating grounded theory does not necessarily require discovering all new categories or ignoring ones previously identified in the literature. Through constant comparison, researchers can compare concepts emerging from the data with similar concepts from existing theory or research to evaluate which parts have emergent fit with the theory being generated.

## Strauss and Corbin's Approach

The Strauss and Corbin (1998) approach to grounded theory analysis differs from the original Glaser and Strauss method with regard to method, processes, and outcomes. Table 16.3 summarizes major analytic differences between these two grounded theory analysis methods.

Glaser (1978) stressed that to generate a grounded theory, the basic problem must emerge from the data—it must be discovered. The theory is, from the very start, grounded

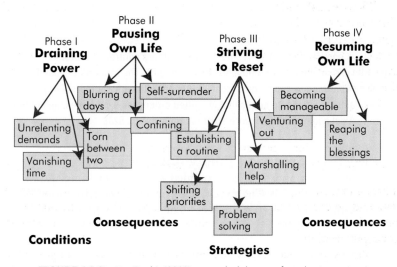

**FIGURE 16.2** ● Beck's (2002) grounded theory of mothering twins.

**TABLE 16.3  Comparison of Glaser's and Strauss/Corbin's Methods**

| | Glaser | Strauss & Corbin |
|---|---|---|
| Initial data analysis | Breaking down and conceptualizing data involves comparison of incident to incident so patterns emerge | Breaking down and conceptualizing data includes taking apart a single sentence, observation and incident |
| Types of coding | Open, selective, theoretical | Open, axial, selective |
| Connections between categories | 18 coding families (plus others added subsequently) | Paradigm model (conditions, contexts, action/interactional strategies, and consequences) |
| Outcome | Emergent theory (discovery) | Conceptual description (verification) |

in the data, rather than starting with a preconceived problem. Strauss and Corbin, however, argued that the research itself is only one of four possible sources of a research problem. Research problems can, for example, come from the literature or a researcher's personal and professional experience.

The Strauss and Corbin method involves three types of coding: open, axial, and selective. In **open coding**, data are broken into parts and compared for similarities and differences. In open coding, the researcher focuses on generating categories and their properties and dimensions. In **axial coding**, the analyst systematically develops categories and links them with subcategories. Strauss and Corbin used "axial" to describe this type of coding because coding was viewed as occurring around the axis of a category. What is called the *paradigm* is used to help identify linkages among categories. The basic components of the paradigm include conditions, actions/interactions, and consequences. **Selective coding** is the process in which the findings are integrated and refined. The first step in integrating the findings is to decide on the **central category** (sometimes called the *core category*), which is the main category of the research.

The outcome of the Strauss and Corbin approach is a full conceptual description. The original grounded theory method, by contrast, generates a theory that explains how a basic social problem that emerged from the data is processed in a social setting.

> **Example of Strauss and Corbin grounded theory analysis:**
> Copeland and Heilemann (2011) studied how mothers confront the problem of housing their adult children with mental illness and a history of violence. The researchers used the Strauss and Corbin analytic approach to coding data from interviews with eight mothers. They used open coding "to break each sentence into codes that identified processes, similarities, and differences present in the data… Axial coding involved more abstract analysis" (p. 523).

## Constructivist Grounded Theory Approach

The constructivist approach to grounded theory is in some ways similar to a Glaserian approach. According to Charmaz (2006), in constructivist grounded theory the "coding generates the bones of your analysis. Theoretical integration will assemble these bones into a working skeleton" (p. 45). Charmaz offered guidelines for different types of coding: word-by-word coding, line-by-line coding, and incident-to-incident coding. Unlike Glaser and Strauss' grounded theory approach in which theory is discovered from data separate from the researcher, Charmaz's position is that researchers construct grounded theories by means of their past and current involvements and interactions with individuals and research practices.

Charmaz distinguished initial coding and **focused coding**. In initial coding, the pieces of data (e.g., words, lines, segments, incidents) are studied so the researcher can learn what the participants view as problematic. In focused coding, the analysis is directed towards identifying the most significant initial codes, which are then theoretically coded. An example of an analysis using the constructivist approach is presented at the end of the chapter.

> 👉 **TIP:** Grounded theory researchers often present conceptual maps or models to summarize their results, such as the one in Figure 16.2, especially when the central phenomenon is a dynamic or evolving process.

# CRITIQUING QUALITATIVE ANALYSIS

Evaluating a qualitative analysis is not easy to do. Readers do not have access to the information they would need to assess whether researchers exercised good judgment and critical insight in coding the narrative materials, developing a thematic analysis, and integrating materials into a meaningful whole. Researchers are seldom able to include more than a handful of examples of actual data in a journal article. Moreover, the process they used to inductively abstract meaning from the data is difficult to describe and illustrate.

A major focus of a critique of qualitative analyses is whether the researchers have adequately documented the analytic process. The report should provide information about the approach used to analyze the data. For example, a report for a grounded theory study should indicate whether the researchers used the Glaserian, Straussian, or constructivist approach.

Another aspect of a qualitative analysis that can be critiqued is whether the researchers have documented that they have used one approach consistently and have been faithful to the integrity of its procedures. Thus, for example, if researchers say they are using the Glaserian approach to grounded theory analysis, they should not also include elements from the Strauss and Corbin method. An even more serious problem occurs when, as sometimes happens, the researchers "muddle" traditions. For example, researchers who describe their study as a grounded theory study should not present *themes*, because grounded theory analysis does not yield themes. Researchers who attempt to blend elements from two traditions may not have a clear grasp of the analytic precepts of either one. For example, a researcher who claims to have undertaken an ethnography using a grounded theory approach to analysis may not be well informed about the underlying goals and philosophies of these two traditions.

Some further guidelines that may be helpful in evaluating qualitative analyses are presented in Box 16.2.

### Box 16.2 Guidelines for Critiquing Qualitative Analyses

1. Was the data analysis approach appropriate for the research design or tradition?
2. Was the category scheme described? If so, does the scheme appear logical and complete?
3. Did the report adequately describe the process by which the actual analysis was performed? Did the report indicate whose approach to data analysis was used (e.g., Glaserian, Straussian, or constructivist in grounded theory studies)?
4. What major themes or processes emerged? Were relevant excerpts from the data provided, and do the themes or categories appear to capture the meaning of the narratives—that is, does it appear that the researcher adequately interpreted the data and conceptualized the themes? Is the analysis parsimonious—could two or more themes be collapsed into a broader and perhaps more useful conceptualization?
5. Was a conceptual map, model, or diagram effectively displayed to communicate important processes?
6. Was the context of the phenomenon adequately described? Did the report give you a clear picture of the social or emotional world of study participants?
7. Did the analysis yield a meaningful and insightful picture of the phenomenon under study? Is the resulting theory or description trivial or obvious?

## RESEARCH EXAMPLES WITH CRITICAL THINKING EXERCISES

☀ Example 1 below is also featured in our *Interactive Critical Thinking Activity* on thePoint website where you can easily record, print, and e-mail your responses to the related questions.

### EXAMPLE 1 ● A Constructivist Grounded Theory Analysis

**Study:** Care transition experiences of spousal caregivers: From a geriatric rehabilitation unit (GRU) to home (Byrne et al., 2011). (This study appears in its entirety in the accompanying *Study Guide*). 📖

**Statement of Purpose:** The purpose of this study was to develop a theory about caregivers' transition processes and experiences during their spouses' return home from a GRU.

**Method:** This grounded theory study involved in-depth interviews with 18 older adult spousal caregivers. Most of the caregivers were interviewed on three occasions: 48 hours prior to discharge from a 36-bed GRU in a Canadian long-term care hospital, 2 weeks postdischarge, and 1 month postdischarge. In addition to the interviews, which lasted between 35 and 120 minutes, the researchers made observations of interactions between spouses and care recipients.

**Analysis:** Analysis began with line-by-line coding by the first author. All authors contributed to focused coding, followed by theoretical coding. They used constant comparison throughout the coding and analysis process and provided a good example: "In the early stages of data collection and analysis, we noticed that caregivers continually used the phrase "I don't know," and thus an open code by this name was created… As data collection and analysis proceeded, we engaged in focused coding using the term *knowing/not knowing* to reflect these instances" (p. 1374). The researchers illustrated with an interview excerpt how they came to understand that knowing/not knowing was part of the process of *navigating*. The researchers also noted that "Moving from line-be-line coding to focused coding was not a linear process. As we engaged with the data, we returned to the data collected to explore new ideas and conceptualization of codes" (p. 1375).

**Key Findings:** The basic problem the caregivers faced was "fluctuating needs," including the physical, emotional, social, and medical needs of their spouses and themselves. The researchers developed a theoretical framework in which *reconciling in response to fluctuating needs* emerged as the basic social process. Reconciling encompassed three subprocesses: navigating, safekeeping, and repositioning. The context that shaped reconciling was a trajectory of prior care transitions and intertwined life events.

## CRITICAL THINKING EXERCISES
1. Answer the relevant questions from Box 16.2 on page 316 regarding this study.
2. Also consider the following targeted questions:
   a. Comment on the researcher's decision to use both interview data and observations.
   b. The authors wrote that "To foster theoretical sensitivity, memos focused on actions and processes, and gradually incorporated relevant literature (e.g., theoretical perspectives on transition)" (p. 1375). Comment on this statement.
3. In what ways do you think the findings could be used in clinical practice?

## EXAMPLE 2 ● A Phenomenological Analysis in Appendix B
- Read the method and results sections from Beck and Watson's phenomenological study ("Subsequent childbirth after a previous traumatic birth") in Appendix B on pages 403–412.

## CRITICAL THINKING EXERCISES
1. Answer the relevant questions from Box 16.2 on page 316 regarding this study.
2. Also consider the following targeted questions:
   a. Comment on the amount of data that had to be analyzed in this study.
   b. Refer to Table 2 in the article, which presents a list of 10 significant statements made by participants. In Colaizzi's approach, the next step is to construct *formulated meanings* (interpretations) from the significant statements. Try to develop your own *formulated meanings* of one or two of these significant statements.

---

**WANT TO KNOW MORE?** A wide variety of resources to enhance your learning and understanding of this chapter are available on thePoint.

- Interactive Critical Thinking Activity
- Chapter Supplement on a Glaserian Grounded Theory Study
- Answers to the Critical Thinking Exercises for Example 2
- Student Review Questions
- Full-text online
- Internet Resources with useful websites for Chapter 16

Additional study aids including eight journal articles and related questions are also available in *Study Guide for Essentials of Nursing Research, 8e.*

# SUMMARY POINTS

- Qualitative analysis is a challenging, labor-intensive activity, guided by few standardized rules.

- A first step in analyzing qualitative data is to organize and index the materials for easy retrieval, typically by coding the content of the data according to a category scheme.

- Traditionally, researchers have organized their data by developing **conceptual files**, which are physical files in which coded excerpts of data for specific categories are placed. Now, however, computer programs (CAQDAS) are widely used to perform basic indexing functions and to facilitate data analysis.

- The actual analysis of data begins with a search for patterns and **themes**, which involves the discovery not only of commonalities across participants but also of natural variation in the data. Some qualitative analysts use *metaphors* or figurative comparisons to evoke a visual and symbolic analogy.

- Another analytic step involves validation of the thematic analysis. Some researchers use **quasi-statistics**, a tabulation of the frequency with which certain themes or relations are supported by the data. In a final step, analysts try to weave the thematic strands together into an integrated picture of the phenomenon under investigation.

- Researchers whose goal is qualitative description often say they used qualitative **content analysis** as their analytic method.

- In ethnographies, analysis begins as the researcher enters the field. One analytic approach is Spradley's method, which involves four levels of analysis: *domain analysis* (identifying **domains**, or units of cultural knowledge), *taxonomic analysis* (selecting key domains and constructing **taxonomies**), *componential analysis* (comparing and contrasting terms in a domain), and a *theme analysis* (to uncover cultural themes).

- There are numerous approaches to phenomenological analysis, including the descriptive methods of Colaizzi, Giorgi, and Van Kaam, in which the goal is to find common patterns of experiences shared by particular instances.

- In Van Manen's approach, which involves efforts to grasp the essential meaning of the experience being studied, researchers search for themes, using a *holistic approach* (viewing text as a whole), a *selective approach* (pulling out key statements and phrases), or a *detailed approach* (analyzing every sentence).

- Central to analyzing data in a hermeneutic study is the notion of the **hermeneutic circle**, which signifies a process in which there is continual movement between the parts and the whole of the text under analysis.

- Diekelmann's team method of hermeneutic analysis calls for the discovery of a **constitutive pattern** that expresses the relationships among themes. Benner's approach consists of three processes: searching for **paradigm cases**, thematic analysis, and analysis of *exemplars*.

- Grounded theory uses the **constant comparative** method of data analysis, a method that involves comparing elements present in one data source (e.g., in one interview) with those in another. *Fit* has to do with how closely concepts fit with incidents they represent, which is related to how thoroughly constant comparison was done.

- One grounded theory approach is the Glaser and Strauss (Glaserian) method, in which there are two broad types of coding: **substantive coding** (in which the empirical substance of the topic is conceptualized) and **theoretical coding** (in which the relationships among the substantive codes are conceptualized).

- Substantive coding involves **open coding** to capture what is going on in the data and then **selective coding**, in which only variables relating to a core category are coded. The **core category**, a behavior pattern that has relevance for participants, is sometimes a **basic social process (BSP)** that involves an evolutionary process of coping or adaptation.

- In the Glaserian method, open codes begin with **level I (in vivo) codes**, which are collapsed into a higher level of abstraction in **level II codes**. Level II codes are then used to formulate **level III codes**, which are theoretical constructs. Through constant comparison, the researcher compares concepts emerging from the data with similar concepts from existing theory or research to see which parts have **emergent fit** with the theory being generated.

- The Strauss and Corbin grounded theory method has full conceptual description as the outcome. This grounded theory approach involves three types of coding: open (in which categories are generated), **axial coding** (where categories are linked with subcategories), and selective (in which the findings are integrated and refined).

- In Charmaz's constructivist grounded theory, coding can be word-by-word, line-by-line, or incident-by-incident. Initial coding leads to **focused coding**, which is then followed by theoretical coding.

# REFERENCES FOR CHAPTER 16

Ackerson, K. (2012). A history of interpersonal trauma and the gynecological exam. *Qualitative Health Research, 22*(5), 679–688.

Beck, C. T. (2002). Releasing the pause button: Mothering twins during the first year of life. *Qualitative Health Research, 12,* 593–608.

Beck, C.T. (2006). Anniversary of birth trauma: Failure to rescue. *Nursing Research, 55,* 381–390.

Becker, H. S. (1970). *Sociological work.* Chicago, IL Aldine.

Benner, P. (1994). The tradition and skill of interpretive phenomenology in studying health, illness, and caring practices. In P. Benner (Ed.), *Interpretive phenomenology* (pp. 99–127). Thousand Oaks, CA: Sage.

Bourbonnais, A., & Ducahrme, F. (2010). The meanings of screams in older people living with dementia in a nursing home. *International Psychogeriatrics, 22,* 1172–1184.

Byrne, K., Orange, J., & Ward-Griffin, C. (2011). Care transition experiences of spousal caregivers: From a geriatric unit to home. *Qualitative Health Research, 21,* 1371–1387.

Charmaz, K. (2006). *Constructing grounded theory: A practical guide to qualitative analysis.* Thousand Oaks, CA: Sage.

Colaizzi, P. (1978). Psychological research as the phenomenologist views it. In R. Valle & M. King (Eds.), *Existential phenomenological alternatives for psychology* (pp. 48–71). New York: Oxford University Press.

Copeland, D., & Heilemann, M. (2011). Choosing "the best of hells": Mothers facing housing dilemmas for their adult children with mental illness and a history of violence. *Qualitative Health Research, 21,* 520–533.

Crotser, C., & Dickerson, S. (2010). Learning about a twist in the road: Perspectives of at-risk relatives learning of potential for cancer. *Oncology Nursing Forum, 37,* 723–733.

Crowe, M., Burrell, B., & Whitehead, L. (2012). Lifestyle risk management: A qualitative analysis of women's descriptions of taking hormone therapy following surgically induced menopause. *Journal of Advanced Nursing, 68,* 1814–1823.

DeSantis, L., & Ugarriza, D. N. (2000). The concept of theme as used in qualitative nursing research. *Western Journal of Nursing Research, 22,* 351–372.

Diekelmann, N. L., Allen, D., & Tanner, C. (1989). *The NLN criteria for appraisal of baccalaureate programs: A critical hermeneutic analysis.* New York: NLN Press.

Doyle, B., Fitzsimons, D., McKeown, P., & McAloon, T. (2012). Understanding dietary decision-making in patients attending a secondary prevention clinic following myocardial infarction. *Journal of Clinical Nursing, 21,* 32–41.

Elfström, M., Karlsson, S., Nilsen, P., Fridlund, B., Svanborg, E., & Broström, A. (2012). Decisive situations affecting partners' support to continuous positive airway pressure-treated patients with obstructive sleep apnea syndrome. *The Journal of Cardiovascular Nursing, 27*(3), 228–239.

Gadamer, H.G. (1975). *Truth and method.* (G. Borden & J. Cumming, trans). London, UK: Sheed & Ward.

Giorgi, A. (1985). *Phenomenology and psychological research.* Pittsburgh, PA: Duquesne University Press.

Glaser, B. G. (1978). *Theoretical sensitivity.* Mill Valley, CA: Sociology Press.

Glaser, B.G. (2005). *The grounded theory perspective III: Theoretical coding.* Mill Valley, CA: Sociology Press.

Glaser, B. G., & Strauss, A. L. (1967). *The discovery of grounded theory: Strategies for qualitative research.* Chicago, IL: Aldine.

Haahr, A., Kirkevold, M., Hall, E., & Ostergaard, K. (2011). Living with advanced Parkinson's disease: A constant struggle with unpredictability. *Journal of Advanced Nursing, 67,* 408–417.

Krippendorff, K. (2013). *Content analysis: An introduction to its methodology* (3rd ed.). Thousand Oaks, CA: Sage.

Leininger, M., & McFarland, M. (2006). *Culture care diversity and universality: A worldwide nursing theory* (2nd ed.). Sudbury, MA: Jones and Bartlett Publishers.

Schumacher, G. (2010). Culture care meanings, beliefs, and practices in rural Dominican Republic. *Journal of Transcultural Nursing, 21*(2), 93–103.

Spradley, J. P. (1979). *The ethnographic interview*. New York: Holt, Rinehart and Winston.

Strauss, A. L., & Corbin, J. M. (1998). *Basics of qualitative research: Techniques and procedures for developing grounded theory* (2nd ed.). Thousand Oaks, CA: Sage.

Sun, H. L., Sinclair, M., Kernohan, G., Chang, T., & Paterson, H. (2011). Sailing against the tide: Taiwanese women's journey from pregnancy loss to motherhood. *MCN: American Journal of Maternal/Child Health, 36*, 127–133.

Thorne, S. & Darbyshire, P. (2005). Land mines in the field: A modest proposal for improving the craft of qualitative health research. *Qualitative Health Research, 15*(8), 1105–1113.

Tzeng, W., Su, P., Chiang, H., Kuan, P., & Lee, J. (2010). A qualitative study of suicide survivors in Taiwan. *Western Journal of Nursing Research, 32*, 185–198.

Van Kaam, A. (1966). *Existential foundations of psychology*. Pittsburgh, PA: Duquesne University Press.

Van Manen, M. (1997). *Researching lived experience* (2nd ed.). London, ON: The Althouse Press.

Yang, J. H., & Yang, B. S. (2011). Alternative view of health behavior: the experience of older Korean women. *Qualitative Health Research, 21*, 324–332.

# Trustworthiness and Integrity in Qualitative Research

## LEARNING OBJECTIVES

*On completing this chapter, you will be able to:*

- Discuss some controversies relating to the issue of quality in qualitative research
- Identify the quality criteria proposed in the Lincoln and Guba framework for evaluating quality and integrity in qualitative research
- Discuss strategies for enhancing quality in qualitative research
- Describe different dimensions relating to the interpretation of qualitative results
- Define new terms in the chapter

## KEY TERMS

| | | |
|---|---|---|
| Audit trail | Inquiry audit | Researcher credibility |
| Authenticity | Member check | Thick description |
| Confirmability | Negative case analysis | Transferability |
| Credibility | Peer debriefing | Triangulation |
| Dependability | Persistent observation | Trustworthiness |
| Disconfirming evidence | Prolonged engagement | |

Integrity in qualitative research is a critical issue for both those doing the research and those considering the use of qualitative evidence.

# PERSPECTIVES ON QUALITY IN QUALITATIVE RESEARCH

Qualitative researchers agree on the importance of doing high-quality research, yet defining "high quality" has been controversial. It is beyond the scope of this book to explain arguments of the debate in detail, but we offer a brief overview.

## Debates about Rigor and Validity

One contentious issue concerns use of the terms *rigor* and *validity*—terms some people shun because they are associated with the positivist paradigm and are viewed as inappropriate goals for constructivist research. For these critics, the concept of rigor is by its nature an empirical analytic term that does not fit into an interpretive paradigm that values insight and creativity.

Others disagree with those opposing the term *validity*. Whittemore and colleagues (2001), for example, argued that validity is an appropriate term in all paradigms, noting that the dictionary definition of validity (the state or quality of being sound, just, and well founded) lends itself equally to qualitative and quantitative research.

The complex debate has given rise to a variety of positions. At one extreme are those who think that validity is an appropriate quality criterion in both qualitative and quantitative studies, although qualitative researchers use different methods to achieve it. At the opposite extreme are those who berate the "absurdity" of validity. A widely adopted stance is what has been called a *parallel perspective*. This position was proposed by Lincoln and Guba (1985), who created standards for the **trustworthiness** of qualitative research that parallel the standards of reliability and validity in quantitative research.

## Generic versus Specific Standards

Another controversial issue concerns whether there should be a generic set of quality standards, or whether specific standards are needed for different types of inquiry—for example, for ethnographers and grounded theory researchers. Many writers subscribe to the idea that research conducted within different qualitative traditions must attend to different concerns, and that techniques for enhancing and demonstrating research integrity vary. Thus, different writers have offered standards for specific forms of qualitative inquiry, such as grounded theory, phenomenology, ethnography, and critical research. Some writers believe, however, that there are some quality criteria that are fairly universal within the constructivist paradigm. For example, Whittemore and colleagues (2001) prepared a synthesis of criteria that they viewed as essential to all qualitative inquiry.

## Terminology Proliferation and Confusion

The result of these controversies is that there is no common vocabulary for quality criteria in qualitative research. Terms, such as *truth value, goodness, integrity, trustworthiness*, and *rigor*, abound, but each proposed term has been deemed inappropriate by some critics.

With regard to actual *criteria* for evaluating quality in qualitative research, dozens (if not hundreds) have been suggested. Establishing a consensus on what the quality criteria for qualitative inquiry should be, and what they should be named, remains elusive, and it is unlikely that a consensus will be achieved in the near future, if ever.

Given the lack of consensus, and the heated arguments supporting and contesting various frameworks, it is difficult to provide guidance about quality standards. We present information about *criteria* from the Lincoln and Guba framework in the next section. We then describe *strategies* that researchers use to strengthen integrity in qualitative research. These strategies should be viewed as points of departure for considering whether a qualitative study is sufficiently rigorous, trustworthy, insightful, or valid.

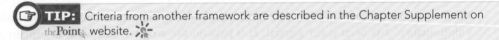
**TIP:** Criteria from another framework are described in the Chapter Supplement on thePoint website.

# LINCOLN AND GUBA'S FRAMEWORK OF QUALITY CRITERIA

Although not without critics, the criteria often viewed as the "gold standard" for qualitative research are those outlined by Lincoln and Guba (1985). These researchers suggested four criteria for developing the *trustworthiness* of a qualitative inquiry: credibility, dependability, confirmability, and transferability. These criteria represent parallels to the positivists' criteria of internal validity, reliability, objectivity, and external validity, respectively. In later writings, responding to criticisms and to their own evolving views, a fifth criterion more distinctively within the constructivist paradigm was added: authenticity (Guba & Lincoln, 1994).

## Credibility

**Credibility** refers to confidence in the truth value of the data and interpretations of them. Qualitative researchers must strive to establish confidence in the truth of the findings for the particular participants and contexts in the research. Lincoln and Guba pointed out that credibility involves two aspects: first, carrying out the study in a way that enhances the believability of the findings, and second, taking steps to *demonstrate* credibility to external readers. Credibility is a crucial criterion in qualitative research that has been proposed in several quality frameworks.

## Dependability

**Dependability** refers to the stability (reliability) of data over time and over conditions. The dependability question is: Would the study findings be repeated if the inquiry were repli-cated with the same (or similar) participants in the same (or similar) context? Credibility cannot be attained in the absence of dependability, just as validity in quantitative research cannot be achieved in the absence of reliability.

## Confirmability

**Confirmability** refers to objectivity, that is, the potential for congruence between two or more independent people about the data's accuracy, relevance, or meaning. This criterion is concerned with establishing that the data represent the information participants provided, and that the interpretations of those data are not imagined by the inquirer. For this criterion to be achieved, the findings must reflect the participants' voice and the conditions of the inquiry, and not the researcher's biases, motivations, or perspectives.

## Transferability

**Transferability**, analogous to generalizability, is the extent to which qualitative findings can be transferred to or have applicability in other settings or groups. Lincoln and Guba noted that the investigator's responsibility is to provide sufficient descriptive data that consum-ers can evaluate the applicability of the data to other contexts: "Thus the naturalist cannot specify the external validity of an inquiry; he or she can provide only the thick description necessary to enable someone interested in making a transfer to reach a conclusion about whether transfer can be contemplated as a possibility" (p. 316).

## Authenticity

**Authenticity** refers to the extent to which researchers fairly and faithfully show a range of different realities. Authenticity emerges in a report when it conveys the feeling tone of participants' lives as they are lived. A text has authenticity if it invites readers into a vicarious experience of the lives being described, and enables readers to develop a heightened sensitiv-ity to the issues being depicted. When a text achieves authenticity, readers are better able to understand the lives being portrayed "in the round," with some sense of the mood, feeling, experience, language, and context of those lives.

# STRATEGIES TO ENHANCE QUALITY IN QUALITATIVE INQUIRY

The criteria for establishing integrity in a qualitative study are complex and challenging. A variety of strategies have been proposed to address these challenges. This section describes some of them in the hope that they will prompt a careful assessment of steps researchers did or not take to enhance integrity.

We have not organized strategies according to criteria (e.g., strategies researchers use to enhance *credibility*) because many strategies simultaneously address multiple criteria. Instead, we have organized strategies according to different phases of a study—data generation, coding and analysis, and report preparation. Table 17.1 indicates how various quality-enhancement strategies map onto Lincoln and Guba's criteria.

**TABLE 17.1    Quality-Enhancement Strategies in Relation to Lincoln and Guba's Quality Criteria for Qualitative Inquiry**

| Strategy | Credibility | Dependability | Confirmability | Transferability | Authenticity |
|---|---|---|---|---|---|
| **Throughout the Inquiry** | | | | | |
| Reflexivity/reflexive journaling | X | | | | X |
| Careful documentation, decision trail | | X | X | | |
| **Data Generation** | | | | | |
| Prolonged engagement | X | | | | X |
| Persistent observation | X | | | | X |
| Comprehensive field notes | X | | | X | |
| Audiotaping and verbatim transcription | X | | | | X |
| Triangulation (data, method) | X | X | | | |
| Saturation of data | X | | | X | |
| Member checking | X | X | | | |
| **Data Coding/Analysis** | | | | | |
| Transcription rigor/data cleaning | X | | | | |
| Intercoder checks; development of a codebook | X | | X | | |
| Quasi-statistics | X | | | | |

TABLE 17.1    **Quality-Enhancement Strategies in Relation to Lincoln and Guba's Quality Criteria for Qualitative Inquiry** *(Continued)*

| Strategy | Credibility | Dependability | Confirmability | Transferability | Authenticity |
|---|---|---|---|---|---|
| **Data Coding/Analysis** *(Continued)* | | | | | |
| Triangulation (investigator, theory, analysis) | X | X | X | | |
| Stepwise replication | | X | X | | |
| Search for disconfirming evidence/ negative case analysis | X | | | | |
| Peer review/debriefing | X | | X | | |
| Inquiry audit | | X | X | | |
| **Presentation of Findings** | | | | | |
| Documentation of quality-enhancement efforts | X | | | X | |
| Thick, vivid description | | | | X | X |
| Impactful, evocative writing | | | | | X |
| Documentation of researcher credentials, background | X | | | | |
| Documentation of reflexivity | X | | | | |

## Quality-Enhancement Strategies During Data Collection

Qualitative researchers use many strategies to enrich and strengthen their studies, some of which are difficult to discern in a report. For example, intensive listening during an interview, careful probing to obtain rich and comprehensive data, and taking pains to gain participants' trust are all strategies to enhance data quality that cannot easily be communicated in a report. In this section, we focus on some strategies that can be described to readers to increase their confidence in the integrity of the study results.

### Prolonged Engagement and Persistent Observation

An important step in establishing integrity in qualitative studies is **prolonged engagement**—the investment of sufficient time collecting data to have an in-depth understanding of the culture, language, or views of the people or group under study, to test for misinformation and distortions, and to ensure saturation of important categories. Prolonged engagement is also essential for building trust and rapport with informants, which in turn makes it more likely that useful and rich information will be obtained.

**Example of prolonged engagement:**

Salt and Peden (2011) studied decision-making relating to treatment for rheumatoid arthritis in a grounded theory study with 30 women. Data were collected over a 13-month period. The researchers noted that "This prolonged engagement assured that the decision-making process was accurately and fully described" (p. 215).

High-quality data collection in qualitative studies also involves **persistent observation**, which concerns the salience of the data being gathered. Persistent observation refers to the researchers' focus on the characteristics or aspects of a situation that are relevant to the phenomena being studied. As Lincoln and Guba (1985) noted, "If prolonged engagement provides scope, persistent observation provides depth" (p. 304).

**Example of persistent observation:**

Ward-Griffin and colleagues (2012) conducted a critical ethnography of the management of dementia home care resources in Ontario. They made detailed observations and conducted multiple interviews with persons with dementia, family caregivers, in-home providers, and case managers in nine dementia care networks over a 19-month period.

### Reflexivity Strategies

Reflexivity involves awareness that the researcher as an individual brings to the inquiry a unique background, set of values, and a social and professional identity that can affect the research process. Reflexivity involves attending continually to the researcher's effect on the collection, analysis, and interpretation of data.

The most widely used strategy for maintaining reflexivity and delimiting subjectivity is to maintain a reflexive journal or diary. Reflexive notes can be used to record, from the outset of the study and in an ongoing fashion, thoughts about the impact of previous life experiences and previous readings about the phenomenon on the inquiry. Through self-interrogation and reflection, researchers seek to be well positioned to probe deeply and to grasp the experience, process, or culture under study through the lens of participants.

 **TIP:** Researchers sometimes begin a study by being interviewed themselves with regard to the phenomenon under study. Of course, this approach usually only makes sense if the researcher has had experience with that phenomenon.

### Data and Method Triangulation

Triangulation refers to the use of multiple referents to draw conclusions about what constitutes truth. The aim of triangulation is to "overcome the intrinsic bias that comes from single-method, single-observer, and single-theory studies" (Denzin, 1989, p. 313). Triangulation can also help to capture a more complete, contextualized picture of the phenomenon under study. Denzin identified four types of triangulation (data triangulation, investigator triangulation, method triangulation, and theory triangulation), and other types have been proposed. Two types are relevant to data collection.

**Data triangulation** involves the use of multiple data sources for the purpose of validating conclusions. There are three types of data triangulation: time, space, and person. **Time triangulation** involves collecting data on the same phenomenon or about the same people at different points in time. Time triangulation can involve gathering data at different times of the day, or at different times in the year. This concept is similar to test–retest reliability assessment—the point is not to study a phenomenon longitudinally to assess how it changes, but to establish the congruence of the phenomenon across time. **Space triangulation** involves collecting data on the same phenomenon in multiple sites, to test for cross-site consistency. Finally, **person triangulation** involves collecting data from different types or levels of people (e.g., individuals, families, communities), with the aim of validating data through multiple perspectives on the phenomenon.

> **Example of person and space triangulation:**
> Miles and colleagues (2011) studied how community responses to HIV play a role in the distress experienced by African Americans with HIV living in the rural south. Data were collected in six communities, and were gathered through focus group and individual interviews with community leaders, service providers, and African Americans with HIV.

**Method triangulation** involves using multiple methods of data collection about the same phenomenon. In qualitative studies, researchers often use a rich blend of unstructured data collection methods (e.g., interviews, observations, documents) to develop a comprehensive understanding of a phenomenon. Multiple data collection methods provide an opportunity to evaluate the extent to which a consistent and coherent picture of the phenomenon emerges.

> **Example of method triangulation:**
> Sloand and colleagues (2012) triangulated multiple data sources in their study of fatherhood and the role of fathers' clubs in promoting child health in Haitian villages. The main data source was personal interviews with 18 fathers from four villages. The researchers triangulated these data with data from interviews with key informants, field notes of meetings with village health agents, and journal entries "to augment the initial analysis findings so that the truest picture could be drawn of fathering in rural Haiti" (p. 490).

## Comprehensive and Vivid Recording of Information

In addition to taking steps to record data from interviews accurately (e.g., via careful transcriptions of audiotaped interviews), researchers should prepare field notes that are rich with descriptions of what transpired in the field. Even if interviews are the only source of data, researchers should record descriptions of the participants' demeanor and behaviors during the interactions, and the interview context. Thoroughness in record-keeping helps readers to develop confidence in the data.

Researchers sometimes specifically develop an **audit trail**, that is, a systematic collection of materials and documentation that would allow an independent auditor to come to conclusions about the data. An adequate audit trail might include the following types of records: the raw data (e.g., interview transcripts); methodologic, theoretic, and reflexive notes; instrument development information (e.g., pilot topic guides); and data reconstruction products (e.g., drafts of the final report). Similarly, the maintenance of a *decision trail* that articulates the researcher's decision rules for categorizing data and making analytic inferences is a useful way to enhance the dependability of the study. When researchers can share some decision trail information in their reports, readers can better evaluate the soundness of the decisions and draw conclusions about the trustworthiness of the findings.

> **Example of an audit trail:**
> In their ethnographic study of anxiety and agitation in mechanically ventilated patients, Tate and colleagues (2012) maintained careful documentation: "An audit trail of methodologic notes and analytic memos was recorded systematically to detail thoughts and establish dependability" (p. 160).

## Member Checking

In a **member check**, researchers give participants feedback about emerging interpretations and then obtain participants' reactions. The argument is that participants should have an opportunity to assess and validate whether the researchers' interpretations are good representations of their realities. Member checking can be carried out as data are being collected (e.g., through deliberate probing to ensure that interviewers have properly interpreted participants' meanings), and more formally after data have been fully analyzed in follow-up interviews or interviews with different participants.

Despite the potential that member checking has for enhancing credibility, it has some potential drawbacks. One issue is that member checks can lead to erroneous conclusions if participants share a common façade or a desire to "cover up." Also, some participants might agree with researchers' interpretations out of politeness or in the belief that researchers are "smarter" or more knowledgeable than they are. Thorne and Darbyshire (2005) cautioned against what they called *adulatory validity*, "a mutual stroking ritual that satisfies the agendas of both researcher and researched" (p. 1110). They pointed out that member checking tends to privilege interpretations that place participants in a charitable light.

Few strategies for enhancing data quality are as controversial as member checking. Nevertheless, it is a strategy that has the potential to enhance credibility if it is done in a manner that encourages candor and critical appraisal by participants.

> **TIP:** Methodologic congruence regarding member checking should be assessed. For example, if Giorgi's phenomenologic methods were used, member checking would not be undertaken, but member checking *is* called for in studies following Colaizzi's approach (see Table 16.1, p. 309).

> **Example of member checking:**
> Chen (2012) conducted a descriptive qualitative study of the life experiences of Taiwanese oral cancer patients during the postoperative period. A sample of 13 patients participated in in-depth interviews. The thematic analysis was reviewed by three study participants and by four patients with oral cancer who had not participated in the study to ensure that the results accurately depicted patients' experiences.

## Strategies Relating to Coding and Analysis

Excellent qualitative inquiry is likely to involve the simultaneous collection and analysis of data, and so several of the strategies described earlier also contribute to analytic integrity. Member checking, for example, can occur in an ongoing fashion as part of the data collection process, but typically also involves participants' review of preliminary analytic constructions. Some analytic validation procedures, such as the use of quasi-statistics, were described in Chapter 16. In this section, we introduce a few additional quality-enhancement strategies associated with the coding, analysis, and interpretation of qualitative data.

## Investigator and Theory Triangulation

During analysis, several types of triangulation are pertinent. **Investigator triangulation** refers to the use of two or more researchers to make data collection, coding, and analytic decisions. The underlying premise is that through collaboration, investigators can reduce the possibility of biased decisions and idiosyncratic interpretations.

Conceptually, investigator triangulation is analogous to inter-rater reliability in quantitative studies, and is a strategy that is often used in coding qualitative data. Some researchers take formal steps to compare two or more independent category schemes or independent coding decisions.

> **Example of independent coding:**
> Skär and Söderberg (2012) studied men's complaints about their encounters with the health care system in Sweden. Both researchers independently coded the transcripts of interviews with nine men who had lodged a complaint, using a category system that had been jointly developed after a preliminary review of the data. The authors discussed their coding until consensus was reached.

If investigators bring to the analysis task a complementary blend of skills and expertise, the analysis and interpretation can potentially benefit from divergent perspectives. Blending diverse methodologic, disciplinary, and clinical skills also can contribute to other types of triangulation.

> **Example of investigator triangulation:**
> Drach-Zahavy and colleagues (2012) studied psychiatric hospital staff's perceptions of and reactions to aggressive patient behavior. Data from in-depth interviews with 11 health care professionals in an Israeli psychiatric hospital were content analyzed separately by all four researchers. "We then comparatively examined our individual analyses, by both the themes' content and the interpretation of their meanings" (p. 46).

One form of investigator triangulation is called **stepwise replication**, a strategy most often mentioned in connection with Lincoln and Guba's dependability criterion. This technique involves having a research team that can be divided into two groups. These groups deal with data sources separately and conduct, essentially, independent inquiries through which data can be compared.

With **theory triangulation**, researchers use competing theories or hypotheses in the analysis and interpretation of their data. Qualitative researchers who develop alternative hypotheses while still in the field can test the validity of each because the flexible design of qualitative studies provides ongoing opportunities to direct the inquiry. Theory triangulation can help researchers to rule out rival hypotheses and to prevent premature conceptualizations.

## Searching for Disconfirming Evidence and Competing Explanations

A powerful verification procedure involves a systematic search for data that will challenge a categorization or explanation that has emerged early in the analysis. The search for **disconfirming evidence** occurs through purposive or theoretical sampling methods. Clearly, this strategy depends on concurrent data collection and data analysis: researchers cannot look for disconfirming data unless they have a sense of what they need to know.

> **Example of searching for disconfirming evidence:**
> Enarsson and colleagues (2007) conducted a grounded theory study to examine common approaches among staff toward patients in long-term psychiatric care. The researchers found that all the categories they were discovering were negative in nature. To assess the integrity of their categories, the researchers performed a specific search for data reflecting common staff approaches that related to positive experiences. No such positive episodes could be found either in interviews or observations.

Lincoln and Guba (1985) discussed the related activity of **negative case analysis**. This strategy (sometimes called *deviant case analysis)* is a process by which researchers revise their interpretations by including cases that appear to disconfirm earlier hypotheses. The goal of this procedure is to continuously refine a hypothesis or theory until it accounts for *all* cases.

> **Example of a negative case analysis:**
> Ching and colleagues (2012) explored coping among Chinese women afflicted with breast cancer. The researchers explained that they "derived hypotheses when relationships between the codes were identified in one interview and verified or modified in the subsequent interviews, illustrating similar responses, different responses, and negative cases" (p. 251).

## Peer Review and Debriefing

Another quality-enhancement strategy involves external validation. **Peer debriefing** involves sessions with peers to review and explore aspects of the inquiry. Peer debriefing exposes researchers to the searching questions of others who are experienced in either the methods of constructivist inquiry, the phenomenon being studied, or both.

In a peer-debriefing session, researchers might present written or oral summaries of the data that have been gathered, categories and themes that are emerging, and researchers' interpretations of the data. In some cases, taped interviews might be played. Among the questions that peer debriefers might address are the following:

- Is there evidence of researcher bias?
- Do the gathered data adequately portray the phenomenon? Have all important themes or categories been identified?
- If there are important omissions, what strategies might remedy this problem?
- Are there any apparent errors of fact or possible errors of interpretation?
- Are there competing interpretations or more parsimonious interpretations?
- Are the themes and interpretations knit together into a cogent, useful, and creative conceptualization of the phenomenon?

> **Example of peer debriefing:**
> Van Dover and Pfeiffer (2012) conducted a grounded theory study of the process that patients of parish nurses experience when they receive spiritual care. The two researchers developed codes and categories separately and then reached consensus. An independent researcher then reviewed the analysis when links among theoretical elements were under construction.

## Inquiry Audits

A similar, but more formal, approach is to undertake an inquiry audit, a procedure that is a means of enhancing a study's dependability and confirmability. An **inquiry audit** involves a scrutiny of the data and relevant supporting documents by an external reviewer. Such an audit requires careful documentation of all aspects of the inquiry. Once the audit trail materials are assembled, the inquiry auditor proceeds to audit, in a fashion analogous to a financial audit, the trustworthiness of the data and the meanings attached to them. Such audits are a good tool for persuading others that qualitative data are worthy of confidence.

**Example of an inquiry audit:**
Rotegård and colleagues (2012) studied cancer patients' experiences and perceptions of their personal strengths through their illness and recovery in four focus group interviews with 26 participants. A partial audit was undertaken by having an external researcher review a sample of transcripts and interpretations. ☀

## Strategies Relating to Presentation

This section describes some aspects of the qualitative report itself that can help to persuade readers of the high quality of the inquiry.

### Thick and Contextualized Description

**Thick description** refers to a rich, thorough, and vivid description of the research context, the people who participated in the study, and the experiences and processes observed during the inquiry. Transferability cannot occur unless investigators provide sufficient information to permit judgments about contextual similarity. Lucid and textured descriptions, with the judicious inclusion of verbatim quotes from study participants, also contribute to the authenticity of a qualitative study.

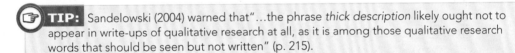

**TIP:** Sandelowski (2004) warned that"...the phrase *thick description* likely ought not to appear in write-ups of qualitative research at all, as it is among those qualitative research words that should be seen but not written" (p. 215).

In high-quality qualitative studies, descriptions typically need to go beyond a faithful rendering of information. Powerful description is evocative and has the capacity for emotional impact. Qualitative researchers should, however, avoid misrepresenting their findings by sharing only the most dramatic or sensational stories. Thorne and Darbyshire (2005) cautioned against what they called *lachrymal validity*, a criterion for evaluating research according to the extent to which the report can wring tears from its readers! At the same time, they observed that the opposite problem with some reports is that they are "bloodless." Bloodless findings are characterized by a tendency of some researchers to "play it safe in writing up the research, reporting the obvious...(and) failing to apply any inductive analytic spin to the sequence, structure, or form of the findings" (p. 1109).

### Researcher Credibility

Another aspect of credibility is **researcher credibility**. In qualitative studies, researchers *are* the data collecting instruments—as well as creators of the analytic process—and so their qualifications, experience, and reflexivity are relevant in establishing confidence in the data. Patton (2002) has argued that trustworthiness is enhanced if the report contains information about the researchers, including information about credentials and any personal connections the researchers had to the people, topic, or community under study. For example, it is relevant for a reader of a report on the coping mechanisms of AIDS patients to know that the researcher is HIV positive. Researcher credibility is also enhanced when reports describe the researchers' efforts to be reflexive and to take their own prejudices and perspectives into account.

> **Example of researcher credibility:**
> Nilvarangkul and colleagues (2011) did an action study to explore and enhance the health-related quality of life of Laotian migrant workers in Thailand. They included a paragraph describing their qualifications for the research. All four researchers were Thai health care professionals (three were nurses) with a focus on workplace health and safety.

# INTERPRETATION OF QUALITATIVE FINDINGS

It is difficult to describe the interpretive process in qualitative studies, but there is considerable agreement that the ability to "make meaning" from qualitative texts depends on researchers' immersion in and closeness to the data. **Incubation** is the process of *living* the data, a process in which researchers must try to understand their meanings, find their essential patterns, and draw well-grounded, insightful conclusions. Another key ingredient in interpretation and meaning-making is researchers' self-awareness and the ability to reflect on their own world view and perspectives—that is, reflexivity. Creativity also plays an important role in uncovering meaning in the data. Researchers need to give themselves sufficient time to achieve the *aha* that comes with making meaning beyond the facts.

For *readers* of qualitative reports, interpretation is hampered by having limited access to the data and no opportunity to "live" the data. Researchers are necessarily selective in the amount and types of information to include in their reports. Nevertheless, you should strive to consider some of the same interpretive dimensions for qualitative studies as for quantitative ones (Chapter 13). In the discussion that follows, we discuss five dimensions.

## The Credibility of Qualitative Results

As with quantitative reports, you should consider whether the results of a qualitative inquiry are believable. It is reasonable to expect authors of qualitative reports to provide *evidence* of the credibility of the findings. Because consumers are exposed to only a portion of the data, they must rely on researchers' efforts to corroborate findings through such mechanisms as peer debriefings, member checks, audits, triangulation, and negative cases analysis. They must also rely on researchers' honesty in acknowledging known limitations.

In considering the believability of qualitative results, it makes sense to adopt the posture of a person who needs to be persuaded about the researcher's conceptualization, and to expect the researcher to marshal evidence with which to persuade you. It is also appropriate to consider whether the researcher's conceptualization of the phenomenon is consistent with common experiences and with your own clinical insights.

## The Meaning of Qualitative Results

From the point of view of researchers themselves, interpretation and analysis of qualitative data occur virtually simultaneously, in an iterative process. Efforts to validate the qualitative analysis are necessarily efforts to validate interpretations as well. Thus, unlike quantitative analyses, the meaning of the data flows directly from qualitative analysis.

Nevertheless, prudent qualitative researchers hold their interpretations up for closer scrutiny—self-scrutiny as well as review by peers and outside reviewers. Even when researchers have undertaken peer debriefings and other strategies described in this chapter, these procedures do not constitute proof that interpretations are correct. For both qualitative and quantitative researchers, it is important to consider possible alternative explanations for the findings and to take into account methodologic or other limitations that could have affected study results.

**TIP:** Interpretation in qualitative studies sometimes yields hypotheses that can be tested in more controlled quantitative studies. Qualitative studies are well suited to generating causal hypotheses, but not to testing them in a rigorous fashion.

## The Importance of Qualitative Results

Qualitative research is especially productive when it is used to describe and explain poorly understood phenomena. The scantiness of prior research on a topic is not, however, a sufficient barometer for deciding whether the findings can contribute to nursing knowledge. The phenomenon must be one that merits scrutiny.

You should also consider whether the findings themselves are trivial. Perhaps the topic is worthwhile, but you may feel after reading a report that nothing has been learned beyond what is common sense or everyday knowledge—this can happen when the data are too "thin" or when the conceptualization is shallow. Readers, like researchers, want to have an *aha* experience when they read about the lives and concerns of clients and their families. Qualitative researchers often attach catchy labels to their themes and processes, but you should ask yourself whether the labels have really captured an insightful construct.

## The Transferability of Qualitative Results

Although qualitative researchers do not strive for generalizability, the possible application of the results to other settings and contexts is important to evidence-based practice. Thus, in interpreting qualitative results, you should consider how transferable the findings are. In what other types of settings and contexts would you expect the phenomena under study to be manifested in a similar fashion? Of course, to make such an assessment, the researchers must have described in sufficient detail the participants and the context in which the data were collected. Because qualitative studies are context bound, it is only through a careful analysis of the key parameters of the study context that the transferability of results can be assessed.

## The Implications of Qualitative Results

If the findings are judged to be believable and important, and if you are satisfied with the interpretation of the results, you can begin to consider what the implications of the findings might be. First, you can consider implications for further research: Should a similar study be undertaken in a different setting? Has an important construct been identified that merits the development of a formal measuring instrument? Do the results suggest hypotheses that could be tested through controlled quantitative research? Second, do the findings have implications for nursing practice? For example, could the health-care needs of a subculture (e.g., the homeless) be addressed more effectively as a result of the study? Finally, do the findings shed light on fundamental processes that could play a role in nursing theories?

# CRITIQUING INTEGRITY AND INTERPRETATIONS IN QUALITATIVE STUDIES

For qualitative research to be judged trustworthy, investigators must earn the trust of their readers. Many qualitative reports do not provide much information about the researchers' efforts to ensure that their research is strong with respect to the quality criteria described in this chapter. In a world that is very conscious about the quality of research evidence, qualitative researchers need to be proactive in doing high-quality research and persuading others that they were successful.

Clearly, demonstrating integrity to others involves providing a good description of the quality-enhancement activities that were undertaken. Yet some qualitative reports do not address the topic of rigor, integrity, or trustworthiness at all. Others pay lip service to validity concerns, simply noting, for example, that an audit trail was maintained. Just as clinicians seek *evidence* for clinical decisions, research consumers need evidence that findings are believable and true. Researchers should include enough information about their quality-enhancement strategies for readers to draw conclusions about study quality. The research example at the end of this chapter is exemplary in this regard.

Part of the difficulty that qualitative researchers face in demonstrating trustworthiness and authenticity is that page constraints in journals impose conflicting demands. It takes a precious amount of space to present quality-enhancement strategies adequately and convincingly. Using space for such documentation means that there is less space for the thick description of context and rich verbatim accounts that support authenticity and vividness. Qualitative research is often characterized by the need for critical compromises. It is well to keep such compromises in mind in critiquing qualitative research reports.

An important point in thinking about quality in qualitative inquiry is that attention needs to be paid to both "art" and "science," and to interpretation and description. Creativity and insightfulness need to be attained, but not at the expense of soundness. And the quest for soundness cannot sacrifice inspiration and elegant abstractions, or else the results are likely to be "perfectly healthy but dead" (Morse, 2006, p. 6). Good qualitative work is both descriptively accurate and explicit, and interpretively rich and innovative. Some guidelines that may be helpful in evaluating qualitative methods and analyses are presented in Box 17.1.

---

### BOX 17.1  Guidelines for Evaluating Trustworthiness and Integrity in Qualitative Studies

1. Does the report discuss efforts to enhance or evaluate the quality of the data and the overall inquiry? If so, is the description sufficiently detailed and clear? If not, is there other information that allows you to draw inferences about the quality of the data, the analysis, and the interpretations?
2. Which specific techniques (if any) did the researcher use to enhance the trustworthiness and integrity of the inquiry? What quality-enhancement strategies were *not* used? Would additional strategies have strengthened your confidence in the study and its evidence?
3. Has the researcher adequately represented the multiple realities of those being studied? Do the findings seem *authentic*?
4. Given the efforts to enhance data quality, what can you conclude about the study's validity/integrity/rigor/trustworthiness?
5. Did the report discuss any study limitations and their possible effects on the credibility of the results or on interpretations of the data? Were results interpreted in light of findings from other studies?
6. Did the researchers discuss the study's implications for clinical practice or future research? Were the implications well grounded in the study evidence, and in evidence from earlier research?

## RESEARCH EXAMPLES WITH CRITICAL THINKING EXERCISES

Example 1 below is also featured in our *Interactive Critical Thinking Activity* on thePoint website where you can easily record, print, and e-mail your responses to the related questions.

### EXAMPLE 1 ● Trustworthiness in a Grounded Theory Study

**Study:** Moving to place: Childhood cancer treatment decision making in single-parent and repartnered family structures (Kelly & Ganong, 2011)

**Statement of Purpose:** The purpose of this study was to address this overarching question: "How do parents who no longer live together make treatment decisions for their children with cancer?"

**Method:** The grounded theory study involved in-depth interviews with 15 custodial parents, nonresident parents, and step-parents from eight families that included a child with cancer. The interviews included such grand tour questions as the following: "Please tell me everything you can remember about what it was like for you making the (specific treatment decision)" (p. 351). The audiotaped interviews were transcribed, and analyzed using the Strauss and Corbin approach.

**Quality Enhancement Strategies:** The researchers' report provided good detail about the efforts the researchers made to enhance the trustworthiness and integrity of their study. They stated that they undertook prolonged engagement with participants, that they triangulated data by gathering information from family members with different perspectives, and that they made efforts to include a diverse sample in terms of family structure and disease experiences. They noted that they reached theoretical saturation with 12 interviews, but conducted three additional interviews to confirm the evolving theory. In these member-check interviews, "parents endorsed the elements of the paradigm model and offered no additional commentary" (p. 351). The first author conducted all the fieldwork, and the second author reviewed her decision trail and ongoing analysis. "Both authors reviewed all the transcripts, category coding decisions, and accompanying memos" (p. 352). They made efforts to maintain objectivity by "thinking comparatively, comparing incident to incident, and staying grounded in the data" (p. 352). At critical points in their analysis, they consulted another grounded theory researcher who had studied parental treatment decision making regarding their conceptualizations. The report also included explicit statements regarding researcher credibility and transferability.

**Key Findings:** The researchers concluded that "moving to place" was the central psychosocial process by which parents in complex and nontraditional family structures negotiated their involvement in treatment decision making. The process was grounded by a focus on the ill child. Parents used the actions of stepping up, stepping back, being pushed, and stepping away to respond to the need for treatment decision making.

### CRITICAL THINKING EXERCISES
1. Answer the relevant questions from Box 17.1 on page 334 regarding this study.
2. Also consider the following targeted questions:
   a. Which quality-enhancement strategy used by Kelly and Ganong gave you the *most* confidence in the integrity and trustworthiness of their study? Why?
   b. Think of an additional type of triangulation that the researchers could have used in their study and describe how this could have been operationalized.
3. In what ways do you think the findings could be used in clinical practice?

### EXAMPLE 2 ● Trustworthiness in the Phenomenologic Study in Appendix B
- Read the method and results sections from Beck and Watson's phenomenological study ("Subsequent childbirth after a previous traumatic birth") in Appendix B on pages 403–412.

### CRITICAL THINKING EXERCISES
1. Answer the relevant questions from Box 17.1 on page 334 regarding this study.
2. Also consider the following targeted questions:
   a. Suggest one or two ways in which triangulation could have been used in this study.
   b. Which quality-enhancement strategy used by Beck and Watson gave you the *most* confidence in the integrity and trustworthiness of their study? Why?

**WANT TO KNOW MORE?** A wide variety of resources to enhance your learning and understanding of this chapter are available on thePoint.

- Interactive Critical Thinking Activity
- Chapter Supplement on Whittemore and Colleagues' Framework of Quality Criteria in Qualitative Research
- Answers to the Critical Thinking Exercises for Example 2
- Student Review Questions
- Full-text online
- Internet Resources with useful websites for Chapter 17

Additional study aids including eight journal articles and related questions are also available in *Study Guide for Essentials of Nursing Research, 8e.*

## SUMMARY POINTS

- One of several controversies regarding *quality* in qualitative studies involves terminology. Some argue that *rigor* and *validity* are quantitative terms that are not suitable as goals in qualitative inquiry, but others believe these terms are appropriate. Other controversies involve what criteria to use as indicators of integrity and whether there should be generic or study-specific criteria.

- One prominent evaluative framework is that of Lincoln and Guba, who identified five criteria for evaluating **trustworthiness** in qualitative inquiries: credibility, dependability, confirmability, transferability, and authenticity.

- **Credibility**, which refers to confidence in the truth value of the findings, has been viewed as the qualitative equivalent of internal validity. **Dependability**, the stability of data over time and over conditions, is somewhat analogous to reliability in quantitative studies. **Confirmability** refers to the objectivity of the data. **Transferability**, the analog of external validity, is the extent to which findings can be transferred to other settings or groups. **Authenticity** is the extent to which researchers faithfully show a range of different realities and convey the feeling tone of lives as they are lived.

- Strategies for enhancing quality during qualitative data collection include **prolonged engagement**, which strives for adequate scope of data coverage; **persistent observation**, which is aimed at achieving adequate depth; comprehensive recording of information (including maintenance of an **audit trail**); triangulation, and **member checks** (asking study participants to review and react to study data and emerging conceptualizations).

● **Triangulation** is the process of using multiple referents to draw conclusions about what constitutes the truth. This includes **data triangulation** (using multiple data sources to validate conclusions) and **method triangulation** (using multiple methods to collect data about the same phenomenon).

● Strategies for enhancing quality during the coding and analysis of qualitative data include **investigator triangulation** (independent coding and analysis of some of the data by two or more researchers), **theory triangulation** (use of competing theories or hypotheses in the analysis and interpretation of data), **stepwise replication** (dividing the research team into two groups that conduct independent inquiries that can be compared and merged), searching for **disconfirming evidence**, searching for rival explanations and undertaking a **negative case analysis** (revising interpretations to account for cases that appear to disconfirm early conclusions), external validation through **peer debriefings** (exposing the inquiry to the searching questions of peers), and launching an **inquiry audit** (a formal scrutiny of audit trail documents by an independent auditor).

● Strategies that can be used to convince readers of reports of the high quality of qualitative inquiries include using **thick description** to vividly portray contextualized information about study participants and the central phenomenon, and making efforts to be transparent about researcher credentials and reflexivity so that **researcher credibility** can be established.

● Interpretation in qualitative research involves "making meaning"—a process that is difficult to describe or critique. Yet interpretations in qualitative inquiry need to be reviewed in terms of credibility, importance, transferability, and implications.

# REFERENCES FOR CHAPTER 17

Chen, S. C. (2012). Life experiences of Taiwanese oral cancer patients during the postoperative period. *Scandinavian Journal of Caring Sciences, 26*(1), 98–103.

Ching, S., Martinson, I., & Wong, T. (2012). Meaning making: psychological adjustment to breast cancer by Chinese women. *Qualitative Health Research, 22*, 250–262.

Denzin, N. K. (1989). *The research act* (3rd ed.). New York: McGraw-Hill.

Drach-Zahavy, A., Goldblatt, H., Granot, M., Hirschmann, S., & Kostintski, H. (2012). Control: Patients' aggression in psychiatric settings. *Qualitative Health Research, 22*, 43–53.

Enarsson, P., Sandman, P-O., & Hellzen, O. (2007). The preservation of order: The use of common approaches among staff toward clients in long-term psychiatric care. *Qualitative Health Research, 17*, 718–729.

Guba, E., & Lincoln, Y. (1994). Competing paradigms in qualitative research. In N. Denzin & Y. Lincoln (Eds.), *Handbook of qualitative research*, (pp. 105–117). Thousand Oaks, CA: Sage.

Kelly, K. P., & Ganong, L. (2011). Moving to place: Childhood cancer treatment decision making in single-parent and repartnered family structures. *Qualitative Health Research, 21*, 349–364.

Lincoln, Y. S., & Guba, E. G. (1985). *Naturalistic inquiry*. Newbury Park, CA: Sage.

Miles, M. S., Isler, M., Banks, B., Sengupta, S., & Corbie-Smith, G. (2011). Silent endurance and profound loneliness: Socioemotional suffering in African Americans living with HIV in the rural south. *Qualitative Health Research, 21*, 489–501.

Morse, J. M. (2006). Insight, inference, evidence, and verification: Creating a legitimate discipline. *International Journal of Qualitative Methods, 5*(1), Article 8. Retrieved August 7, 2012 from http://www.ualberta.ca/ijqm/.

Nilvarangkul, K., McCann, T., Rungreangkulkij, S., & Wongprom, J. (2011). Enhancing a health-related quality of life model for Laotian migrant workers in Thailand. *Qualitative Health Research, 21*, 312–332.

Patton, M. Q. (2002). *Qualitative evaluation and research methods* (3rd ed.). Thousand Oaks, CA: Sage.

Rotegård, A., Fagermoen, M., & Ruland, C. (2012). Cancer patients' experiences of their personal strengths through illness and recovery. *Cancer Nursing, 35*, E8–E17.

Salt, E., & Peden, A. (2011). The complexity of the treatment: The decision-making process among women with rheumatoid arthritis. *Qualitative Health Research, 21*, 214–222.

Sandelowski, M. (2004). Counting cats in Zanzibar. *Research in Nursing & Health, 27*, 215–216.

Skär, L., & Söderberg, S. (2012). Complaints with encounters in healthcare—men's experiences. *Scandinavian Journal of Caring Science, 26*(2), 279–286.

Sloand, E., Gebrian, B., & Astone, N. M. (2012). Fathers' beliefs about parenting and fathers' clubs to promote child health in rural Haiti. *Qualitative Health Research, 22*, 488–498.

Tate, J. A., Dabbs, A., Hoffman, L., Milbrandt, E., & Happ, M. (2012). Anxiety and agitation in mechanically ventilated patients. *Qualitative Health Research, 22*, 157–173.

Thorne, S. & Darbyshire, P. (2005). Land mines in the field: A modest proposal for improving the craft of qualitative health research. *Qualitative Health Research, 15*, 1105–1113.

Van Dover, L., & Pfeiffer, J. (2012). Patients of parish nurses experience renewed spiritual identity: A grounded theory study. *Journal of Advanced Nursing, 68*, 1824–1833.

Ward-Griffin, C., Hall, J., DeForge, R., St-Amant, O., McWilliam, C., Oudshoorn, A., et al. (2012). Dementia home care resources: How are we managing? *Journal of Aging Research, 2012*, 590–724.

Whittemore, R., Chase, S. K., & Mandle, C. L. (2001). Validity in qualitative research. *Qualitative Health Research, 11*, 522–537.

# part 5

# Special Topics in Research

## chapter 18

# Mixed Methods and Other Special Types of Research

## LEARNING OBJECTIVES

*On completing this chapter, you will be able to:*

- Identify several advantages of mixed methods research and describe specific applications
- Describe strategies and designs for conducting mixed methods research
- Identify the purposes and some of the distinguishing features of specific types of research (e.g., clinical trials, evaluations, surveys)
- Define new terms in the chapter

## KEY TERMS

| | | |
|---|---|---|
| Clinical trial | Exploratory design | Nursing intervention research |
| Concurrent design | Health services research | Outcomes research |
| Convergent parallel design | Impact analysis | Pragmatism |
| Economic (cost) analysis | Intervention theory | Process analysis |
| Embedded design | Methodologic research | Secondary analysis |
| Evaluation research | Mixed methods (MM) | Sequential design |
| Explanatory design | research | Survey research |

In this final part of the book, we explain several special types of research. We begin by discussing mixed methods (MM) research that combines qualitative and qualitative approaches.

## MIXED METHODS RESEARCH

A growing trend in nursing research is the planned collection and integration of qualitative and quantitative data within single studies or coordinated clusters of studies. This section discusses the rationale for such **mixed methods research** and presents a few applications.

## Rationale for Mixed Methods Research

The dichotomy between quantitative and qualitative data represents a key methodologic distinction. Some argue that the paradigms that underpin qualitative and quantitative research are fundamentally incompatible. Most people, however, now believe that many areas of inquiry can be enriched through the judicious triangulation of qualitative and quantitative data. The advantages of an MM design include the following:

- *Complementarity*. Qualitative and quantitative approaches are complementary. By using MM, researchers can possibly avoid the limitations of a single approach.
- *Practicality*. Given the complexity of phenomena, it is practical to use whatever methodological tools are best suited to addressing pressing research questions, and to not have one's hands tied by rigid adherence to a single approach.
- *Incrementality*. Progress on a topic tends to be incremental. Qualitative findings can generate hypotheses to be tested quantitatively, and quantitative findings may need clarification through in-depth probing. It can be productive to build such a feedback loop into the design of a study.
- *Enhanced validity*. When a hypothesis or model is supported by multiple and complementary types of data, researchers can be more confident about their inferences. Triangulation of methods can provide opportunities for testing alternative interpretations of the data and for examining the extent to which the context helped to shape the results.

Perhaps the strongest argument for MM research, however, is that some questions *require* MM. **Pragmatism**, a paradigm often associated with MM research, provides a basis for a position that has been stated as the "dictatorship of the research question" (Tashakkori & Teddlie, 2010, p. 21). Pragmatist researchers consider that it is the research question that should drive the inquiry, and its design and methods. They reject a forced choice between the traditional postpositivists' and constructivists' modes of inquiry.

## Purposes and Applications of Mixed Methods Research

In MM research, there is typically an overarching goal, but there are inevitably at least two research questions, each of which requires a different type of approach. For example, MM researchers may simultaneously ask exploratory (qualitative) questions and confirmatory (quantitative) questions. In an MM study, researchers can examine causal *effects* in a quantitative component, but can shed light on causal *mechanisms* in a qualitative component.

Creswell and Plano Clark (2011) identified several types of research situations that are especially well suited to MM research, including the following:

1. The concepts are poorly understood, and qualitative exploration is needed before more formal, structured methods can be used
2. The findings from one approach can be greatly enhanced with a second source of data
3. Neither a qualitative nor a quantitative approach, by itself, is adequate in addressing the complexity of the problem
4. The quantitative results are difficult to interpret, and qualitative data can help to explain them

As this list suggests, mixed methods research can be used in various situations, a few of which are described here.

### Developmental Work

When a construct is new, qualitative research can help to capture its full complexity and dimensionality. Nurse researchers sometimes gather qualitative data as the basis for developing formal instruments—that is, for generating and wording the questions on quantitative scales that are subsequently subjected to rigorous testing. Similarly, qualitative research is playing an increasingly important role in the development of promising nursing interventions and in efforts to assess their efficacy.

**Example of intervention development:**

Zoffman and Kirkevold (2012) described how their grounded theory studies on barriers to empower-ment among patients with diabetes led to the development of a problem-solving intervention called Guided Self-Determination (GSD). The intervention was subsequently evaluated in a randomized controlled trial (RCT).

## Hypothesis Generation and Testing

In-depth qualitative studies are often fertile with insights into constructs or relationships among them. These insights then can be tested and confirmed with larger samples in quantitative studies. This often happens in the context of discrete mono-method investi-gations. One problem, however, is that it usually takes years to do a study and publish the results, which means that considerable time may elapse between the qualitative insights and the formal quantitative testing of hypotheses based on those insights. A researcher can undertake a coordinated set of MM studies that has hypothesis generation and testing as an explicit goal.

**Example of hypothesis generation and testing:**

Elstad and colleagues (2011) undertook a mixed methods study of how individuals with lower urinary tract symptoms (LUTS) use fluid manipulation to self-manage their symptoms. Quantitative data came from a random sample of over 5,000 adults participating in a community health survey. Qualitative data came from in-depth interviews and focus group interviews with 152 of the survey participants who had LUTS. Themes from the qualitative data were used as the basis for hypotheses that were then tested statistically using the quantitative data.

## Explication

Qualitative data are sometimes used to explicate the *meaning* of quantitative descriptions or relationships. Quantitative methods can demonstrate that variables are systematically related but may fail to provide insights into *why* they are related. Such explications help to clarify important concepts, corroborate findings from statistical analyses, and give guidance to the interpreting results.

**Example of explication with qualitative data:**

Smyth and colleagues (2011) studied nursing practices associated with the administration of pro re nata (PRN) analgesics to children postoperatively. They used records data to quantify analgesia practices (e.g., doses, routes, time of day) for 95 children. Then, using in-depth interviews and par-ticipant observation, they explored nurses' decisions to administer PRN analgesia.

## Theory Building, Testing, and Refinement

An ambitious application of mixed methods research is in the area of theory construction. A theory gains acceptance as it escapes disconfirmation, and the use of multiple methods provides great opportunity for potential disconfirmation of a theory. If the theory can survive these assaults, it can provide a stronger context for the organization of clinical and intellectual work.

**Example of theory building:**
Gibbons (2009) conducted a theory-validating and theory-synthesizing mixed methods study of *self-neglect*. Qualitative and quantitative data were used to describe characteristics and behaviors of self-neglect among older adults in early stages of the phenomenon and to explain the influence of several variables in the clinical evolution of self-neglect.

## Mixed Methods Designs and Strategies

In designing MM studies, researchers make many important decisions. We briefly describe a few.

### Design Decisions and Notation

Two critical decisions in MM research concern sequencing and prioritization. There are three options for sequencing components of a mixed methods study: qualitative data are collected first, quantitative data are collected first, or both types are collected simultaneously. When the data are collected at the same time, the design is **concurrent**. The design is **sequential** when the two types of data are not collected at the same time. In well-conceived sequential designs, the analysis and interpretation in one phase informs the collection and analysis of data in the second.

In terms of prioritization, researchers usually decide which approach—qualitative or quantitative—to emphasize. One option is that the two components are given equal, or roughly equal, weight. Usually, however, one approach is given priority. The distinction is sometimes referred to as *equal status* versus *dominant status*.

Janice Morse (1991), a prominent nurse researcher, made an important contribution to the MM literature by proposing a widely used notation system for sequencing and prioritization. In this system, priority is designated by upper case and lower case letters: QUAL/quan designates a mixed methods study in which the dominant approach is qualitative, while QUAN/qual designates the reverse. If neither approach is dominant (i.e., both are equal), the notation stipulates QUAL/QUAN. Sequencing is indicated by the symbols + or →. The arrow designates a sequential approach. For example, QUAN → qual is the notation for a primarily quantitative MM study in which qualitative data collection occurs in phase 2. When both approaches occur concurrently, a plus sign is used (e.g., QUAL + quan). Creswell and Plano Clark (2011) have suggested a modification of Morse's notation to include the use of parentheses, which designate an embedded design structure. The notation QUAN (qual) indicates a design in which the qualitative methods are embedded within a quantitative design.

### Specific Mixed Methods Designs

Numerous design typologies have been proposed by different MM methodologists. We illustrate a few basic designs described by Cresswell and Plano Clark (2011).

The purpose of a **convergent parallel design** (also called a *triangulation design*) is to obtain different, but complementary, data about the central phenomenon under study. The goal of this design is to converge on "the truth" about a problem or phenomenon by allowing the limitations of one approach to be offset by the strengths of the other. In this design, qualitative and quantitative data are collected simultaneously, with equal priority (QUAL + QUAN).

**Example of a convergent parallel design:**
Latter and colleagues (2010) used a QUAL + QUAN triangulation design in their study of the effects of an intervention for nurse prescribers to promote medication compliance among diabetic patients. The quantitative data were derived from structured coding of audiotaped consultations, and the qualitative data came from in-depth interviews with the nurses. The triangulation of approaches "illuminated how the intervention was implemented in practice contexts" (p. 1126).

In an **embedded design,** one type of data is used in a supportive capacity in a study based primarily on the other data type. Either qualitative or quantitative data can be dominant—although qual is often supportive of QUAN in embedded designs. Sequencing is often concurrent. The notation for embedded designs uses parentheses: QUAL(quan) or QUAN(qual).

**Example of an embedded design:**
Tluczek and colleagues (2011) used a concurrent QUAL (quan) embedded design to study the psychosocial consequences of false-positive newborn screens for cystic fibrosis. The data were collected by means of in-depth interviews with 87 parents of 44 infants. The qualitative data were content analyzed, yielding 13 categories of consequences. Logistic regression was then used to explore parental characteristics that predicted different consequences.

**Explanatory designs** are sequential designs with quantitative data collected in the first phase, followed by qualitative data collected in the second phase. In explanatory designs, the quantitative strand has priority—that is, the design notation is QUAN → qual. Qualitative data from the second phase are used to build on or explain the quantitative data from the initial phase. This design is especially suitable when the quantitative results are complicated and tricky to interpret.

**Example of an explanatory design:**
Beery and colleagues (2011) used a QUAN → qual explanatory design to study sports participation decisional conflict in youth with cardiac pacemakers. In phase 1, 35 youth completed the Decisional Conflict Scale. In phase 2, semistructured interviews were conducted with 19 participants. The researchers found that the scale did not capture all decisional conflict and that the qualitative data added enriched perspectives on the youth's struggles with sports participation.

**Exploratory designs** are also sequential MM designs, but qualitative data are collected first. The design has as its central premise the need for initial in-depth exploration of a concept. Usually, the first phase focuses on detailed exploration of a poorly understood phenomenon, and the second phase is focused on measuring it or classifying it. In an exploratory design, the qualitative phase is typically dominant (QUAL → quan), although in many studies the two strands have equal priority (QUAL → QUAN).

**Example of an exploratory design:**
Dilles and colleagues (2011) used an exploratory design (QUAL → QUAN) to develop and administer a survey to nurses in Belgian nursing homes. In the first phase, 12 expert nurses convened in small groups to brainstorm barriers that nurses faced with regard to safe medication management in nursing homes. The thematic analysis of these data formed the basis for the survey that was completed by more than 500 nurses and nurse assistants in 20 nursing homes.

## Sampling and Data Collection in Mixed Methods Research

Sampling and data collection in MM studies are often a blend of approaches described in earlier chapters. A few special issues for MM studies merit brief discussion.

Mixed methods researchers can combine sampling designs in various creative ways. The quantitative component is likely to rely on a sampling strategy that enhances the researcher's ability to generalize from the sample to a broader population. For the qualitative component, MM researchers usually adopt purposive sampling methods to select information-rich cases who are good informants about the phenomenon of interest. Sample sizes are also likely to be different in the qualitative and quantitative components in ways one might expect—i.e., larger samples for the quantitative component. A unique sampling issue in MM studies concerns whether the same people will be in both the qualitative and quantitative strands. The best strategy depends on the study purpose and the research design, but using overlapping samples can be advantageous. Indeed, a particularly popular strategy is a *nested* approach in which a subset of participants from the quantitative strand is used in the qualitative strand.

> **Example of nested sampling:**
> As part of a mixed methods inquiry, Shim and colleagues (2012) conducted a qualitative inquiry focused on the experiences of spousal caregivers of people with dementia. In the quantitative component, 187 caregivers were randomly assigned to a control group or to an intervention designed to increase caregiver preparedness. From the full sample, 21 caregivers were selected for in-depth interviews about their experiences at three points in time.

In terms of data collection, all of the data collection methods discussed previously can be creatively combined and triangulated in MM studies. Thus, possible sources of data include group and individual interviews, psychosocial scales, observations, biophysiological measures, records, diaries, and so on. Mixed methods studies can involve *intramethod mixing* (e.g., structured and unstructured self-reports), and *intermethod mixing* (e.g.,, biophyisologic measures and unstructured observation). A fundamental issue concerns the methods' complementarity—that is, having the limitations of one method be balanced and offset by the strengths of the other.

> ☞ **TIP:** One of the greatest challenges in doing mixed methods research concerns how best to analyze the qualitative and quantitative data. The real benefits of MM research cannot be realized if there is no attempt to merge results from the two strands and to develop interpretations and practice recommendations based on integrated understandings. It is, however, beyond the scope of this book to discuss the complex topic of data analysis in MM research.

# OTHER SPECIAL TYPES OF RESEARCH

The remainder of this chapter briefly describes types of research that vary by study purpose rather than by research design or tradition.

## Intervention Research

In Chapter 9, we discussed RCTs and other experimental and quasi-experimental designs for testing the effects of interventions. In actuality, intervention research is often more complex than a simple experimental–control group comparison of outcomes—indeed, intervention research often relies on mixed methods to develop, refine, test, and understand the intervention.

Different disciplines have developed their own approaches and terminology in connection with intervention efforts. *Clinical trials* are associated with medical research, *evaluation research* is linked to the fields of education and public policy, and nurses are developing their own tradition of intervention research. We briefly describe these three approaches.

## Clinical Trials

**Clinical trials** are designed to assess clinical interventions. Clinical trials undertaken to test an innovative therapy or drug are often designed in a series of phases:

- *Phase I* of the trial is designed to establish safety, tolerance, and dose with a simple design (e.g., before–after with no control group). The focus is on developing the best treatment.
- *Phase II* is a pilot test of treatment effectiveness. Researchers see if the treatment holds promise, look for possible side effects, and identify possible refinements. This phase is designed as a small-scale experiment or a quasi-experiment.
- *Phase III* is a full experimental test of the treatment—an RCT with random assignment to treatment conditions under controlled conditions. The objective is to develop evidence about the treatment's *efficacy*—i.e., whether the innovation is more efficacious than usual care or another alternative. When the term *clinical trial* is used in the nursing literature, it most often is referring to a phase III trial.
- *Phase IV* of clinical trials involves studies of the *effectiveness* of an intervention in the general population. The emphasis in effectiveness studies is on the external validity of an intervention that has demonstrated efficacy under controlled (but artificial) conditions.

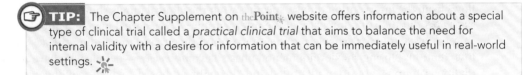

**TIP:** The Chapter Supplement on thePoint website offers information about a special type of clinical trial called a *practical clinical trial* that aims to balance the need for internal validity with a desire for information that can be immediately useful in real-world settings.

## Evaluation Research

**Evaluation research** focuses on developing useful information about a program or policy—information that decision makers need on whether to adopt, modify, or abandon a program.

Evaluations are undertaken to answer various questions. Questions about program effectiveness rely on experimental or quasi-experimental designs, but other questions do not. Many evaluations are MM studies with distinct components.

For example, a **process analysis** is often undertaken to obtain descriptive information about the process by which a program gets implemented and how it actually functions. A process analysis is designed to address such questions as the following: What exactly *is* the program or intervention and how does it differ from traditional practices? What are the barriers to successful program implementation? How do staff and clients feel about the intervention? Qualitative data play a big role in process analyses.

In an **impact analysis** component of an evaluation, researchers seek to identify the program's *net impacts*, that is, impacts that can be attributed to the program, over and above the effects of usual care. Impact analyses, analogous to phase III clinical trials, use an experimental or strong quasi-experimental design because the aim is to make a causal inference about the benefits of a special program.

Program evaluations may also include an **economic (or cost) analysis** to assess whether the program's benefits outweigh its monetary costs. Administrators make decisions about resource allocation for health services not only on the basis of whether something "works," but also based on economic viability. Often, cost analyses are done in conjunction with impact analyses—that is, when researchers are also evaluating program efficacy.

**Example of an economic analysis:**
Hansen and colleagues (2011) examined the effects and total costs associated with the implementation of telemonitoring programs in rural home health agencies.

## Nursing Intervention Research

Both clinical trials and evaluations involve *interventions*. However, the term **intervention research** is increasingly being used by nurse researchers to describe a research approach distinguished not so much by research methodology as by a distinctive *process* of planning, developing, testing, and disseminating interventions. Proponents of the process are critical of the simplistic and atheoretical approach that is often used to design and evaluate interventions. The recommended process involves an in-depth understanding of the problem and the people for whom the intervention is being developed; careful, collaborative planning with a diverse team; and the development or adoption of a theory to guide the inquiry.

Similar to clinical trials, nursing intervention research that focuses on the development of a complex intervention involves several phases: (1) basic developmental research, (2) pilot research, (3) efficacy research, and (4) effectiveness research.

Conceptualization, a major focus of the development phase, is supported through collaborative discussions, consultations with experts, critical literature reviews, and in-depth qualitative research to understand the problem. The construct validity of the emerging intervention is enhanced through efforts to develop an **intervention theory** that clearly articulates what must be done to achieve desired outcomes. The intervention design, which flows from the intervention theory, specifies what the clinical inputs should be, and also such aspects as duration and intensity of the intervention. A conceptual map (Chapter 8) is often a useful visual tool for articulating the intervention theory and for guiding the design of the intervention. During the developmental phase, key *stakeholders*—people who have a stake in the intervention—are often identified and "brought on board," which may involve participatory action research. Stakeholders include potential beneficiaries of the intervention and their families, advocates and community leaders, and agents of the intervention.

The second phase of nursing intervention research is a pilot test of the intervention, typically using simple quasi-experimental designs. The central activities during the pilot test are to secure preliminary evidence of the intervention's benefits, to refine the intervention theory and intervention protocols, and to assess the feasibility of a rigorous test. The feasibility assessment should involve an analysis of factors that affected implementation during the pilot (e.g., recruitment, retention, and adherence problems). Qualitative research may be used to gain insight into how the intervention should be refined.

As in a classic clinical trial, the third phase involves a full experimental test of the intervention, and the final phase focuses on effectiveness and utility in real-world clinical settings. This full model of intervention research is, at this point, more of an ideal than an actuality. For example, effectiveness studies in nursing research are rare. A few research teams have begun to implement portions of the model, and efforts are likely to expand.

> **Example of nursing intervention research:**
> Van Hecke and colleagues (2011) described the careful and systematic development of a multifaceted nursing intervention to promote adherence to self-care for patients with leg ulcers. Extensive qualitative research and a theoretical perspective on behavior change contributed to the development and validation of the intervention.

## Health Services and Outcomes Research

**Health services research** is the broad interdisciplinary field that studies how organizational structures and processes, health technologies, social factors, and personal behaviors affect access to health care, the cost and quality of health care, and, ultimately, people's health and well-being.

**Outcomes research,** a subset of health services research, comprises efforts to understand the end results of particular health care practices and to assess the effectiveness of health care services. Outcomes research represents a response to the increasing demand from policy makers and the public to justify care practices in terms of improved patient outcomes and costs.

Many nursing studies evaluate patient outcomes, but efforts to appraise the quality of nursing care—as distinct from care provided by the overall health care system—are less common. A major obstacle is attribution—that is, linking patient outcomes to specific nursing actions, distinct from those of other members of the health care team. It is also often difficult to ascertain a causal connection between outcomes and health care interventions because factors outside the health care system (e.g., patient characteristics) affect outcomes in complex ways.

Donabedian (1987), whose pioneering efforts created a framework for outcomes research, emphasized three factors in appraising quality in health care services: structure, process, and outcomes. The *structure* of care refers to broad organizational and administrative features. Nursing skill mix, for example, is a structural variable that has been found to be related to patient outcomes. *Processes* involve aspects of clinical management, decision making, and clinical interventions. *Outcomes* refer to the specific clinical end results of patient care. There have been several suggested modifications to Donabedian's framework for appraising health care quality, the most noteworthy of which is the Quality Health Outcomes Model developed by the American Academy of Nursing (Mitchell et al., 1998). This model is less linear and more dynamic than Donabedian's original framework and takes client characteristics (e.g., illness severity) and system characteristics into account.

Outcomes research usually concentrates on studying various linkages within such models, rather than on testing the overall model. Some studies have examined the effect of health care structures on various health care processes and outcomes, for example. Most outcomes research in nursing, however, has focused on the process–patient–outcomes nexus. Examples of nursing process variables include nursing actions such as nurses' problem-solving skills, clinical decision making, clinical competence and leadership, and specific activities or interventions (e.g., communication, touch).

> **Example of outcomes research:**
> Unruh and Zhang (2012) used 9 years of data from 124 hospitals in Florida to examine the relationship between *changes* in RN staffing and patient safety events.

## Survey Research

A **survey** obtains quantitative information about the prevalence, distribution, and interrelations of variables within a population. Political opinion polls, such as those conducted by Gallup, are examples of surveys. Survey data are used primarily in correlational studies, and are most often used to gather information from nonclinical populations (e.g., college students, nurses, community residents).

Surveys obtain information about people's actions, knowledge, intentions, opinions, and attitudes by self-report. Surveys, which yield quantitative data primarily, may be cross-sectional or longitudinal. Any information that can reliably be obtained by direct questioning can be gathered in a survey, although surveys include mostly questions that require brief responses (e.g., yes/no, always/sometimes/never).

Survey data can be collected in several ways, but the most respected method is through personal interviews in which interviewers meet in person with respondents to ask them questions. Personal interviews are expensive because they involve a lot of personnel time, but they yield high-quality data and the refusal rate tends to be low. Telephone interviews are less costly, but when the interviewer is unknown, respondents may be uncooperative on the phone. Self-administered questionnaires (especially those delivered over the Internet) are an economical approach to doing a survey, but are not appropriate for surveying certain populations (e.g., the elderly, children) and tend to yield low response rates.

The greatest advantage of surveys is their flexibility and broadness of scope. Surveys can be used with many populations, can focus on a wide range of topics, and can be used for many purposes. The information obtained in most surveys, however, tends to be relatively superficial: surveys rarely probe deeply into such complexities as contradictions of human behavior and feelings. Survey research is better suited to extensive rather than in-depth analysis.

**Example of a survey:**
Mealer and colleagues (2012) conducted a survey of intensive care unit (ICU) nurses in the United States. Questionnaires, mailed to a random sample of 3,500 ICU nurses, included measures of resilience, anxiety and depression, and symptoms of psychological distress.

## Secondary Analysis

**Secondary analysis** involves using data gathered in a previous study to address new questions. In most studies, researchers collect far more data than are actually analyzed. Secondary analysis of existing data is efficient and economical because data collection is typically the most time-consuming and expensive part of a study. Nurse researchers have used secondary analysis with both large national data sets and smaller localized sets, and with both qualitative and quantitative data. Outcomes research frequently involves secondary analyses of large clinical datasets.

A number of avenues are available for making use of an existing set of quantitative data. For example, variables and relationships among variables that were previously unanalyzed can be examined (e.g., a dependent variable in the original study could become the independent variable in the secondary analysis). In other cases, a secondary analysis focuses on a particular subgroup of the full original sample (e.g., survey data about health habits from a national sample of adults could be reanalyzed to examine the smoking behavior of rural men).

The use of available data makes it possible to bypass time-consuming and costly steps in the research process, but there are some disadvantages in working with existing data. In particular, secondary analysts may face many "if only" problems: if only an additional question had been asked, or if only a variable had been measured differently. Nevertheless, existing data sets present exciting opportunities for expanding the base of evidence in an economical way.

**Example of a quantitative secondary analysis:**
Cho and colleagues (2012) studied the effects of informal caregivers on the functioning of older adults in home health care (HHC), using data from a computerized patient care database, the Outcome and Assessment Information Set, from an HHC agency in New York.

**Example of a qualitative secondary analysis:**
Rush and colleagues (2011) analyzed previously collected qualitative data from 15 community-dwelling older adults who had participated in in-depth interviews focusing on the meaning of *weakness* in the elderly. The researchers used a theory (selective optimization with compensation) as a lens for examining the elders' adaptations made in response to mobility changes.

## Methodologic Research

**Methodologic research** entails investigations of the methods for conducting rigorous research. Methodologic studies address the development, validation, and evaluation of research tools or methods. The growing demands for sound and reliable outcome measures, for rigorous tests of interventions, and for sophisticated procedures for obtaining data have led to an increased interest in methodologic research by nurse researchers.

Many methodologic studies focus on the development of new instruments. Instrument development research often involves complex and sophisticated research methods, including the use of MM designs. Occasionally, researchers use an experimental design to test competing methodologic strategies.

**Example of a quantitative methodologic study:**
Goshin and Byrne (2012), as part of their longitudinal intervention study of incarcerated women, explored factors that predicted retention in the study following the women's release from prison. Their goal was to learn about variation in retention so they could shed light on possible strategies for retaining such study participants.

In qualitative research, methodologic issues often arise within the context of a substantive study, rather than having a study originate as a methodologic endeavor. In such instances, the researcher typically performs separate analyses designed to highlight a methodologic issue and to generate strategies for solving a methodologic problem.

**Example of a qualitative methodologic study:**
Cook (2012) conducted an in-depth study to explore what the diagnosis of a viral sexually transmitted infection means to women's lives. They wrote a methodologic paper that focused on the use of online recruitment and email interviewing as an approach to recruiting a diverse, multinational sample of vulnerable women.

Methodologic research may seem less compelling than substantive clinical research, but it is virtually impossible to conduct rigorous and useful research on a substantive topic without adequate research methods.

# CRITIQUING STUDIES DESCRIBED IN THIS CHAPTER

It is difficult to provide guidance on critiquing the types of studies described in this chapter, because they are so varied and because many of the fundamental methodologic issues require a critique of the overall design. Guidelines for critiquing design-related issues were presented in previous chapters.

You should, however, consider whether researchers took appropriate advantage of the possibilities of a MM design. Collecting both qualitative and quantitative data is not always necessary or practical, but in critiquing studies, you can consider whether the study would have been strengthened by triangulating different types of data. In studies in which MM were used, you should carefully consider whether the inclusion of both types of data was justified and whether the researcher really made use of both types of data to enhance knowledge on the research topic. Box 18.1 offers a few specific questions for critiquing the types of studies included in this chapter.

> **BOX 18.1 Guidelines for Critiquing Studies Described in Chapter 18**
>
> 1. Is the study exclusively qualitative or exclusively quantitative? If so, could the study have been strengthened by incorporating both approaches?
> 2. If the study used a mixed methods (MM) design, did the inclusion of both approaches contribute to enhanced validity? In what other ways (if any) did the inclusion of both types of data strengthen the study and further the aims of the research?
> 3. If the study used an MM approach, what was the design—how were the components sequenced, and which had priority? Was this design appropriate?
> 4. If the study was a clinical trial or intervention study, was adequate attention paid to developing an appropriate intervention? Was there a well-conceived intervention theory that guided the endeavor? Was the intervention adequately pilot tested?
> 5. If the study was a clinical trial, evaluation, or intervention study, was there an effort to understand how the intervention was implemented (i.e., a process-type analysis)? Were the financial costs and benefits assessed? If not, should they have been?
> 6. If the study was outcomes research, which segments of the structure–process–outcomes model were examined? Would it have been desirable (and feasible) to expand the study to include other aspects? Do the findings suggest possible improvements to structures or processes that would be beneficial to patient outcomes?
> 7. If the study was a survey, was the most appropriate method used to collect the data (i.e., in-person interviews, telephone interviews, mail or Internet questionnaires)?
> 8. If the study was a secondary analysis, to what extent was the chosen dataset appropriate for addressing the research questions? What were the limitations of the dataset, and were these limitations acknowledged and taken into account in interpreting the results?

## RESEARCH EXAMPLES WITH CRITICAL THINKING EXERCISES

The nursing literature abounds with studies of the types described in this chapter. Here we describe an important example.

Example 1 below is also featured in our *Interactive Critical Thinking Activity* on the Point website where you can easily record, print, and e-mail your responses to the related questions.

### EXAMPLE 1 ● Clinical Trial, Methodological Research, and Secondary Analysis

**Studies:** Testing an intervention for preventing osteoporosis in postmenopausal breast cancer survivors (Waltman et al., 2003); The effect of weight training on bone mineral density and bone turnover in postmenopausal breast cancer survivors with bone loss (Waltman et al., 2010); Development of an instrument to measure adherence to strength training in postmenopausal breast cancer survivors (Huberty et al., 2009); Intervention components promoting adherence to strength training exercise in breast cancer survivors with bone loss (McGuire et al., 2011).

**Background and Purpose:** Dr. Nancy Waltman has, together with an interdisciplinary team of researchers, pursued a program of research focused on bone loss in breast cancer survivors. For over a decade, these researchers conducted exploratory studies and then developed an intervention designed to prevent osteoporosis in women who had been treated for breast cancer. The intervention had components that were based on Bandura's social cognitive theory.

**Phase II Clinical Trial:** Waltman and colleagues (2003) conducted a pilot test of a 12-month multi-component intervention for preventing and treating osteoporosis in women who had completed treatment for breast cancer. The intervention involved home-based strength and weight training exercises, a regimen of calcium and vitamin D, and facilitative efforts to promote adherence to the intervention. The intervention was tested with 21 women using a one-group pretest–posttest design. The researchers learned that adherence was high and that the women had significant improvements on several important outcomes, including bone mass density (BMD).

**Phase III Clinical Trial:** Based on results from the pilot test indicating that the intervention was both feasible and had good potential for effectiveness, Waltman and colleagues (2010) launched a multisite trial using an RCT design. A sample of 223 women was randomly assigned to either a 24-month medication-only control group (risedronate, calcium, vitamin D) or to a 24-month medication plus weight-training group. Both groups had significant improvement over time on some BMD measures (total hip, spine). Women in the exercise group had additional increases in BMD in some locations. In addition to outcome data, the researchers carefully collected process information regarding how much of a "dose" of the intervention participants received.

**Methodological Research:** A subsample (N = 85) of the women participating in the phase III clinical trial also participated in a substudy designed to develop a theory-based instrument for assessing barriers and motivation to engaging in strength- or weight-training exercise among women with measurable bone loss after their treatment for cancer. Items for the 47-item Likert scale were based on Bandura's theory, published research, and interview data from the women regarding why they were or were not adherent to the intervention. The reliability estimates for four subscales of the scale ranged from .70 to .82 (Huberty et al., 2009).

**Secondary Analysis:** McGuire, Waltman, and Zimmerman (2011) did a secondary analysis using data from the clinical trial to study factors that predicted adherence to the exercise program among the women in the experimental group. Regression analysis was used to predict adherence (percentage of strength-training exercises performed), using demographic variables (e.g., marital status), clinical variables (e.g., comorbidities), and frequency of receipt of intervention components (e.g., feedback) as the predictors. Participants receiving more frequent feedback were significantly more adherent to exercise.

## CRITICAL THINKING EXERCISES
1. Answer the relevant questions from Box 18.1 on page 350 regarding this study.
2. Also consider the following targeted questions:
   a. Was the secondary analysis experimental or nonexperimental?
   b. In language associated with evaluation research, could any part of this research be described as a process analysis? Impact analysis? Cost analysis?
   c. Suggest a qualitative component that could have been added to this research and describe its potential utility. Specify how this component would be sequenced and identify the design.
3. If the results of this study are valid, in what ways do you think the findings could be used in clinical practice?

## EXAMPLE 2 ● Mixed Methods Study in Appendix D
• Read the report of the mixed methods study by Sawyer and colleagues (2010) in Appendix D on pages 441–466 and then address the following suggested activities.

## CRITICAL THINKING EXERCISES
1. Answer Question 3 in Box 18.1 on page 350 regarding this study.
2. The appendix includes our critique of this study. Before reading our critique, either write your own critique or prepare a list of what you think are the major strengths and weaknesses of the study. Pay particular attention to issues relating to the validity and trustworthiness of the study. Then contrast your critique with ours. Remember that you (or your instructor) do not necessarily have to agree with all of the points made in our critique, and that you may identify strengths and weaknesses that we overlooked. You may find the broad critiquing guidelines in Table 4.1 on page 69 and Table 4.2 on page 70 helpful.
3. Suppose that Sawyer and colleagues had only collected qualitative data. Comment on how this might have affected the results and the overall quality of the evidence. Then suppose they had collected all of their data in a structured, quantitative manner. How might this have changed the results and affected the quality of the evidence?

**WANT TO KNOW MORE?** A wide variety of resources to enhance your learning and understanding of this chapter are available on thePoint.

- Interactive Critical Thinking Activity
- Chapter Supplement on Practical (Pragmatic) Clinical Trials
- Answers to the Critical Thinking Exercises for Example 2
- Student Review Questions
- Full-text online
- Internet Resources with useful websites for Chapter 18

Additional study aids including eight journal articles and related questions  are also available in *Study Guide for Essentials of Nursing Research, 8e.*

## SUMMARY POINTS

- For many research purposes, MM studies are advantageous. **Mixed methods (MM) research** involves the collection, analysis, and integration of both qualitative and quantitative data within a study or series of studies, often with an overarching goal of achieving both discovery and verification.

- MM research has numerous advantages, including the complementarity of qualitative and quantitative data and the practicality of using methods that best address a question. MM research has many applications, including the development and testing of instruments, theories, and interventions.

- The paradigm most often associated with MM research is **pragmatism**, which has as a major tenet "the dictatorship of the research question."

- Key decisions in designing a MM study involve how to sequence the components and which strand (if either) will be given priority. In terms of sequencing, MM designs are either **concurrent** (both strands occurring in one simultaneous phase) or **sequential** (one strand occurring prior to and informing the second strand).

- Notation for MM research often designates priority—all capital letters for the dominant strand and all lower-case letters for the nondominant strand—and sequence. An arrow is used for sequential designs, and a "+" is used for concurrent designs. Parentheses show an embedded structure. QUAL → quan, for example is a sequential, qualitative-dominant design; QUAN (qual) shows a qualitative strand embedded in a quantitative study.

- Specific MM designs include the **convergent parallel design** (QUAL + QUAN), **embedded design** (e.g., QUAL [quan]), **explanatory design** (e.g., QUAN → qual), and **exploratory design** (e.g., QUAL → quan).

- Sampling in MM studies can involve the same or different people in the different components. *Nesting* is a common sampling approach in which a subsample of the participants in the quantitative strand also participates in the qualitative component.

- Different disciplines have developed different approaches to (and terms for) efforts to evaluate interventions. **Clinical trials**, which are studies designed to assess the effectiveness of clinical interventions, often involve a series of phases. *Phase I* is designed to finalize features of the intervention. *Phase II* involves seeking preliminary evidence of efficacy and opportunities for refinements. *Phase III* is a full experimental test of treatment *efficacy*.

In *Phase IV*, the researcher focuses primarily on generalized *effectiveness* and evidence about costs and benefits.

- **Evaluation research** assesses the effectiveness of a program, policy, or procedure to assist decision makers in choosing a course of action. Evaluations can answer a variety of questions. **Process analyses** describe the process by which a program gets implemented and how it functions in practice. **Impact analyses** test whether an intervention caused any *net impacts* relative to the counterfactual. **Economic (cost) analyses** seek to determine whether the monetary costs of a program are outweighed by benefits.

- **Nursing intervention research** is a term sometimes used to refer to a distinctive *process* of planning, developing, testing, and disseminating interventions. The construct validity of an emerging intervention is enhanced through efforts to develop an **intervention theory** that articulates what must be done to achieve desired outcomes.

- **Outcomes research** (a subset of **health services research**) is undertaken to document the quality and effectiveness of health care and nursing services. A model of health care quality encompasses several broad concepts, including *structure* (e.g., nursing skill mix), *process* (nursing interventions and actions), and *outcomes* (the specific end results of patient care in terms of patient functioning).

- **Survey research** examines people's characteristics, behaviors, intentions, and opinions by asking them to answer questions. Surveys can be administered through personal interviews, telephone interviews, or self-administered questionnaires.

- **Secondary analysis** refers to studies in which researchers analyze previously collected data—either quantitative or qualitative. Secondary analyses are economical, but it is sometimes difficult to identify an appropriate existing dataset.

- In **methodologic research**, the investigator is concerned with the development, validation, and assessment of methodologic tools or strategies.

# REFERENCES FOR CHAPTER 18

Beery, T., Smith, C., Kudel, I., & Knailans, T. (2011). Measuring sports participation decisional conflict in youth with cardiac pacemakers and/or ICDs. *Journal of Advanced Nursing, 67*, 821–828.

Cho, E., Kim, E., & Lee, N. (2012). Effects of informal caregivers on function of older adults in home health care. *Western Journal of Nursing Research*, PubMed ID 22068282.

Cook, C. (2012). Email interviewing: Generating data with a vulnerable population. *Journal of Advanced Nursing, 68*(6), 1330–1339.

Creswell, J. W., & Plano Clark, V. L. (2011). *Designing and conducting mixed methods research* (2nd ed.). Thousand Oaks, CA: Sage.

Dilles, T., Elseviers, M., Van Rompaey, B., Van Bortel, L., & Stichele, E. (2011). Barriers for nurses to safe medication management in nursing homes. *Journal of Nursing Scholarship, 32*, 171–180.

Donabedian, A. (1987). Some basic issues in evaluating the quality of health care. In L. T. Rinke (Ed.), *Outcome measures in home care* (Vol. I, pp. 3–28). New York: National League for Nursing.

Elstad, E., Maserejian, N., McKinlay, J., & Tennstedt, S. (2011). Fluid manipulation among individuals with lower urinary tract symptoms: A mixed methods study. *Journal of Clinical Nursing, 20*, 156–165.

Gibbons, S. W. (2009). Theory synthesis for self-neglect: A health and social phenomenon. *Nursing Research, 58*, 194–200.

Goshin, L. S., & Byrne, M. W. (2012). Predictors of post-release research retention and subsequent reenrollment for women recruited while incarcerated. *Research in Nursing & Health, 35*, 94–104.

Hansen, D., Golbeck, A., Noblitt, V., Pinsonneault, J., & Christner, J. (2011). Cost factors in implementing tele-monitoring programs in rural home health agencies. *Home Healthcare Nurse, 29*, 375–382.

Huberty, J., Vener, J., Waltman, N., Ott, C., Twiss, J., Gross, G., et al. (2009). Development of an instrument to measure adherence to strength training in postmenopausal breast cancer survivors. *Oncology Nursing Forum, 36*, E266–E273.

Latter, S., Sibley, A., Skinner, T., Cradock, S., Zinken, K., Lussier, M. et al. (2010). The impact of an intervention for nurse prescribers on consultations to promote patient medicine-taking in diabetes. *International Journal of Nursing Studies, 47*, 1126–1138.

McGuire, R., Waltman, N., & Zimmerman, L. (2011). Intervention components promoting adherence to strength training exercise in breast cancer survivors with bone loss. *Western Journal of Nursing Research, 33*, 671–689.

Mealer, M., Jones, J., Newman, J., McFann, K., Rothbaum, B., & Moss, M. (2012). The presence of resilience is associated with a healthier psychological profile in intensive care (ICU) nurses: Results of a national survey. *International Journal of Nursing Studies, 49,* 292–299.

Mitchell, P., Ferketich, S., & Jennings, B. (1998). Quality health outcomes model. *Image: The Journal of Nursing Scholarship, 30,* 43–46.

Morse, J. M. (1991). Approaches to qualitative-quantitative methodological triangulation. *Nursing Research, 40,* 120–123.

Rush, K., Watts, W., & Stanbury, J. (2011). Mobility adaptations of older adults. *Clinical Nursing Research, 20,* 81–100.

Shim, B., Barroso, J., & Davis, L. (2012). A comparative qualitative analysis of stories of spousal caregivers of people with dementia. *International Journal of Nursing Studies, 49,* 220–229.

Smyth, W., Toombes, J., & Usher, K. (2011). Children's postoperative pro re nata (PRN) analgesia: Nurses' administration practices. *Contemporary Nurse, 37,* 160–172.

Tashakkori, A., & Teddlie, C. (2010). *Handbook of mixed methods in social and behavioral research* (2nd ed.). Thousand Oaks, CA: Sage.

Tluczek, A., Orland, K., & Cavanagh, L. (2011). Psychosocial consequences of false-positive newborn screens for cystic fibrosis. *Qualitative Health Research, 21,* 174–186.

Unruh, L., & Zhang, N. (2012). Nurse staffing and patient safety in hospitals: New variable and longitudinal approaches. *Nursing Research, 61,* 3–12.

Van Hecke, A., Verhaeghe, S., Grypdonck, M., Beele, H., Flour, M., & DeFloor, T. (2011). Systematic development and validation of a nursing intervention: The case of lifestyle adherence promotion in patients with leg ulcers. *Journal of Advanced Nursing, 67,* 662–676.

Waltman, N., Twiss, J., Ott, C., Gross, G., Lindsey, A., Moore, T., et al. (2003). Testing an intervention for preventing osteoporosis in postmenopausal breast cancer survivors. *Journal of Nursing Scholarship, 35,* 333–338.

Waltman, N., Twiss, J., Ott, C., Gross, G., Lindsey, A., Moore, T., et al. (2010). The effect of weight training on bone mineral density and bone turnover in postmenopausal breast cancer survivors with bone loss. *Osteoporosis International, 21,* 1361–1369.

Zoffmann, V., & Kirkevold, M. (2012). Realizing empowerment in difficult diabetes care: A guided self-determination intervention. *Qualitative Health Research, 22,* 103–118.

# 19 Systematic Reviews: Meta-Analysis and Metasynthesis

## LEARNING OBJECTIVES

*On completing this chapter, you will be able to:*

- Discuss alternative approaches to integrating research evidence, and advantages to using systematic methods of reviewing research
- Describe key decisions and steps in doing a meta-analysis and metasynthesis
- Critique key aspects of a written systematic review
- Define new terms in the chapter

## KEY TERMS

| | | |
|---|---|---|
| Fixed effects model | Meta-ethnography | Sensitivity analysis |
| Forest plot | Meta-summary | Standardized mean |
| Frequency effect size | Metasynthesis | difference |
| Intensity effect size | Primary study | Statistical heterogeneity |
| Manifest effect size | Publication bias | Subgroup analysis |
| Meta-analysis | Random effects model | Systematic review |

In Chapter 7, we described major steps in conducting a literature review. This chapter also discusses reviews of existing evidence but focuses on systematic reviews in the form of **meta-analyses** and **metasyntheses**. Systematic reviews, a cornerstone of evidence-based practice (EBP), are inquiries that follow many of the same rules as those for **primary studies**, i.e., original research investigations. This chapter provides guidance to help you understand and evaluate systematic research integration.

# RESEARCH INTEGRATION AND SYNTHESIS

Nurses seeking to adopt EBP must take into account as much of the research evidence as possible, organized and synthesized in a diligent manner. A **systematic review** is a review that methodically integrates research evidence about a specific research question using careful sampling and data collection procedures that are spelled out in advance in a protocol. The review process is disciplined and largely transparent, so that readers of a systematic review can assess the conclusions.

About 20 years ago, systematic reviews usually involved narrative integration, using nonstatistical methods to synthesize research findings. Narrative reviews continue to be published in the nursing literature, but meta-analytic techniques that use statistical integration are being increasingly used. Most reviews in the Cochrane Collaboration, for example, are meta-analyses. Statistical integration, however, is not always appropriate, as we shall see.

Qualitative researchers also are developing techniques to integrate findings across studies. Many terms exist for such endeavors (e.g., meta-study, meta-method, meta-summary, metaethnography, qualitative meta-analysis, formal grounded theory), but the one that appears to be emerging as the leading term among nurse researchers is *metasynthesis*.

The field of research integration is expanding rapidly. This chapter provides a brief introduction to this extremely important and complex topic.

# META-ANALYSES

Meta-analyses of randomized controlled trials (RCTs) are at the pinnacle of traditional evidence hierarchies (see Figure 2.1, p. 23). The essence of a meta-analysis is that information from different studies is used to compute a common metric, an *effect size*. Effect sizes are averaged across studies, yielding not only information about the *existence* of a relationship between variables in many studies but also an estimate of its *magnitude* across studies.

## Advantages of Meta-Analyses

Meta-analysis offers a simple advantage as an integration method: *objectivity*. It is difficult to draw objective conclusions about a body of evidence using narrative methods when results are disparate, as they often are. Narrative reviewers make subjective decisions about how much weight to give findings from different studies, and so different reviewers may reach different conclusions about the evidence in reviewing the same studies. Meta-analysts also make decisions, but the decisions are explicit and open to scrutiny. The integration itself also is objective because it uses statistical formulas. Readers of a meta-analysis can be confident that another analyst using the same data set and making the same analytic decisions would come to the same conclusions.

Another advantage of meta-analysis concerns *power*, i.e., the probability of detecting a true relationship between variables (Chapter 12). By combining effects across multiple studies, power is increased. Indeed, in a meta-analysis it is possible to conclude, at a given probability, that a relationship is real (e.g., an intervention is effective), even when a series of small studies yielded nonsignificant findings. In a narrative review, 10 nonsignificant findings would almost surely be interpreted as lack of evidence of a true effect, which could be an erroneous conclusion.

Despite these advantages, meta-analysis is not always appropriate. Indiscriminate use has led critics to warn against potential abuses.

## Criteria for Using Meta-Analytic Techniques in a Systematic Review

Reviewers need to decide whether it is appropriate to use statistical integration. One basic criterion is that the research question being addressed should be nearly identical across studies. This means that the independent and dependent variables, and the study populations, are sufficiently similar to merit integration. The variables may be operationalized differently, to be sure. A nurse-led intervention to promote weight loss among diabetics could be a 4-week, clinic-based program in one study and a 6-week, home-based intervention in another, for example. However, a study of the effects of a 1-hour lecture to discourage eating "junk food" among overweight adolescents would be a poor candidate to include in this meta-analysis. This is frequently referred to as the "apples and oranges" or "fruit" problem. Meta-analyses should not be about *fruit*—i.e., a broad encompassing category—but rather about specific questions that have been addressed in multiple studies—i.e., "apples," or, even better, "Granny Smith apples."

A second criterion concerns whether there is a sufficient base of knowledge for statistical integration. If there are only a few studies, or if all of the studies are weakly designed and harbor extensive bias, it usually would not make sense to compute an "average" effect.

One final issue concerns the consistency of the evidence. When the same hypothesis has been tested in multiple studies and the results are highly conflicting, meta-analysis is likely not appropriate. As an extreme example, if half the studies testing an intervention found benefits for those in the intervention group, but the other half found benefits for the controls, it would be misleading to compute an average effect. In this situation, it would be better to do an in-depth narrative analysis of *why* the results are conflicting.

**Example of inability to conduct a meta-analysis:**
Fronteria and Ferrinho (2011) did a systematic review of the literature on nurses' physical health compared to other health workers. They determined that, although there were many relevant studies (*N* = 187), there was too much diversity to undertake a meta-analysis.

## Steps in a Meta-Analysis

We begin by describing major steps in a meta-analysis so that you can understand the decisions a meta-analyst makes—decisions that affect the quality of the review and need to be evaluated.

### Problem Formulation

A systematic review begins with a problem statement and a research question or hypothesis. As with a primary study, reviewers need to develop research questions that are clearly worded. Questions for a meta-analysis are usually narrow, focusing, for example, on a particular type of intervention and specific outcomes. Key constructs should be conceptually defined—the definitions are critical for deciding whether a primary study qualifies for the synthesis.

**Example of research question from a systematic review:**
Ndosi and colleagues (2011) conducted a meta-analysis that addressed the following question: Are clinical outcomes of nurse-led care for patients with rheumatoid arthritis (RA) similar to those produced by usual care? In this example, receipt of nurse-led versus usual care was the independent variable; clinical outcomes, such as RA disease activity, functional status, pain, fatigue, and quality of life, were the outcomes. Patients with RA constituted the population.

### The Design of a Meta-Analysis

One critical design issue concerns sampling. In a systematic review, the sample consists of the primary studies that have addressed the research question. Reviewers must state exclusion or inclusion criteria, which are often based on substantive, methodologic, and practical considerations. Substantively, the criteria stipulate key variables and the population. For example, if the reviewer is integrating material about the effectiveness of an intervention, which outcomes variables *must* the researchers have studied? With regard to the population, will (for example) certain age groups be excluded? Methodologically, the criteria might specify that only studies that used a randomized experimental design will be included. On practical grounds, the criteria might exclude, for example, reports written in a language other than English. Another decision is whether both published and unpublished reports will be included in the review.

> **Example of sampling criteria:**
> McInnes and colleagues (2012) did a meta-analysis that examined evidence on the effectiveness of pressure-redistributing support surfaces in preventing pressure ulcers. Intervention studies (both RCTs and quasi-experiments) that compared "beds, mattresses, mattress overlays, and cushions in any setting, on any clinical population, of any age, with any condition" and that measured the incidence of new pressure ulcers were included. Trials that used subjective measures of the outcome (e.g., skin condition was "worse") were excluded.

A related issue is the quality of the primary studies, a topic that has stirred some controversy. Researchers sometimes use quality as a sampling criterion, either directly or indirectly. Screening out studies of lower quality can occur indirectly if the meta-analyst excludes studies that did not use a randomized design or studies that were not published in a peer-reviewed journal. More directly, each potential primary study can be rated for quality, and excluded if the quality score falls below a certain threshold. Alternatives to handling study quality are discussed in a later section. Suffice it to say, however, that evaluations of study quality are inevitably part of the integration process, and so analysts need to decide how to assess quality and what to do with assessment information.

Another design issue concerns the **statistical heterogeneity** of results in the primary studies. For each study, meta-analysts compute an index to summarize the strength and direction of relationship between an independent variable and a dependent variable. Just as there is inevitably variation *within* studies (not all people in a study have identical scores on the outcome measures), so there is inevitably variation in effects *across* studies. If the results are highly variable (e.g., results are conflicting across studies), a meta-analysis may be inappropriate. But if the results differ modestly, an important design decision concerns exploration of the source of variation. For example, the effects of an intervention might be systematically different for men and women. Researchers often plan for subgroup analyses during the design phase of the project.

## The Search for Evidence in the Literature

Reviewers must decide whether their review will cover published and unpublished findings. There is some disagreement about whether reviewers should limit their sample to published studies or should cast as wide a net as possible and include *grey literature*—that is, studies with a more limited distribution, such as dissertations, unpublished reports, and so on. Some people restrict their sample to reports in peer-reviewed journals, arguing that the peer review system is an important, tried-and-true screen for findings worthy of consideration as evidence.

The limitations of excluding nonpublished findings, however, have increasingly been noted. The primary issue concerns **publication bias**—the tendency for published studies to systematically over-represent statistically significant findings (sometimes called the *bias against the null hypothesis*). This bias is widespread: authors often refrain from submitting manuscripts with nonsignificant findings, reviewers and editors tend to reject such reports when they are submitted, and users of evidence tend to ignore the findings if they are published. The exclusion of grey literature in a systematic review can lead to bias, notably the overestimation of effects.

Meta-analysts can use various search strategies to locate grey literature, in addition to the usual methods for a literature review. These include *hand searching* journals known to publish relevant content, contacting key researchers in the field to see if they have done studies that have not (yet) been published, and contacting funders of relevant research.

> ☞ **TIP:** There are statistical procedures to detect and correct for publication biases, but opinions vary about their utility. A brief explanation of methods for assessing publication bias is included in the Chapter Supplement on thePoint website. ☀—

**Example of a search strategy from a systematic review:**
Klainin-Yobas and colleagues (2012) did a meta-analysis of the effectiveness of mindfulness-based interventions on depressive symptoms among people with mental disorders. Their search strategy included a search of published and unpublished studies in nine databases, scrutiny of the bibliographies of relevant studies, and a search through journals that commonly publish articles in this domain.

## Evaluations of Study Quality

In systematic reviews, the evidence from primary studies needs to be evaluated to assess how much confidence to place in the findings. Rigorous studies should be given more weight than weaker ones in coming to conclusions about a body of evidence. In meta-analyses, evaluations of study quality sometimes involve overall quantitative ratings of evidence quality for each study. Hundreds of rating instruments exist, but the use of an overall scale has been criticized. Quality criteria vary from instrument to instrument, and the result is that study quality can be rated differently with different assessment instruments—or by different raters using the same tool. Also, when an overall scale score is used, there is a lack of transparency to users of the review regarding what the scores mean.

The Cochrane *Handbook* (Higgins & Greene, 2009) recommends a *domain-based evaluation*, that is, a *component approach*, as opposed to a *scale approach*. Individual features are given a separate rating or code for each study. So, for example, a researcher might code for such design elements as whether randomization was used, whether participants were blinded, the extent of attrition from the study, and so on.

Quality assessments of primary studies, whether they are assessments of individual study features or overall ratings, should be done by two or more qualified individuals. If there are disagreements between the raters, there should be a discussion until a consensus has been reached or other raters should be asked to help resolve the difference. Indexes of inter-rater reliability are often calculated to demonstrate to readers that rater agreement on study quality was adequate.

**Example of a quality assessment:**
Bryanton and Beck (2010) completed a Cochrane review of RCTs testing the effects of structured postnatal education for parents. They used the Cochrane domain approach to capture elements of trial quality. Both reviewers completed assessments, and disagreements were resolved by discussion.

## Extraction and Encoding of Data for Analysis

The next step in a meta-analysis is to extract and record relevant information about the findings, methods, and study characteristics of each study in the analysis. The goal is to produce a data set amenable to statistical analysis.

Basic source information about each study must be recorded, such as year of publication and country where data were collected. In terms of methodologic information, sample size is especially critical. Other important attributes include whether participants were randomized to treatments, whether blinding was used, rates of attrition, and the period of follow-up. Characteristics of participants must be encoded as well (e.g., their mean age). Finally, information about findings must be extracted. Reviewers must either calculate effect sizes (discussed in the next section) or must record sufficient statistical information that they can be computed by a program.

As with other decisions, extraction and coding of information should be completed by two or more people, at least for a portion of the studies in the sample. This allows for an assessment of inter-rater agreement, which should be sufficiently high to persuade readers of the review that the recorded information is accurate.

### Example of intercoder agreement:

Conn and colleagues (2011), in their meta-analysis of interventions to increase physical activity in healthy adults, coded numerous participant and intervention characteristics. Two thoroughly trained coders independently extracted all data. Codes were then compared to achieve 100% agreement. A third coder verified the extracted effect size information.

## Calculation of Effects

Meta-analyses depend on the calculation of an index that encapsulates in a single number the relationship between the independent and outcome variables in each study. Effects are captured differently depending on the level of measurement of variables. The three most common scenarios for meta-analysis involve comparisons of two groups such as an experimental versus a control group on a continuous outcome (e.g., blood pressure), comparisons of two groups on a dichotomous outcome (e.g., stopped smoking vs. continued smoking), or correlations between two continuous variables (e.g., between blood pressure and anxiety scores).

The first scenario, comparison of two group means, is especially common. When the outcomes across studies are on identical scales (e.g., all outcomes are measures of weight in pounds), the effect is captured by simply subtracting the mean for one group from the mean for the other. For example, if the mean post-intervention weight in an intervention group were 182.0 pounds and that for a control group were 194.0 pounds, the effect would be –8.0. More typically, however, outcomes are measured on different scales (e.g., different scales to measure stress). Mean differences across studies cannot in such situations be combined and averaged—researchers need an index that is neutral to the original metric. Cohen's *d*, the effect size index most often used, transforms all effects into standard deviation units (Chapter 12). If *d* were computed to be .50, it means that the group mean for one group was one half a standard deviation higher than the mean for the other group—regardless of the original measurement scale.

**TIP:** The term *effect size* is widely used for *d* in the nursing literature, but the preferred term for Cochrane reviews is **standardized mean difference** or SMD.

When the outcomes in the primary studies are dichotomous meta-analysts have a choice of effect index, including the odds ratio (OR) and risk ratio (RR). In nonexperimental studies, a common effect size statistic is Pearson's *r*, which indicates the magnitude and direction of effect.

## Data Analysis

After an effect size is computed for each study, as just described, a pooled effect estimate is computed as a *weighted average* of the individual effects. The bigger the weight given to any study, the more that study will contribute to the weighted average. One widely used approach is called the *inverse variance method* which involves using the standard error to calculate a weight. Larger studies, which have smaller standard errors, are given greater weight than smaller ones.

An important decision that meta-analysts make concerns how to deal with the heterogeneity of findings—i.e., differences from one study to another in the magnitude and direction of the effect size. Heterogeneity should be formally tested, and meta-analysts should report their results in their reports.

Visual inspection of heterogeneity usually relies on the construction of **forest plots**, which are often included in meta-analytic reports. A forest plot graphs the effect size for each study, together with the 95% CI around each estimate. Figure 19.1 illustrates forest plots for situations in which there is low heterogeneity (A) and high heterogeneity (B) for five studies.

In panel A, all effect size estimates (here, OR) favor the intervention group; the CI information indicates the intervention effect is statistically significant (does not encompass 1.0, the OR value indicating no difference) for studies 2, 4, and 5. In panel B, by contrast, the results are "all over the map." Two studies favor controls at significant levels (studies 1 and 5) and two favor the treatment group (studies 2 and 4). Meta-analysis is not appropriate for the situation in panel B. Heterogeneity can be evaluated using statistical methods that test the null hypothesis that heterogeneity across studies represents random fluctuations.

Heterogeneity affects not only whether a meta-analysis is appropriate but also which of two statistical models should be used in the analysis. Although this is too complex a topic for this book, suffice it to say that when heterogeneity is low, the researchers may use a *fixed effects model*. When results are more varied, it is better to use a *random effects model*. Some argue that a random effects model is usually more tenable. One solution is to perform a **sensitivity analysis**—which, in general, refers to an effort to test how sensitive the results of an analysis are to changes in the way the analysis was done. In this case, it would involve using *both* statistical models to see how the results are affected. If the results differ, estimates from the random effects model would be preferred.

Many meta-analysts seek to understand the determinants of effect size heterogeneity through formal analyses. Variation across studies could reflect systematic differences with regard to important clinical or methodologic characteristics. For example, in intervention

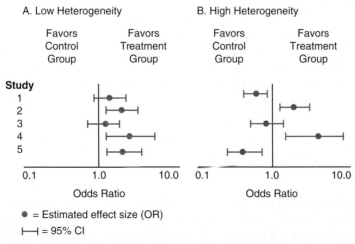

**FIGURE 19.1** ● Two forest plots of different heterogeneity.

studies, variation in effects could reflect who the agents were (e.g., nurses vs. others), how long the intervention lasted, and whether or not the intervention was individualized. Or, variation in results could be explained by differences in participant characteristics (e.g., men vs. women).

One strategy for exploring moderating effects on effect size is to do **subgroup analyses**, which involve splitting effect size information into distinct categorical groups—for example, men and women. Effects for studies with all-male (or predominantly male) samples could be compared to those for studies with all or predominantly female samples.

**Example of a subgroup analysis:**
Hodnett and colleagues (2011) assessed the effects of continuous, one-to-one intrapartum support on birth and labor outcomes. They found positive overall effects for such outcomes as use of analgesia, time in labor, and caesarean birth. Subgroup analyses were conducted to examine whether differences in effects were observed for subgroups defined by the provider's relationship to the hospital and to the women, type of routine practices in the setting, and time of onset of the support.

Another analytic issue concerns study quality. There are four basic strategies for dealing with study quality in a meta-analysis. One, as previously noted, is to establish a quality threshold for study inclusion (e.g., omitting studies with a low score on a quality assessment scale).

**Example of excluding low-quality studies:**
DeNiet and colleagues (2009) did a meta-analysis of the effects of music-assisted relaxation interventions to improve sleep quality in adults with sleep complaints. They used a nine-item quality assessment list, and only studies with a score of at least five were included in the review.

A second strategy is to undertake sensitivity analyses to determine whether the exclusion of lower-quality studies changes the results of analyses based only on the most rigorous studies. Another approach is to consider quality as the basis for exploring variation in effects. For example, do randomized designs yield different average effect size estimates than quasi-experimental designs? Do effects vary as a function of the study's score on a quality assessment scale? A fourth strategy is to *weight* studies according to quality criteria. Most meta-analyses routinely give more weight to larger studies, but effect sizes can also be weighted by quality scores, thereby placing more weight on the estimates from rigorous studies. A mix of strategies, including appropriate sensitivity analyses, is probably the most prudent approach to dealing with variation in study quality.

**Example of a quality-related sensitivity analysis:**
Jin and colleagues (2011) did a meta-analysis of 13 trials that tested the effects of warmed irrigation fluid on core body temperatures during endoscopic surgeries. The researchers undertook sensitivity analyses "when there were different designs, methods, or methodological quality problems potentially interfering with the results of the review" (p. 307).

# METASYNTHESES

Integration of qualitative findings is a burgeoning but rapidly evolving field for which there are no standard procedures. Indeed, five leading thinkers on qualitative integration noted the "terminological landmines" (p. 1343) that complicate the field, and the challenges of working in "an era of metamadness" (p. 1357) (Thorne, Jensen, Kearney, Noblit, and Sandelowski, 2004).

## Metasynthesis Defined

Terminology relating to qualitative integration is diverse and complex. Thorne and colleagues (2004) acknowledged the diversity and used the term metasynthesis as an umbrella term, with metasynthesis broadly representing "a family of methodological approaches to developing new knowledge based on rigorous analysis of existing qualitative research findings" (p. 1343).

Many writers on this topic are fairly clear about what a metasynthesis is *not*. Metasynthesis is not a literature review—i.e., a summary of research findings—nor is it a concept analysis. Schreiber and colleagues (1997) offered a definition that has often been used for what metasynthesis *is*, "...the bringing together and breaking down of findings, examining them, discovering the essential features and, in some way, combining phenomena into a transformed whole" (p. 314). A common view is that metasyntheses are products that are more than the sum of the parts—they offer new insights and interpretations of findings. Most methods of qualitative synthesis involve a transformational process.

Metasynthesis has had its share of controversies, one of which concerns whether to integrate studies based on different research traditions and methods. Some researchers have argued against combining studies from different epistemological perspectives, and have recommended separate analyses using groupings from different traditions. Others, however, advocate combining findings across traditions and methodologies. Which path to follow is likely to depend on several factors, including the focus of the inquiry, its intent vis-à-vis theory development, and the nature of the available evidence at the time the metasynthesis is undertaken.

## Steps in a Metasynthesis

Many of the steps in a metasynthesis are similar to ones we described in connection with a meta-analysis, and so some details will not be repeated here. However, we point out some distinctive issues relating to qualitative integration that are relevant in the various steps.

### Problem Formulation

In metasynthesis, researchers begin with a research question or focus of investigation, and a key issue concerns the scope of the inquiry. Finfgeld (2003) recommended a strategy that balances breadth and utility. She advised that the scope be broad enough to fully capture the phenomenon of interest, but focused enough to yield findings that are meaningful to clinicians, other researchers, and public policy makers.

> **Example of a statement of purpose in a metasynthesis:**
> Finfgeld-Connett and colleagues (2012) stated that the aim of their metasynthesis was "to articulate new insights relating to the most efficient and effective means of helping homeless women with substance abuse problems to enhance their well-being and become more stably housed" (p. 417).

### The Design of a Metasynthesis

Like a quantitative systematic review, a metasynthesis requires considerable advance planning. Having a team of at least two researchers to design and implement the study is often advantageous because of the highly subjective nature of interpretive efforts. Just as in a primary study, the design of a qualitative metasynthesis should involve efforts to enhance integrity and rigor, and investigator triangulation is one such strategy.

> **☞ TIP:** Meta-analyses often are undertaken by researchers who did not do one of the primary studies in the review. Metasyntheses, by contrast, are often done by researchers whose area of interest has led them to do both original studies and metasyntheses on the same topic. Prior work in an area offers advantages in terms of researchers' ability to grasp subtle nuances and to think abstractly about a topic, but a disadvantage may be a certain degree of partiality toward one's own work.

Like meta-analysts, metasynthesists must also make upfront sampling decisions. For example, they face the same issue of opting to include only findings from peer-reviewed journals in the analysis. One advantage of including alternative sources, in addition to wanting a more inclusive sample, is that journal articles tend to be constrained by space limitations. Finfgeld (2003) noted that in her metasynthesis on *courage*, she used dissertations even when a peer-reviewed journal article was available from the same study because the dissertation offered richer information. Another sampling decision, as previously noted, involves whether to search for qualitative studies about a phenomenon in multiple traditions. Finally, a researcher may decide to exclude studies in which the reported findings are not adequately supported with direct quotes from participants.

> **Example of sampling decisions:**
> Flores and Pellico (2011) conducted a metasynthesis of studies on the postincarceration experiences of women reentering the community. They searched for published and unpublished studies on women's experiences written in the past decade. Relevant studies were drawn from all qualitative traditions. Of the 10 primary studies, 3 were phenomenological, 3 were grounded theory studies, and the others were descriptive qualitative.

### The Search for Data in the Literature

It is generally more difficult to find qualitative than quantitative studies using mainstream approaches, such as searching electronic databases. For example, "qualitative" became a MeSH (medical subject heading) term in MEDLINE in 2003, but it is risky to assume that all qualitative studies (e.g., ethnographies) are coded as qualitative.

> **☞ TIP:** Sample sizes in nursing metasyntheses are highly variable, ranging from a very small number—e.g., four primary studies on person-centered nursing in the metasynthesis by McCormack and colleagues (2010)—to nearly 300 in Paterson's (2001) synthesis of qualitative studies on chronic illness. Sample size is likely to vary as a function of scope of the inquiry, the extent of prior research, and type of metasynthesis undertaken. As with primary studies, one guideline for sampling adequacy is whether categories in the metasynthesis are saturated.

### Evaluations of Study Quality

Formal evaluations of primary study quality are not as common in metasynthesis as in meta-analysis. Yet, it is often useful for reviewers to perform some type of quality assessment of primary studies, if for no other purpose than to be able to describe the sample of studies in the review. In recent years, nurse researchers have increasingly used the 10-question assessment tool from the Critical Appraisal Skills Programme (CASP) of the Centre for Evidence-Based Medicine in the United Kingdom (http://www.phru.nhs.uk/Pages/PHD/CASP.htm).

Although some reviews exclude low-quality studies from their metasynthesis, not everyone agrees that quality ought to be a criterion for study inclusion. Some have argued that a flawed study does not necessarily invalidate the rich data from those studies. Noblit and Hare (1988), whose ethnographic approach is widely used by nurse researchers, advocated including all relevant studies, but also suggested giving more weight to higher-quality studies. A more systematic application of assessments in a metasynthesis is to use quality information in a sensitivity analysis that explores whether interpretations are altered when low-quality studies are removed.

> **Example of a sensitivity analysis:**
> Bridges and colleagues (2010) synthesized studies on the experiences of older people and relatives in acute care settings. Primary studies were appraised using the CASP criteria. A total of 42 primary studies and a previous synthesis were included in the review. A sensitivity analysis revealed that the findings and interpretations were robust to the removal of the nine low-quality studies.

## Extraction of Data for Analysis

Information about various features of each study need to be abstracted and coded as part of the project. Just as in quantitative integration, the metasynthesist records features of the data source (e.g., year of publication), characteristics of the sample (e.g., age), and methodologic features (e.g., research tradition). Most important, information about the study findings must be extracted and recorded—typically the key themes, metaphors, or categories from each study.

As Sandelowski and Barroso (2002) noted, however, *finding* the findings is not always easy. Qualitative researchers intermingle data with interpretation and findings from other studies with their own. Noblit and Hare (1988) advised that just as primary study researchers must read and reread their data before they can proceed with a meaningful analysis, metasynthesists must read the primary studies multiple times to fully grasp the categories or metaphors being explicated.

## Data Analysis and Interpretation

Strategies for metasynthesis diverge most markedly at the analysis stage. We briefly describe three approaches. Regardless of approach, metasynthesis is a complex interpretive task that involves "carefully peeling away the surface layers of studies to find their hearts and souls in a way that does the least damage to them" (Sandelowski et al., 1997, p. 370).

### The Noblit and Hare Approach

Noblit and Hare (1988), whose approach to integration is called **meta-ethnography** argued that integration should be interpretive and not aggregative—i.e., that the synthesis should focus on constructing interpretations rather than descriptions. Their approach for synthesizing qualitative studies includes seven phases that overlap and repeat as the metasynthesis progresses, the first three of which are preanalytic: (1) deciding on the phenomenon, (2) deciding which studies are relevant for the synthesis, and (3) reading and rereading each study. Phase 7 involves writing up the synthesis, but phases 4 through 6 concern the analysis:

- *Phase 4*: Deciding how the studies are related. In this phase, the researcher makes a list of the key metaphors (or themes/concepts) in each study and their relation to each other. Studies can be related in three ways: *reciprocal* (directly comparable), *refutational* (in opposition to each other), or in a *line of argument* rather than either reciprocal or refutational.

- *Phase 5*: Translating the qualitative studies into one another. Noblit and Hare noted that "translations are especially unique syntheses because they protect the particular, respect holism, and enable comparison. An adequate translation maintains the central metaphors and/or concepts of each account in their relation to other key metaphors or concepts in that account" (p. 28).

○ *Phase 6*: Synthesizing translations. Here the challenge for the researcher is to make a whole into more than the individual parts imply.

**Example of Noblit and Hare's approach:**

Schmeid and colleagues (2011) used Noblit and Hare's approach in their meta-ethnography of 31 studies on women's perceptions and experiences of professional breast-feeding support. The meta-synthesis resulted in four categories comprising 20 themes. The synthesis indicated that support for breast-feeding occurred along a continuum from authentic presence at one end to disconnected encounters at the other.

### The Paterson, Thorne, Canam, and Jillings Approach

The method developed by Paterson and a team of Canadian colleagues (2001) involves three components: *meta-data* analysis, *meta-method* and meta-theory. A *meta-data* analysis involves the study of the results of reported research in a specific substantive area by analyzing the "processed data." *meta-method* is the study of the methodologic rigor of the studies included in the metasynthesis. Lastly, *meta-theory* refers to the analysis of the theoretical underpinnings on which the studies are grounded. The end product is a metasynthesis that results from bringing back together the findings of these three *meta-study* components.

**Example of the Paterson et al. approach:**

Bench and Day (2010) used the Paterson framework in their metasynthesis focusing on the specific problems faced by patients and relatives immediately following discharge from a critical care unit to another hospital unit.

### The Sandelowski and Barroso Approach

The strategies developed by Sandelowski and Barroso (2007) are likely to inspire metasynthesis in the years ahead. In their multiyear methodologic project, they dichotomized integration efforts based on level of synthesis and interpretation. Primary studies are called summaries if they yield descriptive synopses of the qualitative data, usually with lists and frequencies of themes, without any conceptual reframing. Syntheses, by contrast, are more interpretive and involve conceptual or metaphorical reframing. Sandelowski and Barroso have argued that only findings that are syntheses should be used in a metasynthesis.

Both summaries and syntheses can, however, be used in a **meta-summary**, which can lay a foundation for a metasynthesis. Sandelowski and Barroso provided an example of a meta-summary, using studies of mothering within the context of HIV infection. The first step, extracting findings, resulted in almost 800 complete sentences from 45 reports and represented a comprehensive inventory of findings. The 800 sentences were then reduced to 93 thematic statements or abstracted findings.

The next step involved calculating **manifest effect sizes**, i.e., effect sizes calculated from the manifest content pertaining to mothering in the context of HIV, as represented in the 93 abstracted findings. (Qualitative effect sizes are not to be confused with effects in a meta-analysis). Two types of effect size can be created from the abstracted findings. A **frequency effect size**, which indicates the magnitude of the findings, is the number of reports that contain a given finding, divided by all reports (excluding those with duplicated findings from the same data). For example, Sandelowski and Barroso calculated an overall frequency effect size of 60% for the finding of mothers' struggle about disclosing their HIV status to their children. In other words, 60% of the 45 primary studies had a finding of this nature. Effect size information can be calculated for subgroups of studies—e.g., for published versus unpublished studies, for ones in different research traditions, and so on.

An **intensity effect size** indicates the concentration of findings *within* each report. It is calculated by calculating the number of different findings in a given report, divided by the total number of findings in all reports. As an example, one primary study in Sandelowski and Barroso's meta-summary had 29 out of the 93 total findings, for an intensity effect size of 31%.

Metasyntheses can build upon metasummaries, but require findings that are more interpretive, i.e., from reports that are characterized as syntheses. The purpose of a metasynthesis is not to summarize, but to offer novel interpretations of qualitative findings. Such interpretive integrations require metasynthesists to piece the individual syntheses together to craft a new coherent explanation of a target event or experience.

**Example of Sandelowski and Barroso's approach:**
Draucker and colleagues (2009) conducted a metasynthesis to identify the essence of healing from sexual violence, as described by adults who experienced it as children or as adults. Meta-summary techniques were used to aggregate findings from 51 reports, and metasynthesis techniques were used to interpret the findings. A total of 11 meta-findings with frequency effect sizes over 15% were abstracted and summarized in a table.

# CRITIQUING SYSTEMATIC REVIEWS

Reports for systematic reviews, including meta-analyses and metasyntheses, typically follow a similar format as for a report for a primary study. There is usually an introduction, method section, results section, and discussion, and full citations for the entire sample of studies included in the review (often identified separately from other citations by using asterisks).

The method section is especially important. Readers of the review need to assess the validity of the findings, and so methodologic and statistical strategies, and their rationales, should be adequately described. For example, if reviewers of quantitative studies decided that a meta-analysis was not justified, the rationale for this decision should be made clear. Tables and figures typically play a key role in reports of systematic reviews. For meta-analyses, forest plots are often presented, showing effect size and 95% CI information for each study, as well as for the overall pooled result. There is often a table showing the characteristics of studies included in the review.

Metasynthesis reports are similar to meta-analytic reports, except that the results section contains the new interpretations rather than quantitative findings. When a metasummary has been done, however, the meta-findings would typically be presented in a table. The method section of a metasynthesis report should contain a detailed description of the sampling criteria, the search procedures, and efforts made to enhance the integrity and rigor of the integration.

A thorough discussion section is crucial in systematic reviews. The discussion should include the reviewers' assessment about the strengths and limitations of the body of evidence, suggestions on further research needed to improve the evidence base, and the implications of the review for clinicians. The review should also discuss the consistency of findings across studies and provide an interpretation of why there might be inconsistency.

Like all studies, systematic reviews should be critiqued before the findings are deemed trustworthy and relevant to clinicians. Box 19.1 offers guidelines for evaluating systematic reviews. Although these guidelines are fairly broad, not all questions apply equally well to all types of systematic reviews. In particular, we have distinguished questions about analysis separately for meta-analyses and metasyntheses. The list of questions in Box 19.1 is not necessarily comprehensive. Supplementary questions might be needed for particular types of review.

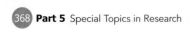 

Box 19.1 GUIDELINES FOR CRITIQUING SYSTEMATIC REVIEWS

**The Problem**
- Did the report clearly state the research problem and/or research questions? Is the scope of the project appropriate? Were concepts, variables, or phenomena adequately defined?
- Was the approach to integration adequately described, and was the approach appropriate?

**Search Strategy**
- Did the report describe criteria for selecting primary studies, and are the criteria defensible?
- Were the bibliographic databases used by the reviewers identified, and are they appropriate and comprehensive? Were keywords identified, and are they exhaustive?
- Did the reviewers use adequate supplementary efforts to identify relevant studies?

**The Sample**
- Did the search strategy yield a good and thorough sample of studies?
- If an original report was lacking key information, did reviewers attempt to contact the original researchers for additional information—or did the study have to be excluded?

**Quality Appraisal**
- Did the reviewers appraise the quality of the primary studies? Did they use a well-defined set of criteria or a well-validated quality appraisal scale?
- Did two or more people do the appraisals, and was interrater agreement reported?
- Was appraisal information used appropriately in selecting studies or analyzing results?

**Data Extraction**
- Was adequate information extracted about the study design, sample characteristics, and study findings?
- Were steps taken to enhance the integrity of the dataset (e.g., were two or more people used to extract and record information for analysis)?

**Data Analysis—General**
- Did the reviewers explain their method of pooling and integrating the data?
- Was the analysis of data thorough and credible?
- Were tables, figures, and text used effectively to summarize findings?

**Data Analysis—Quantitative**
- If a meta-analysis was not performed, was there adequate justification for using narrative integration? If a meta-analysis *was* performed, was this justifiable?
- For meta-analyses, did the report describe how effect sizes were computed? Were procedures for computing effect size estimates appropriate?
- Was heterogeneity of effects assessed? Was the decision to use a random effects model versus a fixed effects model sound? Were appropriate subgroup analyses undertaken—or was the absence of subgroup analyses justified?

**Data Analysis—Qualitative**
- In a metasynthesis, did the reviewers describe the techniques they used to compare the findings of each study, and did they explain their method of interpreting their data?
- If a meta-summary was done, were appropriate methods used to compute effect sizes? Was information presented effectively?
- In a metasynthesis, did the synthesis achieve a fuller understanding of the phenomenon to advance knowledge? Do the interpretations seem well grounded? Was there a sufficient amount of data included to support the interpretations?

Box 19.1 GUIDELINES FOR CRITIQUING SYSTEMATIC REVIEWS (*Continued*)

**Conclusions**
- Did the reviewers draw reasonable conclusions about the quality, quantity, and consistency of evidence relating to the research question?
- Are limitations of the review/synthesis noted?
- Are implications for nursing practice and further research clearly stated?

Color key

      All systematic reviews

      Systematic reviews of quantitative studies

      Metasyntheses

## RESEARCH EXAMPLES WITH CRITICAL THINKING EXERCISES

We conclude this chapter with a description of two systematic reviews. Additionally, a meta-analysis and a metasynthesis appear in their entirety in the *Study Guide* that accompanies this book.

Examples 1 and 2 below are also featured in our *Interactive Critical Thinking Activity* on thePoint website where you can easily record, print, and e-mail your responses to the related questions.

### EXAMPLE 1 ● A Meta-Analysis

**Study:** Use of weaning protocols for reducing duration of mechanical ventilation in critically ill adult patients: Cochrane systematic review and meta-analysis (Blackwood et al., 2011)

**Purpose:** The purpose of the meta-analytic study was to examine the effects of standardized weaning protocols on the total duration of mechanical ventilation, mortality, adverse events, weaning duration, and length of stay of critically ill adults in intensive care units (ICUs).

**Eligibility Criteria:** A primary study was included if it examined the effect of using a formal weaning protocol (compared to usual weaning practice) on patient outcomes using an experimental or quasi-experimental design. The population comprised adult patients who were receiving invasive mechanical ventilation with a nasotrachial or orotracheal tube.

**Search Strategy:** The strategy involved a search of multiple databases, including Medline, Embase, CINAHL, Web of Science, and LILACS. The researchers also searched reference lists of all identified reports and searched registries of ongoing trials. No language restrictions were applied. The search terms included mechanical ventilation; ventilators, mechanical; ventilators, negative pressure; ventilator weaning; and weaning protocol.

**Sample:** Two authors independently scanned possible studies identified in the search for inclusion in the meta-analysis. The search had retrieved 6,016 citations. Ultimately, only 11 trials met all inclusion criteria. The trials involved a total of 1,971 participants, ranging from 15 to 357 per trial. The studies had been conducted in the United States, Brazil, Italy, Germany, and Australia.

**Data Extraction:** Using a data extraction form adapted from the Cochrane Anesthesia Review Group, three authors independently extracted data to record study design and sample characteristics, intervention features, and patient outcomes. Disagreements were resolved through consultation with a fourth author.

**Quality Assessments:** Each study was assessed with regard to its risk of bias, using the Cochrane Collaboration's domain-based evaluation. The researchers coded for six risks (e.g., adequacy of generating the random allocation sequence, blinding of outcome assessors). A table in the report showed how the 11 studies were coded for each bias risk. No studies were eliminated based on quality.

**Effect Size Calculation:** The outcomes of interest included both dichotomous measures (e.g., mortality) and continuous measures (e.g., duration of mechanical ventilation). For dichotomous outcomes, the OR was used as the effect size index (e.g., the odds of dying in the protocol group relative to the odds of dying in the usual care group). For continuous outcomes, the standardized mean difference ($d$) comparing the two groups was used as the effect size index.

**Statistical Analyses:** The researchers used a fixed effects model for the meta-analysis. When statistical heterogeneity was detected, however, a random effects model was used. Subgroup analyses were performed to examine whether effect size results varied by the approach to delivering the protocol (professional led vs computer driven) or type of ICU (medical, surgical, neurological). Sensitivity analyses were performed to assess the impact of excluding studies with high risk of bias. Publication bias does not appear to have been formally assessed.

**Key Findings:** Results were presented in tables and a series of forest plots. Compared to usual care, the mean duration of mechanical ventilation when a formal protocol was used was reduced by 25% (95% CI = 9% to 39%). Duration of weaning itself was reduced by 78%, and length of stay in the ICU was significantly reduced by 10%. There were no significant differences in terms of mortality, adverse events, or length of stay in the hospital. There was significant heterogeneity for total duration of mechanical ventilation, but subgroup analyses could not account for differences among studies. In terms of the sensitivity analysis, the exclusion of six studies with at least one bias risk did not change the observed beneficial effects of the protocol.

**Discussion:** The researchers concluded that the evidence points to the benefits of using a formal weaning protocol, but noted that the substantial variation among studies and the small number of studies in the meta-analysis make it difficult to understand circumstances under which a standardized protocol is most effective.

## CRITICAL THINKING EXERCISES

1. Answer the relevant questions from Box 19.1 on page 368 regarding this study.
2. Comment on the authors' decision to not conduct a publication bias analysis.
3. In what ways do you think the findings could be used in clinical practice?

## EXAMPLE 2 ● A Metasynthesis

**Study:** A systematic review and meta-ethnography of the qualitative literature: Experiences of the menarche (Chang, Hayter, & Wu, 2010)

**Purpose:** The purpose of the meta-ethnography was to synthesize qualitative studies on women's lived experience of the menarche, and to explore the factors affecting how it is experienced.

**Eligibility Criteria:** A primary study was included if it used a qualitative approach, was published in English, and described women' experiences of menarche.

**Search Strategy:** An expert panel guided the review process. The authors searched nine databases (e.g., MEDLINE, CINAHL, EMBASE, Web of Science), using a broad range of keywords, which they listed in a table of their report. An ancestry search was also conducted, using the reference lists of eligible studies.

**Sample:** The report presented a flow chart showing the researchers' sampling decisions. Of the 2377 studies initially identified by title, 125 abstracts were screened and 22 full papers were examined for eligibility. Some were rejected after full reading or as a result of critical appraisal. In all, 14 papers, mostly of descriptive qualitative studies, were included in the analysis. The combined sample of participants in the primary studies included 483 women, mostly adolescents, from the United States, United Kingdom, and Zimbabwe.

**Data Extraction and Analysis:** Two reviewers independently assessed and extracted information from the studies. Quality assessment was performed using the CASP critical appraisal criteria. Four studies were deemed to be of insufficient quality and were excluded. Data were extracted using an extraction protocol. Disagreements between reviewers were resolved by consensus. Noblit and Hare's approach was used to analyze, compare, and synthesize study findings.

**Key Findings:** The five cross-cutting themes were: (1) Preparing for menarche; (2) the response of significant others; (3) the physical experience of menarche; (4) the psychological experience of menarche; and (5) sociocultural perspectives.

**Discussion:** The reviewers concluded that the menarche experience had a major impact on women. They felt their findings were of particular importance to school nurses, and could provide a framework for interventions aimed at helping adolescents make the transition to womanhood.

## CRITICAL THINKING EXERCISES

1. Answer the relevant questions from Box 19.1 on page 368 regarding this study.
2. Also consider the following targeted questions:
   a. Do you think it would have been possible for the researchers to compute frequency and intensity effect sizes with their sample of studies?
   b. Do you think the researchers should have searched for studies written in other languages? Why or why not?
3. In what ways do you think the findings could be used in clinical practice?

**WANT TO KNOW MORE?** A wide variety of resources to enhance your learning and understanding of this chapter are available on thePoint.

- Interactive Critical Thinking Activity
- Chapter Supplement on Publication Bias in Meta-Analyses
- Student Review Questions
- Full-text online
- Internet Resources with useful websites for Chapter 19

Additional study aids including eight journal articles and related questions are also available in *Study Guide for Essentials of Nursing Research, 8e.*

# SUMMARY POINTS

- Evidence-based practice relies on rigorous integration of research evidence on a topic through **systematic reviews** of research findings.

- Systematic reviews often involve statistical integration of findings through **meta-analysis**, a procedure whose advantages include objectivity and enhanced power. Yet, meta-analysis is not appropriate for broad questions or when there is substantial inconsistency of findings.

- The steps in both quantitative and qualitative integration are similar and involve formulating the problem, designing the study (including establishing sampling criteria), searching the literature for a sample of **primary studies**, evaluating study quality, extracting and encoding data for analysis, analyzing the data, and reporting the findings.

● There is no consensus on whether integrations should include the *grey literature*—i.e., unpublished reports; in quantitative studies, a concern is that there is a *bias against the null hypothesis*, a **publication bias** stemming from the underrepresentation of nonsignificant findings in published reports.

● In meta-analysis, findings from primary studies are represented by an **effect size** index that quantifies the magnitude and direction of relationship between the independent and dependent variables. The most common effect size indexes in nursing are *d* (the *standardized mean difference*), the odds ratio, and correlation coefficients.

● Effects from individual studies are pooled to yield an estimate of the population effect size by calculating a weighted average of effects, often using a procedure that gives greater weight to larger studies

● **Statistical heterogeneity** (diversity in effects across studies) is a major issue in meta-analysis, and affects decisions about using a **fixed effects model** (which assumes a single true effect size) or a **random effects model** (which assumes a distribution of effects). Heterogeneity can be examined using a **forest plot**.

● Nonrandom heterogeneity can be explored through **subgroup analyses** (*moderator analyses)*, the purpose of which is to identify clinical or methodologic features systematically related to differences in effects.

● Quality assessments (which may involve formal quantitative ratings of methodologic rigor) are sometimes used to exclude weak studies from reviews, but they can also be used to differentially weight studies or in **sensitivity analyses** to determine if including or excluding weaker studies changes conclusions.

● **Metasyntheses** are more than just summaries of prior qualitative findings; they involve a discovery of essential features of a body of findings and a transformation that yields new interpretations.

● Numerous approaches to metasynthesis (and many terms related to qualitative integration) have been proposed. Metasynthesists grapple with such issues as whether to combine findings from different research traditions and whether to exclude poor-quality studies.

● One approach to qualitative integration, **meta-ethnography** as proposed by Noblit and Hare, involves listing key themes or metaphors across studies and then translating them into each other.

● Paterson and colleagues' metastudy method integrates three components: (1) *meta-data analysis*, the study of results in a specific substantive area through analysis of the "processed data;" (2) *meta-method*, the study of the studies' methodologic rigor, and (3) *meta-theory*, the analysis of the theoretical underpinnings on which the studies are grounded.

● A **meta-summary**, a method developed by Sandelowski and Barroso, involves listing abstracted findings from the primary studies and calculating **manifest effect sizes**. A **frequency effect size** is the percentage of reports that contain a given findings. An **intensity effect size** indicates the percentage of all findings that are contained in any given report.

● In the Sandelowski and Barroso approach, a meta-summary can lay the foundation for a metasynthesis, which can use a variety of qualitative approaches to analysis and interpretations (e.g., constant comparison).

# REFERENCES FOR CHAPTER 19

Bench, S., & Day, T. (2010). The user experience of critical care discharge: A meta-synthesis of qualitative research. *International Journal of Nursing Studies, 47*, 487–499.

Blackwood, B., Alderdice, F., Burns, K., Cardwell, C., Lavery, G., & O'Halloran, P. (2011). Use of weaning protocols for reducing duration of mechanical ventilation in critically ill adult patients. *British Medical Journal, 342c*, 7237.

Bridges, J., Flatley, M., & Meyer, J. (2010). Older people's and relatives' experiences in acute care settings: Systematic review and synthesis of qualitative studies. *International Journal of Nursing Studies, 47*, 89–107.

Bryanton, J., & Beck, C. T. (2010). Postnatal parental education for optimizing infant general health and parent-infant relationships. *Cochrane Database of Systematic Reviews, 1*, CD004068.

Chang, Y., Hayter, M., & Wu, S. (2010). A systematic review and meta-ethnography of the qualitative literature: Experiences of the menarche. *Journal of Clinical Nursing, 19*, 447–460.

Conn, V., Hafdahi, A., & Mehr, D. (2011). Interventions to increase physical activity among health adults: Meta-analysis of outcomes. *American Journal of Public Health, 101*, 751–759.

DeNiet, G., Tiemens, B., Lendemeijer, B., & Hutschemaekers, G. (2009). Music-assisted relaxation to improve sleep quality: Meta-analysis. *Journal of Advanced Nursing, 65*, 1356–1364.

Draucker, C., Martsolf, D., Ross, R., Cook, C., Stidham, A., & Mweemba, P. (2009). The essence of healing from sexual violence. *Research in Nursing and Health, 32*, 366–378.

Finfgeld, D. (2003). Metasynthesis: The state of the art—so far. *Qualitative Health Research, 13*, 893–904.

Finfgeld-Connett, D., Bloom, T., & Johnson, E. (2012). Perceived competency and resolution of homelessness among women with substance abuse problems. *Qualitative Health Research, 22*, 416–427.

Flores, J., & Pellico, L. (2011). A meta-synthesis of women's postincarceration experiences. *Journal of Obstetric, Gynecologic, and Neonatal Nursing, 40*, 486–496.

Fronteria, I., & Ferrinho, P. (2011). Do nurses have a different physical health profile? A systematic review of experimental and observational studies on nurses' physical health. *Journal of Clinical Nursing, 20*, 2404–2424.

Higgins, J., & Greene, S. (Eds.). (2009). *Cochrane handbook for systematic reviews of interventions*. Chichester, UK: Wiley-Blackwell.

Hodnett, E., Gates, S., Hofmeyr, G., Sakala, C., & Weston, J. (2011). Continuous support for women during childbirth. *Cochrane Database of Systematic Reviews, (2)*, CD003766.

Jin, Y., Tian, J., Sun, M., & Yang, K. (2011). A systematic review of randomized controlled trials of the effects of warmed irrigation fluid on core body temperature during endoscopic surgeries. *Journal of Clinical Nursing, 20*, 305–316.

Klainin-Yobas, P., Cho, M., & Creedy, D. (2012). Efficacy of mindfulness-based intervention on depressive symptoms among people with mental disorders: A meta-analysis. *International Journal of Nursing Studies, 49*, 109–121.

McCormack, B., Karlsson, B., Dewing, J., & Lerdal, A. (2010). Exploring person-centredness: A qualitative meta-synthesis of four studies. *Scandinavian Journal of Caring Sciences, 24*, 620–634.

McInnes, E., Jammali-Blasi, A., Bell-Syer, S., Dumville, J., & Cullum, N. (2012). Preventing pressure ulcers—are pressure-redistributing support surfaces effective? A Cochrane systematic review and meta-analysis. *International Journal of Nursing Studies, 49*(3), 345–359.

Ndosi, M., Vinall, K., Hale, C., Bird, H., & Hill, J. (2011). The effectiveness of nurse-led care in people with rheumatoid arthritis: A systematic review. *International Journal of Nursing Studies, 48*, 642–654.

Noblit, G., & Hare, R. D. (1988). *Meta-ethnography: Synthesizing qualitative studies*. Newbury Park, CA: Sage.

Paterson, B. (2001). The shifting perspectives model of chronic illness. *Journal of Nursing Scholarship, 33*, 57–62.

Paterson, B. L., Thorne, S. E., Canam, C., & Jillings, C. (2001). *Meta-study of qualitative health research*. Thousand Oaks, CA: Sage.

Sandelowski, M., Docherty, S., & Emden, C. (1997). Qualitative metasynthesis: Issues and techniques. *Research in Nursing and Health, 20*, 365–377.

Sandelowski, M., & Barroso, J. (2002). Finding the findings in qualitative studies. *Journal of Nursing Scholarship, 34*, 213–219.

Sandelowski, M., & Barroso, J. (2007). *Synthesizing qualitative research*. New York: Springer Publishing Company.

Schmeid, V., Beake, S., Sheehan, A., McCourt, C., & Dykes, F. (2011). Women's perceptions and experiences of breastfeeding support: A metasynthesis. *Birth, 38*, 49–60.

Schreiber, R., Crooks, D., & Stern, P. N. (1997). Qualitative meta-analysis. In J. M. Morse (Ed.), *Completing a qualitative project* (pp. 311–326). Thousand Oaks, CA: Sage.

Thorne, S., Jensen, L., Kearney, M., Noblit, G., & Sandelowski, M. (2004). Qualitative metasynthesis: Reflections on methodological orientation and ideological agenda. *Qualitative Health Research, 14*, 1342–1365.

# Glossary

**Note:** A few entries in this glossary were not explained in this book, but are included here because you might come across them in the research literature.

## A

**Absolute risk (AR)** The proportion of people in a group who experienced an undesirable outcome.

**Absolute risk reduction (ARR)** The difference between the absolute risk in one group (e.g., those exposed to an intervention) and the absolute risk in another group (e.g., those not exposed).

**Abstract** A brief description of a study, usually located at the beginning of a report.

**Accessible population** The population available for a study, often a nonrandom subset of the target population.

**Acquiescence response set** A bias in self-report instruments, especially in psychosocial scales, created when participants characteristically agree with statements ("yea-say"), independent of content.

**After-only design** An experimental design in which data are collected from participants only after an intervention has been introduced.

**Alpha (α)** (1) In tests of statistical significance, the significance criterion—the risk the researcher is willing to accept of making a Type I error; (2) in assessments of internal consistency, a reliability coefficient, Cronbach's alpha.

**Analysis** The organization and synthesis of data so as to answer research questions and test hypotheses.

**Analysis of covariance (ANCOVA)** A statistical procedure used to test mean differences among groups on an outcome variable, while controlling for one or more covariates.

**Analysis of variance (ANOVA)** A statistical procedure for testing mean differences among three or more groups by comparing variability between groups to variability within groups, yielding an $F$-ratio statistic.

**Ancestry approach** In literature searches, using citations from relevant studies to track down earlier research upon which the studies were based (the "ancestors").

**Anonymity** Protection of participants' confidentiality such that even the researcher cannot link individuals with the data they provided.

**Applied research** Research designed to find a solution to an immediate practical problem.

**Assent** The affirmative agreement of members of a vulnerable group (e.g., children) to participate in a study.

**Associative relationship** An association between two variables that cannot be described as causal.

**Assumption** A principle that is accepted as being true based on logic or reason, without proof.

**Asymmetric distribution** A distribution of data values that is skewed, with two halves that are not mirror images of each other.

**Attention control group** A control group that gets a similar amount of attention to the intervention group, without the "active ingredients" of the treatment.

**Attrition** The loss of participants over the course of a study, which can create bias by changing the composition of the sample initially drawn.

**Audit trail** The systematic documentation of material that allows an independent auditor of a qualitative study to draw conclusions about trustworthiness.

**Authenticity** The extent to which qualitative researchers fairly and faithfully show a range of different realities in the collection, analysis, and interpretation of their data.

**Autoethnography** An ethnographic study in which a researcher studies his or her own culture or group.

**Axial coding** The second level of coding in a Strauss and Corbin grounded theory study, involving the process of categorizing and condensing first-level codes by connecting a category and its subcategories.

## B

**Baseline data** Data collected prior to an intervention, including pretreatment measures of the outcomes.

**Basic research** Research designed to extend the base of knowledge in a discipline for the sake of knowledge production or theory construction, rather than for solving an immediate problem.

**Basic social process (BSP)** The central social process emerging through analysis of grounded theory data.

**Before–after design** An experimental design in which data are collected from participants both before and after the introduction of an intervention.

**Beneficence** An ethical principle that seeks to maximize benefits for study participants, and prevent harm.

**Beta (β)** (1) In multiple regression, the standardized coefficients indicating the relative weights of the predictor variables in the equation; (2) in statistical testing, the probability of a Type II error.

**Bias** Any influence that distorts the results of a study and undermines validity.

**Bimodal distribution** A distribution of data values with two peaks (high frequencies).

**Bivariate statistics** Statistical analysis of two variables to assess the empirical relationship between them.

**Blind review** The review of a manuscript or a research proposal such that neither the author nor the reviewer is identified to the other party.

**Blinding** The process of preventing those involved in a study (participants, intervention agents, or data collectors) from having information that could lead to a bias, e.g., knowledge of which treatment group a participant is in; also called *masking*.

**Bracketing** In phenomenological inquiries, the process of identifying and holding in abeyance any preconceived beliefs and opinions about the phenomena under study.

## C

**Carry-over effect** The influence that one treatment can have on subsequent treatments, notably in a crossover design.

**Case-control design** A nonexperimental design that compares "cases" (i.e., people with a specified condition, such as lung cancer) to matched controls (similar people without the condition).

**Case study** A method involving a thorough, in-depth analysis of an individual, group, or other social unit.

**Categorical variable** A variable with discrete values (e.g., sex) rather than values along a continuum (e.g., weight).

**Category system** In studies involving observation, the prespecified plan for recording the behaviors and events under observation; in qualitative studies, a system used to sort and organize the data.

**Causal modeling** The development and statistical testing of an explanatory model of hypothesized causal relationships among phenomena.

**Causal (cause-and-effect) relationship** A relationship between two variables wherein the presence or value of one variable (the "cause") determines the presence or value of the other (the "effect").

**Cause-probing research** Research designed to illuminate the underlying causes of phenomena.

**Cell** (1) The intersection of a row and column in a table with two or more dimensions; (2) in an experimental design, the representation of an experimental condition in a schematic diagram.

**Central (core) category** The main category or pattern of behavior in grounded theory analysis using the Strauss and Corbin approach.

**Central tendency** A statistical index of the "typicalness" of a set of scores, derived from the center of the score distribution; indices of central tendency include the mode, median, and mean.

**Chi-square test** A statistical test used in various contexts, most often to assess differences in proportions, symbolized as $\chi^2$.

**Clinical practice guidelines** Practice guidelines that are evidence based, combining a synthesis and appraisal of research evidence with specific recommendations for clinical decisions.

**Clinical research** Research designed to generate knowledge to guide health care practice.

**Clinical trial** A study designed to assess the safety, efficacy, and effectiveness of a new clinical intervention, sometimes involving several phases, one of which (Phase III) is a *randomized controlled trial* (RCT) using an experimental design.

**Closed-ended question** A question that offers respondents a set of mutually exclusive response options.

**Cochrane Collaboration** An international organization that aims to facilitate well-informed decisions about health care by preparing systematic reviews of the effects of health care interventions.

**Code of ethics** The fundamental ethical principles established by a discipline or institution to guide researchers' conduct in research with human (or animal) study participants.

**Coding** The process of transforming raw data into standardized form for data processing and analysis; in quantitative research, the process of attaching numbers to categories; in qualitative research, the process of identifying recurring words, themes, or concepts within the data.

**Coefficient alpha (Cronbach's alpha)** A reliability index that estimates the internal consistency of a measure comprised of several items or subparts.

**Coercion** In a research context, the explicit or implicit use of threats (or excessive rewards) to gain people's cooperation in a study.

**Cohen's *d*** An effect size for comparing two group means, computed by subtracting one mean from the other and dividing by the pooled standard deviation; also called *standardized mean difference (SMD)*.

**Cohort design** A nonexperimental design in which a defined group of people (a cohort) is followed over time to study outcomes for subsets of the cohorts; also called a *prospective design*.

**Comparison group** A group of study participants whose scores on an outcome variable are used to evaluate the outcomes of the group of primary interest (e.g., nonsmokers as a comparison group for smokers); term often used in lieu of *control group* when the study design is not a true experiment.

**Concealment** A tactic involving the unobtrusive collection of research data without participants' knowledge or consent, used to obtain an accurate view of naturalistic behavior when the known presence of an observer would distort the behavior of interest.

**Concept** An abstraction based on observations of behaviors or characteristics (e.g., fatigue, pain).

**Conceptual definition** The abstract or theoretical meaning of a concept under study.

**Conceptual file** A manual method of organizing qualitative data, by creating file folders for each category in the coding scheme and inserting relevant excerpts from the data.

**Conceptual map** A schematic representation of a theory or conceptual model that graphically represents key concepts and linkages among them.

**Conceptual model** Interrelated concepts or abstractions assembled together in a rational scheme by virtue of their relevance to a common theme; sometimes called *conceptual framework*.

**Concurrent design** A study design for a mixed methods study in which the qualitative and quantitative strands of data are collected simultaneously; notated with a plus sign, as in QUAL + QUAN.

**Concurrent validity** The degree to which scores on an instrument are correlated with scores on an external criterion, measured at the same time.

**Confidence interval (CI)** The range of values within which a population parameter is estimated to lie, at a specified probability (e.g., 95% CI).

**Confidence limit** The upper limit (UL) or lower limit (LL) of a confidence interval.

**Confidentiality**  Protection of study participants so that data provided are never publicly divulged.

**Confirmability**  A criterion for integrity in a qualitative inquiry, referring to the objectivity or neutrality of the data and interpretations.

**Confounding variable**  A variable that is extraneous to the research question and that confounds understanding of the relationship between the independent and dependent variables; confounding variables can be controlled in the research design or through statistical procedures.

**Consecutive sampling**  The recruitment of *all* people from an accessible population who meet the eligibility criteria over a specific time interval or for a specified sample size.

**Consent form**  A written agreement signed by a study participant and a researcher concerning the terms and conditions of voluntary participation in a study.

**CONSORT guidelines**  Widely adopted guidelines (Consolidated Standards of Reporting Trials) for reporting information for a randomized controlled trial, including a checklist and flow chart for tracking participants through the trial, from recruitment through data analysis.

**Constant comparison**  A procedure used in a grounded theory analysis wherein newly collected data are compared in an ongoing fashion with data obtained earlier, to refine theoretically relevant categories.

**Constitutive pattern**  In hermeneutic analysis, a pattern that expresses the relationships among relational themes and is present in all the interviews or texts.

**Construct**  An abstraction or concept that is deliberately invented (constructed) by researchers for a scientific purpose (e.g., health locus of control).

**Construct validity**  The validity of inferences from *observed* persons, settings, and interventions in a study to the constructs that these instances might represent; for a measuring instrument, the degree to which it measures the construct under investigation.

**Constructivist grounded theory**  An approach to grounded theory, developed by Charmaz, in which the grounded theory is constructed from shared experiences and relationships between the researcher and study participants and interpretive aspects are emphasized.

**Constructivist paradigm**  An alternative paradigm (also called *naturalistic paradigm*) to the positivist paradigm that holds that there are multiple interpretations of reality, and that the goal of research is to understand how individuals construct reality within their context; associated with qualitative research.

**Contamination**  The inadvertent, undesirable influence of one treatment condition on another treatment condition, as when members of the control group receive the intervention.

**Content analysis**  The process of organizing and integrating narrative, qualitative information according to emerging themes and concepts.

**Content validity**  The degree to which the items in an instrument adequately represent the universe of content for the concept being measured.

**Content validity index (CVI)**  An index of the degree to which an instrument is content valid, based on ratings of a panel of experts; content validity for individual items and the overall scale can be assessed.

**Contingency table**  A two-dimensional table in which the frequencies of two categorical variables are cross-tabulated.

**Continuous variable**  A variable that can take on an infinite range of values along a specified continuum (e.g., height).

**Control**  The process of holding constant confounding influences on the dependent variable (the outcome) under study.

**Control group**  Subjects in an experiment who do not receive the experimental intervention and whose performance provides a baseline against which the effects of an intervention can be measured.

**Controlled trial**  A trial of an intervention that includes a control group, with or without randomization.

**Convenience sampling**  Selection of the most readily available persons as participants in a study.

**Convergent parallel design**  A concurrent, equal-priority mixed methods design in which different but complementary data, qualitative and quantitative, are gathered about a central phenomenon under study; symbolized as QUAL + QUAN; also called a triangulation design.

Core category (variable) In a grounded theory study, the central phenomenon that is used to integrate all categories of the data.

Correlation A bond or association between variables, with variation in one variable systematically related to variation in another.

Correlation coefficient An index summarizing the degree of relationship between variables, ranging from +1.00 (a perfect positive relationship) through 0.0 (no relationship) to –1.00 (a perfect negative relationship).

Correlation matrix A two-dimensional display showing the correlation coefficients between all pairs of a set of variables.

Correlational research Research that explores the interrelationships among variables of interest without researcher intervention.

Cost (economic) analysis An analysis of the relationship between costs and outcomes of alternative nursing or other health care interventions.

Counterbalancing The process of systematically varying the order of presentation of stimuli or treatments to control for ordering effects, especially in a crossover design.

Counterfactual The condition or group used as a basis of comparison in a study, embodying what would have happened *to the same people* exposed to a causal factor if they *simultaneously* were *not* exposed to the causal factor.

Covariate A variable that is statistically controlled (held constant) in ANCOVA, typically a confounding influence on the outcome variable, or a preintervention measure of the outcome.

Credibility A criterion for evaluating integrity and quality in qualitative studies, referring to confidence in the truth of the data; analogous to internal validity in quantitative research.

Criterion-related validity The degree to which scores on an instrument are correlated with an external criterion.

Criterion sampling A purposive sampling approach used by qualitative researchers that involves selecting cases that meet a predetermined criterion of importance.

Critical ethnography An ethnography that focuses on raising consciousness in the group or culture under study in the hope of effecting social change.

Critical incident technique A method of obtaining data from study participants by in-depth exploration of specific incidents and behaviors related to the topic under study.

Critical theory An approach to viewing the world that involves a critique of society, with the goal of envisioning new possibilities and effecting social change.

Cronbach's alpha A widely used reliability index that estimates the internal consistency of a measure composed of several subparts; also called *coefficient alpha*.

Crossover design An experimental design in which one group of subjects is exposed to more than one condition or treatment, in random order.

Cross-sectional design A study design in which data are collected at one point in time; sometimes used to infer change over time when data are collected from different age or developmental groups.

Cross-tabulation A calculation of frequencies for two variables considered simultaneously—e.g., sex (male/female) cross-tabulated with smoking status (smoker/nonsmoker).

Cutoff point The score on a screening or diagnostic instrument used to distinguish *cases* (e.g., people with depression) and *noncases* (people without it).

# D

*d* A widely used effect size index for comparing two group means, computed by subtracting one mean from the other and dividing by the pooled standard deviation; also called *Cohen's d*.

Data The pieces of information obtained in a study (singular is *datum*).

Data analysis The systematic organization and synthesis of research data and, in quantitative studies, the testing of hypotheses using those data.

Data collection protocols The formal guidelines researchers develop to give direction to the collection of data in a standardized fashion.

**Data saturation** See *saturation*.

**Data set** The total collection of data on all variables for all study participants.

**Data triangulation** The use of multiple data sources for the purpose of validating conclusions.

**Debriefing** Communication with study participants after participation is complete regarding aspects of the study (e.g., explaining the study purpose more fully).

**Deception** The deliberate withholding of information, or the provision of false information, to study participants, usually to reduce potential biases.

**Deductive reasoning** The process of developing specific predictions from general principles (see also *inductive reasoning*).

**Degrees of freedom** (*df*) A statistical concept referring to the number of sample values free to vary (e.g., with a given sample mean, all but one value would be free to vary).

**Delayed treatment design** A design for an intervention study that involves putting control group members on a waiting list for the intervention until follow-up data are collected; also called a *wait-list design*.

**Dependability** A criterion for evaluating integrity in qualitative studies, referring to the stability of data over time and over conditions; analogous to reliability in quantitative research.

**Dependent variable** The variable hypothesized to depend on or be caused by another variable (the *independent variable*); the outcome of interest.

**Descendancy approach** In literature searches, finding a pivotal early study and searching forward in citation indexes to find more recent studies ("descendants") that cited the key study.

**Descriptive research** Research that typically has as its main objective the accurate portrayal of people's characteristics or circumstances and/or the frequency with which certain phenomena occur.

**Descriptive statistics** Statistics used to describe and summarize data (e.g., means, percentages).

**Descriptive theory** A broad characterization that thoroughly accounts for a phenomenon.

**Determinism** The belief that phenomena are not haphazard or random, but rather have antecedent causes; an assumption in the positivist paradigm.

**Dichotomous variable** A variable having only two values or categories (e.g., gender).

**Directional hypothesis** A hypothesis that makes a specific prediction about the direction of the relationship between two variables.

**Disconfirming case** A concept used in qualitative research that concerns a case that challenges the researchers' conceptualizations; sometimes used in a sampling strategy.

**Domain** In ethnographic analysis, a unit or broad category of cultural knowledge.

**Double-blind experiment** A clinical trial in which neither the participants nor those who administer the treatment know who is in the experimental or control group.

## E

**Economic analysis** An analysis of the relationship between costs and outcomes of alternative health care interventions.

**Effect size** A statistical expression of the magnitude of the relationship between two variables, or the magnitude of the difference between groups on an attribute of interest; also used in metasummaries of qualitative research to characterize the salience of a theme or category.

**Effectiveness study** A clinical trial designed to shed light on intervention effectiveness under ordinary conditions, usually with an intervention already found to be efficacious in an efficacy study.

**Efficacy study** A tightly controlled trial designed to establish the efficacy of an intervention under ideal conditions, using a design that stresses internal validity.

**Element** The most basic unit of a population for sampling purposes, typically a human being.

**Eligibility criteria** The criteria designating the specific attributes of the target population, by which people are selected for inclusion in a study.

**Embedded design** A particular mixed methods design in which one strand is primarily in a supportive role to the other strand; symbolized with brackets, as in QUAL(quan).

**Emergent design** A design that unfolds in the course of a qualitative study as the researcher makes ongoing design decisions reflecting what has already been learned.

**Emic perspective** An ethnographic term referring to the way members of a culture themselves view their world; the "insider's view."

**Empirical evidence** Evidence rooted in objective reality and gathered using one's senses as the basis for generating knowledge.

**Error of measurement** The deviation between hypothetical true scores and obtained scores of a measured characteristic.

**Estimation procedures** Statistical procedures that estimate population parameters based on sample statistics.

**Ethics** A system of moral values that is concerned with the degree to which research procedures adhere to professional, legal, and social obligations to the study participants.

**Ethnography** A branch of human inquiry, associated with anthropology, that focuses on the culture of a group of people, with an effort to understand the world view and customs of those under study.

**Ethnonursing research** The study of human cultures, with a focus on a group's beliefs and practices relating to nursing care and related health behaviors.

**Etic perspective** In ethnography, the "outsider's" view of the experiences of a cultural group.

**Evaluation research** Research aimed at learning how well a program, practice, or policy is working.

**Event sampling** A sampling plan that involves the selection of integral behaviors or events to be observed.

**Evidence-based practice (EBP)** A practice that involves making clinical decisions on the best available evidence, with an emphasis on evidence from disciplined research.

**Evidence hierarchy** A ranked arrangement of the validity and dependability of evidence based on the rigor of the method that produced it; the traditional evidence hierarchy is appropriate primarily for cause-probing research, especially Therapy questions.

**Exclusion criteria** The criteria specifying characteristics that a population does *not* have.

**Experiment** A study in which the researcher controls (manipulates) the independent variable and randomly assigns subjects to different conditions; randomized controlled trials use experimental designs.

**Experimental group** The study participants who receive the experimental treatment or intervention.

**Explanatory design** A sequential mixed methods design in which quantitative data are collected in the first phase and qualitative data are collected in the second phase to build on or explain quantitative findings; symbolized as QUAN → qual or quan → QUAL.

**Exploratory design** A sequential mixed methods design in which qualitative data are collected in the first phase and quantitative data are collected in the second phase based on the initial in-depth exploration; symbolized as QUAL → quan or qual → QUAN.

**External validity** The degree to which study results can be generalized to settings or samples other than the one studied.

**Extraneous variable** A variable that confounds the relationship between the independent and dependent variables and that needs to be controlled either in the research design or through statistical procedures; often called *confounding variable*.

**Extreme case sampling** A qualitative sampling approach that involves the purposeful selection of the most extreme or unusual cases.

**Extreme response set** A bias in psychosocial scales created when participants select extreme response alternatives (e.g., "strongly agree"), independent of the item's content.

**F**

*F*-ratio The statistic obtained in several statistical tests (e.g., ANOVA) in which score variation attributable to different sources (e.g., between groups and within groups) is compared.

**Face validity** The extent to which an instrument looks as though it is measuring what it purports to measure.

**Feminist research** Research that seeks to understand, typically through qualitative approaches, how gender and a gendered social order shape women's lives and their consciousness.

**Field diary** A daily record of events and conversations in the field; also called a log.

**Field notes** The notes taken by researchers to record the unstructured observations made in the field, and the interpretation of those observations.

**Field research** Research in which the data are collected "in the field" from individuals in their normal roles, with the aim of understanding the practices, behaviors, and beliefs of individuals or groups as they normally function in real life.

**Fieldwork** The activities undertaken by qualitative researchers to collect data out in the field, i.e., in natural settings.

**Findings** The results of the analysis of research data.

**Fit** An element in Glaserian grounded theory analysis in which the researcher develops categories of a substantive theory that fit the data.

**Fixed alternative question** A question that offers respondents a set of prespecified response options.

**Fixed effects model** In meta-analysis, a model in which studies are assumed to be measuring the same overall effect; a pooled effect estimate is calculated under the assumption that observed variation between studies is attributable to chance.

**Focus group interview** An interview with a group of individuals assembled to answer questions on a given topic.

**Focused interview** A loosely structured interview in which an interviewer guides the respondent through a set of questions using a topic guide.

**Follow-up study** A study undertaken to determine the outcomes of individuals with a specified condition or who have received a specified treatment.

**Forest plot** A graphic representation of effects across studies in a meta-analysis, permitting a visual assessment of heterogeneity.

**Framework** The conceptual underpinnings of a study—e.g., a *theoretical framework* in theory-based studies, or *conceptual framework* in studies based on a specific conceptual model.

**Frequency distribution** A systematic array of numeric values from the lowest to the highest, together with a count of the number of times each value was obtained.

**Frequency effect size** In a metasummary of qualitative studies, the percentage of reports that contain a given thematic finding.

**Full disclosure** The communication of complete, accurate information to potential study participants.

**Functional relationship** A relationship between two variables in which it cannot be assumed that one variable caused the other.

**Funnel plot** In a meta-analysis, a graphical display of some measure of study precision (e.g., sample size) plotted against effect size that can be used to explore the possibility of publication bias.

**G**

**Gaining entrée** The process of gaining access to study participants through the cooperation of key actors in the selected community or site.

**Generalizability** The degree to which the research methods justify the inference that the findings are true for a broader group than study participants; in particular, the inference that the findings can be generalized from the sample to the population.

**Grand theory** A broad theory aimed at describing large segments of the physical, social, or behavioral world; also called a *macrotheory*.

**Grand tour question** A broad question asked in an unstructured interview to gain a general overview of a phenomenon, on the basis of which more focused questions are subsequently asked.

**Grey literature** Unpublished, and thus less readily accessible, research reports.

**Grounded theory** An approach to collecting and analyzing qualitative data that aims to develop theories about social psychological processes grounded in real-world observations.

**H**

**Hand searching** The planned searching of a journal "by hand," to identify all relevant reports that might be missed by electronic searching.

**Hawthorne effect** The effect on the dependent variable resulting from subjects' awareness that they are participants under study.

**Hermeneutic circle**  In hermeneutics, the methodologic process in which, to reach understanding, there is continual movement between the parts and the whole of the text being analyzed.

**Hermeneutics**  A qualitative research tradition, drawing on interpretive phenomenology, that focuses on the lived experiences of humans, and on how they interpret those experiences.

**Heterogeneity**  The degree to which objects are dissimilar (i.e., characterized by variability) on an attribute.

**Historical research**  Systematic studies designed to discover facts and relationships about past events.

**History threat**  The occurrence of events external to an intervention but concurrent with it, which can affect the dependent variable and threaten the study's internal validity.

**Homogeneity**  (1) In terms of the reliability of an instrument, the degree to which its subparts are internally consistent (i.e., are measuring the same critical attribute). (2) More generally, the degree to which objects are similar (i.e., characterized by low variability).

**Hypothesis**  A statement of predicted relationships between variables or predicted outcomes.

**I**

**Impact analysis**  An evaluation of the effects of a program or intervention on outcomes of interest, net of other factors influencing those outcomes.

**Implementation potential**  The extent to which an innovation is amenable to implementation in a new setting, an assessment of which is often made in an evidence-based practice project.

**Implied consent**  Consent to participate in a study that a researcher assumes has been given based on participants' actions, such as returning a completed questionnaire.

**IMRAD format**  The organization of a research report into four main sections: the Introduction, Method, Results, and Discussion sections.

**Incidence**  The rate of new cases with a specified condition, determined by dividing the number of new cases over a given period of time by the number at risk of becoming a new case (i.e., free of the condition at the outset of the time period).

**Independent variable**  The variable that is believed to cause or influence the dependent variable; in experimental research, the manipulated (treatment) variable.

**Inductive reasoning**  The process of reasoning from specific observations to more general rules (see also *deductive reasoning*).

**Inference**  In research, a conclusion drawn from the study evidence, taking into account the methods used to generate that evidence.

**Inferential statistics**  Statistics that permit inferences about whether results observed in a sample are likely to occur in the larger population.

**Informant**  An individual who provides information to researchers about a phenomenon under study, usually in qualitative studies.

**Informed consent**  An ethical principle that requires researchers to obtain people's voluntary participation in a study, after informing them of possible risks and benefits.

**Inquiry audit**  An independent scrutiny of qualitative data and relevant supporting documents by an external reviewer, to determine the dependability and confirmability of qualitative data.

**Insider research**  Research on a group or culture—usually in an ethnography—by a member of that group or culture.

**Institutional Review Board (IRB)**  In the United States, a group of people affiliated with an institution who convene to review proposed and ongoing studies with respect to ethical considerations.

**Instrument**  The device used to collect research data (e.g., a questionnaire, test, observation schedule, etc.).

**Intensity effect size**  In a metasummary of qualitative studies, the percentage of all thematic findings that are contained in any given report.

**Intention to treat**  A strategy for analyzing data in an intervention study that includes participants with the group to which they were assigned, whether or not they received or completed the treatment associated with the group.

**Interaction effect** The effect of two or more independent variables acting in combination (interactively) on an outcome.

**Intercoder reliability** The degree to which two coders, working independently, agree on coding decisions.

**Internal consistency** The degree to which the subparts of an instrument are measuring the same attribute or dimension, as a measure of the instrument's reliability.

**Internal validity** The degree to which it can be inferred that the experimental treatment (independent variable), rather than confounding factors, is responsible for observed effects on the outcome.

**Interrater (interobserver) reliability** The degree to which two raters or observers, operating independently, assign the same ratings or values for an attribute being measured or observed.

**Interval estimation** A statistical estimation approach in which the researcher establishes a range of values that are likely, within a given level of confidence, to contain the true population parameter.

**Interval measurement** A measurement level in which an attribute of a variable is rank ordered on a scale that has equal distances between points on that scale (e.g., Fahrenheit degrees).

**Intervention** In experimental research (clinical trials), the experimental treatment.

**Intervention fidelity** The extent to which the implementation of a treatment is faithful to its plan.

**Intervention protocol** The specification of exactly what the intervention and alternative (control) treatment conditions are, and how they should be administered.

**Intervention research** Research involving the development, implementation, and testing of an intervention.

**Intervention theory** The conceptual underpinning of a health care intervention, which articulates the theoretical basis for what must be done to achieve desired outcomes.

**Interview** A data collection method in which an interviewer asks questions of a respondent, either face-to-face, by telephone, or over the Internet.

**Interview schedule** The formal instrument that specifies the wording of all questions to be asked of respondents in structured self-report studies.

**Intuiting** The second step in descriptive phenomenology, which occurs when researchers remain open to the meaning attributed to the phenomenon by those who experienced it.

**Inverse relationship** A relationship characterized by the tendency of high values on one variable to be associated with low values on the second variable; also called a *negative relationship*.

**Inverse variance method** In meta-analysis, the use of the inverse of the variance of the effect estimate (one divided by the square of its standard error) as the weight to calculate a weighted average of effects.

**Investigator triangulation** The use of two or more researchers to analyze and interpret a data set, to enhance validity.

**Item** A single question on an instrument, or a single statement on a scale.

**J**

**Journal article** A report appearing in professional journals such as *Research in Nursing & Health*.

**Journal club** A group that meets regularly in clinical settings to discuss and critique research articles appearing in journals.

**K**

**Key informant** A person knowledgeable about the phenomenon of research interest and who is willing to share information and insights with the researcher (often an ethnographer).

**Keyword** An important term used to search for references on a topic in a bibliographic database.

**Known-groups technique** A technique for estimating the construct validity of an instrument through an analysis of the degree to which the instrument separates groups predicted to differ based on known characteristics or theory.

## L

**Level of measurement** A system of classifying measurements according to the nature of the measurement and the type of permissible mathematical operations; the levels are nominal, ordinal, interval, and ratio.

**Level of significance** The risk of making a Type I error in a statistical analysis, established by the researcher beforehand (e.g., the .05 level).

**Likelihood ratio (LR)** For a screening or diagnostic instrument, the relative likelihood that a given result is expected in a person with (as opposed to one without) the target attribute; LR indexes summarize the relationship between specificity and sensitivity in a single number.

**Likert scale** A composite measure of an attribute involving the summation of scores on a set of items that respondents typically rate for their degree of agreement or disagreement.

**Literature review** A critical summary of research on a topic, often prepared to put a research problem in context or to summarize existing evidence.

**Log** In participant observation studies, the observer's daily record of events and conversations.

**Logical positivism** The philosophy underlying the traditional scientific approach; see also *positivist paradigm.*

**Logistic regression** A multivariate regression procedure that analyzes relationships between one or more independent variables and a categorical dependent variable and yields an odds ratio.

**Longitudinal study** A study designed to collect data at more than one point in time, in contrast to a cross-sectional study.

## M

**Macrotheory** A broad theory aimed at describing large segments of the physical, social, or behavioral world; also called a *grand theory.*

**Manipulation** The introduction of an intervention or treatment in an experimental or quasi-experimental study to assess its impact on the dependent (outcome) variable.

**MANOVA** See *multivariate analysis of variance.*

**Masking** See *Blinding*

**Matching** The pairing of participants in one group with those in a comparison group based on their similarity on one or more dimension, to enhance overall group comparability.

**Maturation threat** A threat to the internal validity of a study that results when changes to the outcome (dependent) variable result from the passage of time.

**Maximum variation sampling** A sampling approach used by qualitative researchers involving the purposeful selection of cases with a wide range of variation.

**Mean** A measure of central tendency, computed by summing all scores and dividing by the number of cases.

**Measurement** The assignment of numbers to objects according to specified rules to characterize quantities of some attribute.

**Median** A descriptive statistic that is a measure of central tendency, representing the exact middle value in a score distribution; the value above and below which 50% of the scores lie.

**Mediating variable** A variable that mediates or acts like a "go-between" in a causal chain linking two other variables.

**Member check** A method of validating the credibility of qualitative data through debriefings and discussions with informants.

**MeSH** Medical Subject Headings, used to index articles in MEDLINE.

**Meta-analysis** A technique for quantitatively integrating the results of multiple studies addressing the same or a highly similar research question.

**Metasummary** A process that lays the foundation for a metasynthesis, involving the development of a list of abstracted findings from primary studies and calculating manifest effect sizes (frequency and intensity effect size).

**Metasynthesis** The grand narratives or interpretive translations produced from the integration or comparison of findings from qualitative studies.

**Method triangulation** The use of multiple methods of data collection about the same phenomenon, to enhance validity.

**Methodologic research** Research designed to develop or refine methods of obtaining, organizing, or analyzing data.

**Methods (research)** The steps, procedures, and strategies for gathering and analyzing data in a study.

**Middle-range theory** A theory that focuses on a limited piece of reality or human experience, involving a selected number of concepts (e.g., a theory of stress).

**Minimal risk** Anticipated risks that are no greater than those ordinarily encountered in daily life or during the performance of routine tests or procedures.

**Mixed methods (MM) research** Research in which both qualitative and quantitative data are collected and analyzed, to address different but related questions.

**Moderator variable** A variable that affects (moderates) the relationship between the independent and dependant variables.

**Mode** A measure of central tendency; the value that occurs most frequently in a distribution of scores.

**Model** A symbolic representation of concepts or variables and interrelationships among them.

**Mortality threat** A threat to the internal validity of a study, referring to differential attrition (loss of participants) from different groups.

**Multimodal distribution** A distribution of values with more than one peak (high frequency).

**Multiple comparison procedures** Statistical tests, normally applied after an ANOVA indicates statistically significant group differences, that compare different pairs of groups; also called *post hoc tests*.

**Multiple correlation coefficient** An index that summarizes the degree of relationship between two or more independent variables and a dependent variable; symbolized as $R$.

**Multiple regression analysis** A statistical procedure for understanding the effects of two or more independent (predictor) variables on a dependent variable.

**Multistage sampling** A sampling strategy that proceeds through a set of stages from larger to smaller sampling units (e.g., from states, to census tracts, to households).

**Multivariate analysis of variance (MANOVA)** A statistical procedure used to test the significance of differences between the means of two or more groups on two or more dependent variables, considered simultaneously.

**Multivariate statistics** Statistical procedures designed to analyze the relationships among three or more variables (e.g., multiple regression, ANCOVA).

**N**

$N$ The symbol designating the total number of subjects (e.g., "the total $N$ was 500").

$n$ The symbol designating the number of subjects in a subgroup or cell of a study (e.g., "each of the four groups had an $n$ of 125, for a total $N$ of 500").

**Narrative analysis** A type of qualitative approach that focuses on the story as the object of the inquiry.

**Naturalistic paradigm** An alternative paradigm (also called *constructivist paradigm*) to the positivist paradigm that holds that there are multiple interpretations of reality, and that the goal of research is to understand how individuals construct reality within their natural context; associated with qualitative research.

**Naturalistic setting** A setting for the collection of research data that is natural to those being studied (e.g., homes, places of work, and so on).

**Negative case analysis** The refinement of a theory or description in a qualitative study through the inclusion of cases that appear to disconfirm earlier hypotheses.

**Negative relationship** A relationship between two variables in which there is a tendency for high values on one variable to be associated with low values on the other (e.g., as stress increases, emotional well-being decreases); also called an *inverse relationship*.

**Negative results** Results that fail to support the researcher's hypotheses.

**Negatively skewed distribution** An asymmetric distribution of data values with a disproportionately high number of cases at the upper end; when displayed graphically, the tail points to the left.

**Network sampling** The sampling of participants based on referrals from others already in the sample; also called *snowball sampling*.

**Nominal measurement** The lowest level of measurement involving the assignment of characteristics into categories (e.g., males, category 1; females, category 2).

**Nondirectional hypothesis** A research hypothesis that does not stipulate the expected direction of the relationship between variables.

**Nonequivalent control group design** A quasi-experimental design involving a comparison group that was not created through random assignment.

**Nonexperimental research** Studies in which the researcher collects data without introducing an intervention; also called *observational research*.

**Nonparametric tests** A class of statistical tests that do not involve stringent assumptions about the distribution of variables in the analysis.

**Nonprobability sampling** The selection of sampling units (e.g., people) from a population using nonrandom procedures (e.g., convenience and quota sampling).

**Nonresponse bias** A bias that can result when a nonrandom subset of people invited to participate in a study decline to participate.

**Nonsignificant result** The result of a statistical test indicating that group differences or an observed relationship could have occurred by chance, at a given level of significance; sometimes abbreviated as NS.

**Normal distribution** A theoretical distribution that is bell shaped and symmetrical: also called a *normal curve* or a *Gaussian distribution*.

**Null hypothesis** A hypothesis stating no relationship between the variables under study; used primarily in statistical testing as the hypothesis to be rejected.

**Number needed to treat (NNT)** An estimate of how many people would need to receive an intervention to prevent one undesirable outcome, computed by dividing one by the value of the absolute risk reduction.

**Nursing research** Systematic inquiry designed to develop knowledge about issues of importance to the nursing profession.

## O

**Objectivity** The extent to which two independent researchers would arrive at similar judgments or conclusions (i.e., judgments not biased by personal values or beliefs).

**Observational notes** An observer's in-depth descriptions about events and conversations observed in naturalistic settings.

**Observational research** Studies that do not involve an experimental intervention—i.e., nonexperimental research; also, research in which data are collected through direct observation.

**Observed (obtained) score** The actual score or numerical value assigned to a person on a measure.

**Odds** A way of expressing the chance of an event—the probability of an event occurring to the probability that it will not occur, calculated by dividing the number of people who experienced an event by the number for whom it did not occur.

**Odds ratio (OR)** The ratio of one odds to another odds, e.g., the ratio of the odds of an event in one group to the odds of an event in another group; an odds ratio of 1.0 indicates no difference between groups.

**Open-ended question** A question in an interview or questionnaire that does not restrict respondents' answers to preestablished response alternatives.

**Open coding** The first level of coding in a grounded theory study, referring to the basic descriptive coding of the content of narrative materials.

**Operational definition** The definition of a concept or variable in terms of the procedures by which it is to be measured.

**Operationalization** The translation of research concepts into measurable phenomena.

**Ordinal measurement** A measurement level that rank orders phenomena along some dimension.

**Outcome variable** The dependent variable; a measure that captures the outcome of an intervention.

**Outcomes research** Research designed to document the effectiveness of health care services and the end results of patient care.

# P

**p value** In statistical testing, the probability that the obtained results are due to chance alone: the probability of a Type I error.

**Pair matching** See *matching*.

**Paradigm** A way of looking at natural phenomena that encompasses a set of philosophical assumptions and that guides one's approach to inquiry.

**Paradigm case** In a hermeneutic analysis following the precepts of Benner, a strong exemplar of the phenomenon under study, often used early in the analysis to gain understanding of the phenomenon.

**Parameter** A characteristic of a population (e.g., the mean age of all U.S. citizens).

**Parametric tests** A class of statistical tests that involve assumptions about the distribution of the variables and the estimation of a parameter.

**Participant** See *study participant*.

**Participant observation** A method of collecting data through the participation in and observation of a group or culture.

**Participatory action research (PAR)** A research approach based on the premise that the use and production of knowledge can be political and used to exert power.

**Path analysis** A regression-based procedure for testing causal models, typically using correlational data.

**Pearson's *r*** A correlation coefficient designating the magnitude of relationship between two interval- or ratio-level variables; also called *the product–moment correlation*.

**Peer debriefing** Meetings with peers to review and explore various aspects of a study, used to enhance trustworthiness in a qualitative study.

**Peer reviewer** A researcher who reviews and critiques a research report or proposal, and who makes a recommendation about publishing or funding the research.

**Pentadic dramatism** An approach for analyzing narratives, developed by Burke, that focus on five key elements of a story: act (what was done), scene (when and where it was done), agent (who did it), agency (how it was done), and purpose (why it was done).

**Per-protocol analysis** Analysis of data from a randomized controlled trial that excludes participants who did not obtain the protocol to which they were assigned.

**Perfect relationship** A correlation between two variables such that the values of one variable can perfectly predict the values of the other; designated as 1.00 or – 1.00.

**Persistent observation** A qualitative researcher's intense focus on the aspects of a situation that are relevant to the phenomena being studied.

**Person triangulation** The collection of data from different levels of persons, with the aim of validating data through multiple perspectives on the phenomenon.

**Personal interview** An in-person, face-to-face interview between an interviewer and a respondent.

**Personal notes** In field studies, written comments about the observer's own feelings during the research process.

**Phenomenon** The abstract concept under study; a term sometimes used by qualitative researchers in lieu of the term *variable*.

**Phenomenology** A qualitative research tradition, with roots in philosophy and psychology, that focuses on the lived experience of humans.

**Photo elicitation** An interview stimulated and guided by photographic images.

**PICO question** A well-worded question for evidence-based practice that identifies the population, intervention, comparison, and outcome of interest.

**Pilot study** A small scale version, or trial run, done in preparation for a major study or to assess feasibility.

**Placebo** A sham or pseudointervention, often used as a control group condition.

**Placebo effect** Changes in the dependant variable attributable to the placebo.

**Point estimation** A statistical procedure that uses information from a sample (a statistic) to estimate the single value that best represents the population parameter.

**Population** The entire set of individuals or objects having some common characteristics (e.g., all RNs in New York); sometimes called *universe*.

**Positive relationship** A relationship between two variables in which high values on one variable tend to be associated with high values on the other (e.g., as physical activity increases, pulse rate increases).

**Positive results** Research results that are consistent with the researcher's hypotheses.

**Positively skewed distribution** An asymmetric distribution of values with a disproportionately high number of cases at the lower end; when displayed graphically, the tail points to the right.

**Positivist paradigm** The paradigm underlying the traditional scientific approach, which assumes that there is an orderly reality that can be objectively studied; often associated with quantitative research.

*Post hoc* **test** A test for comparing all possible pairs of groups following a significant test of overall group differences (e.g., in an ANOVA).

**Poster session** A session at a professional conference in which several researchers simultaneously present visual displays summarizing their studies, while conference attendees circulate around the room perusing the displays.

**Posttest** The collection of data after introducing an intervention.

**Posttest-only design** An experimental design in which data are collected from participants only after the intervention has been introduced; also called an *after-only design*.

**Power** The ability of a design or analysis strategy to detect true relationships that exist among variables.

**Power analysis** A procedure for estimating either the needed sample size for a study or the likelihood of committing a Type II error.

**Practical (pragmatic) clinical trial** Trials that address practical questions about the benefits, risks, and costs of an intervention as they would unfold in routine clinical practice, using less rigid controls than in typical efficacy trials.

**Precision** The degree to which an estimated population value (a statistic) clusters closely around the estimate, usually expressed in terms of the width of the confidence interval.

**Prediction** The use of empirical evidence to make forecasts about how variables will behave with a new group of people.

**Predictive validity** The degree to which an instrument can predict a criterion observed at a future time.

**Pretest** (1) The collection of data prior to the experimental intervention; sometimes called baseline data. (2) The trial administration of a newly developed instrument to identify potential weaknesses.

**Pretest–posttest design** An experimental design in which data are collected from research subjects both before and after introducing an intervention; also called a *before–after design*.

**Prevalence** The proportion of a population having a particular condition (e.g., fibromyalgia) at a given point in time.

**Primary source** First-hand reports of facts or findings; in research, the original report prepared by the investigator who conducted the study.

**Primary study** In a systematic review, an original study whose findings are used as the data in the review.

**Priority** A key issue in mixed methods research, concerning which strand (qualitative or quantitative) will be given more emphasis; in notation, the dominant strand is in all capital letters, as QUAL or QUAN, and the nondominant strand is in lower case, as qual or quan.

**Probability sampling** The selection of sampling units (e.g., participants) from a population using random procedures (e.g., simple random sampling).

**Probing** Eliciting more useful or detailed information from a respondent in an interview than was volunteered in the first reply.

**Problem statement** An expression of a dilemma or disturbing situation that needs investigation.

**Process analysis** A descriptive analysis of the process by which a program or intervention gets implemented and used in practice.

**Process consent** In a qualitative study, an ongoing, transactional process of negotiating consent with participants, allowing them to collaborate in the decision making about their continued participation.

**Product moment correlation coefficient** ($r$) A correlation coefficient designating the magnitude of relationship between two variables measured on at least an interval scale; also called *Pearson's r*.

**Prolonged engagement** In qualitative research, the investment of sufficient time during data collection to have an in-depth understanding of the group under study, thereby enhancing credibility.

**Proposal** A document communicating a research problem, proposed procedures for solving the problem, and, when funding is sought, how much the study will cost.

**Prospective design** A study design that begins with an examination of a presumed cause (e.g., cigarette smoking) and then goes forward in time to observe presumed effects (e.g., lung cancer): also called a *cohort design*.

**Psychometric assessment** An evaluation of the quality of an instrument, primarily in terms of its reliability and validity.

**Psychometrics** The theory underlying principles of measurement and the application of the theory in the development of measuring tools.

**Publication bias** The tendency for published studies to systematically overrepresent statistically significant findings, reflecting the tendency of researchers, reviewers, and editors to not publish nonsignificant results; also called a *bias against the null hypothesis*.

**Purposive (purposeful) sampling** A non-probability sampling method in which the researcher selects participants based on personal judgment about who will be most informative.

# Q

**Q sort** A data collection method in which participants sort statements into piles (usually 9 or 11) according to some bipolar dimension (e.g., most helpful/least helpful).

**Qualitative analysis** The organization and interpretation of narrative data for the purpose of discovering important underlying themes, categories, and patterns.

**Qualitative data** Information collected in narrative (nonnumeric) form, such as the dialogue from a transcript of an unstructured interview.

**Qualitative research** The investigation of phenomena, typically in an in-depth and holistic fashion, through the collection of rich narrative materials using a flexible research design.

**Quantitative analysis** The manipulation of numeric data through statistical procedures for the purpose of describing phenomena or assessing the magnitude and reliability of relationships among them.

**Quantitative data** Information collected in a quantified (numeric) form.

**Quantitative research** The investigation of phenomena that lend themselves to precise measurement and quantification, often involving a rigorous and controlled design.

**Quasi-experimental design** A design for testing an intervention in which participants are not randomly assigned to treatment conditions; also called a *nonrandomized trial* or a *controlled trial without randomization*.

**Quasi-statistics** An "accounting" system used to assess the validity of conclusions derived from qualitative analysis.

**Questionnaire** A document used to gather self-report data via self-administration of questions.

**Quota sampling** A nonrandom sampling method in which "quotas" for certain subgroups based on sample characteristics are established to increase the representativeness of the sample.

# R

$r$ The symbol for a bivariate correlation coefficient, summarizing the magnitude and direction of a relationship between two variables measured on an interval or ratio scale.

$R$ The symbol for the multiple correlation coefficient, indicating the magnitude (but not direction) of the relationship between a dependent variable and multiple independent variables, taken together.

$R^2$ The squared multiple correlation coefficient, indicating the proportion of variance in the dependent variable explained by a group of independent variables.

**Random assignment** The assignment of participants to treatment conditions in a random manner (i.e., in a manner determined by chance alone); also called *randomization*.

**Random effects model** In meta-analysis, a model in which studies are not assumed to be measuring the same overall effect, but rather reflect a distribution of effects; often preferred to a fixed effect model when there is extensive variation of effects across studies.

**Random number table** A table displaying hundreds of digits (from 0 to 9) in random order; each number is equally likely to follow any other.

**Random sampling** The selection of a sample such that each member of a population has an equal probability of being included.

**Randomization** The assignment of subjects to treatment conditions in a random manner (i.e., in a manner determined by chance alone); also called *random assignment*.

**Randomized controlled trial (RCT)** A full experimental test of an intervention, involving random assignment to treatment groups; often, an RCT is phase III of a full clinical trial.

**Randomness** An important concept in quantitative research, involving having certain features of the study established by chance rather than by design or personal preference.

**Range** A measure of variability, computed by subtracting the lowest value from the highest value in a distribution of scores.

**Rating scale** A scale that requires ratings of an object or concept along a continuum.

**Ratio measurement** A measurement level with equal distances between scores and a true meaningful zero point (e.g., weight).

**Raw data** Data in the form in which they were collected, without being coded or analyzed.

**Reactivity** A measurement distortion arising from the study participant's awareness of being observed, or, more generally, from the effect of the measurement procedure itself.

**Readability** The ease with which materials (e.g., a questionnaire) can be read by people with varying reading skills, often determined through readability formulas.

**Reflexive notes** Notes that document a qualitative researcher's personal experiences, reflections, and progress in the field.

**Reflexivity** In qualitative studies, critical self-reflection about one's own biases, preferences, and preconceptions.

**Regression analysis** A statistical procedure for predicting values of a dependent variable based on one or more independent variables.

**Relationship** A bond or a connection between two or more variables.

**Relative risk (RR)** An estimate of risk of "caseness" in one group compared to another, computed by dividing the absolute risk for one group (e.g., an exposed group) by the absolute risk for another (e.g., the nonexposed); also called the *risk ratio*.

**Reliability** The degree to which a measurement is free from measurement error--its accuracy and consistency.

**Reliability coefficient** A quantitative index, usually ranging in value from .00 to 1.00, that provides an estimate of how reliable an instrument is (e.g., Cronbach's alpha).

**Repeated-measures ANOVA** An analysis of variance used when there are multiple measurements of the dependent variable over time.

**Replication** The deliberate repetition of research procedures in a second investigation for the purpose of determining if earlier results can be confirmed.

**Representative sample** A sample whose characteristics are comparable to those of the population from which it is drawn.

**Research** Systematic inquiry that uses orderly methods to answer questions or solve problems.

**Research control** See *control*.

**Research design** The overall plan for addressing a research question, including strategies for enhancing the study's integrity.

**Research hypothesis** The actual hypothesis a researcher wishes to test (as opposed to the *null hypothesis*), stating the anticipated relationship between two or more variables.

**Research methods** The techniques used to structure a study and to gather and analyze information in a systematic fashion.

**Research misconduct** Fabrication, falsification, plagiarism, or other practices that deviate from those that are commonly accepted within the scientific community for conducting or reporting research.

**Research problem** A disturbing or perplexing condition that can be investigated through disciplined inquiry.

**Research question** A specific query the researcher wants to answer to address a research problem.

**Research report** A document (often a journal article) summarizing the main features of a study, including the research question, the methods used to address it, the findings, and the interpretation of the findings.

**Research utilization** The use of some aspect of a study in an application unrelated to the original research.

**Researcher credibility** The faith that can be put in a researcher, based on his or her training, qualifications, and experiences.

**Respondent** In a self-report study, the person responding to questions posed by the researcher.

**Response rate** The rate of participation in a study, calculated by dividing the number of persons participating by the number of persons sampled.

**Response set bias** The measurement error resulting from the tendency of some individuals to respond to items in characteristic ways (e.g., always agreeing), independently of item content.

**Results** The answers to research questions, obtained through an analysis of the collected data.

**Retrospective design** A study design that begins with the manifestation of the outcome variable in the present (e.g., lung cancer), followed by a search for a presumed cause occurring in the past (e.g., cigarette smoking).

**Risk–benefit ratio** The relative costs and benefits, to an individual subject and to society at large, of participation in a study; also, the relative costs and benefits of implementing an innovation.

**Risk ratio** *See* Relative risk

**Rival hypothesis** An alternative explanation, competing with the researcher's hypothesis, for interpreting the results of a study.

**ROC curve** *See* Receiver operating characteristic curve

## S

**Sample** The subset of a population selected to participate in a study.

**Sampling** The process of selecting a portion of the population to represent the entire population.

**Sampling bias** Distortions that arise when a sample is not representative of the population from which it was drawn.

**Sampling distribution** A theoretical distribution of a statistic, using the values of the statistic computed from an infinite number of samples as the data points in the distribution.

**Sampling error** The fluctuation of the value of a statistic from one sample to another drawn from the same population.

**Sampling frame** A list of all the elements in the population, from which a sample is drawn.

**Sampling plan** The formal plan specifying a sampling method, a sample size, and procedures for recruiting subjects.

**Saturation** The collection of qualitative data to the point where a sense of closure is attained because new data yield redundant information.

**Scale** A composite measure of an attribute, involving the combination of several items that have a logical and empirical relationship to each other, resulting in the assignment of a score to place people on a continuum with respect to the attribute.

**Scientific method** A set of orderly, systematic, controlled procedures for acquiring dependable, empirical—and typically quantitative—information; the methodologic approach associated with the positivist paradigm.

**Scientific merit** The degree to which a study is methodologically and conceptually sound.

**Screening instrument** An instrument used to determine whether potential subjects for a study meet eligibility criteria, or for determining whether a person tests positive for a specified condition.

**Secondary analysis** A form of research in which the data collected in one study are reanalyzed in another investigation to answer new questions.

**Secondary source** Second-hand accounts of events or facts; in research, a description of a study prepared by someone other than the original researcher.

**Selection threat (self-selection)** A threat to a study's internal validity resulting from preexisting differences between groups under study; the differences affect the dependent variable in ways extraneous to the effect of the independent variable.

**Selective coding** A level of coding in a grounded theory study that involves selecting the core category, systematically integrating relationships between the core category and other categories, and validating those relationships.

**Self-determination** A person's ability to voluntarily decide whether or not to participate in a study.

**Self-report** A data collection method that involves a direct verbal report by a person being studied (e.g., by interview or questionnaire).

**Semistructured interview** An open-ended interview in which the researcher is guided by a list of specific topics to cover.

**Sensitivity** The ability of a screening instrument to correctly identify a "case," i.e., to correctly diagnose a condition.

**Sensitivity analysis** An effort to test how sensitive the results of a statistical analysis are to changes in assumptions or in the way the analysis was done (e.g., in a meta-analysis, used to assess whether conclusions are sensitive to the quality of the studies included).

**Sequential design** A mixed methods design in which one strand of data collection (qualitative or quantitative) occurs prior to the other, informing the second strand; symbolically shown with an arrow, as QUAL → QUAN.

**Setting** The physical location and conditions in which data collection takes place in a study.

**Significance level** The probability that an observed relationship could be caused by chance; significance at the 0.5 level indicates the probability that a relationship of the observed magnitude would be found by chance only 5 times out of 100.

**Simple random sampling** Basic probability sampling involving the selection of sample members from a sampling frame through completely random procedures.

**Site** The overall location where a study is undertaken.

**Skewed distribution** The asymmetric distribution of a set of data values around a central point.

**Snowball sampling** The selection of participants through referrals from earlier participants; also called *network sampling*.

**Social desirability response set** A bias in self-report instruments created when participants have a tendency to misrepresent their opinions in the direction of answers consistent with prevailing social norms.

**Space triangulation** The collection of data on the same phenomenon in multiple sites, to enhance the validity of the findings.

**Spearman's rank-order correlation (Spearman's rho)** A correlation coefficient indicating the magnitude of a relationship between variables measured on the ordinal scale.

**Specificity** The ability of a screening instrument to correctly identify noncases.

**Standard deviation** The most frequently used statistic for measuring the degree of variability in a set of scores.

**Standard error** The standard deviation of a sampling distribution, such as the sampling distribution of the mean.

**Standardized mean difference (SMD)** In meta-analysis, the effect size for comparing two group means, computed by subtracting one mean from the other and dividing by the pooled standard deviation; also called Cohen's *d*.

**Statement of purpose** A declarative statement of the overall goals of a study.

**Statistic** An estimate of a parameter, calculated from sample data.

**Statistical analysis** The organization and analysis of quantitative data using statistical procedures, including both descriptive and inferential statistics.

**Statistical conclusion validity** The degree to which inferences about relationships and differences from a statistical analysis of the data are accurate.

**Statistical control** The use of statistical procedures to control confounding influences on the dependent variable.

**Statistical heterogeneity** Diversity of effects across primary studies included in a meta-analysis.

**Statistical inference** The process of inferring attributes about the population based on information from a sample, using laws of probability.

**Statistical power** The ability of the research design and analytic strategy to detect true relationships among variables.

**Statistical significance** A term indicating that the results from an analysis of sample data are unlikely to have been caused by chance, at a specified level of probability.

**Statistical test** An analytic tool that estimates the probability that obtained results from a sample reflect true population values.

**Stipend** A monetary payment to individuals participating in a study to serve as an incentive for participation and/or to compensate for time and expenses.

**Strata** Subdivisions of the population according to some characteristic (e.g., males and females); singular is *stratum*.

**Stratified random sampling** The random selection of study participants from two or more strata of the population independently.

**Structured data collection** An approach to collecting data from participants, either through self-report or observations, in which categories of information (e.g., response options) are specified in advance.

**Study participant** An individual who participates and provides information in a study.

**Subject** An individual who participates and provides data in a study; term used primarily in quantitative research.

**Summated rating scale** A scale consisting of multiple items that are added together to yield an overall, continuous measure of an attribute (e.g., a Likert scale).

**Survey research** Nonexperimental research that obtains information about people's activities, beliefs, preferences, and attitudes via direct questioning.

**Symmetric distribution** A distribution of values with two halves that are mirror images of each other.

**Systematic review** A rigorous synthesis of research findings on a particular research question, using systematic sampling and data collection procedures and a formal protocol.

**Systematic sampling** The selection of sample members such that every *kth* (e.g., every 10th) person or element in a sampling frame is chosen.

## T

**Tacit knowledge** Information about a culture that is so deeply embedded that members do not talk about it or may not even be consciously aware of it.

**Target population** The entire population in which a researcher is interested and to which he or she would like to generalize the study results.

**Taxonomy** In an ethnographic analysis, a system of classifying and organizing terms and concepts, developed to illuminate a domain's organization and the relationship among the domain's categories.

**Test statistic** A statistic used to test for the reliability of relationships between variables (e.g., chi-squared, *t*); sampling distributions of test statistics are known for circumstances in which the null hypothesis is true.

**Test–retest reliability** Assessment of the stability of an instrument by correlating the scores obtained on two administrations.

**Theme** A recurring regularity emerging from an analysis of qualitative data.

**Theoretical sampling** In qualitative studies, the selection of sample members based on emerging findings to ensure saturation of important theoretical categories.

**Theory** An abstract generalization that presents a systematic explanation about relationships among phenomena.

**Thick description** A rich, thorough description of the context and participants in a qualitative study.

**Time sampling** In structured observations, the sampling of time periods during which observations will take place.

**Time series design** A quasi-experimental design involving the collection of data over an extended time period, with multiple data collection points both prior to and after an intervention.

**Time triangulation** The collection of data on the same phenomenon or about the same people at different points in time, to enhance validity.

**Topic guide** A list of broad question areas to be covered in a semistructured interview or focus group interview.

**Transferability** The extent to which qualitative findings can be transferred to other settings or groups; analogous to generalizability.

**Treatment** The experimental intervention under study; the condition being manipulated.

**Treatment group** The group receiving the intervention being tested; the experimental group.

**Triangulation** The use of multiple methods to collect and interpret data about a phenomenon, so as to converge on an accurate representation of reality.

**Triangulation design** A concurrent, equal-priority mixed methods design in which different, but complementary data, qualitative and quantitative, are gathered about a central phenomenon under study; symbolized as QUAL + QUAN; also called a convergent parallel design.

**True score** A hypothetical score that would be obtained if a measure were infallible.

**Trustworthiness** The degree of confidence qualitative researchers have in their data and analyses, assessed using the criteria of credibility, transferability, dependability, confirmability, and authenticity.

*t*-test A parametric statistical test for analyzing the difference between two group means.

**Type I error** An error created by rejecting the null hypothesis when it is true (i.e., the researcher concludes that a relationship exists when in fact it does not—a false positive).

**Type II error** An error created by accepting the null hypothesis when it is false (i.e., the researcher concludes that *no* relationship exists when in fact it does—a false negative).

## U

**Unimodal distribution** A distribution of values with one peak (high frequency).

**Unit of analysis** The basic unit or focus of a researcher's analysis—typically individual study participants.

**Univariate statistics** Statistical analysis of a single variable for descriptive purposes (e.g., computing a mean).

**Unstructured interview** An interview in which the researcher asks respondents questions without having a predetermined plan regarding the content or flow of information to be gathered.

**Unstructured observation** The collection of descriptive data through direct observation that is not guided by a formal, prespecified plan for observing or recording the information.

## V

**Validity** A quality criterion referring to the degree to which inferences made in a study are accurate and well-founded; in measurement, the degree to which an instrument measures what it is intended to measure.

**Variability** The degree to which values on a set of scores are dispersed.

**Variable** An attribute that varies, that is, takes on different values (e.g., body temperature, heart rate).

**Variance** A measure of variability or dispersion, equal to the standard deviation squared.

**Vignette** A brief description of an event, person, or situation to which respondents are asked to express their reactions.

**Visual analog scale (VAS)** A scaling procedure used to measure certain clinical symptoms (e.g., pain, fatigue) by having people indicate on a straight line the intensity of the symptom.

**Vulnerable groups** Special groups of people whose rights in studies need special protection because of their inability to provide meaningful informed consent or because their circumstances place them at higher-than-average-risk of adverse effects (e.g., children, unconscious patients).

## W

**Wait-list design** An experimental design that involves putting control group members on a waiting list for the intervention; also called a *delayed treatment design*.

**Web-based survey** The administration of a self-administered questionnaire over the Internet on a dedicated survey website.

Applied Nursing Research 20 (2007) 17–23

Original article

# The relationships among anxiety, anger, and blood pressure in children

Carol C. Howell, PhD, APRN-BC[a],*, Marti H. Rice, PhD, RN[b],
Myra Carmon, EdD, RN, CPNP[a], Roxanne Pickett Hauber, PhD, CNRN[c]

[a]Byrdine F. Lewis School of Nursing, Georgia State University, PO Box 4019, Atlanta, Georgia 30302-4019, USA
[b]School of Nursing, University of Alabama at Birmingham, Birmingham, Alabama 35294-1210, USA
[c]Department of Nursing, University of Tampa, Tampa, FL 33615, USA
Received 15 July 2005; accepted 23 October 2005

**Abstract**

Relationships between anger and anxiety have been examined in adults but less frequently in children. This investigation explored relationships among trait anxiety, trait anger, anger expression patterns, and blood pressure in children. The participants were 264 third- through sixth-grade children from five elementary schools who completed Jacob's Pediatric Anger and Anxiety Scale and Jacob's Pediatric Anger Expression Scale and had their blood pressure measured. Data were analyzed using descriptive and correlational statistics and hierarchical regression. Results have implications for the way in which anxiety and anger are perceived in children and the importance of teaching children to deal with emotions.
© 2007 Elsevier Inc. All rights reserved.

## 1. Introduction

Hypertension affects over 50 million Americans aged 6 and over and is a recognized risk factor for the development of cardiovascular disease (American Heart Association, 2004). Although few children have hypertension or cardiovascular disease, biological and psychosocial risk factors for the development of hypertension in adulthood are estimated to be present in children by the age of 8 (Solomon & Matthews, 1999). With the large number of individuals with hypertension and the progressive nature of cardiovascular disease, it is important to identify and modify risk factors early in life. Although some risk factors are not modifiable, others, such as anger and anxiety, are more amenable to change. The identification and modification of risk factors at an early age might reduce the incidence of hypertension in adulthood (Ewart & Kolodner 1994; Hauber, Rice, Howell, & Carmon, 1998; Meininger, Liehr, Chan, Smith, & Mueller, 2004).

## 2. Review of the literature

Trait anger (Johnson, 1989, 1990; Siegel, 1984), patterns of anger expression (Johnson, 1989; Muller, Grunbaum, & Labarthe, 2001; Seigel, 1984), and trait anxiety (Ewert & Kolodner, 1994; Johnson, 1989; Meininger et al., 2004) are psychological factors that have been associated with high blood pressure in adolescents. Biological factors such as sex, height, and weight have also been significantly associated with high blood pressure (Johnson, 1984, 1989; Meininger et al., 2004; Muller et al., 2001). Although the contribution of these factors to the development of hypertension has been investigated in adults and adolescents (Ewart & Kolodner, 1994; Harburg, Gkeuberman, Russell, & Cooper, 1991; Meininger et al., 2004), much less research has been done with children (Hauber et al., 1998). It is the intent of this study to investigate relationships among psychosocial factors, biological factors, and blood pressure in children.

### 2.1. Psychosocial factors

#### 2.1.1. Trait anger

Trait anger is defined as an emotion that can vary from mild displeasure to rage and reflects a more permanent characteristic than state anger (Speilberger et al., 1985). Anger is thought to lead to an increase in blood pressure through its effect on the sympathetic nervous system (Meininger et al., 2004; Muller

* Corresponding author. Tel.: +1 404 651 3645 (home); +1 404 255 5453; fax: +1 404 255 1086.
*E-mail addresses:* chowell@gsu.edu (C.C. Howell), schauf@uab.edu (M.H. Rice), mcarmon@gsu.edu (M. Carmon), rhauber@ut.edu (R.P. Hauber).

0897-1897/$ – see front matter © 2007 Elsevier Inc. All rights reserved.
doi:10.1016/j.apnr.2005.10.006

et al., 2001; Taylor, Repetti, & Seeman, 1997; Williams & Williams, 1993). Repeated episodes of anger arousal may lead to a chronic state of elevated blood pressure or hypertension (Muller et al., 2001; Williams & Williams, 1993). Researchers have noted an association between anger scores and blood pressure (Hauber et al., 1998; Johnson, 1989, 1990; Siegel, 1984; Siegel & Leitch, 1981).

### 2.1.2. Anger expression patterns

Anger expression patterns include anger out, which implies that anger is openly expressed. Anger suppression or anger in implies that the anger is denied and held in. Anger reflection control involves a cognitive approach to resolving anger (Speilberger et al., 1985).

Siegel (1984) found that subjects who had higher scores on the Frequent Anger Directed Outward factor also had higher systolic (SBP) and diastolic blood pressure (DBP). In contrast, Johnson (1984, 1989) found significant positive correlations between anger suppression and high blood pressures in male and female adolescents. In one of the few studies with children, Hauber et al. (1998), in a study of 230 third-grade children, found significant inverse relationships between anger suppression and DBP and anger reflection/control for both SBP and DBP. Muller et al. (2001) found that anger expression predicted blood pressure in 167 14-year-olds or after controlling ethnicity, height, weight, percent body fat, and maturity. However, the instrument used in this study did not differentiate between anger in and anger out.

### 2.1.3. Trait anxiety

Trait anxiety is defined as a subjective feeling of apprehension, tension, and worry, which is thought to be a relatively stable personality characteristic (Speilberger, Edwards, Lushene, Montuori, & Platzek, 1973). Jonas, Franks, and Ingram (1997) suggested that anxiety contributes to the development of hypertension in two ways. Anxiety has been shown to directly stimulate acute autonomic arousal (Russek, King, Russek, & Russek, 1990) and blood pressure reactivity (Krantz & Manuck, 1984; Suls & Wan, 1993; Waked & Jutai, 1990). Responding to stress- or anxiety-provoking experiences with anger has been shown to contribute to cardiovascular disease (Chang, Ford, Meoni, Wang & Klag, 2002; Wascher, 2002). The presence of anxiety has been associated with high-risk health behaviors such as smoking, drinking, low levels of physical activity, and noncompliance with prescribed medical treatments, which in turn have been associated with elevations in blood pressure (Jonas et al., 1997). In addition, Heker, Whalen, Jamner, and Delfino (2002) found that high-anxiety teenagers expressed higher levels of anger when compared with low-anxiety teenagers.

### 2.2. Biological factors

### 2.2.1. Gender

Research with children and adolescents has shown a differential association between anger, anger expression,

and blood pressure when gender is considered (Hauber et al., 1998; Johnson, 1984, 1989; Muller et al., 2001; Weinrich et al., 2000). In a study with third graders, Hauber et al. (1998) identified a positive correlation between anger reflection/control and SBP in female third graders. In male third graders, however, there was a positive correlation between anger reflection/control and DBP. Starner and Peters (2004) found a significant correlation between anger in and SBP and between anger out and SBP.

### 2.2.2. Height and weight

Among the factors known to influence blood pressure in children are height and weight. Normative tables published by the National Heart, Lung, and Blood Institute (1996) (Task Force Report of High Blood Pressure in Children and Adolescents) list blood pressure standards based on height, weight, and sex in order to include body size to more accurately classify blood pressure norms. However, a more recent report no longer used weight as a factor for calculating normal blood pressure (National High Blood Pressure Education Program Working Group on High Blood Pressure in Children and Adolescents, 2004). However, the increasing occurrence of hypertension in children has been linked to the increase in weight (Couch & Daniels, 2005; Davis et al., 2005; Wyllie, 2005). Overall, the literature supports height and weight as factors that affect blood pressure (Couch & Daniels, 2005; Markovitz, Matthews, Wing, Kuller, & Meilahn, 1991, Muller et al., 2001; Muller, Wiechmann, Helms, Wulff, & Kolenda, 2000).

## 3. Purpose

The purpose of this study was to determine the relationships between trait anxiety, trait anger, height, weight, patterns of anger expression, and blood pressure in a group of elementary school children.

## 4. Research questions

Specific research questions addressed were as follows:

1. What are the bivariate relationships between SBP and DBP and height, weight, and sex, trait anger and patterns of anger expression, and trait anxiety in elementary school children?
2. What is the contribution of height, weight, trait anger, anger expression patterns, and trait anxiety to SBP and DBP in elementary school boys and girls?

## 5. Method

### 5.1. Design

A descriptive correlational design was used in this study.

### 5.2. Sample and setting

A convenience sample of 264 children was recruited from the third through the sixth grades in five public elementary schools serving kindergarten through sixth grade in a large metropolitan city in the southeastern United States. These schools served communities of varying socioeconomic levels in urban and suburban locations.

### 5.3. Instruments

#### 5.3.1. Trait anger

Trait anger was measured by the Trait Anger subscale of the Jacobs Pediatric Anger Scale (Jacobs & Blumer, 1984) (PANG Forms PPS-1 and PPS-2). The PANG is a 10-item self-report inventory developed for use with children. Reliability coefficients for the PANG range from .77 to .84 (Jacobs & Mehlhaff, 1994). A more recent study found the reliability to be .89 (M. Rice, personal communication, November 2004). Items included in the scale are in a Likert format with responses of 1, *hardly ever*; 2, *sometimes*; and 3, *often*. Scores on the PANG range from 10 to 30 and the higher the score, the greater the trait anger.

#### 5.3.2. Anger expression

The 15-item Jacobs Pediatric Anger Expression Scale (PAES) (Jacobs, Phelps, & Rohrs, 1989) was used to measure patterns of anger expression. The instrument contains three scales that have five items each and measure anger-out, anger suppression, and anger reflection/control. Each item is in the form of declarative statements with choices for responses of 1 for *hardly ever*, 2 for *sometimes*, and 3 for *often*. Possible scores for each scale range from 5 to 15. Alpha coefficients for the entire PAES ranged from .57 to .79 (Jacobs et al., 1989). Coefficients for anger out ranged from .66 to .78, for anger suppression from .57 to .76, and for the anger reflection/control scale from .36 to .62 (Jacobs & Mehlhaff, 1994). A more recent study found reliability measure of internal consistency for anger out to be .85, for anger suppression to be .76, and for anger reflection/control to be .70 (M. Rice, personal communication, November 2004).

#### 5.3.3. Trait anxiety

Measurement of trait anxiety was accomplished through use of the Jacob's Pediatric Anxiety Scale (PANX) (Jacobs & Blumer, 1984), a 10-item self-report inventory designed for use with young children. Item to total correlations range from .37 to .53 with an alpha reliability score of .78 for the total scale. A Likert format with three responses was used with a 1 for *hardly ever*, 2 for *sometimes*, and 3 for *often*. Scale scores are calculated by summing the responses on all items so that scores can range from 10 to 30. The higher the score the greater the anxiety. Alpha coefficients on the scale range from .77 to .84 (Jacobs & Mehlhaff, 1994). A more recent study found the reliability to be .80 (M. Rice, personal communication, November 2004).

#### 5.3.4. Blood pressure

The Hawksley's Random Zero sphygmomanometer (W. A. Braum Company Inc., Copiagne, NY), a conventional mercury sphygmomanometer with calibrations 0 to 300 mmHg, was used to obtain blood pressure. This sphygmomanometer is designed to eliminate error variance due to operator and technique by using a shifting zero device. This allows random halting of the mercury between 0 and 20 mmHg so that the operator cannot automatically assume a value. Mercury values must be subtracted from both systolic and diastolic readings to obtain correct blood pressure. The researchers for the study reported here were trained to use the Hawksley. Independent blood pressures on the same participant were taken until a 100% agreement rate was achieved in order to assure interrater reliability. The suggested protocol for measurement of children, including choice of correct cuff size and use of the first reading for nondiagnostic purposes, was followed (National Heart, Lung, and Blood Institute, 1996). Because blood pressure readings were not obtained for the purpose of diagnosing hypertension but for determining the relationships of blood pressure to anger and anxiety scores, only one blood pressure reading was obtained.

#### 5.3.5. Height and weight

Height and weight were measured by a balanced beam scale and the height rod of the balanced beam scale, respectively.

### 5.4. Procedures

The human assurance committee of the university and the research committee of the county school district approved the proposal. A letter explaining the project and requesting consent for the child to participate was sent home to each child's legally designated caregiver 1 month prior to data collection at each school. On the day of data collection, children with returned completed forms were requested to sign assent forms. The assent form was read aloud to the children before they were requested to sign the form. After assent forms were signed by the children, the PANG, PAES, and the PANX instruments were administered. All instruments were administered by the same investigator. Directions were read aloud, and then the children responded.

Every child read and completed the scales independently. Special effort was taken to stress to the children that this was not a test and that there were no "right" or "wrong" answers. When the scales were completed, the children walked to an adjoining room where a blood pressure reading was obtained for each child.

### 6. Results

#### 6.1. Sample characteristics

Of the 264 participants enrolled in the study who indicated gender and ethnicity, 107 were boys, 155 were girls; 189 were Black, 58 were White, and 17 were other ethnicities.

#### 6.2. Scale scores

Table 1 shows scores on the study variables for the entire group and then separately for girls and boys. Boys had

Table 1
Scale scores

| Variable | Total | | Boys | | Girls | |
|---|---|---|---|---|---|---|
| | M | SD | M | SD | M | SD |
| Trait anxiety | 18.66 | 4.16 | 18.13 | 4.23 | 19.0 | 4.11 |
| Trait anger | 17.87 | 4.84 | 18.72 | 4.74 | 17.34 | 4.84 |
| Anger out | 9.00 | 2.61 | 9.50 | 2.62 | 8.69 | 2.57 |
| Anger suppression | 9.28 | 2.27 | 9.30 | 2.23 | 9.29 | 2.31 |
| Anger reflection | 9.98 | 2.42 | 9.55 | 2.22 | 10.32 | 2.47 |
| Systolic BP | 102.58 | 10.96 | 104.66 | 11.03 | 101.16 | 10.75 |
| Diastolic BP | 63.28 | 9.83 | 64.30 | 8.72 | 62.55 | 10.50 |

higher mean anger scores but lower mean anxiety scores than the girls. The girl participants had higher SBP and DBP readings, lower anger out, lower anger suppression, and higher anger reflection/control scores than the boys.

### 6.3. Research Question 1: bivariate correlations

Pearson's product–moment correlations were done in order to address Research Question 1. Table 2 shows correlation results for the children as a group and then separately for boys and girls. For the group as a whole, significant although weak correlations were found between anger reflection/control scores and DBP. Significant and moderately strong correlations were found between height and weight and both SBP and DBP. In addition, there was a significant inverse correlation between height and anger/reflection control scores. Moderate to strong correlations between height and weight and both SBP and DBP were noted for boys and girls.

When correlation analyses were restricted to boys and then girls, different results were obtained. Significant although weak correlations were noted in the boys between DBP and trait anger. A moderate significant correlation was noted between weight and DBP, and a significant although weak correlation was noted between height and DBP in the boys. When girls were considered, a significant although weak negative correlation was found between DBP and anger reflection/control scores.

### 6.4. Research Question 2: hierarchical multiple regression

In order to answer Research Question 2, six separate hierarchical regression analyses were performed. Two regressions were tested with the entire group, for SBP and DBP in turn, followed by two regressions restricted to sample boys and sample girls, again for SBP then DBP. The variables of height, weight, and sex were entered first as a block as these variables were correlated with blood pressure in this study. The next block included the variables of trait anger, anger out, anger reflection control, and anger suppression because links between blood pressure and anger have been widely documented. The anxiety variable was entered last. When SBP was the dependent variable, 24% of the variance was accounted for in the entire group. Only the first block contributed significantly ($p < .001$; $F = 22.58$).

When DBP was the dependent variable, sex, height, and weight together accounted for 12.4% of the variance ($F = 10.21$; $p < .001$). Only the first block contributed significantly to the model.

### 6.4.1. Gender

In the next two multiple regression equations, the contribution of study variables to SBP and DBP was restricted to the boys in the study group. Thirty percent of the variance in SBP was accounted for by height and weight ($F = 18.05$; $p < .001$). Height and weight also accounted for 8% of the variance in DBP in the boys ($F = 3.90$; $p < .001$). In the last two multiple regression equations, the contribution of study variables to SBP and DBP was restricted to the girls in the study group. Here, the first block, sex, height, and weight, accounted for 18% of the variance in SBP ($F = 14.53$; $p < .001$). Neither the anger variables nor the anxiety variable that was added in the next block contributed significantly to the model. Height and

Table 2
Correlation table for the entire group, boys, and girls

| Variable | Trait anger | Anger out | Anger suppression | Anger reflection | Trait anxiety | Height | Weight |
|---|---|---|---|---|---|---|---|
| SBP | | | | | | | |
| Entire group | −.02 | −.04 | −.04 | −.08 | −.07 | .30*** | .46*** |
| Boys | −.04 | −.03 | −.14 | −.13 | −.02 | .45*** | .57*** |
| Girls | −.00 | −.06 | −.04 | −.20* | −.13 | .27** | .45*** |
| DPB | | | | | | | |
| Entire group | −.06 | −.07 | −.04 | −.12* | −.04 | .21** | .34*** |
| Boys | −.19* | .08 | −.07 | −.07 | −.04 | .20 | .27** |
| Girls | −.04 | .07 | −.10 | −.19 | −.05 | .24** | .37*** |

* $p \leq .05$.
** $p \leq .01$.
*** $p \leq .001$.

weight accounted for 13% of the variance in DBP ($F = 10.09$; $p < .001$). Again, neither anger nor anxiety variables made significant contributions to the model.

## 7. Discussion

In this study, support was found for the relationships of some of the identified psychosocial and biological factors and blood pressure in children. Children in the group as a whole who indicated more use of anger reflection/control had lower DBP readings. This is consistent with earlier research reporting an association between anger reflection/control and lower blood pressures in adults and children (Harburg, Blakelock, Roeper, 1979; Harburg et al., 1991; Hauber et al., 1998; Muller et al., 2001).

There were no significant relationships between trait anxiety and blood pressure. Much of the research linking anxiety to blood pressure has been conducted with adult samples. Anxiety is thought to contribute to hypertension through repeated autonomic arousal (Jonas et al., 1997; Russek et al., 1990), blood pressure reactivity (Suls & Wan, 1993; Waked & Jutai, 1990), or through the association of anxiety and high-risk health behaviors. The findings in the current study are consistent with the work of Johnson (1989) who found that anxiety was not a predictor of blood pressure in a group of older adolescents. Perhaps the young participants in the current study, as well as Johnson's study, had not yet experienced the long-term negative effects of anxiety on blood pressure.

In this study, height and weight were significantly correlated with SBP and DBP for the entire group. In boys, height and weight were significantly correlated with SBP but not with DBP. In girls, height and weight were significantly correlated with both SBP and DBP. As noted earlier, this relationship is widely acknowledged. Blood pressure has been found to vary with the height, weight, sex, age, and fitness of an individual (Task Force Report of High Blood Pressure in Children and Adolescents, National Heart, Lung, & Blood Institute, 1996). Although weight is no longer used as a factor for calculating normal blood pressure (National High Blood Pressure Education Program Working Group on High Blood Pressure in Children and Adolescents, 2004), the results of this research strongly suggest a relationship.

A bivariate correlation between height and anger reflection control was found in this study. This implies that the taller the individual, the less anger reflection control is used. Perhaps taller children feel less inhibited about expressing their anger in more aggressive ways because their size protects them somewhat from reprisal.

Boys had significant correlations between trait anger scores and DBP. Similar findings have been reported between trait anger and higher blood pressure in both adolescents and adults (Markovitz et al., 1991; Siegel & Leitch, 1981). Girls in the present study showed negative correlations between both SBP and DBP and anger

reflection/control. Similar findings were obtained in an earlier study with children (Hauber et al., 1998) where an inverse relationship was noted between anger reflection/control and SBP in girls. These findings suggest the importance of gender-specific research in the area of hypertension and cardiovascular disease. In her study of gender and gender-role identity and expression of anger, Thomas (1997) found that gender was an important factor in anger expression. She suggested that masculine sex-role identity was associated with being more anger prone, expressing anger in an outward manner, and being less likely to control anger expression. Female sex role types were less likely to express anger outwardly or to suppress anger and more likely to attempt anger control. Fabes and Eisenberg (1992) found that female preschoolers vented their anger less than their male counterparts. Fuchs and Thelen (1988) suggested that girls were socialized to hide their anger where boys were taught to hide their sadness or any other feeling such as anxiety that could be interpreted as a sign of weakness. Perhaps, even at this young age, anger reflection is a less acceptable choice for males and does not translate into lower blood pressure in male children in this sample. It may be that no particular expression pattern is associated with blood pressure with boys, although the characteristic of trait anger is related.

In the regression models, neither trait anxiety nor any of the other anger expression patterns accounted for any of the variance in blood pressure. Muller et al. (2001) also found that anger variables did not account for any of the variance in blood pressure in a group of 167 adolescents. In their longitudinal study with 541 normotensive middle-aged women, Raikkonen, Matthews, and Kuller (2001) found that baseline levels of anxiety and anger did not predict subsequent hypertension. However, in the 75 women who became hypertensive during this 9-year study, increases in anger and anxiety during follow-up significantly predicted the incidence of hypertension.

When separate analyses were done for boys and girls after controlling for height and weight, no additional variance in SBP or DBP was explained by trait anger, patterns of anger expression, or trait anxiety. These findings were similar to those of Johnson (1990), who identified no overall relationship between anger variables and SBP.

Although neither the anger variables nor anxiety contributed significantly to the regression model in this study, it should be recognized that factors considered in this study are thought to influence blood pressure in adulthood and are risk factors in children for the future development of hypertension. As children with these risk factors move into adulthood, they may develop hypertension due to repeated episodes of anger and anxiety, which continually stimulate the sympathetic–adrenal–medullary system. The end result is damage to cardiovascular health (Muller et al., 2001). It is important to know that these risk factors, if identified as early as childhood, can be modified before hypertension develops (Meininger et al., 2004; Solomon & Matthews, 1999).

## 8. Limitations

Blood pressure readings and anger instruments were administered only once per subject. Multiple measurements could provide a pattern of blood pressure, and tracking participants for a longer period could aid in the identification of patterns across developmental periods.

## 9. Implications and recommendations

Because anger and anxiety are associated with hypertension in adults, a longitudinal study would help identify when anger and anxiety begin to contribute to the explanation of hypertension.

Current results indicate that anger reflection/control patterns are associated with lower levels of blood pressure in girls of this age. This finding is consistent with results of an earlier study with 230 third-grade boys and girls (Hauber et al., 1998) and suggests that children may benefit from anger management interventions aimed at anger control strategies. Identification of factors that influence a child's choice of anger expression patterns, the effect on blood pressure, and the contributions of gender would be helpful when designing intervention programs. The school nurse could be involved in identifying and recommending interventions for children who have frequent anger problems in the classroom or whose parents report frequent angry outbursts in the home environment.

Future research should investigate whether these findings remain consistent across younger age groups, different socioeconomic groups, varying regions of the country, and more varied ethnic groups (Rice & Howell, 2006).

This study supports the belief that certain modifiable risk factors for hypertension are present at an early age. It has been recommended that BP should be monitored by the age of 3 for every child during every scheduled physical examination (National High Blood Pressure Education Program Working Group on High Blood Pressure in Children and Adolescents, 2004). It is important to monitor BP across a period of time to determine any elevations or pattern of BP (Cook, Gillman, Rosner, Taylor, & Hennekens, 2000). This type of assessment is most often performed by a nurse (Hauber et al., 1998). According to Moran, Panzarino, Darden, and Reigart (2003) although the rate of BP screening during well-child checkups has increased, it does not meet current recommendations. If the BP reading is normal (less than 90th percentile for sex, age, and height) it should be rechecked at the next scheduled physical exam and the nurse should encourage adequate sleep and an active lifestyle with healthy meals. A prehypertensive reading is the 90th percentile to less than the 95th percentile. This reading should be rechecked in 6 months. In this instance the nurse should counsel the parents and the child about active lifestyle and diet changes and weight reduction if the child is overweight (National High Blood Pressure Education Program Working Group on High Blood Pressure in Children and Adolescents, 2004). If hypertensive (95th–99th percentile with the addition of 5 mmHg) the reading should be checked again on at least two occasions, usually within a few weeks to confirm the diagnosis of hypertension (National High Blood Pressure Education Program Working Group on High Blood Pressure in Children and Adolescents, 2004).

The nurse may also be the first health care professional to recognize unhealthy patterns of anger and anger expression. The nurse may be able to teach healthier means of expressing anger, such as anger reflection control, physical activity, or cognitive behavioral interventions (Rice & Howell, 2006). It is important to intervene in unhealthy lifestyles early rather than later when the disease becomes evident (Meininger et al., 2004; Solomon & Matthews, 1999). Lifestyle changes are more easily accomplished at early ages before behavior patterns become ingrained. If risk factors for cardiovascular disease are reduced early enough, cardiovascular disease will be delayed or avoided altogether. Early anger management training for children holds promise for preventing the translation of anger into medical and behavioral problems.

## Acknowledgment

This research was supported by grants from the College of Health Sciences, Georgia State University, Atlanta, Georgia.

## References

American Heart Association. (2004). Statistical supplement. Retrieved August 10, 2004, from http://www.americanheart.org.

Chang, P., Ford, D., Meoni, L., Wang, N., & Klag, M. (2002, Apr). Anger in young men and subsequent premature cardiovascular disease. *Archives of Internal Medicine, 162*(8), 901–906.

Cook, N., Gillman, M., Rosner, B., Taylor, J., & Hennekens, C. (2000). Combining annual blood pressure measurements in childhood to improve prediction of young adult blood pressure. *Statistics in Medicine, 19*(19), 2625–2640.

Couch, S., & Daniels, S. (2005). Diet and blood pressure in children. *Current Opinions in Pediatrics, 17*(5), 642–647.

Davis, C., Flickinger, B., Moore, D., Bassali, R., Domel Baxter, S., & Yin, Z. (2005, Aug). Prevalence of cardiovascular risk factors in schoolchildren in a rural Georgia community. *American Journal of Medicine and Science, 330*(2), 53–59.

Ewart, C., & Kolodner, K. (1994). Negative affect, gender and expressive style predict elevated ambulatory blood pressure in adolescents. *Journal of Personality and Social Psychology, 66*(3), 596–605.

Fabes, R., & Eisenberg, N. (1992). Young children's coping with interpersonal anger. *Child Development, 63*, 116–128.

Fuchs, D., & Thelen, M. (1988). Children's expected interpersonal consequences of communicating their affective state and reported likelihood of expression. *Childhood Development, 59*, 1314–1322.

Harburg, E., Blakelock, E., & Roeper, P. (1979). Resentful and reflective coping with arbitrary authority and blood pressure: Detroit. *Psychosomatic Medicine, 41*, 189–202.

Harburg, E., Gleiberman, L., Russell, M., & Cooper, M. (1991). Anger-coping styles and blood pressure in Black and White males: Buffalo, New York. *Psychosomatic Medicine, 41*, 189–202.

Hauber, R., Rice, M., Howell, C., & Carmon, M. (1998). Anger and blood pressure readings in children. *Psychosomatic Medicine, 11*(1), 2–11.

Heker, B., Whalen, C., Jamner, L., & Delfino, R. (2002, June). Anxiety, affect, and activity teenagers: Monitoring daily life with electronic diaries. *Journal of American Academy of Child and Adolescent Psychiatry, 41*(6), 660–670.

Jacobs, G., & Blumer, C. (1984). *The pediatric anger scale*. Vermillion: University of South Dakota, Department of Psychology.

Jacobs, G., & Mehlhaff, C. (1994). *Children's stress and the expression and experience and experience of anger*. Unpublished manuscript, University of South Dakota, Vermillion.

Jacobs, G., Phelps, M., & Rhors, B. (1989). Assessment of anger in children: The pediatric anger scale. *Personality and Individual Differences, 10*, 59–65.

Johnson, E. (1984). *Anger and anxiety as determinants of elevated blood pressure in adolescents: The Tampa study*. Unpublished doctoral dissertation, University of South Florida, Tampa.

Johnson, E. (1989). The role of the experience and expression of anger and anxiety in elevated blood pressure among black and white adolescents. *Journal of the National Medical Association, 81*(5), 573–584.

Johnson, E. (1990). Interrelationships between psychological factors, overweight, and blood pressure in adolescents. *Journal of Adolescent Healthcare, 11*, 310–318.

Jonas, B., Franks, P., & Ingram, D. (1997). Are symptoms of anxiety and depression risk factors for hypertension? *Archives of Family Medicine, 6*, 43–49.

Krantz, D., & Manuck, S. (1984). Acute psychophysiologic reactivity and risk of cardiovascular disease: A review and methodological critique. *Psychological Bulletin, 96*, 535–564.

Markovitz, J. H., Matthews, K., Wing, R. R., Kuller, L. H., & Meilahn, E. N. (1991). Psychological, biological and health behavior predictors of blood pressure changes in middle-aged women. *Journal of Hypertension, 9*, 399–406.

Meininger, J., Liehr, P., Chan, W., Smith, G., & Muller, W. (2004). Developmental, gender, and ethic group differences in moods and ambulatory blood pressure in adolescents. *Annals of Behavioral Medicine, 28*(1), 10–19.

Moran, C., Panzarino, V., Darden, P., & Reigart, J. (2003). Preventive services: Blood pressure checks at well child visits. *Clinical Pediatrics, 42*(7), 627–634.

Muller, W., Grunbaum, J., & Labarthe, D. (2001, Jul–Aug). Anger expression, body fat, and blood pressure in adolescents: Project HeartBeat. *American Journal of Human Biology, 13*(4), 531–538.

Muller, M., Wiechmann, M., Helms, C., Wulff, C., & Kolenda, K. (2000, May). Nutrient intake with low-fat diets in rehabilitation of patients with coronary heart disease. *Zeitschrift fur Kardiologie, 89*(5), 454–464.

National Heart, Lung, and Blood Institute. National Institutes of Health. (1996). *Update on the task force report on high blood pressure in children and adolescents: A working group report from the National High Blood Pressure Education Program (SDHSS Publication No. NIH 96-3790)*. Washington, DC: U.S. Government Printing Office. Children and Adolescents.

National High Blood Pressure Education Program Working Group on High Blood Pressure in Children and Adolescents. (2004). The fourth report on the diagnosis, evaluation, and treatment of high blood pressure in children and adolescents. *Pediatrics, 114*(2), 555–576.

Raikkonen, K., Matthews, K., & Kuller, L. (2001). Trajectory of psychological risk and incident of hypertension in middle-aged women. *Hypertension, 38*(4), 798–802.

Rice, M., & Howell, C. (2006). Differences in trait anger among children with varying levels of anger expression patterns. *Journal of Child and Adolescent Psychiatric Nursing, 19*(2), 51–61.

Russek, L., King, S., Russek, S., & Russek, H. (1990). The Harvard Mastery of Stress Study 35-year follow-up: Prognostic significance of patterns of psychophysiological arousal and adaptation. *Psychosomatic Medicine, 52*, 271–285.

Siegel, J. (1984). Anger and cardiovascular risk in adolescents. *Health Psychology, 3*, 293–313.

Siegel, J., & Leitch, C. (1981). Behavioral factors and blood pressure in adolescence: The Tacoma study. *American Journal of Epidemiology, 113*, 171–181.

Solomon, K., Matthews, K. (1999, March). *Paper presented at the American Psychosomatic Society Annual Meeting*. Vancouver, British Columbia, Canada.

Speilberger, C., Edwards, C., Lushene, R., Montuori, J., & Platzek, D. (1973). *State-trait anxiety inventory for children*. Palo Alto, CA: Consulting Psychologists Press.

Speilberger, C., Johnson, E., Russell, S., Crane, R., Jacobs, G., & Worden, T. (1985). The experience and expression of anger: Construction and validation of an anger expression scale. In M. Chesney, R. Rosenman, (Eds.), *Anger and hostility in cardiovascular and behavioral disorders* (pp. 5–30). Washington, DC: Hemisphere.

Starner, T., & Peters, R. (2004). Anger expression and blood pressure in adolescents. *Journal of School Nursing, 20*(6), 335–342.

Suls, J., & Wan, C. (1993). The relationship between trait hostility and cardiovascular reactivity: A quantitative review and analysis. *Psychophysiology, 30*, 615–626 http://www.nhlbi.nih.gov/meetings/ish/stamler.htm.

Taylor, S., Repetti, R., & Seeman, T. (1997). Health psychology: What is an unhealthy environment and how does it get under the skin? *Annual Review of Psychology, 48*, 411–447.

Thomas, S. (1997). Women's anger: Relationship of suppression to blood pressure. *Nursing Research, 46*(6), 324–330.

Waked, E., & Jutai, J. (1990). Baseline and reactivity measures of blood pressure and negative affect in borderline hypertension. *Physiological Behavior, 47*, 266–271.

Wascher, R. (2002, April). Stay at home dads and risk of cardiovascular disease. *Jewish World Review* 2002, April.

Weinrich, S., Weinrich, M., Hardin, S., Gleaton, J., Pesut, D., & Garrison, C. (2000). Effects of psychological distress on blood pressure in adolescents. *Holistic Nurse Practitioner, 5*(1), 57–65.

Williams, R., & Williams, V. (1993). *Anger kills*. New York: Harper Collins Publishers.

Wyllie, R. (2005). Obesity in childhood: An overview. *Current Opinions Pediatrics, 17*(5), 632–635.

# Subsequent Childbirth After a Previous Traumatic Birth

Cheryl Tatano Beck ▼ Sue Watson

▶ **Background:** Nine percent of new mothers in the United States who participated in the Listening to Mothers II Postpartum Survey screened positive for meeting the *Diagnostic and Statistical Manual of Mental Disorders, Fourth Edition* criteria for posttraumatic stress disorder after childbirth. Women who have had a traumatic birth experience report fewer subsequent children and a longer length of time before their second baby. Childbirth-related posttraumatic stress disorder impacts couples' physical relationship, communication, conflict, emotions, and bonding with their children.

▶ **Objective:** The purpose of this study was to describe the meaning of women's experiences of a subsequent childbirth after a previous traumatic birth.

▶ **Methods:** Phenomenology was the research design used. An international sample of 35 women participated in this Internet study. Women were asked, "Please describe in as much detail as you can remember your subsequent pregnancy, labor, and delivery following your previous traumatic birth." Colaizzi's phenomenological data analysis approach was used to analyze the stories of the 35 women.

▶ **Results:** Data analysis yielded four themes: (a) riding the turbulent wave of panic during pregnancy; (b) strategizing: attempts to reclaim their body and complete the journey to motherhood; (c) bringing reverence to the birthing process and empowering women; and (d) still elusive: the longed-for healing birth experience.

▶ **Discussion:** Subsequent childbirth after a previous birth trauma has the potential to either heal or retraumatize women. During pregnancy, women need permission and encouragement to grieve their prior traumatic births to help remove the burden of their invisible pain.

▶ **Key Words:** phenomenology · posttraumatic stress disorder (PTSD) · subsequent childbirth · traumatic childbirth

I n the United States, 9% of new mothers who participated in the Listening to Mothers II Postpartum Follow-Up Survey screened positive for meeting the *Diagnostic and Statistical Manual of Mental Disorders, Fourth Edition* (American Psychiatric Association, 2000) criteria for posttraumatic stress disorder (PTSD) after childbirth (Declercq, Sakala, Corry, & Applebaum, 2008). In this survey, the mothers' voices revealed a troubling pattern of maternity care.

A large percentage of women giving birth in the United States experienced hospital care that did not reflect the best evidence for practice nor for women's preferences. The Institute of Medicine (2003) identified childbirth as a national healthcare priority for quality improvement. A maternity care quality chasm still exists (Sakala & Corry, 2007).

Researchers and healthcare professionals at an international meeting on current issues regarding PTSD after childbirth recommended the need for research focusing on women's subjective birth experiences (Ayers, Joseph, McKenzie-McHarg, Slade, & Wijma, 2008). Olde, van der Hart, Kleber, and van Son (2006) called for examining the chronic nature of childbirth-related posttraumatic stress lasting longer than 6 months after birth.

The purpose of the current study was to help fill the knowledge gap of one aspect of the chronicity of birth trauma: women's subjective experiences of the subsequent pregnancy, labor, and delivery after a traumatic childbirth.

## Review of Literature

Traumatic childbirth is defined as "an event occurring during the labor and delivery process that involves actual or threatened serious injury or death to the mother or her infant. The birthing woman experiences intense fear, helplessness, loss of control, and horror" (Beck, 2004a, p. 28). For some women, a traumatic birth also involves perceiving their birthing experience as dehumanizing and stripping them of their dignity (Beck, 2004a, 2004b, 2006). After a traumatic childbirth, 2% to 21% of women meet the diagnostic criteria for PTSD (Ayers, 2004; Ayers, Harris, Sawyer, Parfitt, & Ford, 2009), involving the development of three characteristic symptoms stemming from the exposure to the trauma: persistent reexperiencing of the traumatic event, persistent avoiding of reminders of the trauma and a numbing of general responsiveness, and persistent increased arousal (American Psychiatric Association, 2000).

### Risk Factors

Risk factors contributing to women perceiving their childbirth as traumatic can be divided into three categories: prenatal factors, nature and circumstances of the delivery,

*Cheryl Tatano Beck, DNSc, CNM, FAAN, is Distinguished Professor, School of Nursing, University of Connecticut, Storrs.*

*Sue Watson, is Chairperson, Trauma and Birth Stress, Auckland, New Zealand.*

and subjective factors during childbirth (van Son, Verkerk, van der Hart, Komproe, & Pop, 2005). Under the prenatal category are factors such as histories of previous traumatic births, prenatal PTSD (Onoye, Goebert, Morland, Matsu, & Wright, 2009), child sexual abuse, and psychiatric counseling. Factors included in the category of nature and circumstances of the delivery include a high level of medical intervention, extremely painful labor and delivery, and delivery type (Ayers et al., 2009). Subjective risk factors during childbirth can include feelings of powerlessness, lack of caring and support from labor and delivery staff, and fear of dying (Thomson & Downe, 2008).

> *A large percentage of women giving birth in the United States experienced hospital care that did not reflect the best evidence for practice nor for women's preferences.*

▼▼▼

### Long-Term Impact of Traumatic Childbirth

Researchers are uncovering an unsettling gamut of long-term detrimental effects of traumatic childbirth not only on the mothers themselves but also on their relationships with infants and other family members. Mothers' breastfeeding experiences and the yearly anniversary of their birth trauma can also be negatively impacted.

Impaired mother–infant relationships after traumatic childbirth are being confirmed in the literature. For example, in the study of Ayers, Wright, and Wells (2007) of mothers who experienced birth trauma in the United Kingdom, women described themselves as feeling detached and having feelings of rejection toward their infants. Nicholls and Ayers (2007) reported two different types of mother–infant bonding in couples who shared that PTSD after childbirth affected their relationships with their children; they became anxious/overprotective or avoidant/rejecting. Childbirth-related PTSD also impacted their relationships with their partners, including their physical relationship, communication, conflict, emotions, support, and coping.

Long-term detrimental effects of traumatic childbirth can extend also into women's breastfeeding experiences. In their Internet study, Beck and Watson (2008) explored the impact of birth trauma on the breastfeeding experiences of 52 mothers. For some mothers, their traumatic childbirth led to distressing impediments that curtailed their breastfeeding attempts, such as feeling that their breasts were just one more thing to be violated.

Another aspect of the chronic effect of birth trauma was identified in Beck's (2006) Internet study of the anniversary of traumatic childbirth, an invisible phenomenon that mothers struggled with. Thirty-seven women comprised this international sample of mothers from the United States, New Zealand, Australia, United Kingdom, and Canada. Beck concluded that a failure to rescue occurred for women as the anniversary approached, and all others focused on the celebration of the children's birthdays. This failure to rescue led to unnecessary emotional or physical suffering or both.

Catherall (1998) warned of secondary trauma in families living with trauma survivors. The entire family is vulnerable to becoming secondarily traumatized. The long-term impact of trauma does not result necessarily in PTSD symptoms in family members. Catherall stated that it can have a more insidious effect of a disturbing milieu in the family. The members of the family may be close physically, but their ability to express emotions is limited. True closeness in the family is missing, and their problem solving is impaired. Abrams (1999) identified one of the central clinical characteristics of intergenerational transmission of trauma is the silence that happens in families regarding traumatic experiences. Abrams pleaded that the multigenerational impact of trauma should not be underestimated.

### Posttraumatic Growth

Researchers are reporting that traumatic experiences can have positive benefits in a person's life. Posttraumatic growth has been documented in a wide range of people who faced traumatic experiences such as bereaved parents (Engelkemeyer & Marwit, 2008), human immunodeficiency virus caregivers (Cadell, 2007), and homeless women with histories of traumatic experiences (Stump & Smith, 2008). "Posttraumatic growth describes the experience of individuals whose development, at least in some areas, has surpassed what was present before the struggle with the crisis occurred. The individual has not only survived, but has experienced changes that are viewed as important, and that go beyond what was the previous status quo" (Tedeschi & Calhoun, 2004, p. 4). It is not the actual trauma that is responsible for posttraumatic growth but what happens after the trauma. Tedeschi and Calhoun (2004, p. 6) proposed five domains of posttraumatic growth: "greater appreciation of life and changed sense of priorities; warmer, more intimate relationships with others; a greater sense of personal strength; recognition of new possibilities or paths for one's life; and spiritual development."

Childbirth can have an enormous potential to help change how a woman feels about herself and can impact her transition to motherhood (Levy, 2006). Attias and Goodwin (1999, p. 299) noted that a woman who survives a traumatic experience may be able to rebuild her wounded inner self "by having a child, transforming her body from a container of ashes to a container for a new human life." A positive childbirth has the potential to empower a traumatized woman and help her reclaim her life.

One study was located that touched on the positive growth of women after a previous negative birthing experience. In Cheyney's (2008) qualitative study of women in the United States who chose home births after experiencing a negative birth, three integrated conceptual themes emerged from their home birth narratives: knowledge, power, and intimacy. The power of their home births helped heal scars of their past hospital births. Positive growth after birth trauma has yet to be investigated systematically by researchers.

One of the knowledge gaps identified in this literature review focused on an aspect of the long-term effects of birth trauma: mothers' subsequent childbirth. This phenomenological study was designed to answer the research question:

What is the meaning of women's experiences of a subsequent childbirth following a previous traumatic birth?

## Methods

### Research Design

The term *phenomenology* is derived from the Greek word *phenomenon*, which means "to show itself." The goal of phenomenology is to describe human experiences as they are experienced consciously without theories about their cause and as free as possible from the researchers' unexamined presuppositions about the phenomenon under study. In phenomenology, researchers "borrow" other individuals' experiences to better understand the deeper meaning of the phenomenon (Van Manen, 1984).

The existential phenomenological method developed by Colaizzi (1973, 1978) was used in this Internet study. His method is designed to uncover the fundamental structure of a phenomenon, that is, the essence of an experience. An assumption of phenomenology is that for any phenomenon, there are essential structures that comprise that human experience. Only by examining specific experiences of the phenomenon being studied can their essential structures be uncovered.

Colaizzi's (1973, 1978) method includes features of Husserl's and Heidegger's philosophies. Colaizzi maintains that description is the key to discovering the essence and the meaning of a phenomenon and that phenomenology is presuppositionless (Husserl, 1954). Colaizzi, however, holds a Heideggerian view of reduction, the process of researchers bracketing presuppositions and their natural attitude about the phenomenon being studied. For Colaizzi (1978, p. 58), researchers identify their presuppositions regarding the phenomenon under study not to bracket them off to the side but instead to use them to "interrogate" one's "beliefs, hypotheses, attitudes, and hunches" about the phenomenon to help formulate research questions. Colaizzi agrees with Merleau-Ponty (1956, p. 64) that "the greatest lesson of reduction is the impossibility of a complete reduction." Individual phenomenological reflection about the phenomenon being studied is one approach Colaizzi (1973) offers for assisting researchers to decrease the coloring of their presuppositions and biases on their research activity.

Because the phenomenon of subsequent childbirth after a previous traumatic birth had not been examined systematically before this current study, description of the meaning of women's experiences was the focus of this study. Before the start of the study, the researchers undertook an individual phenomenological reflection. They questioned themselves regarding their presuppositions about the phenomenon of subsequent childbirth after a traumatic birth and how these might influence what and how they conducted their research.

### Sample

Thirty-five women participated in the study (Table 1). Saturation of data was achieved easily with this sample size. Their mean age was 33 years (range = 27 to 51 years). All the participants were Caucasian and had two to four children. The length of time since their previous birth trauma to the subsequent birth ranged from 1 to 13 years. Eight of the 35 women (23%) opted for a home birth for their

**TABLE 1. Demographic and Obstetric Characteristics**

| | n | % |
|---|---|---|
| Country | | |
| United States | 15 | 43 |
| United Kingdom | 8 | 23 |
| New Zealand | 6 | 17 |
| Australia | 5 | 14 |
| Canada | 1 | 3 |
| Marital status | | |
| Married | 34 | 98 |
| Divorced | 1 | 2 |
| Single | 0 | 0 |
| Education | | |
| High school | 3 | 9 |
| Some college | 5 | 15 |
| College degree | 13 | 38 |
| Graduate | 7 | 19 |
| Missing | 7 | 19 |
| Delivery | | |
| Vaginal | 25 | 72 |
| Cesarean | 10 | 29 |
| Diagnosed PTSD | | |
| Yes | 14 | 40 |
| No | 19 | 55 |
| Missing | 2 | 5 |
| Currently under care of therapist | | |
| Yes | 8 | 23 |
| No | 22 | 63 |
| Missing | 5 | 15 |

*Note.* PTSD = posttraumatic stress disorder.

subsequent births. Of these 8 mothers who gave birth at home, 4 lived in Australia, 3 in the United States, and 1 in the United Kingdom. Fourteen mothers (40%) had been diagnosed with PTSD after childbirth.

All the birth traumas were self-defined. Women were not asked if they had experienced other traumas before their birth traumas. Therefore, this was not an exclusionary criterion. The most frequently identified traumatic births focused on emergency cesarean deliveries, postpartum hemorrhage, severe preeclampsia, preterm labor, high level of medical interventions (i.e., forceps, vacuum extraction, induction), infant in the neonatal intensive care unit, feeling violated, lack or respectful treatment, unsympathetic, nonsupportive labor and delivery staff, and "emotional torture."

### Procedure

Once institutional review board approval was obtained from the university, recruitment began. Data collection continued for 2 years and 2 months. Women were recruited by means of a notice placed on the Web site of Trauma and Birth Stress (TABS; www.tabs.org.nz), a charitable trust located in New Zealand. The mission of TABS is to support women who have experienced traumatic childbirth and PTSD because of their birth trauma. The sample criteria required that the mother had experienced a traumatic childbirth with a previous labor and delivery, that she was willing to articulate her experience, and that she could read and write English. This international representation of participants was a strength of this recruitment method. A disadvantage, however, was that only women who had access to the Internet and who used TABS for support participated in this study.

Women who were interested in participating in this Internet study contacted the first author at her university e-mail address, which was listed on the recruitment notice. An information sheet and directions for the study were sent by attachment to interested mothers. After reading these two documents, women could e-mail the researcher if they had any questions concerning the study.

Women were asked, "Please describe in as much detail as you can remember your subsequent pregnancy, labor, and delivery following your previous traumatic birth." Women sent their descriptions of their experiences as e-mail attachments to the researcher. The sending of their story implied their informed consent. The length of time varied from when a mother first e-mailed about her interest in the study to when she sent her completed story to the researchers. The shortest turn-around time was 2 days whereas the longest was 9 months. If women did not respond within a certain period, the researchers did not recontact them. The women's wish not to follow through on participation in the study was respected. Throughout this procedure, the first author kept a reflexive journal.

**Data Analysis**

Colaizzi's (1978) method of data analysis was used. The order of his steps is as follows: written protocols, significant statements, formulated meanings, clusters of themes, exhaustive description, and fundamental structure. It should be noted, however, that these steps do overlap. From each participant's description of the phenomenon, significant statements, which are phrases or sentences that directly describe the phenomenon, are extracted (Table 2). For each significant statement, the researcher formulates its meaning. Here, creative insight is called into play. Colaizzi cautioned that in this step of data analysis, the researcher must take a precarious leap from what the participants said to what they mean. Formulated meanings should never sever all connections from the original transcripts. It is in this step of formulating meanings that Colaizzi's connection to Heidegger can be seen. The next step entails organizing all the formulated meanings into clusters of themes. At this point, all the results to date are combined into an exhaustive description. This step is followed by revising the exhaustive description into a more condensed statement of the identification of the fundamental structure of the phenomenon being studied. The fundamental structure can be shared with the participants to validate how well it captured aspects of their experiences. If any participants share new data, they are integrated into the final description of the phenomenon. Member checking was done with one participant who reviewed the themes and

| No. | Significant statements |
|---|---|
| | **TABLE 2. Example of Extracting Significant Statements** |
| 1 | One thing that I'd noticed when I was a child was that when my parents got together with other adults, the talk eventually turned to two things: for my father (a Vietnam veteran) and the other men the talk turned to the war and interestingly, to me as a small child, for my mother and the other women the talk always turned to childbirth. |
| 2 | It was as if, from a young age, for me, the connections between the two were drawn. A man is tested through war, a women is tested through childbirth. |
| 3 | My dad, as abusive as he was, was considered a "good man" because he'd been a good soldier and so, I reasoned forward with a child's intelligence, that all that really mattered for a woman was to be strong and capable in childbirth. |
| 4 | And I failed. In the past, with the previous two births (particularly with the one that resulted in PTSD)—that's what it felt like. I failed at being a woman. |
| 5 | I don't think that I am alone in feeling. I have a sneaking suspicion that this is pretty universal. |
| 6 | Just as a man who "talks" under torture in a POW situation feels as though he's failed, a woman who can't "handle" tortuous situations during childbirth feels like she's failed. It is not true. But it feels true. |
| 7 | My dad received two Purple Hearts and a Bronze Star during Vietnam. He, by most standards, would be considered a hero. Where are my Purple Hearts? My Bronze Star? I've fought a war, no less terrifying, no less destroying but there are no accolades. At least that's what it feels like. |
| 8 | I am viewed as flawed if not down right strange that I find L & D so terrifying. |
| 9 | The medical establishment thinks that I am "mental" and I have no common ground on which to discuss my childbirth experiences with "normal" women. |
| 10 | I know, I've tried. And that makes me feel isolated and inferior. |

*Note.* PTSD = posttraumatic stress disorder.

totally agreed with them. In addition, one mother who had not participated in the study but had experienced the phenomenon being studied reviewed the findings and also agreed with them.

## Results

The researchers reflected on the written descriptions provided by the 35 women to explicate the phenomenon of their experiences of subsequent childbirth after a previous traumatic birth. These reflections yielded 274 significant statements that were clustered into four themes and finally into the fundamental structure that identified the essence of this phenomenon (Table 3).

### Theme 1: Riding the Turbulent Wave of Panic During Pregnancy

Fear, terror, anxiety, panic, dread, and denial were the most frequent terms used to describe the world women lived in during their pregnancy after a previous traumatic birth.

I remember the exact moment I realized what was happening. I was on my lunch break at work, sitting under a large oak tree, watching cars go by my office, talking with my husband. I suddenly knew… I am pregnant again! I remember the exact angle of the sun, the shading of the objects around me. I remember looking into the sun, at that tree, at the windows to the office thinking, "NO! God PLEASE NO!" I felt my chest at once sink inward on me and take on the weight of a 1000 bricks. I was short of breath, my head seared. All I could think of was "NOOOOOOOOOO!"

Another woman described in detail the day she took her pregnancy test.

I took the test and crumpled over the edge of our bed, sobbing and retching hysterically for hours. I was dizzy. I was nauseous. I was sick. I could not breathe. I thought my chest would implode. I had a terrible migraine. I could not move from the spot where I had crumpled. I could not talk to my husband or see our daughter. I felt torn to pieces, shredded as shards of glass. I spent the next 2 trimesters hanging on for my life with suicidal

thoughts but no real desire to carry them out through. I wanted to see my little girl. It was hell on earth.

Some women went into denial during the first trimester of their pregnancy to cope. Throughout her pregnancy, one woman revealed that she "felt numb to my baby." Some women described how they turned their denial of pregnancy into something positive. One multipara explained that after she was in denial for a few months, she then became determined to make things different this next time, and right at the end of her pregnancy she felt empowered by all that she had learned: "After 3 months of ignoring the fact that I was going to have to go through birth again, I decided I would treat my next labor and delivery as a healing and empowering experience."

Other mothers remained in a heightened state of anxiety throughout their pregnancy, and for some this anxiety escalated to panic and terror. Knowing she may have to go through the same "emotional torture" she endured with her previous traumatic birth, one woman shared, "My 9 months of pregnancy were an anxiety filled abyss which was completely marred as an experience due to the terror that was continually in my mind from my experience 8 years earlier." As the delivery date got closer, some mothers reported having panic attacks.

### Theme 2: Strategizing: Attempts to Reclaim Their Body and Complete the Journey to Motherhood

"Well, this time; I told myself *things would be different*. I actually started planning for this birth literally while they were stitching me up from the traumatic first birth." During pregnancy women described a number of different strategies they used to help them survive the 9 months of pregnancy while waiting for what they were dreading: labor and delivery (Table 4). Some women spent time nurturing themselves by swimming, walking, going to yoga classes, and spending time outdoors.

Keeping a journal throughout the pregnancy helped mothers because they had somewhere to write things down, especially if they felt that family and friends did not understand just how difficult this pregnancy, subsequent to their prior traumatic delivery, was. Inspirational quotes were placed around the house to read and motivate women.

---

| TABLE 3. Fundamental Structure of the Phenomenon |
| --- |
| Subsequent childbirth after a previous traumatic birth far exceeds the confines of the actual labor and delivery. During the 9 months of pregnancy, women ride turbulent waves of panic, terror, and fear that the looming birth could be a repeat of the emotional and/or physical torture they had endured with their previous labor and delivery. Women strategized during pregnancy how they could reclaim their bodies that had been violated and traumatized by their previous childbirth. Women vowed to themselves that things would be different and that this time they would complete their journey to motherhood. Mothers employed strategies to try to bring a reverence to the birthing process and rectify all that had gone so wrong with their prior childbirth. The array of various strategies entailed such actions as hiring doulas for support during labor and delivery, becoming avid readers of childbirth books, writing a detailed birth plan, learning birth hypnosis, interviewing obstetricians and midwives about their philosophy of birth, doing yoga, and drawing birthing art. All these well-designed strategies did not ensure that all women would experience the healing childbirth they desperately longed for. For the mothers whose subsequent childbirth was a healing experience, they reclaimed their bodies, had a strong sense of control, and their birth became an empowering experience. The role of caring supporters was crucial in their labor and delivery. Women were treated with respect, dignity, and compassion. Although their subsequent birth was positive and empowering, women were quick to note that it could never change the past. Still elusive for some women was their longed-for healing subsequent birth. |

**TABLE 4. Strategies Used to Cope With Pregnancy and Looming Labor and Delivery**

- Writing a detailed birth plan
- Mentally preparing for birth
- Learning birth hypnosis
- Doing birth art
- Writing positive affirmations
- Preparing for birthing at home
- Hiring a doula for labor and delivery
- Celebrating upcoming birth
- Avoiding ultrasounds
- Trying not to think about upcoming birth
- Reading books on healthy pregnancy and birth
- Mapping out your pelvis
- Learning birthing positions to open up the pelvis
- Practicing hypnosis for labor
- Researching birth centers and scheduling tours
- Interviewing obstetricians and midwives
- Exercising to help baby get in the correct position
- Using Internet support group
- Hiring a life coach
- Painting previous birth experience
- Creating "what if" sheet with all possible concerns and then solutions for them
- Creating "Yes, if necessary No" sheet for labor of what the mother wanted to happen
- Determining role of supporters during birth
- Researching homeopathic remedies to prepare body for labor and birth
- Developing a tool kit to help cope in labor
- Developing trust with healthcare provider

Figure 1 is an illustration of one mother's poster that she put up in her home.

Women strategized how to ensure that their looming labor and delivery was not another traumatic one. As one multipara explained, "I need to bring a reverence to the process so I won't feel like a piece of meat lost in the system." Attempts were made to put into place a plan that would attempt to rectify all that had gone wrong with the previous childbirth. Some women turned to doulas in hopes of being supported during their subsequent labor and delivery. Hypnobirthing was a plan used by some women to keep the first traumatic birth from being repeated.

Women reported reading avidly to understand the birth process fully. The most frequently cited books were *Rebounding from Childbirth* (Madsen, 1994), *Birthing from Within* (England & Horowitz, 1998), and *Birth and Beyond* (Gordon, 2002). Mothers often engaged in birth art exercises.

Toward the end of pregnancy I did the birth art exercises out of the book *Birthing from Within*... I began to trust myself. That will stay with me forever. That is more than

just what I needed to birth the way I wanted to. That is what I needed to become a real woman.

Opening up to their healthcare providers about their previous traumatic births was helpful for some mothers. Once clinicians knew of their history, they would address the mothers' concerns during each prenatal visit. Also sharing with their partners their fears and insecurities around pregnancy and birth helped women's emotional preparedness.

**Theme 3: Bringing Reverence to the Birthing Process and Empowering Women**

Three quarters of the women who participated in this Internet study reported that their subsequent labor and delivery was either a "healing experience" or at least "a lot better" than their previous traumatic birth. Women became more confident in themselves as women and as mothers in that they really did know what was best for their babies and themselves. The role of supporters throughout labor and delivery was crucial. What was it that made a subsequent birth a healing experience? In the mothers' own words:

I was treated with respect, my wishes and those of my husband were listened to. I wasn't made to feel like a piece of meat this time but instead like a woman experiencing one of nature's most wonderful events.

Pain relief was taken seriously. First time around I was ignored. I begged and pleaded for pain relief. Second time it was offered but because I was made to feel in control, I was able to decline.

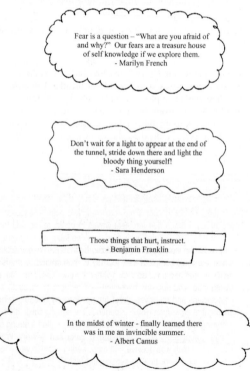

**FIGURE 1.** A poster of inspirational quotes by one mother.

I wasn't rushed! My baby was allowed to arrive when she was ready. When my first was born, I was told "5 minutes or I get the forceps" by the doctor on call. I pushed so hard that I tore badly.

Communication with labor and delivery staff was so much better the second time. The first time the emergency cord was pulled but no one told me why. I thought my baby was dead and no one would elaborate.

Women reclaimed their bodies, had a strong sense of control, and birth became an empowering experience. Only essential fetal monitoring and minimal medical intervention occurred. Women were allowed to start labor on their own and not be induced. Under gentle supervision of caring and supportive healthcare professionals, women were reassured to just do what their body felt like doing and to follow their body's lead. The number of vaginal examinations was kept at a minimum, and women were permitted to walk around and choose the position they felt best laboring in. One mother described her healing birth:

I pushed my baby into the world and I was shocked. I had never dared to dream for such a perfect delivery. They let me push spontaneously and my baby was delivered into my arms. My husband and I both cried with utter relief that I had given birth exactly how I wanted to and my trauma was healed.

For some women, the birth plan they had prepared during their pregnancy was honored by the labor and delivery staff, which helped them feel like they had some control and were a part of the birth and not just a witness.

Eight women opted for home births after their previous traumatic births, and for six of them, it did end in fulfilling their dream.

It was as healing and empowering as I had always hoped for. I did not want any high tech management. My home birth was the proudest day of my life and the victory was sweeter because I overcame so very much to come to it.

Another mother who had a successful home birth labored mostly in her bedroom under candlelight and music playing. She described it as very peaceful being at home surrounded by all her things. Her dog kept vigil by her side. She shared how it was such a gentle way for her baby to be born.

My baby cried for a minute or two as if telling me his birth story and crawled up my body and found my heart and left breast. My heart swelled with so many emotions—love, joy, happiness, pride, relief, and wonderment.

A couple of women explained that their subsequent birth was healing, but at the same time they mourned what they had missed out with their prior birth. The following quote illustrates this.

Even though it was an enormously healing experience, the expectations I had were unrealistic. What I went through during and after my first delivery cannot be erased from memory. If anything with this second birth being so wonderful, it makes dealing with my first birth harder. It makes it sadder and me angrier as before I had nothing to compare it to. I didn't know how different it could be or

how special those first few moments are. I didn't fully understand what I had missed out on. So now 3 years later I find myself grieving again for what we went through, how I was treated and what I missed out on.

Other mothers admitted that although their subsequent births were healing, they could never change the past.

All the positive, empowering births in the world won't ever change what happened with my first baby and me. Our relationship is forever built around his birth experience. The second birth was so wonderful I would go through it all again, but it can never change the past.

### Theme 4: Still Elusive: The Longed-for Healing Birth Experience

Sadly, some mothers did not experience the healing subsequent birth they had hoped for. Two women chose to try a home birth after their previous traumatic birth but did not end up with the healing experience they longed for. One mother did deliver at home, but because of postpartum hemorrhage, she was transported by ambulance to the hospital, terrified she would not live to raise her baby. After laboring at home, another multipara who attempted a vaginal birth after cesarean needed to be transported by ambulance for a repeat cesarean birth after she failed to progress.

When the ambulance arrived I felt rescued. I have never been so grateful that hospitals exist. The blue light ambulance journey was terrifying and I was in excruciating pain. By this point I was trying to detach my head from my body, as I had done years earlier when I was being raped.

She went on to vividly describe that as she lay on the operating table:

…with my legs held in the air by 2 strangers while a third mopped the blood between my legs I felt raped all over again. I wanted to die. I had failed as a woman. My privacy had been invaded again. I felt sick.

One multipara shared that although this birth had been a better experience, she would not say it was healing in relation to her first birth that had been so traumatic. "The contrast in the way I was treated just emphasized how bad the first one was. I had no sense of healing until 30 years later when I received counseling for PTSD."

### Discussion

Healthcare professionals' failure to rescue women during their previous traumatic childbirth can result in a troubling effect on mothers as they courageously face another pregnancy, labor, and delivery. Subsequent childbirth after a previous birth trauma provides clinicians with not only a golden opportunity but also a professional responsibility to help these traumatized women reclaim their bodies and complete their journey to motherhood.

To help women prepare for a subsequent childbirth after a previous traumatic birth, clinicians first need to identify who these women are. There are instruments available to screen women for posttraumatic stress symptoms due to birth trauma. An essential part of initial prenatal visits should be taking time to discuss with women their previous births. Traumatized women need permission and encouragement to grieve their prior traumatic births to help remove the burden of their invisible pain. Pregnancy is a valuable time for healthcare professionals to help women recognize and deal with unresolved, buried, or traumatic issues. Women should be asked about their hopes and fears for their impending labor and delivery and how they envision this birth. If a woman is exploring the possibility of a home birth, clinicians should question the mother about her previous births. Opting for a home birth may be an indication of a prior traumatic birth (Cheyney, 2008). If women need mental health follow-up during their pregnancy, cognitive behavior therapy and eye movement desensitization reprocessing treatment are two options for PTSD because of birth trauma. Treatment can be given in conjunction with a woman's family members to address secondary effects of PTSD.

Strategies can be employed to help mothers heal and increase their confidence before labor and delivery. Clinicians can share with mothers the Web site for TABS (www. tabs.org.nz), a charitable trust in New Zealand that provides support for women who have suffered through a traumatic birth. Obstetric care providers can suggest to the women some of the numerous strategies that mothers in this study described using during their pregnancies. Women can be encouraged to write down their previous traumatic birth stories. Mothers can share their written stories with their current obstetric care providers so that they understand these women. Some women who participated in this study revealed that birthing artwork definitely helped them prepare for their subsequent labor and delivery after a traumatic childbirth.

Some women in this study touched on one of Tedeschi and Calhoun's (2004) domains of posttraumatic growth, a sense of personal growth. These women revealed feelings of empowerment and of reclaiming their bodies with their subsequent childbirths. Future research needs to be focused specifically on examining the five domains of posttraumatic growth in women who have experienced a subsequent childbirth after a previous birth trauma.

When women are traumatized during childbirth, this can leave a lasting imprint on their lives. If subsequent childbirth has the potential to either heal or retraumatize women, healthcare professionals need to be carefully aware of the consequences their words and actions during labor and delivery can have (Levy, 2006). ▼

---

Accepted for publication January 27, 2010.

To all the courageous women who shared their most personal and powerful stories of their subsequent childbirth after a previous traumatic birth, the authors are forever indebted.

Corresponding author: Cheryl Tatano Beck, DNSc, CNM, FAAN, School of Nursing, University of Connecticut, 231 Glenbrook Road, Storrs, CT 06269–2026 (e-mail: cheryl.beck@uconn.edu).

## References

Abrams, M. S. (1999). Intergenerational transmission of trauma: Recent contributions from the literature of family systems approaches to treatment. *American Journal of Psychotherapy, 53*(2), 225–231.

American Psychiatric Association. (2000). *Diagnostic and Statistical Manual of Mental Disorders—text revision.* Washington, DC: Author.

Attias, R., & Goodwin, J. M. (1999). A place to begin: Images of the body in transformation (pp. 287–303). In J. M. Goodwin & R. Attias (Eds.). *Splintered reflections.* New York: Basic Books.

Ayers, S. (2004). Delivery as a traumatic event: Prevalence, risk factors, and treatment for postnatal posttraumatic stress disorder. *Clinical Obstetrics and Gynecology, 47*(3), 552–567.

Ayers, S., Harris, R., Sawyer, A., Parfitt, Y., & Ford, E. (2009). Posttraumatic stress disorder after childbirth: Analysis of symptom presentation and sampling. *Journal of Affective Disorders, 119*(1–3), 200–204.

Ayers, S., Joseph, S., McKenzie-McHarg, K., Slade, P., & Wijma, K. (2008). Post-traumatic stress disorder following childbirth: Current issues and recommendations for future research. *Journal of Psychosomatic Obstetrics and Gynaecology, 29*(4), 240–250.

Ayers, S., Wright, D. B., & Wells, N. (2007). Symptoms of posttraumatic stress disorder in couples after birth: Association with the couple's relationship and parent-baby bond. *Journal of Reproductive and Infant Psychology, 25*(1), 40–50.

Beck, C. T. (2004a). Birth trauma: In the eye of the beholder. *Nursing Research, 53*(1), 28–35.

Beck, C. T. (2004b). Posttraumatic stress disorder due to childbirth: The aftermath. *Nursing Research, 53*(4), 216–224.

Beck, C. T. (2006). The anniversary of birth trauma: Failure to rescue. *Nursing Research, 55*(6), 381–390.

Beck, C. T., & Watson, S. (2008). Impact of birth trauma on breast-feeding: A tale of two pathways. *Nursing Research, 57*(4), 228–236.

Cadell, S. (2007). The sun always comes out after it rains: Understanding posttraumatic growth in HIV caregivers. *Health & Social Work, 32*(3), 169–176.

Catherall, D. R. (1998). Treating traumatized families. In C. R. Figley (Ed.). *Burnout in families: The systematic costs of caring* (pp. 187–215). Boca Raton, FL: CRC Press.

Cheyney, M. J. (2008). Homebirth as systems-challenging praxis: Knowledge, power, and intimacy in the birthplace. *Qualitative Health Research, 18*(2), 254–267.

Colaizzi, P. F. (1973). *Reflection and research in psychology: A phenomenological study of learning.* Dubuque, IA; Kendall/Hunt Publishing Company.

Colaizzi, P. F. (1978). Psychological research as the phenomenologist views it. In R. Valle & M. King (Eds.). *Existential phenomenological alternatives for psychology* (pp. 48–71). New York: Oxford University Press.

Declercq, E. R., Sakala, C., Corry, M. P., & Applebaum, S. (2008). *New mothers speak out: National survey results highlight women's postpartum experience.* New York: Childbirth Connection.

Engelkemeyer, S. M., & Marwit, S. J. (2008). Posttraumatic growth in bereaved parents. *Journal of Traumatic Stress, 21*(3), 344–346.

England, P., & Horowitz, R. (1998). *Birthing from within.* Alburquerque, NM: Partera Press.

Gordon, Y. (2002). *Birth and beyond.* London: Vermilion.

Husserl, E. (1954). *The crisis of European sciences and transcendental phenomenology.* The Hague: Martinus Nijhoff.

Institute of Medicine. (2003). *Board on Health Care Services Committee on identifying priority areas for quality improvements.* Washington, DC: National Academy Press.

Levy, M. (2006). Maternity in the wake of terrorism: Rebirth or retraumatization? *Journal of Prenatal and Perinatal Psychology and Health, 20*(3), 221–249.

Madsen, L. (1994). *Rebounding from childbirth: Toward emotional recovery.* Westport, CT: Bergin & Garvey.

Merleau-Ponty, M. (1956). What is phenomenology? *Crosscurrents, 6,* 59–70.

Nicholls, K., & Ayers, S. (2007). Childbirth-related post-traumatic stress disorder in couples: A qualitative study. *British Journal of Health Psychology, 12*(Pt. 4), 491–509.

Olde, E., van der Hart, O., Kleber, R., & van Son, M. (2006). Post-traumatic stress following childbirth: A review. *Clinical Psychology Review, 26*(1), 1–16.

Onoye, J. M., Goebert, D., Morland, L., Matsu, C., & Wright, T. (2009). PTSD and postpartum mental health in a sample of Caucasian, Asian, and Pacific Islander women. *Archives of Women's Mental Health, 12*(6), 393–400.

Sakala, C., & Corry, M. P. (2007). Listening to Mothers II reveals maternity care quality chasm. *Journal of Midwifery & Women's Health, 52*(3), 183–185.

Stump, M. J., & Smith, J. E. (2008). The relationship between post-traumatic growth and substance use in homeless women with histories of traumatic experience. *American Journal on Addictions, 17*(6), 478–487.

Tedeschi, R. G., & Calhoun, L. G. (2004). Posttraumatic growth: Conceptual foundations and empirical evidence. *Psychological Inquiry, 15*(1), 1–18.

Thomson, G., & Downe, S. (2008). Widening the trauma discourse: The link between childbirth and experiences of abuse. *Journal of Psychosomatic Obstetrics and Gynaecology, 29*(4), 268–273.

Van Manen, M. (1984). Practicing phenomenological writing. *Phenomenology + Pedagogy, 2*(1), 36–69.

Van Son, M., Verkerk, G., van der Hart, O., Komproe, I., & Pop, V. (2005). Prenatal depression, mode of delivery and perinatal dissociation as predictors of postpartum posttraumatic stress: An empirical study. *Clinical Psychology & Psychotherapy, 12*(4), 297–312.

Journal of Pain and Symptom Management, 2008, 36(20), 126–140

Original article

# Randomized Controlled Trial of a Psychoeducation Program for the Self-Management of Chronic Cardiac Pain

Michael H. McGillion, RN, PhD, Judy Watt-Watson, RN, PhD, Bonnie Stevens, RN, PhD, Sandra M. LeFort, RN, PhD, Peter Coyte, PhD, and Anthony Graham, MD, FRCPC

*Lawrence S. Bloomberg Faculty of Nursing (M.H.M., J.W.-W., B.S.) and Faculty of Medicine (B.S., P.C., A.G.), University of Toronto, Toronto; and School of Nursing (S.M.L.), Memorial University of Newfoundland, St. John's, Newfoundland, Canada*

## Abstract

*Cardiac pain arising from chronic stable angina (CSA) is a cardinal symptom of coronary artery disease and has a major negative impact on health-related quality of life (HRQL), including pain, poor general health status, and inability to self-manage. Current secondary prevention approaches lack adequate scope to address CSA as a multidimensional ischemic and persistent pain problem. This trial evaluated the impact of a low-cost six-week angina psychoeducation program, entitled The Chronic Angina Self-Management Program (CASMP), on HRQL, self-efficacy, and resourcefulness to self-manage anginal pain. One hundred thirty participants were randomized to the CASMP or three-month wait-list usual care; 117 completed the study. Measures were taken at baseline and three months. General HRQL was measured using the Medical Outcomes Study 36-Item Short Form and the disease-specific Seattle Angina Questionnaire (SAQ). Self-efficacy and resourcefulness were measured using the Self-Efficacy Scale and the Self-Control Schedule, respectively. The mean age of participants was 68 years, 80% were male. Analysis of variance of change scores yielded significant improvements in treatment group physical functioning [F = 11.75(1,114), P < 0.001] and general health [F = 10.94(1,114), P = 0.001] aspects of generic HRQL. Angina frequency [F = 5.57(1,115), P = 0.02], angina stability [F = 7.37(1,115), P = 0.001], and self-efficacy to manage disease [F = 8.45(1,115), P = 0.004] were also significantly improved at three months. The CASMP did not impact resourcefulness. These data indicate that the CASMP was effective for improving physical functioning, general health, anginal pain symptoms, and self-efficacy to manage pain at three months and provide a basis for long-term evaluation of the program.*

This trial was made possible in part by a Canadian Institutes of Health Research Fellowship (No. 452939) and a University of Toronto Centre for the Study of Pain Clinician-Scientist Fellowship.

Portions of the CASMP first appeared in or are derived from the Chronic Disease Self-Management Program Leader's Master Trainer's Guide (1999). Those portions are Copyright 1999, Stanford University.

*Address correspondence to:* Michael Hugh McGillion, RN, PhD, Lawrence S. Bloomberg Faculty of Nursing, University of Toronto, 155 College Street, Suite 130, Toronto, Ontario M5T 1P8, Canada. E-mail: michael.mcgillion@utoronto.ca

*Accepted for publication: September 26, 2007.*

0885-3924/08/$—see front matter
doi:10.1016/j.jpainsymman.2007.09.015

*Key Words*
*Chronic stable angina, self-management, randomized controlled trial, health-related quality of life*

## Introduction

Cardiac pain arising from chronic stable angina (CSA) pectoris is a cardinal symptom of coronary artery disease (CAD), characterized by pain or discomfort in the chest, shoulder, back, arm, or jaw.[1] CSA is a wide-spread clinical problem with a well-documented, major negative impact on health-related quality of life (HRQL), including pain, poor general health status, impaired role functioning, activity restriction, and reduced ability for self-care.[2-14] Limitations in current surveillance systems worldwide have precluded the examination of CSA prevalence in most countries. Available prevalence data estimate CSA prevalence at 6,500,000 (1999–2002) in the United States,[1] and 28/1000 men and 25/1000 women (April 2001–March 2002) in Scotland.[15] With the growing global burden of angina and CAD, nongovernmental organizations in Canada, the United States, and the United Kingdom have stressed the need for developments in secondary prevention strategies.[1,16,17] Current secondary prevention models largely target postacute cardiac event and/or coronary artery bypass patients and, depending on region, can be inaccessible to those with chronic symptoms.[18,19] Consequently, the vast majority of those with CSA and other CAD-related symptoms must manage on their own in the community. Moreover, these models focus predominantly on conventional CAD risk-factor modification to enhance myocardial conditioning and reduce ischemic threshold. However, cumulative basic science and clinical evidence point to the variability of cardiac pain perception for CSA patients, wherein pain can occur in the absence of myocardial ischemia, and conversely, ischemic episodes can be painless.[20-32] Given few alternatives, CSA patients revisit their local emergency departments when uncertain about how to manage their pain.[33,34] There is a critical need for a secondary prevention strategy with adequate scope and complexity to address CSA as a multidimensional ischemic and persistent pain problem, and to help CSA patients learn pain self-management strategies.[33]

Evidence from well-designed randomized controlled trials has demonstrated the effectiveness of psychoeducation for improving the self-management skills, HRQL, self-efficacy, and/or resourcefulness of persons with other chronic pains including arthritis and chronic non-cancer pain.[35-37] Psychoeducation interventions are multimodal, self-help treatment packages that use information and cognitive-behavioral strategies to achieve changes in knowledge and behavior for effective disease self-management.[38] To date, the effectiveness of psychoeducation for enhancing CSA self-management is inconclusive.[39] Although a few small trials over the last decade have demonstrated positive effects to some degree related to pain frequency, nitrate use, and stress,[40-43] numerous methodological problems, particularly inadequate power and the lack of a standard intervention approach, have precluded the generalization of findings.[39] Moreover, more recent and robust psychoeducation trial research has been limited to patients with newly diagnosed angina.[44] Therefore, the purpose of this study was to evaluate the effectiveness of a standardized psychoeducation program, entitled the Chronic Angina Self-Management Program (CASMP), for improving the HRQL, self-efficacy, and resourcefulness of CSA patients.

## Methods

### Study Design

This study was a randomized controlled trial. On completion of demographic and baseline measures, participants were randomly allocated to either 1) the six-week CASMP group or 2) the three-month wait-list control group;

posttest study outcomes were evaluated at three months from baseline. A short-term follow-up period was chosen for this study as it was the inaugural test of the effectiveness of the CASMP and the basis for a future larger-scale trial, with long-term follow-up. Ethical approval for the study was received from a university in central Canada and three university-affiliated teaching hospitals.

*Study Population and Procedure*

This study was conducted in central Canada over an 18-month period. The target population was CSA patients living in the community. Participants had a confirmed medical diagnosis of CAD, CSA for at least six months and were able to speak, read, and understand English. Individuals were excluded if they had suffered a myocardial infarction and/or undergone a coronary artery bypass graft in the last six months, had Canadian Cardiovascular Society (CCS) Class IV angina[45] and/or a major cognitive disorder. Participants were recruited from three university-affiliated teaching hospitals with large cardiac outpatient programs, allowing for timely subject referral. Three recruitment strategies found to be effective in prior psychoeducation trials with community-based samples were used.[36,37,46,47] First, clinicians at designated hospital recruitment sites identified eligible patients in the clinic setting. Second, study information was made available in participating clinicians' offices and hospital recruitment site newsletters. Third, the study was advertised in community newspapers.

Participant eligibility was initially assessed by a research assistant (RA) via telephone. Willing participants were then interviewed by the RA on-site to confirm eligibility and obtain informed consent. Demographic and baseline measures were completed on-site and participants were randomly allocated to either the six-week CASMP group, or the three-month wait-list control group. Randomization was centrally controlled using a university-based tamper-proof, computerized randomization service. Those randomized to the six-week intervention group were invited to participate in the next available program, whereas those randomized to usual care were told that they were in the three-month wait-list control group. Usual care consisted of all nursing, medical, and emergency care services as

needed; those allocated to the control group did not receive the CASMP during the study period.

Participants were contacted by the RA to schedule posttest data collection at three months from baseline. Assiduous follow-up procedures were used to minimize attrition; participants received up to three telephone calls and a follow-up letter regarding collection of their three-month follow-up data. Participants' completion of all study questionnaires was invigilated by the RA blinded to group allocation. Blinding was preserved by informing participants that their questions would be answered after they completed the questionnaire booklet and that a letter explaining their part in the next phase of the project was forthcoming. Those in the wait-list control group were offered entry into the next available CASMP once posttest measures were completed.

*Intervention*

The CASMP is a standardized psychoeducation program given in two-hour sessions weekly, over a six-week period. The goal of the CASMP is to improve HRQL by increasing patients' day-to-day angina self-management skills. The CASMP is an adaptation of Lorig et al.'s Chronic Disease Self-Management Program (CDSMP, © 1999 Stanford University).[47–50] In 2004, McGillion et al. conducted a preliminary study to identify CSA patients' specific pain-related concerns and self-management learning needs.[33] With permission, the results of this study were used to adapt the CDSMP to make it directly applicable to CSA. The principal investigator (PI) was certified as a CDSMP "Master Trainer" at the Stanford Patient Education Research Center to ensure that all tenets of the adapted program were in accordance with the standardized CDSMP psychoeducation format.

The program was delivered by a Registered Nurse using a group format (e.g., 8–15 patients) in a comfortable classroom setting. Program sessions were offered both day and evening and participants were encouraged to bring a family member or friend if they wished. A facilitator manual specified the intervention protocol in detail to ensure consistent delivery of the CASMP across sessions. In addition, all sessions were audio taped and a random sample of these tapes (10%) was externally audited to ensure standard intervention delivery.

The CASMP integrates strategies known to enhance self-efficacy including skills mastery, modeling, and self-talk. Designed to maximize discussion and group problem solving, it encourages individual experimentation with various cognitive-behavioral self-management techniques and facilitates mutual support, optimism, and the self-attribution of success. Key pain-related content includes relaxation and stress management, energy conservation, symptom monitoring and management techniques, medication review, seeking emergency assistance, diet, and managing emotional responses to cardiac pain. Fig. 1 provides an overview of all content covered over the six-week course of the program.

Both the content and process components of the CASMP are grounded in Bandura's Self-Efficacy Theory, which states that self-efficacy is critical to improve health-related behaviors and emotional well-being and that one's self-efficacy can be enhanced through performance mastery, modeling, reinterpretation of symptoms, and social persuasion.[51,52] Throughout the program, participants worked in pairs between sessions to help one another to stay motivated, problem solve, and meet their respective self-management goals. A CASMP workbook was also provided for reinforcement of key material from each session.

| CASMP Program Overview | | | | | | |
|---|---|---|---|---|---|---|
| | Week 1 | Week 2 | Week 3 | Week 4 | Week 5 | Week 6 |
| Overview of Self-management and Chronic Angina | ✓ | | | | | |
| Making an Action Plan | ✓ | ✓ | ✓ | ✓ | ✓ | ✓ |
| Relaxation/Cognitive Symptom Management | ✓ | | ✓ | ✓ | ✓ | ✓ |
| Feedback/Problem-solving | | ✓ | ✓ | ✓ | ✓ | ✓ |
| Common Emotional Responses to Cardiac Pain: Anger/Fear/Frustration | | ✓ | | | | |
| Staying Active/Fitness | | ✓ | ✓ | | | |
| Better Breathing | | | ✓ | | | |
| Fatigue/Sleep Management | | | ✓ | | | |
| Energy Conservation | | | | ✓ | | |
| Eating for a Healthy Heart | | | | ✓ | | |
| Monitoring Angina Symptoms and Deciding when to Seek Emergency Help | | | | ✓ | | |
| Communication | | | | ✓ | | |
| Angina and Other Common Heart Medications | | | | | ✓ | |
| Evaluating New/Alternative Treatments | | | | | ✓ | |
| Cardiac Pain and Depression | | | | | ✓ | |
| Monitoring Angina Pain Symptoms and Informing the Health Care Team | | | | | | ✓ |
| Communicating with Health Care Professionals About Your Cardiac Pain | | | | | | ✓ |
| Future Self-Management Plans | | | | | | ✓ |

Fig. 1. CASMP overview.

## Measures

Sociodemographic information and angina and related clinical characteristics were obtained via a baseline questionnaire developed for the trial. Braden's evidence-based Self-Help Model of Learned Response to Chronic Illness Experience guided our selection of trial outcomes.[53,54] Braden's model emphasizes human resilience and suggests that people can develop enabling skills to enhance their life quality when faced with the adversities of chronic illness.[53,54] Therefore, the primary outcome was life quality, conceptualized as CSA patients' HRQL. The secondary outcome was enabling skill, reflected by CSA patients' self-efficacy and resourcefulness to self-manage their pain.

*Primary Outcome: HRQL.* HRQL was measured using the Medical Outcomes Study 36-Item Short Form (SF-36).[55-57] The SF-36 is a comprehensive, well-established, and psychometrically strong instrument designed to capture multiple operational indicators of functional status including behavioral function and dysfunction, distress and well-being, self-evaluations of general health status.[58,59] Eight subscales are used to represent widely measured concepts of overall quality of life: physical functioning (PF), role limitations due to physical problems (RP), social functioning (SF), bodily pain (BP), mental health (MH), role limitations due to emotional problems (RE), vitality (VT), and general health perception (GH).[57] Raw SF-36 data were submitted to QualityMetric Incorporated's 100% accurate online scoring service. Scoring was according to the method of summated ratings where items for each subscale are summed and divided by the range of scores. Raw scores were transformed to a 0–100 scale where higher scores reflect better functioning.[57] We also used norm-based scoring (NBS) where linear T-score transformations were performed to transform all scores to a mean of 50 and standard deviation (SD) of 10.[57,60] We chose the NBS method to allow our SF-36 scores to be readily comparable to current published SF-36 CSA population norms.[57] (Raw SF-36 scores available on request from the first author.) NBS also guards against subscale ceiling and floor effects; scores below 50 can be understood as below average.[57]

Reliability estimates for all eight SF-36 subscales have exceeded 0.70 across divergent patient populations including CSA[58-61] and exceeded 0.8 in this study: PF (0.87), RP (0.86); BP (0.81); RE (0.87); SF (0.83); VT (0.83); MH (0.85); GH (0.83). SF-36 construct, convergent, and discriminant validities have also been well documented.[57-59,62]

Although the SF-36 has discriminated among patient samples with divergent medical, psychiatric, and psychiatric and other serious medical conditions, some evidence suggests that it may inadequately discriminate among those with differing CCS angina functional class.[61] The potential for the SF-36 to be insensitive to changes in angina class necessitated the use of a second disease-specific instrument, the Seattle Angina Questionnaire (SAQ),[61,63] to evaluate HRQL.

The SAQ is a disease-specific measure of HRQL for patients with CAD, consisting of 19 items that quantify five clinically relevant domains of CAD: physical limitation, angina pain stability and frequency, treatment satisfaction, and disease perception.[63] The SAQ is scored by assigning each response an ordinal value and summing across items within each of the five subscales. Subscale scores are transformed (0–100) by subtracting the lowest score, dividing by the range of the scale, and multiplying by 100.[63] Higher scores for each subscale indicate better functioning; no summary score for the five subscales is derived. SAQ reliability, construct validity, and responsiveness to intervention have been demonstrated in a number of studies.[13,14,61,63-65] Internal consistency reliabilities for the SAQ in this study were PL (0.85), AF (0.71), TS (0.73), and DP (0.68).

*Secondary Outcomes: Self-Efficacy and Resourcefulness.* Self-efficacy to manage angina pain and other symptoms was measured with a modified version of the 11-item "Pain and Other Symptom" scale of Lorig et al.'s Self-Efficacy Scale (SES), originally developed for arthritis intervention studies.[66] This scale assesses people's perceived ability to cope with the consequences of chronic arthritis including pain and related symptoms and functioning[66] via a 10-point graphic rating scale ranging from

10 (very certain) to 100 (very uncertain) for each of its 11 items. A total score for perceived self-efficacy is obtained by summing all items and dividing by the number of items completed; a higher score indicates greater perceived self-efficacy.

SES test-retest stability and construct validity have been reported in large samples.[35,36,67] The SES has also performed consistently with theoretical predictions in a prior psychoeducation trial for chronic pain, having negative correlation with pain (−0.35) and disability (−0.61), and strong positive correlation with role functioning (0.62) and life satisfaction (0.48); internal consistency was 0.90.[37] Permission was received from the SES developer to adapt the SES by replacing the word "arthritis" with "angina." The internal consistency of our adapted version of the SES in this study was 0.94.

Resourcefulness was measured by Rosenbaum's Self-Control Schedule (SCS),[68] designed to assess individual tendencies to use a repertoire of complex cognitive and behavioral skills when negotiating stressful circumstances. Thirty-six items are scored using a six-point Likert scale (−3 to +3) to assess individual tendencies to engage in aspects of self-control behaviors including 1) the use of cognitions and positive self-statements to cope with negative situations, 2) application of problem solving strategies, 3) delay of immediate gratification, and 4) maintenance of a general belief in self when dealing with challenging circumstances.[68] Eleven items are reverse scored, and all items are summed to generate a total score for resourcefulness ranging from −108 to 108; higher scores indicate greater resourcefulness.[68] SCS test-retest stability, internal consistency, and validity are well documented.[37,68–73] The internal consistency for the SCS in this study was 0.80.

All instruments were pilot tested prior to the trial on a sample of six CSA patients (aged 46–68 years) to assess their comprehension of items and response burden; no changes were required.

*Sample Size*

Sample size estimation was based on achievement of a moderate effect size in our primary outcome of HRQL. Cardiac patients have reported minimum 10-point improvements in SF-36 scales up to four years postinvasive intervention.[7,11] Prior trials suggested that psychoeducation can achieve comparable minimal levels of short-term change in a number of SF-36 scales for patients with chronic pain via the acquisition of disease self-management skills and the self-attribution of success.[35,37] We specified a 10-point difference in SF-36 scores as being clinically important and the sample size was set to test for this difference. Based on Chronic Pain Self-Management Program (CPSMP) trial data,[37] we used an estimated SD of 18; comparable SDs for five SF-36 scales including physical functioning, bodily pain, general health, social functioning, and mental health have been reported among cardiac patients aged 44–84 years.[7] Larger SDs however were reported for two role functioning scales of the SF-36 including role emotional and role physical functioning, thus requiring estimated sample sizes beyond the allowable time frame for this study.[7,57] We therefore expected potentially inadequate power to detect meaningful change in these two SF-36 scales. Allowing for an alpha of 0.05 and 80% power, the required sample for each group was 52. Telephone reminders and flexibility in CASMP program offerings were expected to help minimize attrition. However, to allow for losses to follow-up, the final sample estimate for each group was 65, or 130 in total. The statistics program nQuery Advisor 4.0 was used to compute this sample size estimate.

*Data Analysis*

Analyses were based on intention-to-treat principles.[74] Equivalence of groups on baseline demographic characteristics and pretest scores was examined using Chi-squared analysis for discrete level data and the Student *t*-test for continuous level data. Change score analyses were conducted to determine the impact of the CASMP on HRQL, self-efficacy, and resourcefulness to manage symptoms. Significant differences in change scores between treatment and control groups were examined via analysis of variance (ANOVA).[75] To guard against Type I error, multivariate analysis of variance (MANOVA) was conducted prior to ANOVA testing on SF-36- and SAQ-related data, due to the multiple subscales involved.[75] We chose a change score approach as opposed to analysis of covariance (ANCOVA) so that observed differences in change scores between treatment and control groups would be accessible to the reader and therefore the magnitude of any intervention effects would be readily apparent.[75,76] For verification, we reanalyzed our data via ANCOVA; the findings supported our change score approach. All data were cleaned and assessed for outliers and departure from normality; assumptions of all parametric analyses were met.

## Results

### Derivation of the Sample and Attrition

In total, 277 potential participants were assessed for inclusion via telephone during an 18-month period. Of these potential participants, 130 were included and 147 were excluded. Of those excluded, 44% did not meet the inclusion criteria, 30% refused, and 26% missed their initial appointment for consent and completion of baseline questionnaires, despite assiduous follow-up (i.e., three telephone calls and a follow-up letter). Reasons for refusal included: not interested ($n = 18$), too busy to participate ($n = 15$), transportation problems ($n = 6$), and physical limitations precluding travel ($n = 5$). Those who did not arrive for enrollment procedures

were also counted as refusals when determining acceptance rate. The acceptance rate for enrollment among those eligible was 61%. Of the 130 consenting participants, 66 were randomized to the CASMP, and 64 were randomized to the wait-list control group.

Thirteen participants (treatment group, $n = 9$; usual care group, $n = 4$) did not complete posttest measures, yielding a 10% loss to follow-up (LTF) rate. Of these, nine participants LTF dropped out of the study without explanation and could not be contacted and four became ineligible to continue due to hospitalization. One hundred seventeen participants (treatment group, $n = 57$; usual care group, $n = 60$) completed pre- and posttest measures that were used for data analyses (see Fig. 2).

### Participant Characteristics and Comparability of Groups

Baseline sociodemographic- and angina-related characteristics of the treatment and control groups are presented in Tables 1 and 2, respectively. The mean age of the sample was 68 (SD 11), living with CSA for 7 (SD 7) years on average. The majority of the sample was male, married or cohabitating, and Caucasian. Individuals of East Indian and Pakistani origin

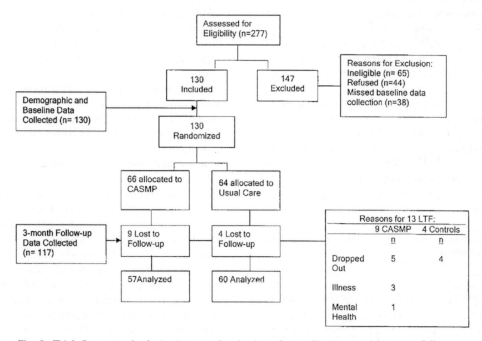

Fig. 2. Trial flow: sample derivation, randomization, data collection, and losses to follow-up.

### Table 1
### Sociodemographic Characteristics by Group

| Characteristic | Treatment ($n = 66$) | Control ($n = 64$) |
|---|---|---|
| Demographics | $n$ (%) | $n$ (%) |
| Mean age (years [SD]) | 67 (11) | 70 (11) |
| Married/cohabitating | 44 (67) | 44 (69) |
| Male | 53 (80) | 50 (78) |
| Working full time | 16 (24) | 15 (23) |
| Retired | 46 (70) | 42 (66) |
| High school | 59 (89) | 55 (86) |
| Postsecondary education | 42 (64) | 44 (69) |
| Caucasian | 48 (73) | 54 (84) |
| Black | 3 (5) | 0 (0) |
| Latin American | 0 (0) | 1 (2) |
| Asian | 2 (3) | 1 (2) |
| East Indian/Pakistani | 11 (17) | 6 (9) |
| Middle Eastern | 3 (5) | 1 (2) |
| Aboriginal | 0 (0) | 1 (2) |

SD = standard deviation.

constituted the second largest racial group enrolled. Most were either retired or working full time. The majority had completed high school and/or had postsecondary education.

### Table 2
### Angina and Related Clinical Characteristics by Group

| Characteristic | Treatment ($n = 66$) | Control ($n = 64$) |
|---|---|---|
| **Angina-related history** | | |
| Mean (SD) years living with angina | 6 (6) | 8 (8) |
| Mean (SD) revascularizations (including CABG, PCI) | 2 (1) | 2 (1) |
| **Comorbid conditions** | $n$ (%) | $n$ (%) |
| Heart failure | 2 (3) | 5 (8) |
| Asthma | 4 (6) | 2 (3) |
| Diabetes | 18 (27) | 9 (14) |
| Emphysema | 1 (2) | 1 (2) |
| Renal failure | 2 (3) | 1 (2) |
| Peptic ulcer | 1 (2) | 3 (5) |
| Thyroid problems | 3 (5) | 7 (11) |
| Other minor medical problem | 34 (52) | 27 (42) |
| **Canadian Cardiovascular Society Functional Class** | | |
| Class I | 23 (35) | 19 (30) |
| Class II | 26 (39) | 29 (45) |
| Class III | 17 (26) | 16 (25) |
| **Medications** | | |
| Ace inhibitors | 33 (50) | 29 (46) |
| Anti-arrhythmics | 3 (5) | 2 (3) |
| Anticoagulants | 57 (86) | 48 (73) |
| Beta-blockers | 40 (61) | 38 (59) |
| Calcium channel blockers | 22 (34) | 20 (32) |
| Cholesterol lowering agents | 49 (74) | 38 (59) |
| Diuretics | 11 (16) | 13 (20) |
| Insulins | 18 (27) | 9 (14) |

SD = standard deviation; CABG = coronary artery bypass graft; PCI = percutaneous coronary intervention.

Approximately half had two prior cardiac revascularization procedures, typically either coronary artery bypass grafting or angioplasty. The majority reported having a comorbid condition, typically a minor medical problem or diabetes. The treatment and control groups were not significantly different on any sociodemographic characteristic, comorbid condition, CCS functional class, number of prior revascularizations, or pretest measure. Comparisons were also made on all sociodemographic characteristics and pretest scores between those LTF ($n = 13$) and those who completed ($n = 117$) the study; no significant differences were found. (All baseline scores available on request from the first author.)

### Intervention Effects: Between-Group Differences in Change Scores

*Primary Outcome: HRQL.* Mean change scores by group, group differences in change scores, and results of MANOVA and ANOVA testing for significant differences in change scores between groups for the SF-36 and SAQ are presented in Tables 3 and 4, respectively. Two omnibus MANOVA tests were performed on the SF-36 data as four subscales reflect mental health aspects of HRQL, and four subscales reflect physical health aspects. MANOVA yielded significantly greater positive change for the treatment group on the overall physical health component of the SF-36 ($F = 4.39$, $P = 0.003$), compared to the usual care group; no significant differences in change were found for the overall mental health component. MANOVA also yielded significantly greater positive change for the treatment group on the SAQ ($F = 3.23$, $P = 0.009$), compared to the usual care group.

Individual-level ANOVA testing on SF-36 subscales indicated significant improvements for the treatment group on physical functioning (PF) [$F = 11.75$ (1,114), $P < 0.001$] and general health (GH) [$F = 10.94$ (1,114), $P = 0.001$]. The Mann-Whitney $U$ test was used to test for significant differences in change between groups for the role physical and role emotional functioning (RP, RE) and bodily pain (BP) subscales, due to their discrete distributions;[75] no significant differences between groups were found. ANOVA also yielded significant improvements for the

*Table 3*
**MANOVA and ANOVA Tests for Significant Differences in SF-36 Change Scores between Groups**

| SF-36 NBS | Change Treatment | Change Control | Difference in Change between Groups | MANOVA | | ANOVA | |
|---|---|---|---|---|---|---|---|
| Range (0–100) | $\Delta(T_2 - T_1)$ M (SD) | $\Delta(T_2 - T_1)$ M (SD) | $(T_\Delta - C_\Delta)$ M (SD) | F (df) | P | F (df) | P |
| Physical health-related items | | | | | | | |
| PF | 5.3 (9.4) | −0.68 (9.3) | 5.95 (9.3) | 4.39 (4, 110) | $0.003^b$ | 11.75 (1, 114) | $<0.001^c$ |
| RP | 4.8 (12.7) | 3.2 (9.6) | 1.66 (11.2) | | | $1.47^a$ | ns |
| BP | 4.4 (8.7) | 2.1 (9.2) | 2.31 (8.95) | | | $1.68^a$ | ns |
| GH | 2.27 (7.7) | −1.6 (6.4) | 4.33 (7.0) | | | 10.94 (1, 114) | $0.001^c$ |
| Mental health-related items | | | | | | | |
| RE | 4.9 (12.2) | 3.6 (12.2) | 1.31 (12.2) | 0.47 (4,108) | ns | $1.49^a$ | ns |
| SF | 2.1 (10.9) | 0.1 (9.5) | 2.04 (10.2) | | | 0.28 (1, 114) | ns |
| VT | 2.3 (8.6) | 0.3 (7.3) | 1.97 (8.0) | | | 1.77 (1, 114) | ns |
| MH | 1.5 (8.8) | 0.9 (7.9) | 0.58 (8.3) | | | 0.14 (1, 114) | ns |

NBS = Norm-based scores; $T_1$ = Time 1; $T_2$ = Time 2; T = treatment; C = controls; $\Delta$ = mean change; $T_\Delta$ = mean change, treatment; $C_\Delta$ = mean change, controls; PF = physical functioning; RP = role physical functioning; BP = bodily pain; GH = general health; RE = role emotional functioning; SF = social functioning; VT = vitality; MH = mental health.
Note: SD of mean change scores expected to be large as range of scores not bound by zero.
[a]Mann-Whitney U test.
[b]$P < 0.05$.
[c]$P \leq 0.01$.
ns = Nonsignificant ($P > 0.05$).

treatment group on two subscales of the SAQ including angina pain frequency (AF) [$F = 5.57$ (1,115), $P = 0.02$] and stability (AS) [$F = 7.37$ (1,115), $P = 0.001$]. At three months, the CASMP resulted in significantly greater improvements in physical functioning and general health, as measured by the SF-36, and significantly greater improvements in angina pain frequency and stability, as measured by the SAQ, compared to usual care.

*Secondary Outcomes: Self-Efficacy and Resourcefulness.* Mean change scores by group, group differences in change scores, and results of ANOVA testing for significant differences in

change in SES and SCS scores between groups are presented in Table 5. ANOVA yielded significant improvement for the treatment group on the SES [$F = 8.45$ (1,115), $P = 0.004$] compared to controls. No significant group differences in SCS change scores were found. Overall, the CASMP resulted in significantly improved self-efficacy scores at three months, compared to usual care. The CASMP did not impact resourcefulness.

*Examination of Intervention Cohort Effects*
Because the CASMP was delivered to the treatment group in six small group cohorts of eight to fifteen participants, we examined for

*Table 4*
**MANOVA and ANOVA Tests for Significant Differences in SAQ Change Scores between Groups**

| SAQ | Change Treatment | Change Control | Difference in Change between Groups | MANOVA | | ANOVA | |
|---|---|---|---|---|---|---|---|
| Range (0–100) | $\Delta(T_2 - T_1)$ M (SD) | $\Delta(T_2 - T_1)$ M (SD) | $(T_\Delta - C_\Delta)$ M (SD) | F (df) | P | F (df) | P |
| AF | 11.4 (23.7) | 2.2 (18.4) | 9.23 (21.2) | 3.23 (5,109) | $0.009^a$ | 5.57 (1,115) | $0.02^a$ |
| AS | 18.0 (35.0) | 2.9 (24.4) | 15.07 (30.0) | | | 7.37 (1,115) | $0.001^b$ |
| DP | 9.9 (23.5) | 3.3 (19.1) | 6.61 (21.4) | | | 2.80 (1,115) | ns |
| PL | 7.1 (16.5) | 1.6 (15.1) | 5.55 (15.8) | | | 3.54 (1,113) | ns |
| TS | 9.7 (24.6) | 4.8 (18.7) | 4.82 (21.8) | | | 1.43 (1,115) | ns |

SAQ = Seattle Angina Questionnaire; $T_1$ = Time 1, $T_2$ = Time 2; T = treatment; C = Controls; $\Delta$ = mean change; $T_\Delta$ = mean change, treatment; $C_\Delta$ = mean change, controls; AF = angina frequency; AS = angina stability; DP = disease perception; PL = physical limitation; TS = treatment satisfaction; SD = standard deviation.
Note: SD of change scores expected to be large as range of scores not bound by zero.
[a]$P < 0.05$.
[b]$P \leq 0.01$.
ns = Nonsignificant ($P > 0.05$).

Reprinted with permission.

*Table 5*

**ANOVA Tests for Significant Differences in SES and SCS Change Scores between Groups**

| Variable (Range) | Change Treatment $\Delta(T_2 - T_1)$ M (SD) | Change Control $\Delta(T_2 - T_1)$ M (SD) | Difference in Change between Groups $(T_\Delta - UC_\Delta)$ M (SD) | ANOVA $F$ (df) | $P$ |
|---|---|---|---|---|---|
| SES (10–100) | 8.4 (17.6) | −0.2 (14.4) | 8.62 (16.1) | 8.45 (1,115) | 0.004[a] |
| SCS (0–100) | 4.2 (26.5) | −1.6 (19.2) | 5.80 (23.0) | 1.60 (1,115) | ns |

$T_1$ = Time 1; $T_2$ = Time 2; T = treatment; C = Controls; $\Delta$ = mean change; $T_\Delta$ = mean change; treatment; $C_\Delta$ = mean change; controls; SES = Self-Efficacy Scale; SCS = Self-Control Schedule; SD = standard deviation.
Note: SD of change scores expected to be large as range of scores not bound by zero.
[a] $P < 0.01$.
ns = Nonsignificant ($P > 0.05$).

significant associations between intervention cohort and differences found in change scores between treatment and control groups. No significant associations between intervention cohort and group differences in change scores were found.

### CASMP Attendance

As a form of process evaluation, an attendance record was kept to track the number of CASMP sessions attended by the treatment group participants. Ninety-three percent of those in the treatment group attended all six program sessions; the remaining 7% attended three or more sessions. The average number of sessions attended overall was 5.8.

## Discussion

Statistically reliable short-term improvements in HRQL and self-efficacy were found for those who participated in the CASMP as compared to the control group; specific components of HRQL significantly improved included overall physical functioning and general health (SF-36) and frequency and stability of angina pain symptoms (SAQ). As no prior psychoeducation-based trials for CSA have used the SF-36 or the SAQ, direct comparisons of our HRQL-related results were not possible. However, our findings generally compare favorably with those of trials that have used other means to evaluate HRQL. We found four psychoeducation trials that reported significant improvements in symptoms including duration, frequency, and severity of cardiac pain.[40–43] Two of these trials also found significant improvements in physical functioning with respect to exercise tolerance and general disability.[40,42] Although our

findings are consistent with these positive trends, comparisons must be viewed with caution due to heterogeneity of methods including design, interventions, timing of outcome measurement, and instrumentation.[39] Nevertheless, sample characteristics across trials are similar to our sample, suggesting that physical functioning and angina symptoms can improve after participation in psychoeducational interventions that target angina pain symptoms, self-management techniques, and physical activity enhancement. Future angina psychoeducation randomized controlled trials (RCT) using robust methods, and standard reliable and valid measures to evaluate HRQL would allow for more direct comparisons to this trial.

Although focused on a different population, LeFort et al.'s CPSMP trial is the only other known study to have used the SF-36 to evaluate the impact of psychoeducation on a persistent pain problem.[37] Comparable to our study with respect to intervention format, design, and sample size, LeFort et al. found that their CPSMP program significantly improved SF-36 role physical functioning, bodily pain, vitality, and mental health for persons with chronic noncancer pain ($P < 0.003$).[37]

LeFort et al.'s significant improvement in a broader array of SF-36 dimensions than those achieved by our program may be attributable to the nature of respective pain problems addressed and participants' corresponding foci for self-management. Participants in LeFort et al.'s study had a number of chronic pain problems, averaging 6.7 somatic locations for pain per participant. Individuals may therefore have focused on a broader range of goals for pain self-management than our sample, leading to improvements across SF-36 physical and mental health components. Participants in our study however were most concerned with reducing their fear of cardiac pain to enhance their physical capacity. Based on pilot data, our program targeted a common misbelief among CSA patients that sedentary behavior will minimize cardiac pain and risks to personal safety.[33] Accordingly, the vast majority of our treatment group identified their fear of physical activity and subsequent pain as a major contributor to deconditioning, poor overall health, fatigue, and obesity. Enhancement of physical activity was therefore their immediate self-management priority. This concentrated self-management focus may account for our treatment group's narrower, although significant, improvements in SF-36 physical functioning and general health. There is also some evidence to suggest that the SF-36 may inadequately discriminate among those with differing CCS angina functional class.[61] Because our sample included those with CCS Classes I–III angina, some SF-36 subscales may not have been sensitive to improvements in angina-induced disability as a result of our program. Finally, baseline scores on all SF-36 dimensions in this study are below Canadian- and U.S. population-adjusted norms.[57,77] Given the deleterious impact of CSA on HRQL, improvement in multiple SF-36 dimensions may be difficult to achieve for CSA patients in the short term.

Prior work has established that a minimum change of 10 points in SAQ subscales reflects clinically meaningful change for angina patients.[13,63,65] In our study, AS and AF scores changed in a positive direction for the treatment group by a mean 18 (35.0) and 11.4 (23.7) points, respectively, and therefore meet this criterion for clinically meaningful change. This finding is consistent with the positive results of recent studies that have tested multifaceted CSA secondary prevention strategies, with some educational components.[65,78] Spertus et al.[65] and Moore et al.[78] reported similar findings resulting from their intervention strategies, featuring combinations of antianginal drug therapy, regional anesthesia, exercise rehabilitation, education sessions, and/or individual counseling. Greater short-term improvement in frequency and stability of angina pain symptoms in our trial as compared to these studies may be due to the self-efficacy enhancing nature of our standardized intervention format. Our significant improvement in treatment group

self-efficacy is consistent with LeFort et al.'s CPSMP trial.[37] and Lorig and Holman's psychoeducation trials for arthritis self-management.[35] Consistent with Bandura' self-efficacy theory, health behavior change by instruction—without addressing self-efficacy—has not shown to be as effective as those interventions that target self-efficacy directly.[79]

Other scores not significantly improved at posttest included SAQ-treatment satisfaction, disease perception and physical limitation, and resourcefulness, as measured by the SCS. As with some SF-36 subscales, a longer-term evaluation period may be required to see significant improvement in these scores for CSA patients. In addition, psychometric properties of the SAQ-physical limitation (PL) scale may account for our lack of a significant finding in this disease-specific HRQL dimension. The SAQ-PL scale was adapted by Spertus et al.[63] from Goldman et al.'s Specific Activity Scale,[80] designed to assess CAD patients' capacity for physical stress. Six of nine total SAQ-PL items examine activities known to increase myocardial oxygen demand including climbing a hill or flight of stairs without stopping, gardening, vacuuming or carrying groceries, walking more than a block at a brisk pace, lifting or moving heavy objects, and participating in strenuous sports.[63] However, as our pilot study suggests, most CSA patients will learn to avoid moderate levels of physical activity due to their fear of pain.[33] Therefore, more strenuous activities captured by the SAQ-PL scale may not be relevant to CSA patients. Notably, Spetrus et al.[65] and Moore et al.[78] also found no significant improvements in SAQ-PL for their chronic angina samples. These data suggest that the responsiveness of the SAQ-PL scale to improvements in mild physical activity for CSA patients, such as walking and household activity, warrants further investigation.

The strengths of our study are the robust methods used to minimize biases and random error including a priori power analysis, centrally controlled randomization, valid and reliable measures, blinding of data collectors, intention-to-treat analyses, and examination for possible intervention cohort effects. In addition, assiduous follow-up procedures and the use of a wait-list control condition guarded against attrition bias, ensuring minimal loss to follow up. Treatment integrity was also maximized using a theoretically sound and standardized intervention protocol, verified by an external auditor via audio recording.

Performance bias cannot be ruled out as it is not possible to blind participants or interveners in a socially based intervention study. Social desirability may also be a possibility due to our use of self-report measures.[81] However, randomization should have equally distributed those prone to socially desirable responses.[74] The risk of sample size bias may be further reduced in a future study by obtaining a larger sample to ensure adequate power for the two SF-36 role functioning scales. Also, our follow-up period was limited to three months after baseline. Therefore, the long-term sustainability of the observed intervention effects is not known. In addition, all CASMP sessions were delivered by a single facilitator. Future studies of this intervention should use multiple facilitators to enhance external validity and include longer-term follow-up. Finally, this study was conducted at a university site in central Canada; the clinical utility and knowledge translation potential of future investigations may be enhanced by examining the effectiveness of the CASMP as an adjunctive component to facets of health care with preexisting infrastructure, such as standard cardiac rehabilitation programs (where applicable), or community health-care programs and facilities.

In conclusion, cumulative evidence supports the deleterious impact of CSA on HRQL. The CASMP was found effective for improving physical functioning, perceived general health, angina pain frequency and stability, and self-efficacy to manage angina at three months posttest. Further research is warranted to determine the capacity of the program to improve other dimensions of generic and disease-specific HRQL, and resourcefulness in the longer term. A subsequent long-term evaluation would also allow for examination of the sustainability of the short-term improvements observed in HRQL and self-efficacy for CSA patients.

## Acknowledgments

We are grateful to the participants of this trial who generously gave their time and effort. We also thank Dr. Kate Lorig, Stanford University Patient Education Research Center, for permission to adapt the Chronic Disease Self-Management Program; Dr. Ellen Hodnett who supported this trial at the Randomized Controlled Trials Unit, Faculty of Nursing, University of Toronto; and Kim Boswell, Julie Kim, Linda Belford, Linda Brubacher, Peter Neilson, Marion Ryujin, and Viola Webster, expert clinicians and administrators who supported trial recruitment.

## References

1. Gibbons RJ, Chatterjee K, Daley J, et al. ACC/AHA-ASIM guidelines for the management of patients with chronic stable angina: executive summary and recommendations [(A report of the American College of Cardiology/American Heart Association Task Force on practice guidelines (Committee on Management of Patients with Chronic Stable Angina)]. Circulation 1999;99:2829–2848.

2. Lyons RA, Lo SV, Littlepage BNC. Comparative health status of patients with 11 common illnesses in Wales. J Epidemiol Community Health 1994;48:388–390.

3. Pocock SJ, Henderson RA, Seed P, Treasure T, Hampton J. Quality of life, employment status, and anginal symptoms after coronary artery bypass surgery: three-year follow-up in the randomized intervention treatment of angina (RITA) trial. Circulation 1996;94:135–142.

4. Erixson G, Jerlock M, Dahlberg K. Experiences of living with angina pectoris. Nurs Sci Res Nord Countries 1997;17:34–38.

5. Miklaucich M. Limitations on life: women's lived experiences of angina. J Adv Nurs 1998;28:1207–1215.

6. Caine N, Sharples LD, Wallwork J. Prospective study of health related quality of life before and after coronary artery bypass grafting: outcome at 5 years. Heart 1999;81:347–351.

7. Brown N, Melville M, Gray D, et al. Quality of life four years after acute myocardial infarction: Short Form 36 scores compared with a normal population. Heart 1999;81:352–358.

8. Gardner K, Chapple A. Barriers to referral in patients with angina: qualitative study. Br Med J 1999;319:418–421.

9. Wandell PE, Brorsson B, Aberg H. Functioning and well-being of patients with type 2 diabetes or angina pectoris, compared with the general population. Diabetes Metab (Paris) 2000;26:465–471.

10. Brorsson B, Bernstein SJ, Brook RH, Werko L. Quality of life of chronic stable angina patients four years after coronary angioplasty or coronary artery bypass surgery. J Intern Med 2001;249:47–57.

11. Brorsson B, Bernstein SJ, Brook RH, Werko L. Quality of life of patients with chronic stable angina before and 4 years after coronary artery revascularization compared with a normal population. Heart 2002;87:140–145.

12. MacDermott AFN. Living with angina pectoris: a phenomenological study. Eur J Cardiovasc Nurs 2002;1:265–272.

13. Spertus JA, Jones P, McDonell M, Fan V, Fihn SD. Health status predicts long-term outcome in outpatients with coronary disease. Circulation 2002;106:43–49.

14. Spertus JA, Salisbury AC, Jones PG, Conaway DG, Thompson RC. Predictors of quality of life benefit after percutaneous coronary intervention. Circulation 2004;110:3789–3794.

15. Murphy NF, Simpson CR, MacIntyre K, et al. Prevalence, incidence, primary care burden, and medical treatment of angina in Scotland: age, sex and socioeconomic disparities: a population-based study. Heart 2006;92:1047–1054.

16. Heart and Stroke Foundation of Canada. The growing burden of heart disease and stroke in Canada 2003. Ottawa: Heart and Stroke Foundation of Canada, 2003.

17. British Cardiac Society, British Hypertension Society, Diabetes UK, et al. JBS 2: Joint British Societies' guidelines on the prevention of cardiovascular disease in clinical practice. Heart 2005; 91(Suppl V):v1–v52.

18. Naylor CD. Summary, reflections and recommendations. In: Naylor CD, Slaughter PM, eds. Cardiovascular health and services in Ontario: An ICES atlas. Toronto: Institute for Clinical Evaluative Sciences, 1999: 355–377.

19. Stone JA, Arthur HM, Austford L, Blair T. Introduction to cardiac rehabilitation. In: Stone JA, Arthur HM, eds. Canadian guidelines for cardiac rehabilitation and cardiovascular disease prevention, 2nd ed. Winnipeg: Can Assoc Cardiac Rehab, 2004: 2–14.

20. Maseri A, Chierchia S, Davies G, Glazier J. Mechanisms of ischemic cardiac pain and silent myocardial ischemia. Am J Med 1985;79(Suppl 3A):7–11.

21. Malliani A. The elusive link between transient myocardial ischemia and pain. Circulation 1986; 73:201–204.

22. Aronow WS, Epstein S. Usefulness of silent myocardial ischemia detected by ambulatory electrocardiographic monitoring in predicting new coronary events in elderly patients. Am J Cardiol 1988;62: 1295–1296.

23. Langer A, Freeman MR, Armstrong PW. ST segment shift in unstable angina: pathophysiology and association with coronary anatomy and hospital outcome. J Am Coll Cardiol 1989;13:1495–1502.

24. Tzivoni D, Weisz G, Gavish A, et al. Comparison of mortality and myocardial infarction rates in stable angina pectoris with and without ischemic episodes during daily activities. Am J Cardiol 1989;63: 273–276.

25. Deedwania PC, Carbajal EV. Silent ischemia during daily life is an independent predictor of mortality in stable angina. Circulation 1990;81:748–756.

26. Yeung AC, Barry J, Orav J, et al. Effects of asymptomatic ischemia on long-term prognosis in chronic stable coronary disease. Circulation 1991;83: 1598–1604.

27. Sylven C. Mechanisms of pain in angina pectoris: a critical review of the adenosine hypothesis. Cardiovasc Drugs Ther 1993;7:745–759.

28. Bugiardini R, Borghi A, Pozzati A, et al. Relation of severity of symptoms to transient myocardial ischemia and prognosis in unstable angina. J Am Coll Cardiol 1995;25:597–604.

29. Cannon RO. Cardiac pain. In: Gebhart GF, ed, Progress in pain research and management, Vol. 5. Seattle: IASP Press, 1995: 373–389.

30. Malliani A. The conceptualization of cardiac pain as a nonspecific and unreliable alarm system. In: Gebhart GF, ed, Progress in pain research and management, Vol. 5. Seattle: IASP Press, 1995: 63–74.

31. Pepine CJ. Does the brain know when the heart is ischemic? Ann Intern Med 1996;124(11): 1006–1008.

32. Procacci P, Zoppi M, Maresca M. Heart, vascular and haemopathic pain. In: Wall P, Melzack R, eds. Textbook of pain, 4th ed. Toronto: Churchill Livingstone, 1999: 621–659.

33. McGillion MH, Watt-Watson JH, Kim J, Graham A. Learning by heart: a focused groups study to determine the psychoeducational needs of chronic stable angina patients. Can J Cardiovasc Nurs 2004;14:12–22.

34. McGillion M, Watt-Watson J, LeFort S, Stevens B. Positive shifts in the perceived meaning of cardiac pain following a psychoeducation for chronic stable angina. Can J Nurs Res 2007;39: 48–65.

35. Lorig K, Holman HR. Arthritis self-management studies: a twelve year review. Health Educ Q 1993;20:17–28.

36. Lorig K, Mazonson P, Holman HR. Evidence suggesting that health education for self-management in patients with chronic arthritis has maintained health benefits while reducing health care costs. Arthritis Rheum 1993;36:439–446.

37. LeFort S, Gray-Donald K, Rowat KM, Jeans ME. Randomised controlled trial of a community based psychoeducation program for the self-management of chronic pain. Pain 1998;74:297–306.

38. Barlow JH, Shaw KL, Harrison K. Consulting the "experts:" children and parents' perceptions of psychoeducational interventions in the context of juvenile chronic arthritis. Health Educ Res 1999;14:597–610.

39. McGillion MH, Watt-Watson JH, Kim J, Yamada J. A systematic review of psychoeducational interventions for the management of chronic stable angina. J Nurs Manag 2004;12:1–9.

40. Bundy C, Carroll D, Wallace L, Nagle R. Psychological treatment of chronic stable angina pectoris. Psychol Health 1994;10(1):69–77.

41. Payne TJ, Johnson CA, Penzein DB, et al. Chest pain self-management training for patients with coronary artery disease. J Psychosom Res 1994;38:409–418.

42. Lewin B, Cay E, Todd I, et al. The angina management program: a rehabilitation treatment. Br J Cardiol 1995;2:221–226.

43. Gallacher JEJ, Hopkinson CA, Bennett ML, Burr ML, Elwood PC. Effect of stress management on angina. Psychol Health 1997;12:523–532.

44. Lewin RJP, Furze G, Robinson J, et al. A randomized controlled trial of a self-management plan for patients with newly diagnosed angina. Br J Gen Pract 2002;52:194–201.

45. Campeau L. The Canadian Cardiovascular Society grading of angina pectoris revisited 30 years later. Can J Cardiol 2002;18:371–379.

46. Lorig K, Lubeck D, Kraines RG, Selenznick M, Holman HR. Outcomes of self-help education for patients with arthritis. Arthritis Rheum 1985;28:680–685.

47. Lorig KR, Sobel DS, Stewart AL, et al. Evidence suggesting that a chronic disease self-management program can improve health status while reducing utilization and costs: a randomized trial. Med Care 1999;37:5–14.

48. Lorig K, Gonzalez V, Laurent D. The chronic disease self-management workshop master trainer's guide 1999. Palo Alto, CA: Stanford Patient Education Research Center, 1999.

49. Lorig KR, Ritter P, Stewart AL, et al. Chronic disease self-management program: two-year health status and health care utilization outcomes. Med Care 2001;39:1217–1223.

50. Lorig KR, Sobel D, Ritter PL, Laurent D, Hobbs M. One-year health status and health care utilization outcomes for a chronic disease self-management program in a managed care setting. Eff Clin Pract 2001;4:256–262.

51. Bandura A. Social foundations of thought and action: A social cognitive theory. Englewood Cliffs: Prentice Hall, 1986.

52. Bandura A. Self-efficacy: The exercise of control. New York: W.H. Freeman, 1977.

53. Braden CJ. A test of the self-help model: learned response to chronic illness experience. Nurs Res 1990;39:42–47.

54. Braden CJ. Research program on learned response to chronic illness experience: self-help model. Holist Nurs Pract 1993;8:38–44.

55. Rand Corporation, Ware J. The Short-Form-36 Health Survey. In: McDowell I, Newell C, eds. Measuring health: A guide to rating scales and questionnaires, 2nd ed. New York: Oxford University Press, 2006: 446–454.

56. Ware JE, Sherbourne CD. The MOS 36-item short-form health survey (SF-36): I Conceptual framework and item selection. Med Care 1992;30:473–483.

57. Ware JE, Snow KK, Kosinski M, Gandek B. SF-36® health survey: Manual and interpretation guide. Lincoln: QualityMetric Incorporated, 2005.

58. McHorney CA, Ware JE, Rachel Lu JF, Sherborne CD. The MOS 36-item short-form health survey (SF-36): III. Tests of data quality, scaling assumptions, and reliability across divergent patient groups. Med Care 1994;32:40–66.

59. Tsai C, Bayliss MS, Ware JE. SF-36® Health survey annotated bibliography. (1988–1996), 2nd ed. Boston: Health Assessment Lab, New England Medical Center, 1997.

60. Ware JE, Snow KK, Kosinski M, Gandek B. SF-36® health survey: Manual and interpretation guide. Boston, MA: The Health Institute, New England Medical Center, 1993.

61. Dougherty C, Dewhurst T, Nichol P, Spertus J. Comparison of three quality of life instruments in stable angina pectoris: Seattle angina questionnaire, Short Form health survey (SF-36), and quality of life index-cardiac version III. J Clin Epidemiol 1998; 51(7):569–575.

62. McHorney CA, Ware JE, Raczek AE. The MOS 36-item short-form health survey (SF-36): II. Psychometric and clinical tests of validity in measuring physical and mental health constructs. Med Care 1993;31:247–263.

63. Spertus JA, Winder JA, Dewhurst TA, et al. Development and evaluation of the Seattle Angina Questionnaire: a new functional status measure for coronary artery disease. J Am Coll Cardiol 1995;25:333–341.

64. Seto TB, Taira DA, Berezin R, et al. Percutaneous coronary revascularization in elderly patients: impact on functional status and quality of life. Ann Intern Med 2000;132:955–958.

65. Spertus JA, Dewhurst TA, Dougherty CM, et al. Benefits of an "angina clinic" for patients with coronary artery disease: a demonstration of health status measures as markers of health care quality. Am Heart J 2002;143:145–150.

66. Lorig K, Chastain RL, Ung E, Shoor S, Holman H. Development and evaluation of a scale

to measure perceived self-efficacy in people with arthritis. Arthritis Rheum 1989;32:37—44.

67. Lorig K, Lubeck D, Selenznick M, et al. The beneficial outcomes of the arthritis self-management course are inadequately explained by behaviour change. Arthritis Rheum 1989;31:91—95.

68. Rosenbaum M. A schedule for assessing self-control behaviours: preliminary findings. Behav Ther 1990;11:109—121.

69. Weisenberg M, Wolf Y, Mittwoch T, Mikulincer M. Learned resourcefulness and perceived control of pain: a preliminary examination of construct validity. J Res Pers 1990;24:101—110.

70. Redden EM, Tucker RK, Young L. Psychometric properties of the Rosenbaum schedule for assessing self control. Psychol Rec 1983;33:77—86.

71. Rosenbaum M, Palmon N. Helplessness and resourcefulness in coping with epilepsy. J Consult Clin Psychol 1984;52:244—253.

72. Richards PS. Construct validation of the self-control schedule. J Res Pers 1985;19:208—218.

73. Clanton L, Rude S, Taylor C. Learned resourcefulness as a moderator of burnout in a sample of rehabilitation providers. Rehabil Psychol 1992;37: 131—140.

74. Meinart CL. Clinical trials: Design, conduct and analysis. New York: Oxford University Press, 1986.

75. Norman GR, Streiner DL. Biostatistics: The bare essentials, 2nd ed. Hamilton: BC Decker Inc., 2000.

76. Bonate P. Analysis of pretest-posttest designs. Boca Raton: Chapman & Hall/CRC, 2000.

77. Hopman WM, Towheed T, Anastassiades T, et al. Canadian normative data for the SF-36 health survey. Can Med Assoc J 2000;163:265—271.

78. Moore RK, Groves D, Bateson S, et al. Health related quality of life of patients with refractory angina before and one year after enrolment onto a refractory angina program. Eur J Pain 2005;9:305—310.

79. Marks R, Allegrante JP, Lorig K. A review and synthesis of research evidence for self-efficacy enhancing interventions for reducing chronic disability: implications for health education practice (Part II). Health Promot Pract 2005;6:148—156.

80. Goldman L, Hashimoto B, Cook EF, Loscalzo MS. Comparative reproducibility and validity of systems for assessing cardiovascular functional class: advantages of a new specific activity scale. Circulation 1981;22:1227—1234.

81. Sackett DL. Bias in analytic research. J Chronic Dis 1979;32:51—63.

# Critique of McGillion et al.'s (2008) Study "*Randomized Controlled Trial of a Psychoeducation Program for the Self-Management of Chronic Cardiac Pain*"

## OVERALL SUMMARY

Overall, this was an extremely well-done study that tested a promising intervention to promote better outcomes among patients with chronic stable angina (CSA). The researchers used a strong research design and implemented stringent strategies to enhance the study's internal validity. They provided evidence that neither selection bias nor attrition bias affected their conclusions. They paid careful attention to such issues as blinding data collectors, reducing attrition, standardizing the intervention, and monitoring intervention fidelity. The instruments they used to measure the outcomes demonstrated strong validity and reliability. The study results indicated significant (and clinically important) improvements for those in the intervention group for many important outcomes. The researchers' power analysis led them to recruit a sample sufficiently large to detect moderate intervention effects, but a larger sample would likely have yielded evidence of even further program benefits—this limitation on statistical power was one that the researchers themselves acknowledged. The researchers provided excellent suggestions for further research on the promising psychoeducation intervention that they studied.

## TITLE

The title of this report was excellent. It communicated or implied the research design (a randomized controlled trial or RCT), the independent variable (participation vs. nonparticipation in a special program), the nature of the intervention (psychoeducational program, involving self-management), a dependent variable (self-management of pain), and the study population (patients with chronic pain from cardiac disease). All this information was conveyed succinctly—only 14 words were used. It could be argued that something about health-related quality of life (HRQL) (the primary outcome variable) should have been included in the title, but this would have made the title quite long. The authors did, however, list HRQL as a keyword for indexing purposes.

# ABSTRACT

The abstract, written in the traditional abstract style without subheadings, was excellent, summarizing all major features of the study. The abstract presented a summary of the problem, described the intervention, outlined crucial aspects of the research designs and study methods, described the study sample, summarized major findings, and stated the conclusion that the findings warrant further research on the long-term effects of the intervention. Despite its strength, the abstract could perhaps have been shorter without diminishing its informativeness. For example, statistical details (all of the information about the $F$ statistics and the actual probability values) were not necessary. Names of the specific instruments that measured the outcomes (e.g., the Medical Outcomes Study 36-Item Short Form) could also have been omitted. People review abstracts to determine whether the full article is of interest, and methodologic details can be excessive to busy readers.

# INTRODUCTION

The introduction to this study was short—briefer than is typical, in fact. Yet, the introduction covered a lot of ground in a concise and admirable fashion, thus leaving more space in the article for details about the researchers' methods and findings.

The very first sentence, which stated that cardiac pain from CSA is a cardinal symptom of coronary artery disease, introduced the problem. Later sentences indicated that this clinical problem has not been satisfactorily addressed with secondary prevention strategies. Consequences of the problem were summarized (i.e., that CSA has repercussions for HRQL, including pain, poor general health status, impaired role functioning, reduced ability for self-care, and activity restriction). Ample citations supporting these assertions were provided. Next, the researchers presented information about the prevalence of CSA—that is, about the scope of the problem.

McGillion and colleagues then laid the groundwork for the testing of a new intervention. They noted that existing models of secondary prevention are not necessarily accessible to those managing their chronic symptoms in the community. They identified a potential model of self-management for helping patients with CSA—psychoeducation interventions, which they defined as "multimodal, self-help treatment packages that use information and cognitive-behavioral strategies to achieve changes in knowledge and behavior for effective disease management" (p. 414). They described existing evidence about the utility of such interventions for improving outcomes for patients with other types of chronic pain, but stated that the evidence of the effectiveness of psychoeducation for CSA self-management is inconclusive. They briefly noted some of the methodologic problems with existing studies (e.g., inadequate power, lack of a standardized intervention). McGillion and other colleagues themselves undertook a systematic review of this literature, which they cited, so they were well poised to critique the existing body of work.[1]

The researchers' argument led logically to the undertaking of this study, in that it highlighted the need for a well-designed test of a psychoeducation intervention for CSA patients. Their statement of purpose, placed as the last sentence of the introduction, was: "to

---

[1] Note that the researchers' presentation of the problem covered all six components we discussed in connection with problem statements in Chapter 6 of the textbook.

evaluate the effectiveness of a standardized psychoeducation program, entitled the Chronic Angina Self-Management Program (CASMP) for improving the HRQL, self-efficacy, and resourcefulness of CSA patients" (p. 414). Although the researchers did not explicitly state a hypothesis, the clear implication is that the researchers expected that patients who participated in the CASMP intervention would have better outcomes than patients who did not. The introduction to this article indicates that the researchers targeted a problem of considerable clinical significance to the health care community.

Overall, the introduction was well written and clearly organized. It concisely communicated the rationale for the study, and interwove supporting literature nicely, rather than having a separate literature review section. One comment about the literature cited, however, is that the majority of studies were fairly old. Of the 81 citations, fully 53 were published before the year 2000 and 16 were published before 1990. Without knowing this literature, we cannot determine whether the researchers were zealous and thorough (and therefore included studies comprehensively, including many older ones) or were not up-to-date in the current literature and therefore relied on older literature. We strongly suspect the former to be the case, but we wonder whether the space devoted to listing older citations in the reference list could have been better used, inasmuch as page constraints for this journal article must have been an issue (see below for some suggested additions to the introduction). On a very positive note, the researchers did a nice job of citing an interdisciplinary mix of studies from medical, nursing, other health care, and psychological journals.

Although the succinctness of the introduction is in many respects laudable, a few additional paragraphs might have better set the stage for readers. Here are some possible supplementary topics that could have strengthened the introduction:

- The authors stated several of the consequences of CSA, but did not document any economic implications (e.g., lost time from work for patients, increased costs from treatment for depression, costs associated with care in emergency departments). Given that psychoeducation programs such as the one tested involve an investment of resources, a more convincing argument for its utility might involve outlining how such an intervention might be cost-effective.

- The theoretical basis of the psychoeducation intervention was not alluded to in the introduction (it is briefly mentioned later in the article). It would be useful to have a brief upfront theoretical rationale for why a psychoeducation intervention might translate into improved psychosocial and physical outcomes.

- Relatedly, the introduction did not articulate a rationale for the researchers' selection of intervention outcomes. Several of the consequences of CSA that were mentioned in the first paragraph (e.g., activity restrictions, impaired role functioning) were apparently not specifically viewed as targets for improvement in this study. Also, certain outcomes stated in the purpose statement (self-efficacy, resourcefulness) were not described earlier as being relevant to either the clinical problem or the intervention model. Perhaps if there had been a better description of the theoretical framework in the introduction, the rationale for selecting these outcomes would have been clearer.

- The purpose statement indicated that the study would be tested on an existing structured intervention, CASMP. The introduction should perhaps have provided readers with a one- to two-sentence description of what prior research had found concerning the effectiveness of this specific intervention.

# METHOD

The method section was nicely organized, with numerous subheadings so that readers could easily locate specific elements of the design and methods. The method section included important and useful information about how the researchers designed and implemented their study.

## Research Design

McGillion and colleagues' clinical trial involved a very strong research design—a pretest–posttest experimental design that involved random assignment of study participants to an experimental (E) group that received the 6-week CASMP program or a control (C) group that received only "usual care" during the study period. Data were collected from all sample members at baseline and then again 3 months later. The researchers chose an ethically strong control group strategy of wait-listing controls for 3 months so that, after the posttest data were collected, control group members could opt to receive the intervention. One of the shortcomings of such a "delay of treatment" design is that it precludes long-term follow-up. That is, once the Cs are allowed to enroll in the intervention, E–C comparisons no longer provide a valid basis for inferring program effects. The researchers were fully aware of this, and noted that their intent in this research was to seek evidence of short-term (3-month) effects as a basis for launching a larger-scale trial with longer follow-up. (The researchers' rationale for collecting posttest data at 3 months—as opposed to, say, 2 months or 4 months, was not stated). As discussed later in this critique, the research design is one that has the potential for strong internal validity—that is, for permitting inferences about whether the intervention *caused* beneficial outcomes.

## Study Population and Procedures

The researchers provided a good description of the study population, recruitment strategies, inclusion and exclusion criteria, methods of screening for eligibility, and procedures for obtaining informed consent. This subsection also did an extraordinarily good job of describing the randomization process and methods the researchers used to eliminate certain biases and validity threats. The researchers used a tightly controlled randomization process to ensure proper allocation to treatment, and used "assiduous follow-up procedures" (p. 415) to minimize attrition, which is the single biggest threat to internal validity in experimental studies. As is always true in interventions wherein both the program participants and the agents know who is in the experimental group, traditional blinding was not possible. Commendably, however, the researchers did take steps to ensure that the research assistant collecting the data was blinded to participants' group status.

The researchers also stated that usual care "consisted of all nursing, medical, and emergency care services as needed" (p. 415) and that Cs did not receive CASMP during the study period. It is noteworthy that the researchers mentioned what *usual care* means—"usual care" is often stated without further elaboration. This section further noted that wait-listed controls were offered entry into the next available CASMP once posttest data were collected. It cannot be ascertained from this article whether there was any possibility of contamination—that is, whether Cs could have been exposed to any part of the intervention during the study period, either through contact with Es being treated at the same hospitals or by the same clinicians, or through more direct contact with intervention agents. Judging from the care the researchers took in implementing the study, contamination likely was not a problem.

## Intervention

The CASMP intervention—a psychoeducation program given in 6 weekly sessions of 2 hours in a small classroom-type setting with 8 to 15 patients—was described in this section. The research team had undertaken preliminary research on CSA, and had adapted the CASMP program to increase its relevance to their study population.

The researchers selected an intervention that was standardized, meaning that the independent variable was presumably the same from one session to the next. Moreover, the nurse who delivered the program used a formal facilitator's manual to ensure consistent delivery. It is noteworthy that the researchers made efforts to assess intervention fidelity: all program sessions were audiotaped, and there was an external audit of a random sample of 10% of the tapes. Presumably, these audits provided reassurance to the research team that the intervention was appropriately implemented.

The intervention itself was succinctly but adequately described as an integrated approach using strategies "known to enhance self-efficacy, including skills mastery, modeling, and self-talk." Major strategies included discussion, group problem solving, individual experimentation with self-management techniques, and paired problem solving between sessions to enhance motivation. Figure 1 (p. 416) provided a nice overview of the content covered in the 6 weekly sessions.

In the description of the intervention, the authors noted that both the content and process aspects of CASMP are "grounded in Bandura's Self-Efficacy Theory" (p. 416), which posits that self-efficacy is critical to improving health-related behaviors. Although space constraints likely limited the researchers' ability to include a well-formulated conceptual map linking program components to mediating effects (such as self-efficacy) and to ultimate outcomes, such a map (or a verbal description of the theoretical pathway) would have been useful in understanding some of the researchers' decisions, including their selection of outcome variables.

## Measures

The researchers stated that their selection of outcomes was guided by Braden's Self-Help Model of Learned Response to Chronic Illness Experience. According to the authors, this model emphasizes human resilience and that people can develop skills to enhance life quality in the face of chronic illness. The relationship between this model and Bandura's Self-Efficacy Theory, and the link between Braden's model and CASMP is not explicated, and so the conceptual basis of the study remains a bit cloudy. Again, a conceptual map would be useful. The report stated that the primary outcome was HRQL and the secondary outcome was enabling skill (patients' self-efficacy and resourcefulness to manage their pain).

HRQL was measured using the 36-item Medical Outcome Study Short Form (SF-36). The SF-36 has eight subscales used to represent various aspects of health (e.g., physical functioning, bodily pain, vitality), and is a well-respected instrument with strong psychometric properties. The researchers reported that the reliability estimates for the SF-36 in this study (presumably internal consistency estimates as calculated by coefficient alpha) were all above .80, which is excellent. Commendably, because of some evidence that the SF-36 may not adequately discriminate patients with differing angina function, they administered a supplementary scale, the Seattle Angina Questionnaire (SAQ). This scale has five subscales (e.g., pain stability, physical limitation), and in this study the reliabilities ranged from .68 to .85.

The secondary outcome of self-efficacy was measured by an adapted 11-item Self-Efficacy Scale (SES), and resourcefulness was measured by Rosenbaum's 36-item Self Control Schedule (SCS). The known psychometric characteristics of these two scales were good, and the researchers found that internal consistency in this study was .94 for the SES and .80 for the SCS, both very strong.

It is also admirable that the researchers pretested their instrument package with a small sample of patients from the study population. They found that no changes were needed.

Overall, except for some ambiguity about the researchers' rationale for including particular constructs as outcomes (especially resourcefulness) and not including other potential constructs (e.g., ability for self-care, mentioned in the introduction as a documented consequence of CSA), the researchers' data collection plan seems sound and the specific measures they selected had excellent reliability and validity.

## Sample Size

The researchers' discussion about their sample size was very good. They assumed a moderate effect size for the effect of the program on their primary outcome, HRQL, and also offered a standard for clinical importance. They provided empirical support from other studies about the viability of their assumption of a moderate effect. Based on their assumption, they projected a need for 52 participants in each study group, to achieve a power of .80 with an alpha of .05. Even though their research plan included methods to keep attrition to a minimum, they built a cushion into their sample size estimates, and therefore sought to enroll 65 participants in each group. This was the total number of patients randomized, with 66 being enrolled in CASMP and 64 put in the wait-list control group.

## Data Analysis

The researchers' data analysis strategy was explained in some detail, with information about both analytic strategies and the rationale for analytic decisions.

The first sentence indicated that the intention-to-treat (ITT) principle was used in the analyses, the approach that is considered the gold standard for the analysis of RCT data. Randomization to treatment groups is a critical ingredient in permitting causal inferences to be made about the effect of the intervention on outcomes of interest. Randomization creates groups presumed to be equal in every respect, except that one group gets the intervention and the other does not. Group equivalence is lost, however, whenever there is attrition: people withdrawing from a study cannot be assumed to be a random subset of the original groups. Therefore, the preferred method of analysis is to keep all original participants in the analysis, whether they remained in the study or not. Study dropouts by definition do not provide posttest data, and so researchers using an ITT approach must use some method to estimate (or *impute*) the posttest values for people whose data are missing. ITT yields conservative estimates of program effects because it includes people who may not have actually received the treatment, but it is the only accepted way of preserving randomization and minimizing an important threat to internal validity—the nonequivalence of the groups being compared. In other words, the researchers stated that they adopted the most widely accepted approach to analysis.

It is not clear, however, that ITT *was* used. As indicated in the excellent CONSORT-type flow chart (Figure 2, p. 419), 130 participants were randomized, but 13 dropped out of the study (Nine Es and four Cs). Follow-up data were collected from 117. Judging from the degrees of freedom in Tables 3 through 5 (degrees of freedom can be used to determine how many people were in the analysis), the final analysis was based on the people who actually provided posttest data, not the full sample of 130 who were randomized. Moreover, if the researchers had estimated values for the missing posttest data for the 13 patients who withdrew, they presumably would have explained their method of imputation. In sum, it does not appear that a true ITT was actually used.

The data analysis section provided an excellent explanation of the researchers' primary statistical analyses. The results reported in this paper involved comparisons of the *change scores* for the E versus the C group. That is, for every person, the difference between his or her posttest score and baseline score (for all scale and subscale scores) was used as the dependent variable, so that readers could see directly how much improvement had occurred. The report indicated that an alternative analytic method, ANCOVA, was also used and that the results were totally consistent with that reported. (In ANCOVA, posttest scores, rather than change scores were used as the dependent variables, and baseline scores were used as covariates, so that baseline values would be statistically controlled). Because the researchers had multiple dependent variables—multiple subscale scores for the SF-36, for example—multivariate analysis of variance was used. The tables show results for both ANOVA and MANOVA. The researchers' statistical approach was very strong.

# RESULTS

The results section provided useful information about how many people were recruited and what the flow of participants was in this study. Attrition in this study was fairly low, with follow-up data obtained from 90% of the patients randomized.

An excellent early subsection of the results was devoted to analyzing potential biases and threats to internal validity. The researchers presented two tables showing the baseline characteristics of the Es and Cs, and reported that none of the baseline group differences was statistically significant at conventional levels. These tables not only demonstrated the initial comparability of the groups (in terms of demographic and clinical variables), they also communicated vital information about the study population, which is extremely important to readers considering whether the CASMP intervention might be appropriate for their own clients. The researchers also reported their analysis of attrition bias: for all of the demographic and clinical characteristics measured at baseline, people who remained in the study were not significantly different from those who dropped out. (The researchers probably also looked at comparability of the groups in terms of baseline performance on the outcome variables, but these results were not, unfortunately, reported).

The key results were reported in a subsection labeled *Intervention Effects*. The tables summarizing the results were inherently complex, but they were well organized and clear, with good footnotes to help interpret the symbols and abbreviations used. Text was used judiciously to highlight the main findings. The results indicated that improvements were significantly greater for Es than Cs on several important outcome measures. For the SF-36 outcome measure, differences in change scores were significantly better for those who were in the intervention group with regard to physical functioning and general health—but not bodily pain, nor any of the mental health subscales. On the SAQ, significant improvements were observed for both angina frequency and angina stability. In terms of secondary outcomes, the program had significant effects on improving SES scores, but not resourcefulness. One comment is that it would have been desirable to present information about the precision of the change score differences using confidence intervals and (especially) effect size estimates. It is possible, however, that page limitations constrained the researchers' ability to include this information.

The researchers also included very valuable information about cohort effects—results that are seldom noted in RCT reports. When an intervention unfolds over time, as many do, it is useful to see if the intervention effects are consistent over time. Changes in the degree of improvement might occur if, for example, sample characteristics change over time or if the implementation of the program changes over time (for example, improves as a result of early experiences or declines because of waning enthusiasm of the facilitator). McGillion and colleagues noted that there were six cohorts of patients, and that differences in the amount of improvement among the Es in the six cohorts were not significant.

Finally, the researchers provided some information about actual program participation using data from their process evaluation. It is reassuring that the vast majority of patients assigned to the intervention group (93%) actually attended all six sessions. This is a remarkably high rate of participation, and shows a very high "dose" of the treatment for almost all participants. Thus, the report indicated that not only was the *delivery* of the independent variable standardized, its *receipt* was fairly uniform as well.

# DISCUSSION

McGillion and colleagues offered a thoughtful discussion of their findings. They began by providing a context, comparing their study findings to findings from other studies of the effects of psychoeducation interventions for CSA patients and patients with slightly different chronic pain problems. They offered some plausible interpretations of differences and similarities in the results. The results of these studies are broadly consistent, in that positive effects on indicators of quality of life were observed in all studies, though on slightly different dimensions (or measures) of HRQL.

The authors also discussed the clinical significance of their findings. That is, in addition to achieving statistically significant program effects, they argued that the amount of improvement demonstrated by the intervention group is sufficiently large to be considered clinically significant.

The authors discussed the strengths of their study, which were considerable. They also noted some possible limitations, which included the following: lack of blinding of participants and intervention agents, which could have led to possible performance bias (i.e., people performing at their best because of their awareness of being in the intervention); the possibility that there was inadequate power to detect group differences for some of the outcomes for which program effects were more modest; the short-term follow-up of participants, making it impossible to draw conclusions about the program's longer-term effects; the use of a single facilitator, which could adversely affect the generalizability of the results; and the setting of the study in a university site, which again has implications for the external validity of the findings. It was admirable and insightful of the investigators to have noted these shortcomings, and they offered suggestions for addressing them in subsequent research.

# GENERAL COMMENTS

## Presentation

This report was well written and well organized and provided an unusually good amount of detail about the researchers' decisions and their rationales. The primary presentational shortcoming concerned the limited elaboration of the conceptual basis of the study. We suspect that the ambiguity about the linkages between the theories/models and the intervention are not conceptual flaws, but rather communication issues. Given the great care that was taken in the design and execution of the study, the researchers likely had a fully developed conceptualization, but opted to abbreviate their presentation.

## Ethical Aspects

The authors did not provide much information about steps they took to ensure that participants were treated ethically—which does not mean that there were ethical transgressions.

For example, no mention was made of having the study approved by a human subject committee (in Canada, a Research Ethics Board). The only relevant information in the report was a statement about obtaining informed consent. There is no indication in the report that the participants were harmed, deceived, or mistreated in any way. And, indeed, their wait-list design is ethically commendable.

## Validity Issues

McGillion and colleagues undertook an extremely rigorous study, and they are to be commended for the excellence of their work. They used a powerful research design and made exemplary efforts to reduce or eliminate serious validity threats. Many of the limitations of this excellent study were noted by the authors themselves.

The study was quite strong in terms of internal validity: we can be reasonably confident that the CASMP program had beneficial effects on the participants' perceptions of self-efficacy and on aspects of their quality of life. Participants were carefully randomized, and the authors presented evidence that randomization was successful in creating two groups that were comparable at the outset of the study. Thus, a key threat to internal validity—selection bias—was adequately addressed. There is no reason to suspect that threats such as history, maturation, or testing played a role in influencing the results. The major plausible internal validity threat in experimental designs is mortality—i.e., differential attrition from study groups. Attrition was modestly higher among the Es than the Cs, but overall attrition was low. The authors reported that those who dropped out of the study were not significantly different than those who stayed in the study in terms of baseline characteristics.

In terms of statistical conclusion validity, the fact that the researchers found highly significant group differences for several outcomes indicates that statistical conclusion validity was good—but it was not excellent, as the authors themselves noted. If one looks at Tables 3 through 5, the differences in change scores favored Es over Cs *for every single outcome*, but not always at statistically significant levels. This suggests that, with a larger sample (i.e., greater statistical power), more E–C differences would likely have been statistically significant.

It might be noted however, that the positive and significant intervention effects, while likely "real," might possibly be somewhat inflated, given the fact that an ITT analysis does not appear to have been done (or at least, was not the one reported). People who dropped out of the study might have been patients for whom the CASMP program might not have "worked", for example, because of low motivation, interest, or need. We did a rough calculation that suggests that even with the dropouts included in the analysis, the group differences favoring Es would have continued to be large and almost certainly significant. For example, the first outcome in Table 3 (p. 421) is for the physical functioning subscale of the SF-36. On average, Es improved by 5.3 points on the scale over the 3-month study period, while Cs *deteriorated* by .68 points (mean change = –.68). Based on the degrees of freedom, it appears that the analysis was done with 116 participants (1 + 114 + 1); we will assume that the averages shown are for 57 Es and 59 Cs, for a total of 116. (There is no information about why this number is 116 and not 117, as suggested in Figure 2). The original E group included 66 patients, not 57. So, if we assume conservatively that the average change score for the 9 Es who dropped out of the study was –.68 (i.e., if we imputed the average missing change scores as identical to the average change among the Cs who, like program dropouts, did not get the intervention), and we compute a new average for all 66 Es, the value would

---

[2] Here is how we arrived at the calculation. First, we multiplied .68 × 9 (the number of Es who dropped out) = 6.12. Then, we multiplied the mean of 5.3 × 57 (the number of Es in the analysis) = 302.1. Next, because the change for the C group was negative, we subtracted 6.12 from 302.1 = 295.98. Finally, this overall sum of change scores was divided by the original number of Es (66), to yield the new average of 4.485, which we rounded to 4.5.

drop from 5.3 to 4.5—still considerably better than the -.68 for Cs.[2] In sum, we think that the evidence is persuasive that participation in the program was associated with significant improvement in outcomes.

In terms of construct validity, we have already noted that the researchers could have better communicated information about their conceptualization of the intervention. Performance bias—bias stemming from participants' and researchers' awareness of an innovation, and having the awareness rather than the actual intervention affect outcomes—is another construct validity issue that the authors acknowledged. It seems more plausible to us, however, that the *intervention* itself had beneficial effects on, say, angina frequency and physical functioning, than that *awareness* caused these improvements. This is probably more likely to be the case because the posttest outcomes were measured 6 weeks after the end of program sessions, at which point program awareness likely would have waned.

Finally, external validity in this study is an issue that needs to be addressed in subsequent research. The researchers noted some of the factors limiting the generalizability of the findings (e.g., the use of a single facilitator, and the setting for the intervention in a university site in Canada). Other limiting factors include the relatively small sample, the exclusion of very high-risk patients, and the refusal of about 20% of eligible patients to participate. As is almost invariably true in clinical trials, the viability of the intervention for broader groups of CSA patients depends on replications. It may also depend on the ability of future researchers to demonstrate the cost-effectiveness of psychoeducation interventions for this population.

# RESPONSE FROM THE MCGILLION TEAM AND FURTHER COMMENTS:

Dr. McGillion and his team graciously accepted our invitation to review this critique. Many of their comments confirmed that journal page constraints were the reason that some of the additional details or discussion points were absent from their paper. Here, for example, is their comment about conceptual framing (personal communication, June 23, 2008):

> We appreciate the critical importance of a clear conceptual framing that provides the rationale for outcome selection and related measures. Journal style and limitations imposed on length were again factors in why this particular level of detail was left out of the manuscript. The primary outcome for this trial was HRQOL. Secondary outcomes included self-efficacy and resourcefulness. The conceptual framework that guided examination of these outcomes was Braden's Self-Help Model *(references were provided, but are omitted here)*. The effectiveness of the CASMP was tested for improving scores in HRQOL, self-efficacy, and resourcefulness for CSA patients. Braden's Self-Help Model reflects the dynamics of a learned self-management response to chronic illness and was applied in order to link these variables together through the concept of enabling skill. Enabling skill, or one's perceived ability to manage adversity, was the proposed mediating variable by which one learns a self-help capacity, thereby experiencing enhanced life quality.

The authors also commented on our critique of their ITT analysis. This is what they wrote (personal communication, June 23, 2008):

> Regarding intention to treat (ITT) analysis: We do not agree that an analysis conducted according to ITT principles necessarily involves the imputation of posttest values for those participants lost to attrition. Rather, we would argue that ITT is commonly used as an umbrella term for two

separate issues: a) treatment group [i.e. treatment or control] adherence and b) missing data. We state that we have analyzed our data according to ITT because we analyzed the data according to how participants were randomized–control participants remained in the control group and treatment group's participants remained in the treatment group. When data were missing, they were missing; we did not use any method to impute or estimate missing data. There are several methods to impute or estimate missing data such as 'last observation carried forward', or propensity scores. We felt that the use of such imputation techniques for an intervention study was inappropriate, as they are all means of estimating what missing outcome data 'might' have been.

We respectfully disagree with parts of this comment. The more appropriate term for the type of analysis that these researchers did is a *per protocol* analysis (analyzing people in groups according to the protocol to which they were randomized). This is the analytic approach that virtually all researchers follow. Very few researchers actually do a true ITT analysis that maintains all randomized participants in the analysis.

We do agree with the authors, however, that there is a lot of confusion about ITT in the research literature, and outright disagreement about how to (or even whether to) impute missing values. The "state of the art" at the moment is to use sophisticated statistical procedures to "fill in" missing outcome data, and to then test how different procedures affect the results. (The technical term for this is a *sensitivity analysis*, which we talked about in the textbook in the chapter on meta-analysis).

In the McGillion et al. study, we are reasonably confident that if they had performed a true ITT analysis with imputation of outcome data for dropouts, the conclusions that the intervention had positive effects would have remained the same. Our crude demonstration of "imputation" supports this view. Given the low rate of attrition and the analysis indicating that dropouts were similar to those who remained in the study, it is perhaps understandable that the researchers did not undertake time-consuming and challenging analyses with imputations. The main problem, in our view, is that they used a term that implies a type of analysis they did not pursue.

Despite our disagreement with the authors about this point, the fact remains that this research team took extraordinary steps to ensure the integrity of their study. There is little doubt that their study is extremely high on internal validity—one of the best examples we have seen in the nursing research literature.

# Differences in Perceptions of the Diagnosis and Treatment of Obstructive Sleep Apnea and Continuous Positive Airway Pressure Therapy Among Adherers and Nonadherers

Amy M. Sawyer • Janet A. Deatrick •
Samuel T. Kuna • Terri E. Weaver

▶ **Abstract:** Obstructive sleep apnea (OSA) patients' consistent use of continuous positive airway pressure (CPAP) therapy is critical to realizing improved functional outcomes and reducing untoward health risks associated with OSA. We conducted a mixed methods, concurrent, nested study to explore OSA patients' beliefs and perceptions of the diagnosis and CPAP treatment that differentiate adherent from nonadherent patients prior to and after the first week of treatment, when the pattern of CPAP use is established. Guided by social cognitive theory, themes were derived from 30 interviews conducted postdiagnosis and after 1 week of CPAP use. Directed content analysis, followed by categorization of participants as adherent/nonadherent from objectively measured CPAP use, preceded across-case analysis among 15 participants with severe OSA. Beliefs and perceptions that differed between adherers and nonadherers included OSA risk perception, symptom recognition, self-efficacy, outcome expectations, treatment goals, and treatment facilitators/barriers. Our findings suggest opportunities for developing and testing tailored interventions to promote CPAP use.

▶ **Key Words:** Adherence · compliance · content analysis · decision making · health behavior · mixed methods · sleep disorders · social cognitive theory

Obstructive sleep apnea (OSA), characterized by repetitive nocturnal upper airway collapse resulting in intermittent oxyhemoglobin desaturation and sleep fragmentation, contributes to significant disabling sequelae, including daytime sleepiness, impaired cognitive and executive function, mood disturbances, and increased cardiovascular and metabolic morbidity (Al Lawati, Patel, & Ayas, 2009; Harsch et al., 2004; Nieto, et al.

*Qualitative Health Research*, 2010; 20(7):873–892. Copyright © 2010. Reprinted by permission of SAGE Publications.

2000; Peppard, Young, Palta, & Skatrud, 2000). The prevalence of OSA, based on minimal diagnostic criteria (apnea/hypopnea index [AHI] of 5 events/hour), has been estimated at 2% in women and 4% in men in the United States (Young et al., 1993). More recently, large U.S.-cohort studies have provided additional evidence of the prevalence of OSA, estimating that approximately one in five adults with a mean body mass index (BMI) of at least 25 kg/m$^2$ has at least mild OSA, defined as an apnea-hypopnea index (AHI) $\geq$ 5 events/hour; and one in 15 adults with a mean BMI of at least 25 kg/m$^2$ has at least moderate OSA (i.e., AHI $\geq$ 15 events/hour; Young, Peppard, & Gottlieb, 2002). Continuous positive airway pressure (CPAP) therapy is the primary medical treatment for adults with OSA, eliminating repetitive, nocturnal airway closures; normalizing oxygen levels; and effectively improving daytime impairments (Gay, Weaver, Loube, & Iber, 2006; Sullivan, Barthon-Jones, Issa, & Eves, 1981; Weaver & Grunstein, 2008).

Nonadherence to CPAP is recognized as a significant limitation in the effective treatment of OSA, with average adherence rates ranging from 30% to 60% (Engleman, Martin, & Douglas, 1994; Kribbs et al., 1993; Krieger, 1992; Reeves-Hoche, Meck, & Zwillich, 1994; Sanders, Gruendl, & Rogers, 1986; Weaver, Kribbs, et al., 1997). Nonadherent users begin skipping nights of CPAP use during the first week of treatment, and their hourly use of CPAP on days used is significantly shorter than those who apply CPAP consistently (Aloia, Arndt, Stanchina, & Millman, 2007; Weaver, Kribbs, et al., 1997). Patients who are nonadherent during early treatment generally remain nonadherent over the long term (Aloia, Arndt, Stanchina, et al., 2007; Krieger, 1992; McArdle et al., 1999; Weaver, Kribbs, et al., 1997). The return of symptoms and other manifestations of OSA with even one night of nonuse underscores the critical nature of adherence to CPAP (Grunstein et al., 1996; Kribbs et al., 1993).

Many studies have explored what factors predict adherence to CPAP (Engleman et al., 1996; Engleman, Martin, et al., 1994; Kribbs et al., 1993; Massie, Hart, Peralez, & Richards, 1999; McArdle et al., 1999; Meurice et al., 1994; Reeves-Hoche et al., 1994; Rosenthal et al., 2000; Schweitzer, Chambers, Birkenmeier, & Walsh, 1997; Sin, Mayers, Man, & Pawluk, 2002). Self-reported side effects of CPAP do not distinguish between adherers and non-adherers to CPAP. Subjective sleepiness, severity of OSA as determined by apnea-hypopnea index, and severity of nocturnal hypoxia are inconsistently identified as correlates, albeit weak, of CPAP adherence (Weaver & Grunstein, 2008). The majority of these studies have focused on physiological variables and patient characteristics as predictors of adherence. Over the past 10 years, studies have identified psychological and social factors and cognitive perceptions, such as self efficacy, risk perception, and outcome expectancies, as determinants of CPAP use (Aloia, Arnedt, Stepnowsky, Hecht, & Borrelli, 2005; Lewis, Seale, Bartle, Watkins, & Ebden, 2004; Russo-Magno, O'Brien, Panciera, & Rounds, 2001; Stepnowsky, Bardwell, Moore, Ancoli-Israel, & Dimsdale, 2002; Stepnowsky, Marler, & Ancoli-Israel, 2002; Wild, Engleman, Douglas, & Espie, 2004). Social and situational variables have also been suggested as influential on CPAP adherence, with those who live alone, who have had a recent life event, and who experienced problems with CPAP on the first night of exposure having lower adherence to CPAP therapy (Lewis et al., 2004). Support group attendance has also been identified as contributing to higher CPAP use in older men (Russo- Magno et al., 2001). Findings of both of these studies suggest that social support is an important factor influencing decisions to use CPAP, yet the sociostructural context of accepting and adhering to CPAP treatment has not been described from the perspective of the patient in the extant literature. Other studies have identified that early experiences with CPAP (i.e., during the first week) are an important influence on patients' perceptions and beliefs about the OSA diagnosis and treatment with CPAP (Aloia, Arnedt, Stepnowsky, et al., 2005; Stepnowsky, Bardwell, et al., 2002).

From the collective published evidence, early experiences with CPAP, combined with patients' perceptions and beliefs about OSA and CPAP and the balance of their sociostructural facilitators/barriers, are critical factors that influence patients' decisions to use CPAP. To date, there are relatively few studies that have systematically examined the influence of disease and treatment perceptions and beliefs on CPAP adherence. Because the first week of CPAP treatment is critically influential on OSA patients' decisions to use CPAP, it is imperative that the contextual experiences and underlying beliefs and perceptions of the diagnosis and treatment be described. There are no published studies that have addressed this significant gap in the scientific literature. Furthermore, no study has directly explored patient perspectives, employing qualitative methodology, both at diagnosis and with treatment, to more fully describe contextual factors that differentiate CPAP adherers and nonadherers. Our study addressed several important questions: (a) What are adult OSA patients' beliefs and perceptions about OSA, the associated risks, and treatment with CPAP prior to treatment use? (b) What are the consequences of these beliefs and perceptions on the use of CPAP? (c) What are the beliefs and perceptions of adults with OSA after 1 week of CPAP use, including perceived benefits of treatment, effect of treatment on health, and perceived ability to adapt to CPAP? and (d) Do differences exist between adherers and nonadherers with regard to their beliefs and perceptions at diagnosis and with treatment use that might, in part, explain differences in CPAP adherence outcomes? To our knowledge, our study findings provide the first published description of beliefs of those who adhere and those who choose not to adhere to CPAP treatment. These findings contribute to understanding patient treatment decisions regarding CPAP use, suggest opportunities for identifying those at risk for nonadherence

to CPAP, and contribute toward developing tailored interventions to promote CPAP use.

# ■ Conceptual Framework

Acceptance and consistent use of CPAP is influenced by a multitude of factors, as is evidenced in previous studies examining predictors of CPAP adherence (Weaver & Grunstein, 2008). It is therefore important to approach the phenomenon of CPAP adherence from a multifactorial perspective that addresses the complex nature of this particular health behavior. The application of social cognitive theory has been widely applied in studies of adoption, initiation, and maintenance of health behaviors (Bandura, 1977, 1992; Schwarzer & Fuchs, 1996). The core determinants of the model include knowledge, perceived self-efficacy, outcome expectations, health goals, and facilitators/barriers. The model posits that health promoting behaviors are primarily influenced by patients' self-efficacy, or their belief in their ability to exercise control over personal health habits, which influences other critical determinants: knowledge, outcome expectations, goals, and perceived facilitators and impediments (Bandura, 2004; see Figure 1). Knowledge of health risks and specific benefits relative to health behaviors is a necessary determinant for health behaviors, but rarely does knowledge alone promote change in behaviors. Outcome expectations, or the expectancies one holds for investing in a particular health behavior, are evaluated by the individual in terms of costs and benefits, including physical, social, and psychological. Individuals who anticipate that the benefits of a health behavior outweigh the costs are more inclined to perceive the health behavior as favorable, and more inclined to set short- and long-term personal goals to guide adoption of that health behavior. This cascade of health behavior determinants does not occur in isolation, but is influenced by barriers and facilitators that derive from personal, social,

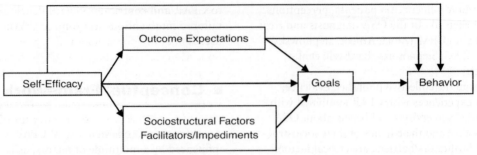

**Figure 1.** Social cognitive theory health determinants: Pathways of influence of self-efficacy on health behaviors. From Bandura, A. (2004). Health promotion by social cognitive means. *Health Education & Behavior, 31*(2), 146. Copyright 2004 by Sage Publications. Reprinted with permission of the publisher.

and environmental circumstances. As individuals identify facilitators for the health behavior and overcome barriers, their belief in their ability to successfully change or adopt a health behavior (i.e., perceived self-efficacy) increases.

Recognizing that individuals exist within a collective agency or community, the construct of self-efficacy is not confined solely to personal capabilities. Although commonalities in the basic concepts of self-efficacy exist across cultures, the "cultivated identities, values, belief structures, and agentic capabilities are the psychosocial systems through which experiences are filtered" (Bandura, 2002, p. 273). Bandura suggested that the application of social cognitive theory must be situated in context, recognizing that "human behavior is socially situated, richly contextualised, and conditionally expressed" (2002, p. 276). From this conceptual perspective and in a predominantly qualitative research paradigm, we examined patients' perceptions, beliefs, and experiences within their own context to permit an explicit description of salient factors that influenced OSA patients' decisions to use or not use CPAP.

# ■ Method

## DESIGN

Using a concurrent nested, mixed method design, we conducted a longitudinal study extending from initial diagnosis through the first week of home CPAP treatment of newly diagnosed OSA patients. We conducted two individual interviews with participants and collected first-week CPAP adherence data. In contrast to a triangulation design, the concurrent nested study design emphasizes one methodology, and the data are mixed at the analysis phase of the study (Creswell, Plano Clark, Gutmann, & Hanson, 2003). Nesting the less dominant quantitative method within the predominant qualitative method permitted an enriched description of the participants and a more in-depth analysis of the overall phenomenon of interest: CPAP adherence (Creswell et al., 2003).

## PARTICIPANTS

Adults with suspected OSA were recruited from a sleep clinic at an urban Veterans Affairs medical center during a 5-month enrollment period. One sleep specialist referred potential participants who were clinically likely to have OSA to the study. Our purposive sampling strategy was to include patients who (a) provided detailed information during their initial clinical visit and were willing to openly discuss their health and health care; (b) had at least moderate OSA (AHI ≥ 15 events/hour; American Academy of Sleep Medicine Task Force, 1999) and were prescribed CPAP treatment; (c) initially accepted CPAP for home use; and (d) were able to speak and understand English. To ensure that participants would be prescribed CPAP treatment based on Veterans Health Administration CPAP prescribing guidelines in place during study enrollment, patients with mild OSA (AHI < 15 events/hour) were excluded. We also excluded participants who had current or historical treatment with CPAP or any other treatment for OSA, a previous diagnosis of OSA, refusal of CPAP treatment by the participant prior to any CPAP exposure (i.e., in-laboratory CPAP titration sleep study), and those who required supplemental oxygen in addition to CPAP and/or bilevel positive airway pressure therapy for treatment of sleep-disordered breathing during their in-laboratory CPAP titration sleep study.

Previous studies have identified that decisions to adhere to CPAP emerge by the second to fourth day of treatment (Aloia, Arnedt, Stanchina, et al., 2007; Weaver, Kribbs, et al., 1997). Therefore, it is possible that patients' beliefs, perceptions, and experiences during the first several experiences with CPAP might significantly influence short- and long-term CPAP adherence patterns. For this reason, we did not include individuals who refused CPAP treatment prior to any CPAP experience, because we sought to describe salient factors preceding and during initial CPAP exposure. The protocol was approved by the research site and the affiliated university's institutional review boards. All participants provided informed consent prior to participating in any study activities.

## PROCEDURE

After study enrollment, each participant had two in-laboratory, full-night sleep studies (i.e., polysomnograms). The first sleep study was a diagnostic study and the second sleep study was to determine the therapeutic CPAP pressure necessary to eliminate obstructive sleep apnea events. All sleep studies were performed and scored using standard criteria (American Academy of Sleep Medicine Task Force, 1999; Rechtschaffen & Kales, 1968). The AHI, a

measure of disease severity in OSA, was computed from the diagnostic polysomnogram as the number of apneas and/or hypopneas per hour of sleep. The therapeutic CPAP pressure, the pressure required to eliminate hypopneas and apneas, was determined on a manual CPAP titration polysomnogram performed about 1 week ($7.9 \pm 6.9$ days) after the diagnostic polysomnogram.

**Semistructured Interviews.** Semistructured interviews, conducted by one study investigator, were scheduled with participants at two intervals: within 1 week following diagnosis but prior to the CPAP titration sleep study, and after the first week of CPAP treatment at home (see Figure 2). All interviews were conducted in an informal, private room at the medical center to ensure privacy, participant comfort, and promote open sharing of information (Streubert Speziale & Carpenter, 2003). To minimize attrition, participants were offered the opportunity to participate in interviews at an alternative location or by telephone if transportation difficulties or ambulatory limitations precluded study participation.

Interview guides, consisting of specific questions and probes (i.e., prompts to encourage focus on the particular issue of interest) were used for each interview to ensure that a consistent sequence and set of questions were addressed across participants. A funnel approach was used in the development and execution of the interview guides. This approach begins with broad questions and gradually progresses to focused questions specific to the phenomenon of interest to promote sharing of experiences by the participants (Tashakkori & Teddlie, 1989). The first interview focused on perceptions of the diagnosis, perceived health effects of the diagnosis, pretreatment perceptions of CPAP, and the social and cultural precedents that led to the participant seeking medical care for their sleep problems (see Table 1). The second interview focused on perceived effects of treatment with CPAP, supportive mechanisms or barriers to using CPAP, and how beliefs and perceptions about the diagnosis, associated risks of

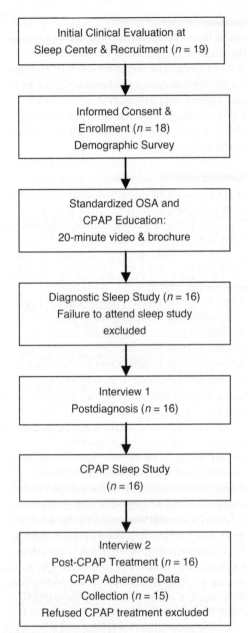

**Figure 2.** Study design.

the diagnosis, and the treatment experience might have affected CPAP adherence (see Table 2). Interviews were digitally audio-recorded and transcribed to an electronic format by a professional transcriptionist not affiliated with the study. Field notes were maintained by the interviewer before and after each interview to describe the environment of the interview, describe the participant at the time of the interview, and note any aberrations from the planned interview guide that occurred and a description of such aberrations. The field notes not only served as a descriptive context of the interview, but also served as interviewer reflexivity notations (i.e., interviewer biases, suppositions, and presuppositions of the research topic). The purpose of maintaining reflexivity notations was to ensure that interviewer-imposed assumptions did not take precedent over the participant's described experience.

**CPAP Adherence.** In accordance with the standard of clinical care at the sleep center, all participants were issued the same model CPAP machine (Respironics Rem- Star Pro®) that records on a data card (SmartCardTM) the time each day that the CPAP circuit is pressurized, an objective measurement of daily CPAP mask-on time. CPAP use was defined as periods when the device was applied for more than 20 minutes at effective pressure. One week of CPAP adherence data were uploaded to a personal computer for software analysis (Respironics EncorePro®) at the time of the second semistructured interview. Graphic adherence data were used as probes to discuss specific occurrences of CPAP nonuse. The objectively measured CPAP adherence data were also used to identify adherent ($\geq$ 6hrs/night CPAP use) and nonadherent participants ($<$ 6hrs/night CPAP use). A cut-off point of 6 hours/night was selected a priori to describe adherers and nonadherers to CPAP treatment, as recent evidence suggests that 6 or more hours of CPAP use per night is necessary to improve both functional and objective sleepiness outcomes (Weaver et al., 2007).

## ANALYSIS

A sequential analysis was conducted, with qualitative-directed content analysis of interview data followed by quantitative descriptive

# Table 1. Postdiagnosis Interview Guide

| Concept | Topic/Question |
|---|---|
| Perceptions and knowledge of diagnosis | How did you know about sleep disorders and the sleep center before coming to your first appointment?<br>Before being told you have OSA,[a] had you heard of OSA? If so, what did you know about OSA?<br>What do you now understand about OSA?<br>After having your sleep study, what are your thoughts about OSA and what it means to you? |
| Perceived effects of diagnosis | How do you believe OSA affects you in your daily life? |
| Sociocultural precedents and influences on health, illness/disease, and care seeking | Do you know anyone else who has been diagnosed with OSA? If so, how did that impact you and your interest in coming to the sleep center?<br>Why did you seek care from the sleep center?<br>Is there anyone who influenced you to seek care for this problem?<br>Is there anyone who has helped you understand what OSA is? If so, how did that information impact your desire to receive treatment?<br>What has you experience with a health care system been to this point?<br>Do sleep, sleeping, and/or the sleep environment have any specific meaning(s) to you? To your family? To your spouse/significant other/bed partner? |

[a]OSA = Obstructive sleep apnea

analysis of the CPAP adherence data. By sequentially analyzing the data, the priority of the individual as informant was emphasized and the investigators were blinded to CPAP adherence until the final analysis procedure, a mixed methods analysis, was conducted (see Figure 3). By dividing the participants into categories of adherent (i.e., ≥ 6 hrs/night CPAP use) and nonadherent (i.e., < 6 hrs/night CPAP use), we examined across-case consistencies in subthemes and themes to describe the contextualized experience of adhering or not adhering to CPAP treatment.

Each transcript was read in its entirety, highlighting, extracting, and condensing text from individual interviews that addressed individual beliefs, perceptions, and/or experiences during diagnosis and early treatment with CPAP. This process of text analysis brought forward the manifest content of the qualitative data (Graneheim & Lundman, 2004). These responses were separated from the interview text, identified by participant identification number, and entered into an analysis table. Abstraction, or the process of taking condensed, manifest data and interpreting the underlying meaning (i.e., latent meaning), followed as participant responses were then described in a condensed format and interpreted for meaning within a thematic coding process. Trustworthiness was enhanced as the likelihood of investigator bias was minimized by first highlighting relevant text for coding, extracting relevant text from complete interviews transcripts, and then coding the meaning units for theory-driven categories or themes and then for subthemes (Hsieh & Shannon, 2005).

*Qualitative Health Research*, 2010; 20(7):873–892.   Copyright © 2010. Reprinted by permission of SAGE Publications.

## Table 2. One Week Post-CPAP Use Interview Guide

| Concept | Topic/Question |
| --- | --- |
| Perceived effects and knowledge of treatment with CPAP | Have you been using CPAP[a] for the treatment of your OSA[b]?<br>How would you describe your use of CPAP?<br>Are you experiencing any improvement in the way that you feel since you have started using CPAP?<br>When did you first learn about CPAP?<br>Who first described CPAP to you?<br>What did you think when you first learned about CPAP? First saw CPAP? First used CPAP in the sleep laboratory?<br>What do you see as the most important reason for using CPAP in the short term? In the long term? |
| Supportive mechanisms or barriers to incorporating CPAP into daily life | How was the first week of CPAP treatment?<br>What kinds of problems are you experiencing using CPAP?<br>What has prevented you from regularly using CPAP?<br>What has been helpful to you in regularly using CPAP? |
| Sociocultural perspectives of health-related decisions to use or not use CPAP | Do you believe CPAP treatment is a treatment you can [continue to] use?<br>Did this belief change since you first learned about your OSA diagnosis? Since starting CPAP?<br>Do you envision yourself using CPAP during the next 3 months? During the next year? During the next 5 years?<br>Do you have any concerns about the CPAP unit? About your sleep [ability or quality]? About your sleep environment that might affect your CPAP use?<br>How does the diagnosis of OSA and treatment with CPAP affect or been affected by those around you? |

[a]CPAP = continuous positive airway pressure.
[b]OSA = obstructive sleep apnea.

The overarching, theory-derived themes were initially determined by applying the broad determinants of health as described in the study's conceptual framework, social cognitive theory (Bandura, 2004). These themes included knowledge, perceived barriers and facilitators, perceived self-efficacy, outcome expectations, and goals. This approach permitted the investigators to examine the applicability of the theoretical framework to the phenomenon of CPAP adherence and elaborate on previous findings suggesting the framework's concepts as measurable predictors of CPAP-related health behaviors (Aloia,

Arnedt, Stepnowsky, et al., 2005; Stepnowsky, Bardwell, et al., 2002; Wild et al., 2004). Emergent subthemes were identified as thematic content analysis progressed. The subthemes were then categorized within the overarching conceptual framework themes (see Table 3). We designed the analysis strategy to be consistent with other recent empirical studies of CPAP adherence while permitting a more robust, narrative description of what these theoretically derived variables mean from the perspective of the OSA patient.

Theme definitions were developed by the investigators and reviewed by an expert

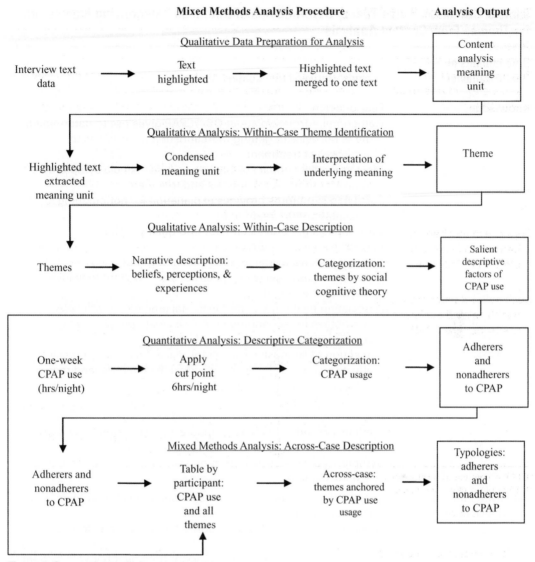

**Figure 3.** Sequential analysis procedure.

qualitative methodologist and an expert in the research application of theoretical constructs. One study investigator, blinded to CPAP adherence data, coded all interview data for the study. Valid application of the themes was examined by an independent expert coder. Coded interviews were independently recoded by the expert coder to establish validity and reliability of the application of the codes to the interview data. All extracted interview data were eligible for recoding; approximately 15% of the data from each total interview were randomly selected for expert recoding. Agreement of the study coder and the expert coder was 94%, meeting the established criteria of 80% agreement for acceptance of the coded data. When differences in application of codes were identified, code definitions were reviewed by coders, discussion of specific application of the code(s) was held, and

## Table 3. Social Cognitive Theory Determinants of Health as Categorizing Framework for Themes From Content Analysis

| Determinants of Health Behavior | Themes[a] Derived From Content Analysis |
| --- | --- |
| Knowledge | Fear of death |
| | Gathering information about OSA/CPAP gives rise to determining the importance of getting to treatment and decisions to accept/reject treatment |
| | Most immediate impact of OSA on daily life [single symptom] as a motivator to pursue diagnosis and treatment |
| | Justifying symptoms provides explanation for not pursuing diagnosis and/or treatment |
| | OSA impacts not only health but also quality of life |
| | Pervasive effects of OSA on life |
| | Sleepiness plays a limited role in life and can be accommodated |
| | Perceived health effects of a disorder are important to valuing diagnosis/treatment |
| | Associating health risks and functional limitations with OSA contributes to recognizing OSA as a health problem with significant effects on overall well-being |
| | Perception of seriousness of symptoms influenced by perceived effects symptoms have on individual [health risks] and those around individual [social network] |
| | Perceived health risks of OSA |
| | Information provided to individual and applicability of information influences individual's assumptions of responsibility for OSA and CPAP treatment |
| | Symptoms of OSA have impact on social roles, functions, and relationships |
| Perceived barriers and facilitators | Social influences as motivators to recognize health problem, seek diagnosis/treatment, and use CPAP |
| | Objective measures of OSA important to health care decision making |
| | Differences in perception of urgency of treatment between patient and provider influences valuing of diagnosis and treatment by patient |
| | Social networks contribute to treatment acceptance but not necessarily to treatment use |
| | Perceived seriousness of symptoms influenced by perceived effects of symptoms on individual [health risks] and those around individual |
| | Social networks provide support, help problem solve health concerns, and are sources of health-related information commonality of symptoms of OSA promotes perception of normalcy: Barrier to seeking diagnosis/treatment |

*(continued)*

## Table 3. *(Continued)*

| Determinants of Health Behavior | Themes[a] Derived From Content Analysis |
|---|---|
| | Social influences as motivators to recognize health problem, seek diagnosis and treatment, and use treatment |
| | Silent symptoms: Fear of what it means if symptoms of OSA are undetectable |
| | Family and social networks contribute to health beliefs about sleep |
| | Expectations of health delivery vs. the actual delivery of health care services impact on the importance individual's place on their health and the value they place on their relationship with health care providers |
| Perceived self-efficacy | Knowledge and information provided to individual and applicability of information influences individual's assumption of responsibility for OSA and CPAP treatment |
| | Early response to CPAP, consistent or inconsistent with outcome expectations, facilitates or is a barrier to treatment use |
| | Early experience with CPAP is a source of support or a barrier to belief in own ability to use treatment |
| | Fitting treatment into life |
| | Problem-solving difficulties/routinization of CPAP responsibilities contribute to disease management |
| Outcome expectations | Understanding why symptoms exist and associating specific symptoms with a diagnosis provides hope that treatment will address experienced symptoms and improve overall quality of life |
| | Expectations of treatment outcomes are facilitators of treatment initiation and use |
| | Early response to CPAP, consistent or inconsistent with outcome expectations, facilitates or is a barrier to using treatment |
| Goals | Problem-solving difficulties/routinization of CPAP responsibilities contribute to disease management |

[a] Themes derived from participant text data were categorized as a determinant of health behavior from social cognitive theory. Themes are not mutually exclusive. Theme definitions were mutually agreed on by investigators of the study and applied to the directed content analysis procedure by a single investigator acting as the primary coder of text data.

mutual agreement was achieved in all instances of coding differences.

After all interview data were coded for themes, the investigators used the average daily CPAP use during the first week of treatment to separate adherers ($\geq$ 6 hours CPAP use/night) and nonadherers ($<$ 6 hours CPAP use/ night). Descriptive statistics were used in the analysis of 1 week of CPAP adherence data (mean $\pm$ standard deviation [SD]).

Across-case analysis of themes and subthemes was then examined from an integrative perspective, using adherent and nonadherent as anchors, or as a unique descriptive qualifier, to identify common perceptions, beliefs, and experiences within the groups of interest. The across-case analysis, including both qualitative and quantitative data sets as complementary within an analysis matrix, gave rise to cases that had common descriptive aspects.

*Qualitative Health Research*, 2010; 20(7):873–892. Copyright © 2010. Reprinted by permission of SAGE Publications.

## RESULTS

With the recurrence of themes in the content analysis phase, data saturation was reached at 15 participants and the sampling procedure was considered complete. The participants were all veterans, predominantly middleaged (53.9 ± 12.7 years) men (88%; see Table 4). The participants were well educated, with

### Table 4. Sample Description

| Characteristic | Frequency (%) (n = 15) |
|---|---|
| Gender | |
| Men | 13 (87%) |
| Women | 2 (13%) |
| Race/ethnicity | |
| African American | 9 (60%) |
| White | 5 (33%) |
| Other | 1 (7%) |
| Marital status | |
| Married | 7 (47%) |
| Single | 3 (20%) |
| Divorced | 3 (20%) |
| Widowed | 2 (13%) |
| Highest education | |
| Middle school | 1 (7%) |
| High school | 7 (47%) |
| 2 yr college | 4 (27%) |
| 4+ yr college | 3 (20%) |
| Shift work | 3 (20%) |
| Employed | 6 (40%) |
| Retired | 6 (40%) |
| | **Mean 6 Standard Deviation** |
| Age, years | 53.9 ± 12.7 |
| Weight, pounds | 248.9 ± 68.7 |
| AHI, events/hour | 53.5 ± 26.5 |
| O2 Nadir, % | 66.4 ± 13.2 |
| CPAP pressure, cmH$_2$O | 10.7 ± 1.6 |
| 1 week CPAP adherence, hours | 4.98 ± 0.5 |

93% (n = 14) of the sample achieving a high school education or higher. The sample, on average, had severe OSA (AHI 53.5 ± 26.5 events/hr), with an oxygen nadir of 66.4% (± 13.2%). The average CPAP pressure setting was 10.7 ± 1.6 cmH20. Average CPAP use during the first 7 days of CPAP treatment was 4.98 ± 0.5 hours/night. Sorting on CPAP adherence (i.e. ≥ 6hrs/night CPAP use and < 6 hrs/ night CPAP use), there were six adherers and nine nonadherers. The interview prior to CPAP exposure was conducted after the diagnostic polysomnogram, on average at Day 9 (range 2 to 28 days), and the second interview was conducted following at least 1 week of CPAP treatment (average number of days from Day 1 of CPAP use, 18; range 7 to 47 days).

## ADHERERS AND NONADHERERS TO CPAP THERAPY

**Knowledge and Perceived Health Risks.**
Knowledge, or the "knowing" an individual has about the health risks and benefits of health behaviors (Bandura, 2004) was a predominant theme in both interviews for all participants. Saturation on nearly every knowledge theme suggests that participants identified that having an understanding of OSA and CPAP is an important part of the experience of being diagnosed with OSA and treated with CPAP. Adherent participants related their knowledge of risks and benefits of CPAP to their own outcome expectations after being diagnosed with OSA. For some participants, knowledge of OSA being simply more than snoring was a first step in recognizing OSA as a syndrome with health implications. One participant described this, saying, "I knew sleep apnea existed, but it just never dawned on me how serious it was in my case. I just didn't pay any attention to it. I just figured I was going to snore for the rest of my life."

For many participants, "putting the whole picture together" after receiving education about OSA and CPAP treatment helped them

*Qualitative Health Research*, 2010;20(7):873–892.   Copyright © 2010. Reprinted by permission of SAGE Publications.

understand that they not only were experiencing symptoms of OSA on a daily basis, but their overall health and quality of life was impacted by OSA. During the first interview, participants were provided with a summary of their diagnostic sleep study results. The combination of education about the OSA diagnosis and treatment with CPAP, and relating their own diagnosis to their daily health and functioning, was important to adherent participants' formulation of accurate beliefs and perceptions of OSA and CPAP. These beliefs served to motivate or facilitate adherent participants' determination to pursue CPAP after diagnosis:

> I didn't know anything really, how the CPAP worked or anything like that. I just knew that there was a disease called sleep apnea and that a lot of people have it and people don't realize it. I really still didn't know anything about it til after I went through the test [diagnostic polysomnogram]. . . . Five [breathing events] is normal and thirty is severe and I'm doing ninety an hour. You know that literally scared the hell right out of me because all I could think of is I'm going to die in my sleep.
> [T]hen when you told me about driving, being tired, I remembered that every time we take off on a long trip, the first hour I got to pull over and rest. So it all came together. So I figured maybe I do have it [OSA].

For many adherent participants, knowledge of health risks associated with OSA was limited to "being sluggish" or "having low energy levels." For some, their perception of OSA was only relative to "falling asleep when I sit down." Participants who "put the whole picture together," relating their diagnosis to their own health status, were motivated to accept CPAP treatment from the outset. For example, one participant said, "It's [OSA] got to take a toll in the long run on a lot of things, like high blood pressure. I'm hoping that it helps me to drop my high blood pressure." These perceptions provided hope for adherent participants that expanded beyond the management of their OSA to other disease and health experiences:

> If I have more energy and I'm not so sluggish— because I go to the local high school track and get in five or six laps, walking around the track—I

will have more energy to do those kinds of things that keep you healthy.

Posttreatment, there was less emphasis on knowledge-based themes among adherent participants. This suggested a shift of emphasis among adherers from knowledge of risks and benefits of OSA to perceptions derived from the actual experience of CPAP treatment.

Nonadherent participants' knowledge at diagnosis was not different from adherent participants' knowledge. However, those with knowledge that served as a barrier, rather than a facilitator, to diagnosis were less likely to pursue a diagnostic sleep study in a timely fashion. This was particularly true for those who had inaccurate knowledge and perceptions of OSA, such as OSA being a condition of simple snoring. Even though many acknowledged they probably had OSA, the snoring was the "problem" that defined OSA, not apneic events and resultant untoward health and functional outcomes. As one participant described,

> My brother does it [snores], and he stopped [breathing] all the time in the middle of the night. My father did it, you know, and I do it. I knew I do it so it's been a while, I mean, I don't remember not being a loud snorer. . . . Like I said, my condition is hereditary. I'm sure my oldest son has it and I'm sure my youngest son is going to end up with it. My brother had it and my father had it, you know, my mother probably had it 'cause she's a snorer. I didn't think it was serious of a problem 'cause it's [snoring, stops in breathing] something that I had experienced for so many years.

Furthermore, describing early knowledge of "having to wear a mask" for the treatment of OSA served as a barrier to both seeking diagnosis and treatment for some. This perception was not consistent among only nonadherers though, as many of the participants expressed concerns about the anticipated treatment of their OSA. CPAP adherers and nonadherers described critically important differences in their own ability to reconcile the following: (a) their OSA diagnosis; (b) their experience of symptoms; (c) their goals for treatment use; and (d) their outcome expectations that were met after treatment exposure. These factors,

*Qualitative Health Research*, 2010; 20(7):873–892. Copyright © 2010. Reprinted by permission of SAGE Publications.

when reconciled by the individual, facilitated overall positive perceptions of the diagnosis and treatment experience.

### Goal Setting and Outcome Expectancies.

Outcome expectancies are the expected or anticipated costs and benefits for healthful habits/behaviors that support or deter from an individual's investment in the behavior (Bandura, 2004). Among the participants, postdiagnosis outcome expectancies that were consistently met were highly influential on participants' decisions to use CPAP. For example, after being diagnosed with OSA, one participant brought all his experienced symptoms into perspective, relating them to his OSA. With treatment, he was hopeful that these symptoms would resolve. He stated, "It seems like sleep apnea basically causes all those problems. So I figure if I can get this taken care of [by wearing CPAP], basically the problems will subside." Making sense of symptoms in terms of treatment outcome expectancies helped adherers commit to trying CPAP and believing that CPAP was going to be a positive experience. One participant summarized his perception of symptoms and outcome expectations like this: "But without me even trying it I know that what I'm experiencing and how it's affected me, and that I want to get better if I can and so there's nothing going to keep me away from getting a CPAP."

A particularly important perception described by participants was their early response to CPAP as influential on future/continued use of CPAP. These early, first experiences were helpful to formulating realistic and personally important outcome expectancies for CPAP use. One participant described his response to CPAP after wearing it for the first time in the sleep laboratory during his second sleep study (i.e., CPAP sleep study):

> But being like I got relief the first night I was at the hospital. I drove home that morning after they woke me up, I went down, I got breakfast, and I'm driving home, I'm saying to myself, gee, I feel great and I only got from one o'clock to six, you know. I feel so much better and I felt so much better that whole day. I felt so good after that five hours of sleep with the machine on that it sold me.

For adherent participants, having a positive response to CPAP during the sleep study night with CPAP was highly motivating for continued CPAP use at home. Furthermore, this early response set the stage for participants to develop an early commitment to the treatment, even when faced with barriers. Persistent, positive responses to CPAP throughout the early treatment period (i.e., 1 week) reinforced participants' outcome expectancies and helped them formulate a perception of the treatment that was conducive to long-term use.

Goals for improved health and for achieving certain health behaviors are an important part of being successful with any health behavior. According to Bandura (2004), individuals set goals for their personal health, including establishing concrete plans or strategies for achieving those goals. Goal setting among adherent CPAP users focused on "how best to adapt to using CPAP" or identifying "solutions to difficulties with use of CPAP." These goals were established so that adherent CPAP users were able to achieve their outcome expectations. Goal setting was not specifically discussed by adherent participants before using CPAP. With exposure to and experience with CPAP, adherent participants first identified that using CPAP was important and, thereafter, identified "tricks and techniques" to successfully use CPAP. Whether these strategies originated from the participant or were a collaborative effort between participant and a support source, having a plan that addressed how best to adapt to CPAP promoted continued effort directed at using CPAP, as described by one adherent participant:

> I guess the first night I put it on I sort of got a little feeling of claustrophobia, but I pushed it out of my mind, saying to myself, "Don't let this [bother you], this is a machine that is going to help you, you got to wear it," so I just put it in my mind that I was going to wear it.

As this participant described, it was important for him to devise a way that he could use the treatment so that he might realize his overall health goals. Similarly, one participant found that he could not fall asleep with CPAP at full

*Qualitative Health Research*, 2010;20(7):873–892. Copyright © 2010. Reprinted by permission of SAGE Publications.

pressure. He emphasized the importance of using CPAP to treat his OSA, but he equated using CPAP to "a tornado blowing through your nose." He recalled being taught about several features on the CPAP machine that might alleviate this sensation. After testing a few tricks on the CPAP machine, he found that he was able to fall asleep on a lower pressure setting while the pressure increased to full pressure setting after he was asleep (i.e., ramp function). By setting an immediate goal to get to sleep while wearing CPAP, he was able to achieve his longer-term goal to wear CPAP each night. The long-term goal of adherent participants was to feel better or sleep better, but the immediate goal was to be able to wear CPAP.

For nonadherers, a negative experience during their CPAP sleep study led them to have an undesirable outlook on CPAP and the overall treatment of OSA. For example, one participant described experiencing no immediate response to CPAP during the CPAP sleep study; therefore, he didn't expect to experience any response to treatment over a more extended period of time:

> I still had the same kind of sleep, I thought. As a matter of fact I thought it took me longer to get to sleep than it did on the first sleep study [without CPAP]. I believe my sleep was still the same type of sleep that I always get, even though, you know, the machine was supposed to make me sleep better. I still woke up in the same condition that I usually wake up in, is what I'm trying to say. I didn't feel any more vigorous or alert or anything after that first night.

Participants' descriptions of their considerations for using CPAP consistently included the question, "What are the down sides of using CPAP?" Combining early negative perceptions of the treatment and early negative experiences with CPAP, nonadherers tended to see the drawbacks of using the treatment as far outweighing any benefits of using the treatment. One participant described both negative perceptions and negative experiences, which caused him to believe that CPAP treatment outcome expectancies were not worth the torment of using the treatment:

> No, I didn't think I couldn't do it from the beginning. I was believing it was gonna do something more than what it did, and it didn't do anything. I'm not getting sleep, I'm still getting up tired. I guess I expected more from it and I didn't get anything, not anything that I could see anyway. No, just a bunch of botheration and I didn't get any sleep.

Among participants who did not adhere, the goal-oriented theme was not present after diagnosis. Nonadherers did not articulate specific goals for attaining treatment and, furthermore, they did not describe strategies to be able to wear CPAP after 1 week of CPAP treatment. For nonadherers, establishing treatment-related goals for use of CPAP was not a priority.

**Facilitators of and Barriers to CPAP use.** Perceived facilitators and barriers can be personal, social, and/or structural. Although perceived facilitators and barriers are influential on health behaviors, this process is mediated by self-efficacy (Bandura, 2004). Therefore, the existence of a barrier, in and of itself, might not be particularly influential on an individual's behavior if their self-efficacy is high. Consistent with this conceptual perspective, some participants identified barriers that were particularly troublesome when using CPAP, but were vigilant users of CPAP despite these barriers. Conversely, those who described numerous facilitators to using CPAP treatment were not necessarily adherent to CPAP.

Adherent participants were less focused on potential or actual facilitators and barriers to using CPAP over time than nonadherers. When adherent participants discussed facilitators and barriers, their overall descriptions were positive, with facilitators being the focus of their experience after using CPAP for 1 week. No adherent participants emphasized barriers to using CPAP after 1 week of treatment. Furthermore, when faced with barriers, adherent participants described perceptions of the treatment as important and identified a belief in their ability to overcome the barrier. For example, one participant experienced a sensation of not being able to breathe during his second night of

*Qualitative Health Research*, 2010; 20(7):873–892.   Copyright © 2010. Reprinted by permission of SAGE Publications.

CPAP use at home, but his ability to use CPAP was influenced by his commitment to "needing" the treatment:

> Because it was like I couldn't breathe and even though the machine was on, it was like I was paralyzed, and this happened every time when I tried to go back to sleep. How many times? Three more times that very same night until I was getting really anxious because every time I would try to go to sleep, after a while I would get that anxiety again. Finally, I prayed. I got up and I prayed real hard, asked God to really help me with this and I was right to sleep. Ever since then, I pray every night and have no problems.

As this example demonstrates, barriers and facilitators are not independent determinants of health behavior. Participants described situations and experiences that were labeled as either a facilitator or barrier, but the actual behavioral outcome of getting to diagnosis and using CPAP was not necessarily reflective of such experiences being a barrier or facilitator.

The facilitating experiences described by adherent participants centered on social interactions that provided motivation and facilitation of their CPAP use. Facilitating experiences included descriptions of social support, shared experiences of CPAP use with other CPAP users, and recognition that their own improvement as a result of CPAP treatment was an important influence on social relationships. Social relationships and the ability to be fully engaged in social interactions during their first week of CPAP use was described by several adherent participants as a facilitator to ongoing treatment:

> I see the difference. People see the difference. My wife sees the difference. My kids see the difference. That helps. I think that's 50% of it. People telling you that you have changed and things are getting better and you look a lot better and you a sound a lot better and you act a lot better, because when you have feedback like that you know it's [CPAP] helping.
>
> Our relationship [with spouse] is getting better and better. I think since the sleep machine it's even been more because some things that irritate me, I would speak on and it would cause like a little bit of friction, as it happens in couples. But since I've had the sleep machine, I've been letting the minor things go, things that irritate me or I would complain about before. . . . Communication, our rela-

tionship, so we've been able to talk more and enjoy each other even more since then [starting CPAP]. Yeah, I like the machine, I really do, and I like what it's doing.

Adherent participants clearly emphasized the importance of improved social relationships as a result of their CPAP treatment. Many recognized such improvements after a close friend or family member suggested the improvement was obvious.

Nonadherent participants emphasized barriers rather than facilitators to using CPAP after being diagnosed with OSA. However, after using CPAP for 1 week, nonadherers identified few, if any, actual barriers to treatment. Unlike adherent participants, nonadherers did not discuss social interactions as an important part of their post- CPAP treatment experience. Nonadherent participants also identified themselves as single, divorced, or widowed, with the exception of one participant. Nonadherers did not discuss their social networks (i.e., friends, family outside of their residence, coworkers) as important to their experiences of being diagnosed with OSA and starting CPAP treatment.

**Perceived Self-Efficacy.** Perceived self-efficacy is the belief that one can exercise control over one's own health habits, producing desired effects by one's own health behaviors (Bandura, 2004). This overarching theme was meaningfully described by participants and represented by several subthemes that were important to both adherers and nonadherers in the study. Within these descriptions, participants offered experiences with being diagnosed with OSA and using CPAP that led to their belief in themselves, or lack thereof, to use or not use the treatment.

Adherers in the sample described generally positive perceived self-efficacy regarding future use of CPAP. Adherers had a positive belief in their ability to use CPAP from the outset, which persisted and became increasingly frequent from diagnosis to early CPAP treatment, even if they first doubted their ability to use the treatment. As one participant described, the first thought of wearing a mask during sleep was not appealing, but with a positive first experience with CPAP, the participant was increasingly confident that CPAP was going to be a part of his life:

> I think I seen the masks sitting there and I thought to myself, I hope I don't have to wear one of those things. Then they came in and said, "Now we're going to put the CPAP on you," and I said, "Okay," and they put the CPAP on me and when they came back into the room I felt great when I woke up at six. They had to wake me up at six o'clock because I was sleeping and you know, I think I felt after that, I didn't care what it was if I got that much sleep from one o'clock to six without getting up. I was going to wear or do whatever I had to do to do it [wear CPAP].

Adherent participants also described that they planned to incorporate CPAP into their daily routine, suggesting an underlying positive belief in their ability to accomplish the health behavior of using CPAP. Recognizing that using CPAP would necessitate additional daily "work," adherers had well-defined plans of incorporating the added demands to their daily schedule:

> I have to just add some things that I have to do in order to keep the CPAP machine clean and to make sure that it's dry and each week I have to disinfect it, but once I did it, once I decided I was gonna do it, I just went in the bathroom, did the whole thing, it only took about twenty minutes, twenty-five minutes, and I was all done. And getting up in the morning and doing the daily cleaning, you know, that's not a negative but it's just something I have to make an adjustment to.

Nonadherent participants described having largely negative experiences with CPAP during the first exposure (i.e., CPAP sleep study) or during the early phase of home CPAP use. Few nonadherent participants experienced benefits with treatment and nonadherers described unsuccessful or a lack of problem-solving efforts with CPAP difficulties. These negative experiences were important areas of concern with regard to their perceived ability to use CPAP over the long term (perceived self-efficacy). For example, one participant had such an extremely negative experience during the first week he was exposed to CPAP that he firmly doubted his ability to ever use it:

> I couldn't breathe in [the mask]. This thing, I had to suck in to get a breath out of it. Last night I got a good night's sleep but I woke up, then I was claustrophobic. I felt like I was stuck under a bed someplace and couldn't get out and then I woke up. When I wore it the whole night through I wasn't sleeping so that's one of the reasons [I won't use CPAP], like I didn't sleep with it on; it was too aggravating.

Each participant described getting used to CPAP during the first several nights of treatment. With unsuccessful experiences during this period, participants either identified resources to help improve their experience or made decisions to use CPAP less or not at all. For all participants, early experiences with CPAP contributed to their belief in their own abilities to get used to the therapy.

Individuals who had difficulty fitting CPAP into their lives were challenged to be adherent to the treatment. When CPAP was seen as not fitting into a life routine, participants offered doubts as to their ability to continue to use the treatment. One participant described having a routine of falling asleep with television. With CPAP, she had difficulty watching television and therefore she experienced more difficulty getting to sleep. Although she continued to try to use CPAP, she expressed that using CPAP was generally annoying to her. The complexities presented by using CPAP within the constraints of her normal routine were likely to increasingly influence doubt in her ability to use CPAP.

## MARRIED AND UNMARRIED CPAP USERS

With the emerging emphasis placed on social support and social networks by adherers in the study, we explored how the social context of daily life impacted on perceptions of OSA and CPAP treatment by examining married ($n = 7$) and unmarried ($n = 8$) participants' responses. Using married and unmarried status from self-reported demographic characteristics as anchors, or as a unique descriptive qualifier, we sorted the subthemes within an analysis matrix to identify common perceptions, beliefs, and experiences within these qualifier groups. We included all participants

*Qualitative Health Research*, 2010; 20(7):873–892.   Copyright © 2010. Reprinted by permission of SAGE Publications.

who identified themselves as married or common-law married as married; all participants who identified themselves as single, divorced, or widowed were included as unmarried.

These groups described different experiences with both diagnosis and CPAP treatment. Married participants offered descriptions of social support resources within immediate proximity that were positive facilitators of seeking diagnosis and starting/staying on treatment. Married participants expressed positive beliefs in their ability to use CPAP with early treatment use, often described in conjunction with a CPAP problem-solving episode that was collaboratively resolved with their partner/spouse. Married participants described overwhelmingly positive early responses and experiences with CPAP treatment. Their outcome expectations were consistent across time. They generally anticipated positive responses to CPAP prior to exposure and experienced positive responses to treatment after 1 week of use. Married participants also identified success in "fitting CPAP into their lives." These participants were able to identify far more benefits from than difficulties with CPAP, benefits that enhanced their ongoing commitment to use of the treatment. Married participants discussed proximate support sources (i.e., spouse, living partner, family members) as important to providing feedback about their response to treatment, trouble-shooting difficulties, and positive reinforcement for persistent use of CPAP.

Unmarried participants commonly identified friends or coworkers as motivating factors (facilitators) to seek diagnosis but less social influence on/facilitation of treatment use after 1 week of CPAP therapy. Without the presence of immediate social support, unmarried participants did not emphasize important social interactions with actual wearing of CPAP. After 1 week of treatment on CPAP, unmarried participants described less confidence in their ability to use CPAP and described less "response" to CPAP than those participants who were married. Unmarried participants described few facilitators of

treatment use during the first week of CPAP therapy. Nearly all unmarried participants identified "self-driven" reasons for pursuing treatment, and there was an absence of social sources of support, or "cheerleaders and helpful problem solvers" while using CPAP during the first week.

## TYPOLOGIES OF ADHERENT AND NONADHERENT CPAP USERS

Described differences in beliefs, perceptions, and experiences of being diagnosed with OSA and early treatment with CPAP were explicit between adherers and nonadherers. Adherers perceived health and functional risks of untreated OSA, had positive belief in their ability to use CPAP from early in the diagnostic process, had clearly defined outcome expectations, had more facilitators than barriers as they progressed from diagnosis to treatment, and identified important social influences and support sources for both pursuing diagnosis and persisting with CPAP treatment. Nonadherers described not knowing the risks associated with OSA, perceived fewer symptoms of their diagnosis, did not have clearly defined outcome expectations for treatment, identified fewer improvements with CPAP exposure, placed less emphasis on social support and socially derived feedback with early CPAP treatment, and perceived and experienced more barriers to CPAP treatment. As a result of the across-case analysis in which consistencies and differences emerged among adherers and nonadherers in the described experience of being diagnosed with OSA and treated with CPAP, we suggest typologies, or descriptive profiles, of persons with CPAP-treated OSA (see Table 5). The typologies we propose are consistent with previous empirical studies of CPAP adherence, in that predictive relationships between risk perception, outcome expectancies, perceived self-efficacy, and social support with CPAP use have been identified. Our study findings extend the previous findings by illuminating the importance of contextual meaning persons

## Table 5. Typologies of Adherent and Nonadherent CPAP Users

| Adherent CPAP Users | Nonadherent CPAP Users |
| --- | --- |
| Define risks associated with OSA | Unable to define risks associated with OSA |
| Identify outcome expectations from outset | Describe few outcomes expectations |
| Have fewer barriers than facilitators | Do not recognize own symptoms |
| Facilitators less important later with treatment use | Describe barriers as more influential on CPAP use than facilitators |
| Develop and define goals and reasons for CPAP use | Facilitators of treatment absent or unrecognized |
| Describe positive belief in ability to use CPAP even with potential or experienced difficulties | Describe low belief in ability to use CPAP |
| Proximate social influences prominent in decisions to pursue diagnosis and treatment | Describe early negative experiences with CPAP, reinforcing low belief in ability to use CPAP<br>Unable to identify positive responses to CPAP during early treatment |

derive from their experiences, beliefs, and perceptions when progressing from diagnosis with OSA to treatment with CPAP. Moreover, the typologies succinctly describe critical differences between these groups of CPAP-treated OSA persons that support the development of patient-centered or -tailored adherence interventions that recognize individual differences.

## ■ Discussion

To our knowledge, this is the first study to apply a predominantly qualitative method to describe individuals' beliefs and perceptions of the diagnosis of OSA and treatment with CPAP relative to short-term CPAP adherence. Our findings are consistent with previous, empirical studies with regard to the overall applicability of social cognitive theory to the phenomenon of CPAP adherence. The findings from our study uniquely extend these previous findings by illuminating the importance of the individual experiences, beliefs, and perceptions as influential on decisions to pursue diagnosis and treatment of OSA. The

described differences between adherers and nonadherers in our study suggest critical tailored or patient-centered intervention opportunities that might be developed and tested among patients who are newly diagnosed with OSA and anticipate CPAP treatment. The major findings of the study include the following: (a) adults described and assigned meaning to being diagnosed with OSA and treated with CPAP, which in turn influenced their decisions to accept or reject treatment and the extent of CPAP use; and (b) differences in beliefs and perceptions at diagnosis and with CPAP treatment were identified among CPAP adherers and nonadherers and also described in the social context of married and unmarried CPAP users. The described differences between these groups provide data to support the first published typology, or descriptive profile, of CPAP adherers and nonadherers.

Theoretically derived variables, such as the determinants of health behaviors described in social cognitive theory and applied in our study, are operational concepts that help us understand OSA patients' perceptions and beliefs about OSA and CPAP, and can guide interventions to improve adherence to CPAP.

Framed by Bandura's social cognitive theory (1977), differences among adherers and non-adherers to CPAP can be defined across social cognitive theory determinants of health behaviors: (a) knowledge, (b) perceived self-efficacy, (c) outcome expectancies and goals, and (d) facilitators and barriers. As previous studies have demonstrated, psychosocial constructs, such as those consistent with social cognitive theory, provide possibly the most explained variance, to date, among adherers and nonadherers (Aloia, Arnedt, Stepnowsky, et al., 2005; Engleman & Wild, 2003; Stepnowsky, Bardwell, et al., 2002; Weaver et al., 2003). Furthermore, recent intervention studies to promote CPAP adherence have applied similar theoretical constructs with some positive findings (Aloia, Arnedt, Millman, et al., 2007; Richards, Bartlett, Wong, Malouff, & Grunstein, 2007). As our study findings suggest, decisions to use CPAP are individualized and at least in part dependent on the patient's support environment and early experiences with and beliefs about CPAP. Because early commitments to use or not use CPAP predict long-term use (Aloia, Arnedt, Stanchina, et al., 2007; Weaver, Kribbs, et al., 1997), it is critically important to understand and examine opportunities to intervene on factors that influence early commitments to use CPAP. This insight will potentiate the development of patient-centered and -tailored interventions to improve CPAP adherence at the individual level while collectively promoting the health outcomes of the OSA population.

Our study confirms that social cognitive theory is applicable to the unique health behavior of using CPAP treatment. Indeed, the interacting determinants of health as described by Albert Bandura (1977) in relationship to decisions to accept and use CPAP were clearly described by our study participants. This affirmation suggests that any one measured domain within the model (i.e., barriers, facilitators, outcome expectancies) is not likely to identify persons at risk for nonadherence to CPAP. Rather, our study findings support the complex and reciprocating nature of the theoretical model as it applies to this

health behavior, and offer clarity to our understanding of CPAP adherence as a multifactorial, iterative decision-making process. It is therefore important to ascertain an understanding of the context of the individual from the initial diagnosis through early treatment use to address the complex nature of the problem of adherence to CPAP and to prospectively identify those likely to be non-adherent to the treatment.

In our study, the experience and perception of symptoms contributed to the participants' motivation to seek diagnosis and treatment and to adhere to CPAP treatment. Although studies that have examined pre-treatment symptoms, particularly subjective sleepiness, have produced inconsistent results with regard to subsequent CPAP use, these studies have measured symptoms on quantitative scales that define specific scenarios of "impairment" related to the symptom of interest (i.e., Epworth Sleepiness Scale (Johns, 1993), Functional Outcomes of Sleep Questionnaire (Weaver, Laizner, et al., 1997), Stanford Sleepiness Scale (MacLean, Fekken, Saskin, & Knowles, 1992; Engleman et al., 1996; Hui et al., 2001; Janson, Noges, Svedberg-Randt, & Lindberg, 2000; Kribbs et al., 1993; Lewis et al., 2004; McArdle et al., 1999; Sin et al., 2002; Weaver, Laizner, et al., 1997). Yet, as our study highlights, perceptions of need relative to one's experience of symptoms were highly individual and significantly influenced decisions to pursue both diagnosis and treatment. Consistent with perceptions that influence medicine-taking behavior (Hansen, Holstein, & Hansen, 2009), particular situations necessitated the pursuit of diagnosis and use of the treatment. The experience of symptoms and the impact of symptoms on daily life were highly variable among participants and not readily amenable to discrete categorization. Understanding particular situations is important insight to explaining adherence to CPAP.

Recognizing and acknowledging that perceived symptoms are part of a disease process and logically linked to the diagnosis of OSA was important to the participants of our study, and to their commitment to move forward from diagnosis to treatment, consistent with Engleman and Wild's findings (2003). A recent intervention study to promote CPAP adherence incorporated specific strategies that address "personalization" of OSA symptoms (Aloia, Arnedt, Riggs, Hecht, & Borrelli, 2004; Aloia, Arnedt, Millman, et al., 2007). Results of this randomized controlled trial showed lower CPAP discontinuation rates among those participants who were in the motivational enhancement and education group when compared with "usual care," suggesting the importance of assisting persons diagnosed with OSA to make the connection between the objectively measured disease/ diagnosis and their lived experience of the disease (Aloia, Arnedt, Millman, et al., 2007). Personalizing symptoms, recognizing the impact of symptoms on daily function, and identifying the meaning of disease in terms of the perception of one's own health were clearly described by participants in our study. Adherent and nonadherent participants clearly expressed differences in their experiences of having OSA, including the impact of functional impairment on social relationships. From these differing perspectives, participants defined outcome expectations and health risks associated with OSA in different ways, possibly influencing their eventual decision to use or discontinue CPAP.

The described importance of participants' early experiences with CPAP and their initial response to CPAP treatment, both during the CPAP sleep study and during the first week of CPAP use, were influential on participants' interest in continuing to use CPAP. Our study results are consistent with Van de Mortel, Laird, and Jarrett's (2000) findings in which nonadherent, CPAP-treated OSA patients had complaints about their sleep study experience and described "major" problems on the night of their CPAP titration. Similarly, Lewis et al. (2004) found that problems identified on the first night of CPAP use, albeit on autotitrating CPAP, were consistent with lower CPAP use. Not only has the initial experience in terms of difficulties with CPAP been identified as

important to subsequent CPAP adherence, but also the patient's response to the first night of CPAP (i.e., degree of sleep improvement) has been correlated with subsequent CPAP adherence (Drake et al., 2003). The importance of promoting a positive initial experience with CPAP and providing anticipatory guidance about outcome expectations is highlighted by our findings.

The significance of social support, both proximate and within the broader social network, was an important facilitator of CPAP use among adherers in our study. Differences between the experiences of married and unmarried individuals with OSA revealed the described importance of an immediate, proximate source of support for CPAP use. Our finding is consistent with previous findings that those CPAP users who lived alone were significantly less likely to use their CPAP than those who lived with someone (Lewis et al., 2004). Not only are immediate sources of support important for continued use of CPAP, but also shared experiences with CPAP from less-immediate social sources. Participants in our study described social relationships as motivators to seek diagnosis, providing positive reinforcement for persisting with treatment use, and a source for sharing tips on managing OSA and CPAP. Studies exploring reasons for nonadherence to antituberculosis drugs have similarly identified the importance of social influences on seeking treatment and using treatment (Naidoo, Dick, & Cooper, 2009). Among CPAP-treated OSA patients, intervention studies that included feedback to participants, positive reinforcement, inclusion of a support person, and assistance with trouble-shooting difficulties resulted in higher CPAP adherence among participants in the intervention groups as compared with placebo or usual-care groups (Aloia et al., 2001; Chervin, Theut, Bassetti, & Aldrich, 1997; Hoy, Vennelle, Kingshott, Engleman, & Douglas, 1999). Confirming the applicability of these intervention strategies, the described experiences of participants in our study provide empirical support for adherence interventions that include a support person, provide early feedback and positive reinforcement to patients, and assist with trouble-shooting difficulties in the early treatment period.

Barriers to subsequent CPAP use that were identified by participants of our study included the process of having to put a mask on every night, aesthetic issues with mask/headgear use, inconvenience of having to use a machine to sleep, and daily routines that were disrupted by CPAP. Consistent with previous studies (Engleman et al., 1994; Hui et al., 2001; Massie et al., 1999; Sanders et al., 1986), side effects of CPAP were not emphasized by participants as barriers to CPAP use. Although identified barriers did not necessitate nonadherence to CPAP in our study, it was important for individuals who experienced such barriers to identify positive reasons to use CPAP and successfully mitigate barriers, often with the help of others.

This study had several limitations. First, although the sample size of 15 was adequate for a qualitative study, there was limited power to conduct any exploratory quantitative analyses. Although not the objective of this study, quantitative exploration of commonly used measures of subjective sleepiness, functional impairment, and adherence to CPAP correlated with descriptive, quantified typologies of adherent and nonadherent CPAP users would support the findings of the study. Study participants included predominantly male veterans with severe OSA who had relatively high educational preparation. Examining this typology in a larger, more heterogeneous sample of OSA patients is needed. As the relationship of gender, disease severity, symptom perception, and disease- specific literacy with CPAP adherence has not been clearly defined, replicating this study in a more diverse sample and expanding concurrently measured quantitative outcomes would be informative and supportive of typology refinement or expansion. Finally, to reduce the potential confounding effect of clinically delivered psychoeducation, we enrolled participants referred to the study from a single clinical provider with limited participant–provider interaction at the first prediagnostic evaluation. However, participants may have had telephone contact with the sleep center staff, or had unscheduled visits at the sleep center that were not controlled for in any way in our study.

Our mixed methods, exploratory study, employing a predominantly qualitative methodology, achieved saturation of themes regarding the diagnosis of OSA and nightly CPAP use during the first week of treatment. The study results are consistent with previous studies of CPAP, even when adherence, in many previous studies, was defined as four hours/night of use rather than six hours/night of use, as in our study. With recent evidence suggesting better outcomes with longer nightly CPAP use (Stradling & Davies, 2000; Weaver et al., 2007; Zimmerman, Arnedt, Stanchina, Millman, & Aloia, 2006), applying a definition of CPAP adherence of six hours vs. four hours likely contributed to more robust differences in described beliefs and perceptions among adherers and nonadherers. To our knowledge, the results of our study provide the first published, narrative descriptions of CPAP adherers and nonadherers that support an overall composite of characteristics that might be useful in identifying specific subgroups of patients who are most likely to benefit from tailored interventions to lessen the risk for subsequent CPAP nonadherence. To date, studies have provided adherence promotion interventions to unselected groups, possibly minimizing variation of response between intervention and control groups. Future randomized controlled trials testing CPAP adherence interventions delivered to participants who are selected based on their risk for treatment failure because of nonadherence are necessary to evaluate intervention effectiveness.

# ■ Acknowledgments

We acknowledge the sleep center staff's commitment to the conduct and completion of the study, and the exemplary transcription services provided by Charlene Hunt at Transcribing4You~Homework4You.

# ■ Declaration of Conflicting Interests

The authors declared a potential conflict of interest (e.g., a financial relationship with the commercial organizations or products discussed in this article) as follows: Dr. Kuna has received contractural support and equipment from Phillips Respironics, Inc. Dr. Weaver has a licensing agreement with Phillips Respironics, Inc., for the Functional Outcomes of Sleep Questionnaire.

# ■ Funding

The authors disclosed receipt of the following financial support for the research and/authorship of this article: The study was supported by award number F31NR9315 (Sawyer) from the National Institute of Nursing Research. The content is solely the responsibility of the authors and does not necessarily represent the official views of the National Institute of Nursing Research or the National Institutes of Health.

## Bios

*Amy M. Sawyer, PhD, RN, is a postdoctoral research fellow at the University of Pennsylvania School of Nursing, Philadelphia, Pennsylvania, and a nurse researcher at the Philadelphia Veterans Affairs Medical Center, Philadelphia, Pennsylvania, USA.*

*Janet A. Deatrick, PhD, RN, FAAN, is an associate professor and associate director, Center for Health Equities Research, at the University of Pennsylvania School of Nursing, Philadelphia, Pennsylvania, USA.*

*Samuel T. Kuna, MD, is an associate professor of medicine at the University of Pennsylvania School of Medicine and chief, Pulmonary, Critical Care and Sleep Medicine, at the Philadelphia Veterans Affairs Medical Center, Philadelphia, Pennsylvania, USA.*

*Terri E. Weaver, PhD, RN, FAAN, is the Ellen and Robert Kapito Professor in Nursing Science, chair, Biobehavioral Health Sciences Division, and associate director, Biobehavioral Research Center, at the University of Pennsylvania School of Nursing, Philadelphia, Pennsylvania, USA.*

## Corresponding Author

Amy M. Sawyer, University of Pennsylvania School of Nursing, Claire M. Fagin Hall, 307b, 418 Curie Blvd., Philadelphia, PA 19104, USA Email: asawyer@nursing.upenn.edu

## REFERENCES

Al Lawati, N. M., Patel, S., & Ayas, N. T. (2009). Epidemiology, risk factors, and consequences of obstructive sleep apnea and short sleep duration. *Progress in Cardiovascular Diseases, 51,* 285–293.

Aloia, M. S., Arnedt, J., Riggs, R. L., Hecht, J., & Borrelli, B. (2004). Clinical management of poor adherence to CPAP: Motivational enhancement. *Behavioral Sleep Medicine, 2*(4), 205–222.

Aloia, M. S., Arnedt, J. T., Millman, R. P., Stanchina, M., Carlisle, C., Hecht, J., et al. (2007). Brief behavioral therapies reduce early positive airway pressure discontinuation rates in sleep apnea syndrome: Preliminary findings. *Behavioral Sleep Medicine, 5,* 89–104.

Aloia, M. S., Arnedt, J. T., Stanchina, M., & Millman, R. P. (2007). How early in treatment is PAP adherence established? Revisiting night-to-night variability. *Behavioral Sleep Medicine, 5,* 229–240.

Aloia, M. S., Arnedt, J. T., Stepnowsky, C., Hecht, J., & Borrelli, B. (2005). Predicting treatment adherence in obstructive sleep apnea using principles of behavior change. *Journal of Clinical Sleep Medicine, 1*(4), 346–353.

Aloia, M. S., Di Dio, L., Ilniczky, N., Perlis, M. L., Greenblatt, D. W., & Giles, D. E. (2001). Improving compliance with nasal CPAP and vigilance in older adults with OAHS. *Sleep and Breathing, 5*(1), 13–21.

American Academy of Sleep Medicine Task Force. (1999). Sleep-related breathing disorders in adults: Recommendations for syndrome definitions and measurement techniques in clinical research. *Sleep, 22,* 667–689.

Bandura, A. (1977). Self-efficacy: Toward a unifying theory of behavioral change. *Psychological Reviews, 84,* 191–215.

Bandura, A. (1992). Exercise of personal agency through the self-efficacy mechanism. In R. Schwarzer (Ed.), *Self-efficacy: Thought control of action* (pp. 3–38). Philadelphia: Hemisphere.

Bandura, A. (2002). Social cognitive theory in cultural context. *Applied psychology: An International Review, 51*(2), 269–290.

Bandura, A. (2004). Health promotion by social cognitive means. *Health Education & Behavior, 31*(2), 143–164.

Chervin, R. D., Theut, S., Bassetti, C., & Aldrich, M. S. (1997). Compliance with nasal CPAP can be improved by simple interventions. *Sleep, 20,* 284–289.

Creswell, J. W., Plano Clark, V. L., Gutmann, M. L., & Hanson, W. (2003). Advanced mixed methods research designs. In A. Tashakkori & C. Teddlie (Eds.), *Handbook of mixed methods in social & behavioral research* (pp. 209–240). Thousand Oaks, CA: Sage.

Drake, C. L., Day, R., Hudgel, D., Stefadu, Y., Parks, M., Syron, M. L., et al. (2003). Sleep during titration predicts continuous positive airway pressure compliance. *Sleep, 26,* 308–311.

Engleman, H. M., Asgari-Jirandeh, N., McLeod, A. L., Ramsay, C. F., Deary, I. J., & Douglas, N. J. (1996). Self-reported use of CPAP and benefits of CPAP therapy. *Chest, 109,* 1470–1476.

Engleman, H. M., Martin, S. E., & Douglas, N. J. (1994). Compliance with CPAP therapy in patients with the sleep apnoea/hypopnoea syndrome. *Thorax, 49,* 263–266.

Engleman, H. M., & Wild, M. (2003). Improving CPAP use by patients with the sleep apnoea/hypopnoea syndrome (SAHS). *Sleep Medicine Reviews, 7*(1), 81–99.

Gay, P., Weaver, T., Loube, D., & Iber, C. (2006). Evaluation of positive airway pressure treatment for sleep related breathing disorders in adults. *Sleep, 29,* 381–401.

Graneheim, U. H., & Lundman, B. (2004). Qualitative content analysis in nursing research: Concepts, procedures and measures to achieve trustworthiness. *Nursing Education Today, 24,* 105–112.

Grunstein, R. R., Stewart, D. A., Lloyd, H., Akinci, M., Cheng, N., & Sullivan, C. E. (1996). Acute withdrawal of nasal CPAP in obstructive sleep apnea does not cause a rise in stress hormones. *Sleep, 19,* 774–782.

Hansen, D. L., Holstein, B. E., & Hansen, E. H. (2009). "I'd rather not take it, but · · ·": Young women's perceptions of medicines. *Qualitative Health Research, 19,* 829–839.

Harsch, I., Schahin, S., Radespiel-Troger, M., Weintz, O., Jahrei, H., Fuchs, S., et al. (2004). Continuous positive airway pressure treatment rapidly improves insulin sensitivity in patients with obstructive sleep apnea syndrome. *American Journal of Respiratory & Critical Care Medicine, 169,* 156–162.

Hoy, C. J., Vennelle, M., Kingshott, R. N., Engleman, H. M., & Douglas, N. J. (1999). Can intensive support improve continuous positive airway pressure use in patients with the sleep apnea/hypopnea syndrome? *American Journal of Respiratory & Critical Care Medicine, 159,* 1096–1100.

Hsieh, H., & Shannon, S. (2005). Three approaches to qualitative content analysis. *Qualitative Health Research, 15,* 1277–1288.

Hui, D., Choy, D., Li, T., Ko, F., Wong, K., Chan, J., et al. (2001). Determinants of continuous positive airway pressure compliance in a group of Chinese patients with obstructive sleep apnea. *Chest, 120,* 170–176.

Janson, C., Noges, E., Svedberg-Randt, S., & Lindberg, E. (2000). What characterizes patients who are unable to tolerate continuous positive airway pressure (CPAP) treatment? *Respiratory Medicine, 94,* 145–149.

Johns, M. (1993). Daytime sleepiness, snoring, and obstructive sleep apnea. The Epworth Sleepiness Scale. *Chest, 103,* 30–36.

Kribbs, N. B., Pack, A. I., Kline, L. R., Smith, P. L., Schwartz, A. R., Schubert, N. M., et al. (1993). Objective measurement of patterns of nasal CPAP use by patients with obstructive sleep apnea. *American Review of Respiratory Diseases, 147,* 887–895.

Krieger, J. (1992). Long-term compliance with nasal continuous positive airway pressure (CPAP) in obstructive sleep apnea patients and nonapneic snorers. *Sleep, 15,* S42–S46.

Lewis, K., Seale, L., Bartle, I. E., Watkins, A. J., & Ebden, P. (2004). Early predictors of CPAP use for the treatment of obstructive sleep apnea. *Sleep, 27,* 134–138.

MacLean, A. W., Fekken, G. C., Saskin, P., & Knowles, J. B. (1992). Psychometric evaluation of the Stanford Sleepiness Scale. *Journal of Sleep Research 1,* 35–39.

Massie, C., Hart, R., Peralez, K., & Richards, G. (1999). Effects of humidification on nasal symptoms and compliance in sleep apnea patients using continuous positive airway pressure. *Chest, 116,* 403–408.

McArdle, N., Devereux, G., Heidarnejad, H., Engleman, H. M., Mackay, T., & Douglas, N. J. (1999). Long-term use of CPAP therapy for sleep apnea/hypopnea syndrome. *American Journal of Respiratory and Critical Care Medicine, 159,* 1108–1114.

Meurice, J. C., Dore, P., Paquereau, J., Neau, J. P., Ingrand, P., Chavagnat, J. J., et al. (1994). Predictive factors of long-term compliance with nasal continuous positive airway pressure treatment in sleep apnea syndrome. *Chest, 105,* 429–434.

Naidoo, P., Dick, J., & Cooper, D. (2009). Exploring tuberculosis patients' adherence to treatment regimens and prevention programs at a public health site. *Qualitative Health Research 19,* 55–70.

Nieto, F., Young, T., Lind, B., Shahar, E., Samet, J., Redline, S., et al. (2000). Association of sleep-disordered breathing, sleep apnea, and hypertension in a large community-based study. *Journal of the American Medical Association, 283,* 1829–1836.

Peppard, P., Young, T., Palta, M., & Skatrud, J. (2000). Prospective study of the association between sleep-disordered breathing and hypertension. *New England Journal of Medicine, 342,* 1378–1384.

Rechtschaffen, A., & Kales, A. (Eds.). (1968). *A manual of standardized terminology, techniques and scoring system for sleep stages in human subjects.* Los Angeles: BIS/BRI. Reeves-Hoche, M. K., Meck, R., & Zwillich, C. W. (1994). Nasal CPAP: An objective evaluation of patient compliance. *American Journal of Respiratory & Critical Care Medicine, 149,* 149–154.

Richards, D., Bartlett, D. J., Wong, K., Malouff, J., & Grunstein, R. R. (2007). Increased adherence to CPAP with a group cognitive behavioral treatment intervention: A randomized trial. *Sleep, 30,* 635–640.

Rosenthal, L., Gerhardstein, R., Lumley, A., Guido, P., Day, R., Syron, M. L., et al. (2000). CPAP therapy in patients with mild OSA: Implementation and treatment outcome. *Sleep Medicine, 1,* 215–220.

Russo-Magno, P., O'Brien, A., Panciera, T., & Rounds, S. (2001). Compliance with CPAP therapy in older men with obstructive sleep apnea. *Journal of American Geriatric Society, 49,* 1205–1211.

Sanders, M. H., Gruendl, C. A., & Rogers, R. M. (1986). Patient compliance with nasal CPAP therapy for sleep apnea. *Chest, 90,* 330–333.

Schwarzer, R., & Fuchs, R. (1996). Self-efficacy and health behaviours. In M. Conner & P. Norman (Eds.), *Predicting health behaviour: Research and practice with social cognition models* (pp. 163–196). Philadelphia: Open Press.

Schweitzer, P., Chambers, G., Birkenmeier, N., & Walsh, J. (1997). Nasal continuous positive airway pressure (CPAP) compliance at six, twelve, and eighteen months. *Sleep Research, 16,* 186.

Sin, D., Mayers, I., Man, G., & Pawluk, L. (2002). Long-term compliance rates to continuous positive airway pressure in obstructive sleep apnea: A population-based study. *Chest, 121,* 430–435.

Stepnowsky, C., Bardwell, W. A., Moore, P. J., Ancoli-Israel, S., & Dimsdale, J. E. (2002). Psychologic correlates of compliance with continuous positive airway pressure. *Sleep, 25,* 758–762.

Stepnowsky, C., Marler, M. R., & Ancoli-Israel, S. (2002). Determinants of nasal CPAP compliance. *Sleep Medicine, 3,* 239–247.

Stradling, J., & Davies, R. (2000). Is more NCPAP better? *Sleep, 23,* S150–S153.

Streubert Speziale, H., & Carpenter, D. (2003). *Qualitative research in nursing* (3rd ed.). Philadelphia: Lippincott Williams & Wilkins.

Sullivan, C., Barthon-Jones, M., Issa, F., & Eves, L. (1981). Reversal of obstructive sleep apnea by continuous positive airway pressure applied through the nares. *Lancet, 1,* 862–865.

Tashakkori, A., & Teddlie, C. (1989). *Mixed methodology: Combining qualitative and quantitative approaches.* London: Sage.

Van de Mortel, T. F., Laird, P., & Jarrett, C. (2000). Client perceptions of the polysomnography experience and compliance with therapy. *Contemporary Nurse, 9,* 161–168.

Weaver, T. E., & Grunstein, R. R. (2008). Adherence to continuous positive airway pressure therapy: The challenges to effective treatment. *Proceedings of the American Thoracic Society, 5,* 173–178.

Weaver, T. E., Kribbs, N. B., Pack, A. I., Kline, L. R., Chugh, D. K., Maislin, G., et al. (1997). Night-to-night variability in CPAP use over first three months of treatment. *Sleep, 20,* 278–283.

Weaver, T. E., Laizner, A. M., Evans, L. K., Maislin, G., Chugh, D. K., Lyon, K., et al. (1997). An instrument to measure functional status outcomes for disorders of excessive sleepiness. *Sleep, 20,* 835–843.

Weaver, T. E., Maislin, G., Dinges, D. F., Bloxham, T., George, C. F. P., Greenberg, H., et al. (2007). Relationship between hours of CPAP use and achieving normal levels of sleepiness and daily functioning. *Sleep, 30,* 711–719.

Weaver, T. E., Maislin, G., Dinges, D. F., Younger, J., Cantor, C., McCloskey, S., et al. (2003). Self-efficacy in sleep apnea: Instrument development and patient perceptions of obstructive sleep apnea risk, treatment benefit, and volition to use continuous positive airway pressure. *Sleep, 26,* 727–732.

Wild, M., Engleman, H. M., Douglas, N. J., & Espie, C. A. (2004). Can psychological factors help us to determine adherence to CPAP? A prospective study. *European Respiratory Journal, 24,* 461–465.

Young, T., Palta, M., Dempsey, J., Skatrud, J., Weber, S., & Badr, S. (1993). The occurrence of sleep-disordered breathing among middle-aged adults. *New England Journal of Medicine, 328,* 1230–1235.

Young, T., Peppard, P., & Gottlieb, D. (2002). Epidemiology of obstructive sleep apnea: A population health perspective. *American Journal of Respiratory & Critical Care Medicine, 165,* 1217–1239.

Zimmerman, M. E., Arnedt, T., Stanchina, M., Millman, R. P., & Aloia, M. S. (2006). Normalization of memory performance and positive airway pressure adherence in memory-impaired patients with obstructive sleep apnea. *Chest, 130,* 1772–1778.

# Critique of Sawyer et al.'s Study (2010) "Differences in Perceptions of the Diagnosis and Treatment of Obstructive Sleep Apnea and Continuous Positive Airway Pressure Therapy among Adherers and Nonadherers"

## OVERALL SUMMARY

This was a well-written, interesting report of a study on a significant topic. The mixed methods QUAL(quan) approach that was used was ideal for combining rich narrative interview data with objective, quantitative measures of adherence to continuous positive airway pressure (CPAP) treatment. The use of a longitudinal design enabled the researchers to gain insights into changes in patients' perceptions from diagnosis to treatment. The study design and methods were described in commendable detail, and the methods themselves were of exceptionally high quality. The authors provided considerable information about how the trustworthiness of the study was enhanced. The results were nicely elaborated, and the researchers incorporated numerous excerpts from the interviews. This was, overall, an excellent paper describing a very strong study.

## TITLE

The title of this report was long, and perhaps a few words could have been omitted (e.g., "differences in" could be removed without affecting readers' understanding of the study). Nevertheless, the title did describe key aspects of the research. The title conveyed the central topic (perceptions about obstructive sleep apnea [OSA] and CPAP therapy). It also communicated the nature of the analysis, which compared perceptions of adherers and nonadherers to CPAP. If this paper had been published in a different journal, it probably would have been desirable to communicate in the title that the study was primarily qualitative, but inasmuch as it was published in *Qualitative Health Research* (QHR), that was not necessary. (However, "qualitative" was not used as a keyword for retrieving this study, either. The keywords included "content analysis" and "mixed methods," but in a search for qualitative studies on OSA or CPAP, this paper might be missed).

# ABSTRACT

As required by QHR, the abstract was written as a traditional abstract (no subheadings) of 150 words or fewer. Although brief, the abstract clearly described major aspects of the study so that readers could quickly learn whether the entire paper might be of interest. The first sentence of the abstract described the significance of the topic. The methods were succinctly presented, covering the overall mixed methods design, the longitudinal nature of the study (two rounds of interviews), the sample (15 OSA patients), the basic type of analysis (content analysis), and the focus on comparing adherent and nonadherent patients using objectively measured CPAP use. The use of social cognitive theory to guide the inquiry was noted. Although specific results were not described, the abstract indicated areas in which differences between adherers and nonadherers were observed. Finally, the last sentence suggests some possible applications for the results in terms of developing tailored interventions to promote CPAP use.

# INTRODUCTION

The introduction to this study was concise and well organized. It began with a paragraph about OSA as an important chronic health problem, describing its prevalence, its effects, and its primary medical treatment, that is, CPAP. This first paragraph helps readers understand the significance of the topic.

Much of the rest of the introduction discussed adherence to CPAP, which has consistently been found to be low. The researchers nicely set the stage for their study by summarizing evidence about rates of adherence and factors predicting adherence. They also described prior research that affected some of their design decisions, such as studies that have found that early experiences with CPAP—that is, in the first week of use—influence patients' perceptions. The studies cited in the introduction include both older studies and ones written very recently, suggesting that the authors were summarizing state-of-the-art knowledge.

The introduction then further set the stage for the new study by describing knowledge gaps: "To date, there are relatively few studies that have systematically examined the influence of disease and treatment perceptions and beliefs on CPAP adherence (p. 443)." The authors stated their four interrelated research questions, which were well suited to an in-depth qualitative approach.

# CONCEPTUAL FRAMEWORK

The article devoted a section to a description of the conceptual framework that underpinned the research. The authors used a conceptual framework that is widely used in health behavior research, Bandura's social cognitive theory. They presented a nice summary of the theory, and included a useful conceptual map (Fig. 1, p. 444). They also noted that Bandura's model is relevant within a qualitative inquiry because of explicit recognition of the role of context: "Bandura suggested that the application of social cognitive theory must be situated in context, recognizing that 'human behavior is socially situated, richly contextualized, and conditionally expressed" (p. 444). One puzzling thing, however, is that both in this section and in the first subsection of the results, considerable attention is paid to the role of *knowledge* in influencing health behaviors. Yet, knowledge is not a component of the theory as depicted in Figure 1.

# METHOD

The method section was well organized into four subsections, and was unusually thorough in providing details about how the researchers conducted this study.

## Design

Sawyer and colleagues used a mixed methods design to study patients' perceptions and beliefs about OSA and CPAP, and to explore differences among adherers and nonadherers. The researchers used terminology that was slightly different than that used in the textbook, which is not unusual because the field of mixed methods research is relatively new and is evolving. They described their design as a concurrent nested mixed methods design, and provided a citation to a paper by Creswell and Plano-Clark (2003), the two authors whose more recent terminology was used in this textbook. (The 2003 paper was probably a recent publication when the Sawyer et al. study was being planned). Using the terminology presented in the textbook, the design would best be described as an embedded QUAL (quan) design. Had Sawyer and colleagues used Morse's notation system, they might have characterized the study as QUAL + quan, which indicates that the data for the two strands were collected concurrently, and that the qualitative component was dominant.

The design section also noted that the design was longitudinal, with data collected both at initial OSA diagnosis and through the first week of CPAP treatment. Such a longitudinal design is an excellent way to track patients' perceptions and beliefs from diagnosis to the early treatment phase. The decision about *when* to collect the two rounds of data was well supported by earlier research. An excellent graphic (Fig. 2, p. 446) illustrated the study design and the timing of key events in the conduct of the study, such as enrollment and collection of demographic data, receipt of treatment education, conduct of the diagnostic sleep study and the CPAP sleep study, and the two interviews.

## Participants

The researchers clearly defined the group of interest and described how participants were recruited into the study. Participants were adults with suspected OSA who were recruited from a Veterans Affairs sleep clinic. To be eligible, patients had to meet various clinical criteria (e.g., had at least moderate OSA, defined as at least 15 apnea or hypopnea events per hour in a sleep study) and practical criteria (had to speak and understand English). Patients were excluded if their responses could have been confounded by prior CPAP experiences, because the researchers were interested in understanding the perceptions and beliefs early in the diagnosis and CPAP treatment transition.

The researchers also excluded individuals who refused CPAP treatment prior to the actual treatment, and Figure 1 suggests that one such person was dropped from the study. That is, 16 patients were interviewed for the pretreatment interview, but only 15 were interviewed a second time, and the analysis was based on responses from 15 patients. (Sample size issues were discussed in a later section).

One comment about this section is that we would have described the sampling approach more as convenience sampling than as purposive sampling. Many qualitative researchers say that their sampling was purposive when they purposefully select people with the characteristic or experience that is the focus of the research. However, we think of these more as eligibility criteria, which need to be identified to ensure that those in the study can provide "expert testimony" about the experience of interest. It would appear that the participants were a convenience sample of those meeting the eligibility criteria, and who were referred by a sleep specialist in one particular clinic. In our view, the term *purposive* connotes conscious and deliberate efforts to sample *particular* exemplars from those who are eligible and who can best meet the conceptual needs of the study. For example, maximum variation sampling is a purposive strategy that involves a deliberate attempt to select participants who not only meet the eligibility criteria but also vary along dimensions thought to be important in understanding the full range of the phenomenon of interest. In this study, the researchers could, for example, have deliberately sampled people with varying degrees of social support, to ensure that this important dimension would have adequate representation. As it turns out, there was variation in social support (marital status) among the study participants, but this does not appear to have been the result of a purposive strategy. With a small sample, and with a goal of looking at differences between adherers and nonadherers, a purposive strategy of sampling patients on dimensions known to differentiate these groups would have increased the likelihood that both groups would be adequately represented.

In terms of the design, the sampling approach for this study would be described as *identical sampling*, a term not mentioned in the textbook. In an identical sample, all study participants provide both qualitative and quantitative data—unlike a nested design, which involves selecting a *subset* of people from the quantitative strand to provide qualitative information.

## Procedures

The section on "Procedures" presented considerable information, focusing primarily on data collection. The section began by describing the two sleep studies that all study participants underwent. In both sleep studies, the patient's Apnea–Hypopnea Index (AHI) was computed via a polysomnogram. The initial AHI provided information that helped to determine study eligibility.

Next, the researchers described the major forms of data collection, which included semistructured interviews and instrumentation to assess CPAP adherence objectively. In the subsection on the in-depth interviews, the article specified that the data were collected by a single investigator at two points in time: within a week following OSA diagnosis but before treatment, and then after the first week of treatment. The authors noted that participants were given choices about where the interviews would take place, in an effort to minimize attrition. And, in fact, there was no attrition in this study.

The interview guides were described in admirable detail. Table 1 (p. 447) listed the questions that guided the initial interview, and Table 2 (p. 448) listed questions for the post-treatment interview. These tables were an excellent way to communicate the nature of the interviews to readers, and the text provided even more detail. For example, a rationale for using a topic guide was provided ("to ensure that a consistent sequence and set of questions were addressed across participants" (p. 445)). Consistency was also enhanced by having a single interviewer responsible for conducting all interviews. To maximize data quality, the interviews were digitally recorded and transcribed by a professional transcriptionist.

The interviewer also maintained field notes before and after each interview. Commendably, these field notes were not only descriptive (i.e., describing participants and the interview environments), but also "served as interviewer reflexivity notations (i.e., interviewer biases, suppositions, and presuppositions of the research topic)" (p. 446).

An important feature of this study was that CPAP adherence was not assessed by self-report. Rather, adherence was objectively determined based on quantitative data from the CPAP machine. A standard definition of "CPAP use" was provided, and a criterion of 6 hours or more per night of CPAP use was established for adherence. The researchers provided a convincing rationale for using the 6-hour limit as the cutoff point for adherence versus nonadherence.

One further note is that the researchers might have considered administering a self-efficacy scale during the course of their study, to anchor their discussion of self-efficacy, which is a key construct in their conceptual model. Although many of the major constructs in the model were ones that merited qualitative exploration, self-efficacy is one that perhaps could have been examined from both a qualitative and quantitative perspective, especially in a study that is explicitly mixed methods in design.

## Data Analysis

The authors are to be congratulated for their detailed description of their data analysis methods. Not only did they carefully explain data analytic procedures in the text, but they also provided a wonderful flow chart (Figure 3, p. 449) illustrating the sequence of steps they followed. It is extremely rare to find such rich information about data analysis in a qualitative or mixed methods study.

The qualitative data were content analyzed, an approach that is appropriate, given that the study was primarily descriptive. That is, this study was not designed to shed light on the lived experience of the patients (phenomenology), nor on their process of adapting to CPAP treatment (e.g., in a grounded theory study). The purpose was to obtain descriptive information at two points in time about participants' perceptions and beliefs relevant to OSA and CPAP. The researchers explained the procedures used in the content analysis, and provided citations for the approach used.

The data analysis section explained how theory-driven themes were extracted in a manner consistent with the broad conceptualization of health behavior articulated in Bandura's theory. The authors offered specific illustrations in Table 3 (p. 450), which listed broad theoretical determinants of health behavior in the first column, and then relevant themes for each determinant as derived from the content analysis. For example, for the broad construct "Perceived self-efficacy," there were five relevant themes, such as "Fitting treatment into life" and "Problem-solving difficulties."

The section on data analysis also included important information about methods the researchers used to enhance trustworthiness—and these methods were strong. For example, one investigator coded all the interview data. Then, an independent expert recoded a randomly selected 15% of the data from each interview. Overall agreement between the study coder and the expert coder was a high 94%. For any differences of opinion about coding, the discrepancy was resolved by consensus. The theme definitions used in the coding, which were developed by the investigative team, were reviewed by two experts, a qualitative methodologist and an expert in the application of the theoretical constructs.

Importantly, the qualitative data were coded and content analyzed for themes by an investigator who was blinded to whether the participant was classified as adherent or non-adherent based on the quantitative data. Only after coding was complete was the adherence status of participants revealed. At that point, across-case analysis was examined "from an integrative perspective, using adherent and nonadherent as anchors…to identify common perceptions, beliefs, and experiences within the groups of interest." The authors used an excellent device—called a *meta-matrix*, to integrate the qualitative and quantitative data.

# RESULTS

The results section began with a description of the study sample, all of whom were military veterans. Table 4 (p. 452) showed basic descriptive statistics on the demographics of the 15 participants, including their gender, race/ethnicity, marital and employment status, educational background, and age. Clinical information (e.g., mean weight, AHI events/hour, and CPAP adherence in terms of hours per night) was also presented. The text stated that the sample included six adherers and nine nonadherers. The introductory paragraph of the results section also noted that data saturation was reached at 15 participants, and that sampling stopped at that point.

Much of the results section was organized according to differences between adherers and nonadherers to CPAP therapy. The differences were nicely organized into major thematic categories, such as "Knowledge and perceived health status," "Goal setting and outcome expectancies," "Facilitators of and barriers to CPAP use," and "Perceived self-efficacy." Key differences between the two groups (and a few areas of overlap) within these major groupings were described and supported with rich excerpts from the interview transcripts.

Social support emerged as an important issue in CPAP adherence, consistent with previous studies. Thus, the researchers performed a useful supplementary analysis in which they examined differences between married and unmarried patients.

The analysis section concluded with a typology (descriptive profiles) of adherent and nonadherent CPAP users, based on an integration of the data across themes. Table 5 (p. 459) nicely summarized their typology.

# DISCUSSION

Sawyer and colleagues offered a thoughtful discussion of their findings. Their discussion highlighted ways in which their findings complement and extend the existing body of evidence on CPAP adherence. The discussion nicely wove together findings from the current study and previous studies and discussed the findings within the context of the theoretical framework.

The authors also noted some of the study's limitations. They pointed out, for example, that study participants were all veterans with fairly high levels of education, and thus exploration with a more diverse population of OSA patients would be desirable. The researchers also pointed out that the small sample size of 15 provided limited power for conducting quantitative analyses of numerical data they had at their disposal, such as measures of subjective sleepiness and functional impairment. They noted that with a larger sample, they could have explored correlations between such quantitative measures and the thematic typology.

Although the discussion is reasonably lengthy, relatively little space was devoted to the implications of the study findings. The researchers noted that "The described differences between adherers and nonadherers in our study suggest critical tailored or patient-centered intervention opportunities…" Indeed, they mentioned the opportunity for tailored interventions several times in connection with their discussion of their theoretically derived themes. A bit more elaboration of how the findings could be used in an intervention might have been helpful.

# GENERAL COMMENTS

## Presentation

This report was clearly written, well organized, and offered an exemplary amount of detail about the research methods. The inclusion of several tables and figures provided readers with explicit and concrete information about aspects of the study that are often ignored or described only briefly. We applaud the authors, and we also applaud the journal, *Qualitative Health Research*, for not having strict page limits.[1] The need for page limits is understandable given the explosion of research that is being undertaken. However, the ability for readers to judge the quality of research evidence is also crucial, and this is sometimes hampered by constraints on researchers' ability to provide thorough information about how the research was conducted.

## Ethical Aspects

The authors briefly stated steps they took to ensure ethical treatment of participants in the subsection labeled "Participants." All participants provided informed consent, and the study protocols were approved by the Institutional Review Boards of the affiliated university and the research site.

# RESPONSE FROM THE SAWYER TEAM

Dr. Sawyer and her colleagues were asked if they wished to comment on this critique. Dr. Sawyer remarked that she was "in near 100% agreement with the draft critique that you provided" and that there was nothing she felt she needed to rebut. Given the generally positive nature of the critique, Dr. Sawyer noted, "I don't know that I have much in the way of response to offer—however, the suggestion to include a self-efficacy instrument is 'spot on.'"

Her email concluded with the following statement: "My study colleagues and I are very pleased with the published paper in QHR and firmly believe the paper is an excellent teaching resource for mixed methods research in health and disease." We agree.

---

[1] The QHR guidelines to authors that were is effect in 2010 state the journal's page limit policy as follows: "There is no predetermined word or page limit. Provided they are "tight" and concise, without unnecessary repetition and/or irrelevant data, manuscripts should be as long as they need to be."

# INDEX

Note: Page numbers followed by "*f*" indicate figures; those followed by "*t*" indicate tables and those followed by "*b*" indicate boxes. Page numbers in bold denote glossary terms.

## A

Absolute risk (AR), 223–224, **374**
Absolute risk reduction (ARR), 225, **374**
Absolute value, 222
Abstract, **374**
  literature search and, 121, 123
  in research reports, 62
Accessible population, 177, **374**
Acquiescence response set bias, 188, 255*t*, **374**
Action research, 277
Active reading, 66
Adaptation Model (Roy), 137
After-only design, **374**
Aim, research, 100, 104
Ajzen's Theory of Planned Behavior, 138–139
Alpha (α), **374**
  reliability (Cronbach's alpha), 203–204
  significance level, 229, 231
American Nurses Association (ANA), 3, 81
American Nurses Credentialing Center, 3
Analysis, 52, 54, **374**. *See also* Data analysis; Qualitative analysis; Quantitative analysis
  content, 275, 306–307, **377**
  cost, 345, **378**
  data, 52, **378**. *See also* Data analysis
  economic, 345, **379**
  impact, 345, **382**
  narrative, 274, **385**
  power, 181, 229, 230, **388**
  process, 345, **388**
  qualitative, 300–317, **389**. *See also* Qualitative analysis
  quantitative, 214–247, **389**. *See also* Quantitative analysis
  statistical, 52, 214–247, **392**. *See also* Quantitative analysis; Statistic(s)
Analysis of covariance (ANCOVA), 166, 239, **374**
  multivariate (MANCOVA), 239
  research design and, 166
Analysis of variance (ANOVA), 233–235, **374**
  multivariate (MANOVA), 239, **385**
Analytic phase of quantitative research, 50*f*, 52
Ancestry approach, 118, **374**
ANCOVA. *See* Analysis of covariance (ANCOVA)
Animal subjects, 91–92
Anonymity, 89, 186, **374**
ANOVA. *See* Analysis of variance (ANOVA)
Applied research, 11, **374**
Appraisal of evidence, 31–33, 32*b*, 35
Appraisal of Guidelines Research and Evaluation (AGREE) instrument, 26

Artistic expressions, phenomenology and, 271, 287, 310
Assent, 90, **374**
Assessment, psychometric, 205
Association of Women's Health, Obstetric and Neonatal Nursing (AWHONN), EBP and, 26
Associative relationship, 46, 47, **374**
Assumptions, **374**
  paradigms and, 7, 7*t*
  parametric tests and, 236
Asymmetric distribution, 216, 218*f*, **374**
Attention control group, 155, **374**
Attrition, 163, 167, **374**
Attrition bias, 168, 255*t*
Audit, inquiry, 325*t*, 330–331
Audit trail, 327–328, **375**
Authenticity, 323, 324*t*–325*t*, **375**
Author search, literature search and, 119
Authorities, as knowledge source, 5
Autoethnography, 269, **375**
Average, 217
Axial coding, 314, **375**

## B

Background questions, 29
Bandura's Social Cognitive Theory, 138, 141
Baseline data, 154, **375**
Basic research, 11, **375**
Basic social process (BSP), 272, 311–312, **375**
Becker's Health Belief Model (HBM), 138
Before-after (pretest-posttest) design, **375**
Being-in-the-world, 270
Bell-shaped curve, 217. *See also* Normal distribution
*Belmont Report*, 81, 83–85
Benchmarking data, 6
Beneficence, 83–84, **375**
Beta (β), 229, **375**
  Type II error and, 229
Bias, 73, 254–255, **375**
  attrition and, 168, 255*t*
  blinding and, 74–75, 151
  credibility and, 254–255
  definition of, 73, 254
  expectation, 151
  full disclosure and, 84
  insider research and, 269–270
  internal validity and, 167–168
  measurement error and, 201
  nonresponse, 183, 255*t*, **386**
  against null hypothesis, 358

Bias (*Continued*)
  observational, 191, 255*t*, 295
  qualitative research and, 266
  publication, 358, **389**
  random, 73
  randomness and, 74
  reflexivity and, 75
  research design and, 154
  response, 183
  response set, 188, 202, **391**
  sampling, 178, 183, **391**
  selection, 161, **392**
  social desirability, 188, 255*t*, **392**
  statement of purpose and, 105
  statistical analysis of, 240–241
  strategies to reduce, 74–75
  systematic, 73, 154
  threats to internal validity, 167–168
  types of, 254, 255*t*
Bibliographic database, 119–123
Bimodal distribution, 216, **375**
Biologic plausibility, causality and, 152
Biophysiologic measures, 51, 184, 192
Bivariate statistics, 221–223, **375**
  descriptive, 221–223. *See also* Descriptive statistics
  inferential, 232–237. *See also* Inferential statistics
  risk indexes and, 223–225
Blind review, 62, **375**
Blinding, 74–75, 79, 151, 156, **375**
Boolean operators, 120
Borrowed theory, 139
Bracketing, 270, 271, **375**
Breach of confidentiality, 89
BSP, 272, 311–312
Burke's pentadic dramatism, 274

**C**

Canadian Nurses Association, 81
CAQDAS, 304
Carryover effect, 155, 166, 255*t*, **375**
Case
  confirming and disconfirming, 285, 288, 329–330
  sensitivity and, 208
Case study, 273–274, **375**
Case-control design, 152*t*, 160, 168, **375**
Categorical variable, 42, **375**
Category scheme, qualitative data and, 301–303
Category system, observational, 190, **375**
Causal modeling, **375**
Causal (cause-and-effect) relationship, 46–47,
    **375**. *See also* Causality
  criteria for, 152
  evidence hierarchy and, 152
  experimental research and, 153, 156
  internal validity and, 167–169, 254
  nonexperimental research and, 159, 161, 260
  quasi-experimental research and, 159
Causality. *See also* Causal (cause-and-effect) relationship
  correlation and, 159, 257
  description of, 151–152
  determinism and, 7

interpretation of, 257, 260–261
  in qualitative research, 267–268
  study goal and, 11
Cause-and-effect relationship. *See* Causal
    (cause-and-effect) relationship
Cause-probing study, 11, 46, 152, **375**
Cell, **375**
  crosstabs table and, 221
  risk indexes and, 223, 224*t*
Central (core) category, 314, **375**. *See also*
    Core category
Central tendency, 217–218, **376**. *See also* Mean
Certificate of Confidentiality, 89
Checklist, observational research, 190
Children, as a vulnerable group, 90
Chi-squared ($\chi^2$) test, 235–236, 238*t*, **376**
CINAHL database, 120–122, 121*f*
Clinical fieldwork, 49–50, 50*f*
Clinical nursing research, 2
Clinical practice guideline, 25–26, 35, **376**
Clinical relevance, 33, 34. *See also* Evidence-based
    practice; Nursing research
Clinical research, 2, 21, **376**. *See also* Nursing research
Clinical significance, 256
Clinical trial, 47, 153, 345, **376**. *See also* Experiment
  practical, 345
  randomized controlled trial (RCT), 22–23, 153, 345
Closed-ended question, 184, **376**
Cochrane Collaboration, 22, 356, **376**
Cochrane Database of Systematic Reviews (CDSR),
    25, 120
Code of ethics, 81, **376**
Codes, in grounded theory
  Charmaz method, 315
  Glaser and Strauss' method, 311–313, 312*t*, 313*f*, 314*t*
  Strauss and Corbin's method, 314, 314*t*
Coding, 52, **376**
  levels of, grounded theory and, 311–315, 312*t*
  qualitative data and, 303, 304*f*, 329
  quantitative data and, 52, 184
Coefficient(s)
  correlation, 222, 236, **378**
  multiple correlation (R), 239, **385**
  product-moment correlation (Pearson's *r*), 222, **388**
  reliability, 202–204, **390**
  validity, 206, 222
Coefficient alpha (Cronbach's alpha), 203–204, **376**
Coercion, 84, **376**
Cohen's *d*, 237, 360, **376**
Cohort design, 152*t*, 160, **376**
Colaizzi's phenomenological method, 308, 309*t*
Comparison
  constant, 272, 302, **377**
  multiple, in ANOVA, 234, **385**
  qualitative studies and, 266–267
  PICO component and, 29–30, 31*t*, 43
  research design, quantitative research and,
    150*t*, 153
  time dimension, 162–163
Comparison group, 157, **376**
Complex hypothesis, 109

Componential analysis, ethnography, 307–308
Composite scale, 187–188, 187*t*
Computer. *See also* Internet
 analysis of qualitative data and, 304
 analysis of quantitative data and, 231
 electronic literature searches and, 119–123
Computer assisted qualitative data analysis software
 (CAQDAS), 304
Concealment, 85, 189, **376**
Concept, 41, 41*t*, 42, **376**
 as component of theories, 133
 concept vs. construct, 42
 conceptual definitions and, 44, 135
 measurement of, 199–200
 models of nursing and, 136
 operational definitions and, 44
Concept analysis, 135
Conceptual definition, 44, 50, 135, **376**
Conceptual description, grounded theory
 and, 272
Conceptual file, 303–304, **376**
Conceptual framework, 135, 142, 142*f*. *See also*
 Conceptual model; Theory
Conceptual integration, 132
Conceptual map, 134, 346, **376**
Conceptual model, 133–134, **376**. *See also* Theory
 models of nursing and, 136–137
 non-nursing models, 138–139
Conceptual phase of research
 qualitative studies and, 53–54
 quantitative studies and, 49–50
Concurrent design, mixed methods and, 342, **376**
Concurrent validity, 206, **376**
Conduct and Utilization of Research in Nursing (CURN)
 Project, 21
Conference, professional, 62
Confidence interval (CI), 32, 227–228, **376**
 correlation coefficients and, 236
 level of significance and, 229–230
 precision and, 32, 256
 proportions and, 236
 *t*-tests and, 233
Confidence limit, 227, **376**
Confidentiality, 89, **377**
Confirmability, 323, 324*t*, 325*t*, **377**
Confirming case, 285, 288
Confounding variable, 73, 151, 152, **377**. *See also*
 Control, research
 analysis of covariance and, 166, 239
 controls for, 73, 151, 164–166
Consecutive sampling, 179, **377**
Consent. *See also* Ethics
 implied, 87, **382**
 informed, 84, 87, 88*f*, **382**
 process, 87–88, **388**
Consent form, 87, 88*f*, **377**
CONSORT flow chart, 252, 253*f*
CONSORT guidelines, 252, **377**
Constancy of condition, 164, 169
Constant, 42
Constant comparison, 272, 302, **377**

Constitutive pattern, 310, **377**
Construct, 42, **377**. *See also* Concept
Construct validity, 169–170, 254, **377**
 credibility and, 254
 interventions and, 346
 measurement and, 206–207
Constructivist grounded theory, 273, 314–315, **377**
Constructivist paradigm, 7*t*, 8, **377**
 methods for, 9–10. *See also* Qualitative research
Consumer of nursing research, 3, 15
Contamination of treatments, 255*t*, **377**
Content analysis, 275, 306–307, **377**
Content validity, 205–206, **377**
Content validity index (CVI), 205, **377**
Contingency table, 221–222, **377**
Continuous variable, 42, **377**
Control group, 153, **377**
 control group condition, 155
 nonequivalent, 157–158
Control, research, 73–74, **377**
 definition of, 73
 evaluation of methods for, 166
 experimental design and, 153–156
 of external confounding factors, 164
 internal validity and, 167–168
 of intrinsic confounding factors, 164–166
 as purpose of research, 13
 qualitative research and, 74
 quasi-experiments and, 158–159
 statistical, 166, 239
 study context and, 164
 validity and. *See* External validity; Internal validity;
 Statistical conclusion validity
Controlled trial, **377**. *See also* Clinical trial; Randomized
 controlled trial
Convenience sampling, 178–179, 284, **377**
Convergent parallel design, mixed methods, 342,
 **377–378**
Core category (variable), 48, 272, 314, **378**
 coding and, 311–312
Corporeality, 270
Correlation, 222, **378**. *See also* Correlation coefficient;
 Relationship
 causation and, 159, 257
 inferential statistics and, 236
 multiple, 239
Correlation coefficient, 222–223, 236, **378**
 multiple (*R*), 239, **385**, **389**
 Pearson's product-moment correlation (*r*), 222, **387**.
 *See also* Pearson's *r*
Correlation matrix, 222–223, **378**
Correlational research, 159–162, **378**
 advantages and disadvantages, 161–162
 internal validity and, 167–169
 interpretation and, 257
 types, 159–160
Corroboration of results, 255
Cost (economic) analysis, 345, **378**
Counterfactual, 151, 155, **378**. *See also* Control group
Covariate, 239, **378**
Covert data collection, 85

Credibility, 323, **378**
  interpretation of quantitative results and, 251–255
  qualitative research and, 72, 323–325, 332
  researcher, 331–332
  trustworthiness and, 72, 323–325, 324t, 325t
Criterion-related validity, 206, **378**
Criterion sampling, 285, **378**
Critical ethnography, 275–276, **378**
Critical incident technique, 291, **378**
Critical theory, 140, 275–276, **378**
Critique, research, 66–75
  analyses, qualitative and, 315, 316b
  analyses, quantitative and, 243, 243b
  credibility of quantitative results and, 251–255
  data collection plan, qualitative and, 295–296, 296b
  data collection plan, quantitative and, 193–194, 194b
  data quality, quantitative studies and, 209, 209b
  ethical issues and, 92–93, 93b
  interpretation of quantitative results and, 260–261, 261b
  literature reviews and, 127, 127b
  meta-analysis and, 367, 368b–369b
  qualitative studies, guideline 68, 70t
  quantitative studies, guideline, 68, 69t
  research design, qualitative and, 277–278, 278b
  research design, quantitative and, 170, 170b
  research problems and, 110, 111b
  sampling plan, qualitative and, 288, 289b
  sampling plan, quantitative and, 182–183, 183b
  systematic reviews and, 367, 368b–369b
  textbook support for, 68–71, 69t, 70t
  theoretical framework and, 143, 143b
  trustworthiness and, 333–334, 334b
Cronbach's alpha, 203, **378**
Crossover design, 154–155, 165, **378**
Cross-sectional design, 151, 162–163, **378**
  qualitative research and, 267
Crosstabs table, 221–222, 221t, 223
Crosstabulation, 221–222, **378**
Cultural theory, ethnography and, 139
Culture, 49, 268. *See also* Ethnography
Cultural issues, nursing research and, 5
Cumulative Index to Nursing and Allied Health Literature
  (CINAHL), 120–122, 121f
CURN Project, 21
Cutoff point, screening instrument, 208, **378**

**D**
*d. See* Cohen's *d*
Data, 45, **378**. *See also* Qualitative data; Quantitative data
  analysis of. *See* Data analysis
  assessment of quality. *See* Data quality
  coding of, 52, 303. *See also* Coding
  collection of. *See* Data collection
  existing vs. original, 183, 184, 348
  extraction and encoding of for meta-analysis, 359–360
  fabrication and falsification of, 92
  narrative, 45. *See also* Qualitative data
  qualitative, 45, **389**. *See also* Qualitative data
  quantitative, 45, **389**. *See also* Quantitative data
  raw, 64, 327, **390**
  saturation of, 55, 286, 324t

Data analysis, 52, **378**. *See also* Qualitative analysis;
    Quantitative analysis
  descriptive statistics, 215–225. *See also* Descriptive
    statistics
  inferential statistics, bivariate, 225–238. *See also*
    Inferential statistics
  meta-analysis and, 359–362
  metasynthesis and, 365–367
  multivariate statistics, 237–240. *See also* Multivariate
    statistics
  qualitative, 300–316. *See also* Qualitative analysis
  quantitative, 52, 215–242. *See also* Quantitative analysis;
    Statistic(s)
Data collection, 51, 183–193, 288–296, **378**. *See also*
    Measurement
  biophysiologic measures, 51, 184, 192
  goal of, 193
  measurement and. *See* Measurement
  mixed methods research and, 343–344
  observational methods, 189–191, 292–295. *See also*
    Observation
  plan for, 51, 192–193
  protocols, **378**
  qualitative research and, 288–296
  quality enhancement, qualitative research and, 325–328
  quantitative research and, 183–193
  self-report methods, 184–189, 290–292. *See also*
    Self-report(s)
  triangulation of methods, 193, 327
Data quality
  critiquing of quantitative data, 209, 209b
  enhancement strategies for, during qualitative data
    collection, 324t, 325–328
  measurement and, 199–200. *See also* Measurement
  qualitative data and, 325–328
  quantitative data and. *See* Reliability; Validity
Data saturation, 55, 286, 324t
Data set, **379**
Data triangulation, 326–327, **379**
Database, bibliographic, 119–123
Debriefing, **379**
  peer, qualitative research and, 325t, 330
  study participant, 90, **379**
Deception, 85, **379**
Decision trail, 324t, 327
Declaration of Helsinki, 81
Deductive reasoning, 42, **379**
  theory testing and, 107, 109, 133, 136
Definition
  conceptual, 44, 50, 135, **376**
  operational, 44, **386**. *See also* Data collection;
    Measurement
Degrees of freedom (*df*), 231, **379**
Delayed treatment design, 155, **379**
Dependability, qualitative integrity and, 323, 324t,
    325t, **379**
Dependent groups *t*-tests, 233
Dependent variable, 43–44, **379**. *See also* Independent
    variable; Outcome variable
  control and, 73
  hypotheses and, 109

keywords and, 119
relationships and, 46
research questions and, 105–106
statistical tests and, 238t, 241t
Descendancy approach, literature search, 118, **379**
Description
as research purpose, 11–12, 12t
conceptual, grounded theory and, 272
thick, 288, 294, 325t, 331, 334, **393**
Descriptive correlational study, 160–161. *See also*
Correlational research
Descriptive notes, 294
Descriptive phenomenology, 270–271, 308, 309t. *See also*
Phenomenology
Descriptive qualitative study, 106–107, 275, 306
Descriptive research, 160, **379**
correlational, 160–161. *See also* Correlational research
qualitative, 106, 275
Descriptive statistics, 215–225, **379**  ✓
bivariate, 221–222. *See also* Bivariate statistics
central tendency and, 217–218
frequency distribution and, 215–217
risk indexes and, 223–225
variability and, 218–221. *See also* Variability
Descriptive theory, 133, **379**
Design. *See* Research design; Sampling
Design phase of quantitative research project, 51–52
Detailed approach, phenomenological analysis,
309–310, 309t
Determinism, 7, **379**
Deviant case analysis, 330
Diary, 269, 290
data collection, 290–291
field, 294
historical research and, 273, 290
Dichotomous question, 185t
Dichotomous variable, **379**
Diekelmann et al. hermeneutic analysis, 310
Diffusion of Innovation Theory (Rogers), 27
Dilemma, ethical, 82
Directional hypothesis, 109, **379**
Disabled people, as a vulnerable group, 90
Disciplinary tradition, qualitative research, 48
Disclosure, full, 84–85
Disconfirming cases, sampling, 285, 287, 288,
329–330, **379**
Disconfirming evidence, 325t, 329–330
Discussion section, research report, 65
critiquing guidelines for, 261
interpretation of results and, 249
Dispersion. *See* Variability
Dissemination of research results, 4, 52–53, 55. *See also*
Research report
internet and, 4
journal article, 61
professional conferences and, 62
qualitative studies, 55
quantitative studies, 52–53
Dissertations, 120, 358, 364
Distribution, 215–217
central tendency and, 217–218
frequency, 215–217. *See also* Frequency distribution
normal (bell-shaped curve ), 217, **386**. *See also* Normal
distribution
sampling, 225–227, 226f, 230f, **391**
theoretical, 230, 231
variability of, 218–221
Documentation
literature reviews and, 123
trustworthiness and, 325t, 327
Domain, 307, **379**
Domain analysis, 307
Donabedian framework, 347
Double-blind experiment, **379**. *See also* Blinding
Duquesne school of phenomenology, 308

**E**

EBP. *See* Evidence-based practice
Economic (cost) analysis, 345, **379**
Effect size, 237, **379**
Cohen's *d*, 237, 360, **376**
interpretation of results and, 256
meta-analysis and, 356, 360–362
metasynthesis and, 366–367
odds ratio, 237, 360
Pearson's *r*, 237, 360
power analysis and, 181–182, 237
Effectiveness study, 345, 346, **379**
Effects
calculation of, in meta-analysis, 360
carryover, 155, 166, 255t, **375**
causality and, 151. *See also* Causality
Hawthorne, 157, **382**
interaction, 234, **383**
magnitude of, 32, 32b, 256. *See also* Effect size
main, 234
meta-analysis and, 360–362
Efficacy study, 345, 346, **379**
Element, sampling and, 177–178, **379**
Eligibility criteria, 177, 284, 285, **379**
EMBASE, 120
Embedded design, mixed methods, 343, **379**
Embodiment, 270
Emergent design, 54, 266, **380**
Emergent fit, 313
Emic perspective, 269, **380**
Empirical evidence, 8, 10, **380**
Empirical phase of quantitative research, 50f, 52
Equivalence, reliability and, 204
Error(s). *See also* Bias
and biases, quantitative studies, 255t
of measurement, 201–202, **380**
sampling, 181, 226, **391**
standard, of the mean, 226, **392**
Type I and Type II, 228–230, 229f, 255t, 258, **394**
Essence, 49, 270. *See also* Phenomenology
Estimation procedure, 227–228, **380**
Ethical dilemma, 82
Ethics, research, 10, 51, 54, 80–96, **380**
animals and, 91–92
code of ethics, 81, **376**
confidentiality procedures, 88–89

Ethics, research (*Continued*)
  critiquing, 92–93, 93*b*
  debriefings and referrals, 90
  ethical principles, 83–86
  external review and, 91
  federal regulations (U.S.) and, 81–82, 91
  feminist research and, 276
  historical background of, 80–81
  informed consent, 84, 87, 88*f*
  Institutional Review Boards and, 91
  Internet research and, 85
  observational research and, 191
  qualitative research and, 54, 87, 89
  research design and, 156, 159
  research misconduct and, 92
  risk/benefit assessments, 86–87, 86*b*
  vulnerable groups and, 90–91
Ethnography, 49, 105, 139, 268–270, **380**. *See also*
    Qualitative research
  autoethnography, 269–270, **375**
  critical, 275–276
  data analysis and, 307–308
  data collection and, 289*t*, 290, 291
  ethnonursing research, 269, 308, **380**
  focused, 268, 269
  interviews and, 290
  literature reviews and, 117
  participant observation and, 287, 292–295
  photo elicitation and, 291
  problem statement and, 104
  research questions and, 106
  sampling in, 287
  statement of purpose and, 104–105
  theoretical framework and, 135, 139
Ethnonursing research, 269, 308, **380**
Etic perspective, 269, **380**
Etiology questions, 14–15, 14*t*, 23*f*, 31*t*,
    152*t*, 160
Evaluation research, 344, 345, **380**
Event sampling, 191, **380**
Evidence
  appraisal of, 31–33, 32*b*, 35
  clinical relevance of, 33
  disconfirming, 329–330
  how to find, 30, 32
  integration of, 33. *See also* Systematic review
  preappraised, 24–26
  quality of, 32, 68, 72, 358, 359, 364
  sources of, 5–6
Evidence-based medicine (EBM), 22
Evidence-based practice (EBP), 2, 4, 20–36, **380**
  challenges, 24
  clinical practice guidelines, 25–26, 35, **376**
  decision-making and, 223–225
  history of EBP movement, 4, 22
  implementation potential, 35, **382**
  Iowa model of, 27, 28*f*, 34
  literature reviews and, 117
  meta-analysis and, 25, 355, 356
  models of, 26–27
  in nursing practice, 27–34

  in organizational context, 34–36
  PICO scheme for formulating questions for, 29–30, 31*t*.
    *See also* PICO components
  research purposes and, 13–15, 14*t*
  research utilization and, 21
  resources for, 24–27
  sources of evidence, 5–6
  steps involved in, 29–34
  systematic reviews and, 4, 22–23, 25, 355
Evidence hierarchy, 22–24, 23*f*, 152*t*, **380**
Exclusion criteria, 177, **380**. *See also* Eligibility
    criteria
Exemplar, hermeneutic analysis, 311
Expectation bias, 151, 255*t*
Expected frequency, 235
Experience
  EBP and, 33
  evidence from, 6
  research problems from, 101
Experiment, 47, 153–159, **380**. *See also* Clinical trial;
    Intervention
  advantages and disadvantages of, 156–157
  characteristics of, 153–154
  clinical trials and, 345
  control and, 165
  control conditions and, 155–156
  designs for, 154–155
  ethical constraints, 156, 159
  evaluation research and, 345
  evidence hierarchy and, 152, 152*t*, 156
  experimental and control conditions, 155–156
  internal validity and, 168–169
  quasi-experiments and, 157–159. *See also*
    Quasi-experiments
  randomized controlled trials, 153–157
  therapy questions and, 152*t*
Experimental group, 153–154, **380**
Experimental intervention (treatment), 153. *See also*
    Intervention
Experimental research, 47–48. *See also* Experiment
Explanation, as research purpose, 11, 12*t*, 13
Explanatory design, mixed methods, 343, **380**
Exploitation, protection from, 83–84
Exploration, as research purpose, 12–13, 12*t*
Exploratory design, mixed methods, 343, **380**
External review, ethical issues and, 91
External validity, 169, 254, **380**. *See also*
    Generalizability
Extraneous variable, 73, 151, **380**. *See also* Confounding
    variable
Extreme case sampling, 285, **380**
Extreme response set bias, 188, 255*t*, **380**

**F**

*F*-ratio, 233–234, **380**
Fabrication of data, 92
Face-to-face (personal) interview, 184, 186, 288, 292.
    *See also* Interview
Face validity, 205, **380**
Factor analysis, construct validity and, 207
Fail-safe number, **380**

Fair treatment, right to, 85
Falsification, 92
Feminist research, 276, **380–381**
Field diary, 294, **381**
Field notes, 294, 295b, 324t, **381**
Field research, **381**. *See also* Ethnography;
    Qualitative research
Fieldwork, **381**
   clinical, 49–50, 50f
   ethnography and, 268–270
Findings, 8, 52, 63, **381**. *See also* Interpretation of results;
    Results
Fit, 311, **381**
Fittingness, **381**
Fixed alternative questions, 184, **381**
Fixed effects model, 361, **381**
Focus group interviews, 290, **381**
Focused coding, 315
Focused interviews, 290, **381**
Follow-up study, 163, **381**
Forced-choice question, 185t
Foreground question, 29. *See also* PICO question
Forest plot, 361, 361f, 367, **381**
Formal grounded theory, 356
Framework, 50, 135, 142–144, **381**. *See also* Conceptual
    model; Theory
   critiquing, 143–144, 143b
Frequency (f), 215–216
   expected vs. observed, 235
   qualitative analysis and, 306
Frequency distribution, 215–217, 216f, **381**. *See also*
    Distribution
   central tendency of, 217–218
   shapes of, 216
   variability of, 218–219, 219f
Frequency effect size, 366, **381**
Frequency polygon, 216, 217f
Full disclosure, 84–85, **381**
Functional relationship, 46, **381**
Funnel plot, **381**

**G**
Gaining entrée, 54, **381**
   participant observation and, 293
Gatekeeper, 54
Generalizability, 8, 75, **381**
   external validity and, 169, 254
   in literature reviews, 125
   in qualitative research, 75, 323
   in quantitative research, 167, 177
   quasi-experiments and, 159
   of results, 260
   sampling and, 169, 177, 254
Giorgi's phenomenological method, 308, 309t
Glaser and Strauss' grounded theory method, 272,
    311–313, 313f, 314t
Grand theory, 133, **381**
Grand tour question, 290, **381**
Grey literature, 358, **381**
Grounded theory, 48, 140, 140f, 145, **381**. *See also*
    Qualitative research

alternative views of, 272–273
constructivist (Charmaz), 273, 314–315
data analysis and, 311–315
data collection and, 289t
formal, 356
Glaser and Strauss' method, 272, 311–314, 313f, 314t
literature reviews and, 117
observation, data collection, 294b–295b
problem statements and, 104
research questions and, 105–106
sampling and, 287–288
statement of purpose and, 105
Strauss and Corbin's method and, 272–273, 313–314
symbolic interactionism and, 140, 272
theory and, 135, 140

**H**
Hand searching, 359, **382**
Harm
   protection from, 83
   studies focused on, 14–15, 14t, 23f, 152t
Hawthorne effect, 157, 255t, **382**
Health as Expanding Consciousness model
    (Newman), 141
Health Belief Model (Becker), 138
Health disparities, nursing research and, 5
Health Insurance Portability & Accountability Act
    (HIPAA), 85–86
Health Promotion Model (Pender), 134–135, 134f, 137,
    144–145
Hermeneutic circle, 271, 310, **382**
Hermeneutics, 271, **382**. *See also* Phenomenology
   data analysis and, 310
Heterogeneity, 219, 358, **382**. *See also* Homogeneity;
    Statistical heterogeneity, meta-analysis;
    Variability
HIPAA, 85–86
Historical research, 273, **382**
History threat, 168, 255t, **382**
Holistic approach, phenomenological analysis, 309
Homogeneity, 165, 219, **382**. *See also* Heterogeneity;
    Variability
   research design and, 165
   of sample, reliability and, 204
Human rights, research subjects and. *See* Ethics, research;
    Rights, human subjects
Human subjects committee, 91
Hypothesis, 50, 50f, 107–110, **382**
   characteristics of, 108–109
   corroboration and, 257
   critique of, 110–111
   deduction and, 107, 109, 133, 136, 141
   function of, 107
   generation of, in qualitative research, 312, 341
   interpretation and, 250, 257–259
   null, 109, 250, **386**
   research, 109, 228, **390**
   rival, 159, **391**
   testing of, 107, 110. *See also* Hypothesis testing
   theories and, 107, 141
   wording of, 109–110

Hypothesis testing, 228–231. *See also* Inferential statistics; Statistic(s)
  level of significance and, 229–230
  mixed methods research and, 341
  null hypothesis and, 228
  overview of procedures for, 231
  parametric and nonparametric tests and, 231, 236
  tests of statistical significance and, 230–231
  Type I and Type II errors and, 228–229, 229*f*

**I**

Ideational theory, 139
Identification, as research purpose, 11–12
Identification (ID) number, 89
Ideological perspectives, research with, 275–277, 276*t*
  critical theory, 275–276
  feminist research, 276
  participatory action research (PAR), 277
Impact analysis, 345, **382**
Implementation potential, EBP and, 35, **382**
Implications of results, 260, 333
Implied consent, 87, **382**
IMRAD format, 62, **382**
In vitro measure, 192
In vivo code, grounded theory, 311
In vivo measure, 192
Incidence, **382**
Inclusion criteria, 177. *See also* Eligibility criteria
Incubation, interpretation and, 332
In-depth interview, 289*t*, 290. *See also* Interview
Independent groups *t*-test, 233
Independent variable, 43–44, **382**. *See also* Dependent variable
  experimental research and, 153
  hypotheses and, 109
  keywords and, 119
  nonexperimental research and, 159
  power and, 167
  PICO components and, 43, 105
  relationships and, 46
  research questions and, 105–106
  statistical tests and, 238*t*, 241*t*
Inductive reasoning, 42, **382**
  theory development and, 136, 140
Inference, **382**
  definition of, 71
  interpretation and, 250, 250*f*, 251*f*, 252*t*, 253*f*
  statistical, 109, 228, **393**. *See also* Inferential statistics
  validity and, 253–254
Inferential statistics, 215, 232–237, **382**. *See also* Hypothesis testing
  analysis of variance, 233–235
  assumptions and, 231
  bivariate, 232–237, 238*t*
  chi-squared test, 235–236
  confidence intervals, 227–228
  correlation coefficients, 236
  effect size indexes, 237
  estimation of parameters, 227–228
  guide to tests, 238*t*, 241*t*
  hypothesis testing and, 228–231. *See also* Hypothesis testing

multivariate, 237–240. *See also* Multivariate statistics
  probability and, 225, 229
  sampling distributions and, 225–227
  *t*-tests, 232–233
Informant, 41, **382**. *See also* Study participant; Subject
  key, 287, **383**
Informed consent, 84, 87, 88*f*, **382**
Inquiry audit, 325*t*, 330–331, **382**
Insider research, 269, **382**
Institutional Review Board (IRB), 91, **382**
Institutionalized people, as a vulnerable group, 90
Instrument, 184, 185, **382**. *See also* Data collection; Measurement; Scale
  assessment of. *See* Data quality; Reliability; Validity
  errors of measurement and, 201–202
  mixed methods research and, 349
  psychometric assessment, 205
  screening, 208, **391**
Integration of qualitative and quantitative designs, 339–344. *See also* Mixed methods research
Integrity, qualitative research and, 321–322
Intensity effect size, 367, **383**
Intention to treat, **383**
Interaction effect, 234, **383**
Intercoder reliability, 204, 324*t*, **383**
Internal consistency, 203–204, **383**
Internal validity, 167–169, 254, 255*t*, **383**
International Council of Nurses (ICN), 81
Internet
  dissemination of research and, 4
  ethics and data collection, 85
  literature searches and, 118
  questionnaires and, 186
  surveys and, 186, 348
Interobserver reliability, 204, 209, **383**
Interpretation of results, 52, 249–261, 332–334
  critiquing of, 260–261, 261*b*, 333–334
  nonexperimental research and, 161–162
  in qualitative research, 332–333
  in quantitative research, 52, 249–264
Interpretive phenomenology, 271. *See also* Hermeneutics; Phenomenology
Interrater reliability, 204, 329, 360, **383**
Interval estimation, 227, **383**
Interval measurement, 200, 238*t*, 241*t*, **383**
Intervention, 150, **383**. *See also* Clinical trial; Experiment; Randomized controlled trial
  clinical trials and, 345
  development of, 341, 346
  ethical constraints and, 156
  experimental research and, 153, 346
  mixed methods research and, 341
  PICO component and, 29, 31*t*, 153
  power and, 167
  protocol for, 51, 346
  qualitative research and, 33, 266
  quasi-experimental research and, 158
  research design and, 150, 150*t*
  theory-based, 141
Intervention fidelity, 164, **383**
Intervention protocol, 51, 155, 346, **383**
Intervention research, 344–346, **383**

Intervention theory, 346, **383**
Interview, **383**. *See also* Self-report(s)
  face-to-face, 184, 186, 288, 292
  focus group, 290, **381**
  focused, 290
  personal (face-to-face), 186, 347, **387**
  photo elicitation, 291
  questionnaire vs., 185–186
  semi-structured, 290
  structured, 184
  telephone, 186, 348
  unstructured, 290, 291–292, **394**
Interview schedule, 184, **383**
Introduction, research report, 62–63
Intuiting, 271, **383**
Inverse relationship, 222, **383**
Inverse variance method, meta-analysis, 361, **383**
Investigation, 40
Investigator, 41, 41*t*
Investigator triangulation, 325*t*, 329, **383**
Iowa Model of Evidence Based Practice, 27, 28*f*, 34
IRB, 91
Item(s), 186–187, **383**. *See also* Question(s); Scale
  internal consistency and, 203–204
  sampling of, errors of measurement and, 202
  scales and, 186–188, 187*t*

**J**

Jargon, research, 40, 65
Journal article, 62–65, **383**. *See also* Research report
  content of, 62–65
  critiquing, 66–71. *See also* Critique, research
  style of, 65–66
  tips on reading, 66
Journal club, 3, 34, 36, **383**
Journal, reflexive, 270, 324*t*
Justice, ethics and, 85–86

**K**

Key informant, 269, 287, **383**
Keyword, 30, 119, **383**
Knowledge-focused trigger, EBP and, 34
Known-groups technique, 207, **384**

**L**

Lazarus and Folkman's Theory of Stress and
  Coping, 139
Leininger's ethnonursing method, 269, 308
Leininger's Theory of Culture-Care Diversity, 269
Level of measurement, 200–201, **384**
  inferential statistics and, 231, 238*t*
  multivariate statistics and, 240, 241*t*
Level of significance, 64, 229–231, **384**
Levels, of coding, grounded theory, 311–315, 312*t*
Likelihood ratio (LR), **384**
Likert scale, 186–188, 187*t*, **384**
Limitations, 10
  constructivist approach and, 9–10
  critiques and, 67, 71
  discussion section and, 65
  interpretation of results and, 251
  scientific approach and, 9

Lincoln and Guba's trustworthiness standards, 72, 322–323
Literary expressions, phenomenology and, 271, 287, 310
Literature review, 49, 54, 116–130, **384**. *See also*
  Systematic review
  abstracting and recording notes for, 123–124, 124*f*
  analysis and evaluation of evidence, 124–125
  bibliographic databases, 119–123
  content of written review, 126
  critiquing, 127–128, 127*b*
  documentation, 122
  electronic literature search, 119–120
  flow of tasks in, 118*f*
  locating sources for, 118–124
  meta-analyses. *See* Meta-analysis
  metasyntheses. *See* Metasynthesis
  organizing, 125
  preparing written review, 125–127
  protocol for, 124, 124*f*
  purposes of, 116–117
  qualitative research and, 54, 117
  research problem source, 101
  search strategies for, 118–119, 358–359
  steps and strategies for, 117–118
  style of written review, 126, 127*t*
  systematic review, 4, 25. *See also* Systematic
    review
  themes in, 125
  types of information to seek in, 117–118
Lived body, 270
Lived human relation, 270
Lived space, 270
Lived time, 270
Log, observational, 294, **384**
Logical positivism, **384**. *See also* Positivism
Logical reasoning, 71, 109, 250, 257. *See also* Inference
Logistic regression, 240, 241*t*, **384**
Longitudinal design, 163–164
  prospective vs., 164
  qualitative studies and, 267
  quantitative studies and, 163–164

**M**

Macroethnography, 268
Macrotheory (grand theory), 133, **384**
Mailed questionnaire, 186. *See also* Questionnaire
Main effect, 234
MANCOVA, 239
Manifest effect size, 366
Manipulation, experimental research and, 153, **384**.
  *See also* Experiment
MANOVA, 239
Map, conceptual, 134, 346, **376**
Mapping, electronic searches and, 119
Masking, 74, 79, **375**
Matching, 165–166, **384**
Materialistic theory, 139
Matrix, correlation, 222–223, 223*t*, **378**
Maturation threat, 168, **384**
Maximum variation sampling, 285, **384**
Mean, 218, **384**
  confidence intervals and, 227–228
  sampling distribution of, 226

Mean (*Continued*)
  standard error of, 226
  testing differences between groups, 232–235
Meaning questions, 14, 14*t*, 23*f*, 31*t*
Measurement, 51, 199–202, **384**. *See also* Data collection;
    Instrument; Measures
  advantages of, 200
  definition, 199–200
  error of, 201–202, **380**
  interval, 201, **383**
  level of, 200–201, **384**. *See also* Level of measurement
  nominal, 200, **386**
  operational definitions and, 44
  ordinal, 200, **386**
  problems of, 9
  ratio, 201, **390**
  reliability of instruments and, 202–205. *See also*
    Reliability
  validity of instruments and, 205–207. *See also* Validity
Measures. *See also* Data collection; Instrument;
    Measurement
  biophysiologic, 51, 192
  observational, 51, 189–191
  psychometric assessment of, 205
  self-report, 51, 184–189
Median, 218, **384**
Mediating variable, 74, **384**
Medical subject headings (MeSH), 122, 364, **384**
MEDLINE database, 119, 122, 364
Member check, 308, 328, **384**
Memos, in qualitative research, 312
MeSH. *See* Medical subject headings (MeSH)
Meta-analysis, 25, 356–362, **384**. *See also* Systematic
    review
  advantages of, 356
  calculation of effects, 360
  criteria for undertaking, 356–357
  critiquing of, 367–369, 368*b*
  data analysis, 361–362
  data extraction and encoding, 359–360
  data searches, 358–359
  definition of, 25
  design of, 357–358
  evidence-based practice and, 25, 355
  power and, 356
  problem formulation, 357
  sampling, 357–358
  steps involved in, 357–362
  study quality in, 359, 362
Metaphor qualitative research and, 305
Metasummary, 366, **384**
Metasynthesis, 25, 362–367, **384**
  controversies regarding, 363
  critiquing of, 367–369, 368*b*
  data analysis, 365–367
  definition of, 25, 363
  description of, 363
  design of, 363–364
  evidence-based practice and, 25, 355
  Noblit and Hare approach, 365–366
  Paterson et al. approach, 366

  problem formulation in, 363
  sampling in, 364
  Sandelowski and Barroso approach, 366–367
  steps in, 363–367
Metatheory, 366
Method section, research reports, 63
Method slurring, qualitative research, 278
Method triangulation, 326–327, **385**
Methodologic notes, 294, 294*b*, **385**
Methodologic research, 349, **385**
Methods, research, 8–10, **385**. *See also* Data collection;
    Measurement; Qualitative analysis; Quantitative
    analysis; Research design; Sampling
Microethnography, 268
Middle-range theory, 133, 137–138, **385**
Minimal risk, 87, **385**
Misconduct, research, 92
Mishel's Uncertainty in Illness Theory, 137–138
Mixed methods (MM) research, 339–344, **385**
  applications of, 340–342
  critiquing, 349–350, 350*b*
  designs and strategies, 342–344
  evaluation research and, 345
  notation for, 342
  purposes of, 340–342
  rationale for, 340
  sampling and, 343
Mixed results, interpretation, 259
Mobile positioning, 293
Mode, 217–218, **385**
Model, 133–135, **385**
  causal, **375**
  conceptual, 133, **376**. *See also* Conceptual model;
    Theory
  of research utilization/EBP, 26–27
  schematic, 134
Moderator, focus group, 290
Moderator variable, **385**
Modernism, 7
Mortality threat, 168, **385**
Multimodal distribution, 216, **385**
Multiple choice question, 185*t*
Multiple comparison procedures, 234, **385**
Multiple correlation, 239
Multiple correlation coefficient (*R*), 239, **385**, **389**
Multiple positioning, 293
Multiple regression, 238–239, **385**
Multisite study, 41
Multistage sampling, 180, **385**
Multivariate analysis of covariance (MANCOVA),
    239, 241*t*
Multivariate analysis of variance (MANOVA), 239–240,
    241*t*, **385**
Multivariate statistics, 237–240, **385**
  guide to, 241*t*

**N**
*N*, 216, **385**
*n*, **385**
Narrative analysis, 274, **385**
Narrative data, 45. *See also* Qualitative data

Narrative literature review. *See* Literature review; Systematic review
National Center for Nursing Research (NCNR), 4
National Guideline Clearinghouse, 26
National Institute for Clinical Excellence (NICE), 26
National Institute of Nursing Research (NINR), 4, 5, 85
National Institutes of Health (NIH), 4, 85
Naturalistic paradigm, 8, **385**
Naturalistic setting, 267, **385**
Nay-sayer, 188, 255*t*
Negative case analysis, 325*t*, 330, **385**
Negative relationship, 222, **385**
Negative results, 258, **385**
Negatively skewed distribution, 216, 218*f*, **385–386**
Nested sampling, mixed methods, 344
Net impact, 345
Network sampling, 284–285, **386**
Newman's Health as Expanding Consciousness model, 141
Nightingale, Florence, 3
NIH. *See* National Institutes of Health (NIH)
NINR. *See* National Institute of Nursing Research (NINR)
Noblit and Hare meta-ethnographic approach, 365–366
Nominal measurement, 200, 238*t*, 241*t*, **386**
Noncase, specificity and, 208
Noncompliance bias, 255*t*
Nondirectional hypothesis, 109, **386**
Nonequivalent control group design, 157–158, 168, **386**
    analysis of covariance and, 239
Nonexperimental research, 47–48, 159–162, **386**
    advantages and disadvantages, 161–162
    correlational research, 159. *See also* Correlational research
    descriptive research, 160
    interpretive issues and, 257, 260–261
    types of, 159–161
Nonparametric statistical test, 231, 236, **386**
Nonprobability sampling, 178–180, 284, **386**. *See also* Sampling
Nonresponse bias, 183, 255*t*, **386**
Nonsignificant results, 231, 258, **386**
Normal distribution, 217, 217*f*, **386**
    hypothesis testing and, 230–231
    sampling distributions and, 226, 226*f*
    standard deviations and, 220, 220*f*
Norms, 268
Notes, observational, 294
Null hypothesis, 109, **386**. *See also* Hypothesis testing
    bias against, 358
    description of, 109, 228–229, 229*f*
    interpretation of results and, 250
Number needed to treat (NNT), **386**
Nuremberg code, 81
Nursing intervention research, 346. *See also* Intervention
Nursing literature, 30, 101, 116–128. *See also* Research report
Nursing practice
    conceptual models of, 136–137. *See also* Conceptual model; Theoretical framework
    evidence-based practice in, 2, 20–39. *See also* Evidence-based practice

as source of research problems, 101
theoretical contexts and, 137–139
utilization of research in, 4, 20–39, 52–53. *See also* Research utilization
Nursing research, 2–15, **386**. *See also* Research
    challenges to utilization of, 24
    clinical, 2, 6
    conceptual models for, 136–139. *See also* Conceptual model; Theory
    consumer-producer continuum, 3
    evidence-based practice and, 2–3, 20–39. *See also* Evidence-based practice
    funding for, 3, 4
    future directions in, 4–5
    history of, 3–4
    importance of, 2–3
    paradigms for, 6–11
    priorities for, 5, 110
    purposes of, 11–15
    quantitative vs. qualitative, 8–10
    sources of evidence and, 5–6
    utilization of, 4, 20–39. *See also* Research utilization

## O

Objectives, research, 100, 104
Objectivity, 7, **386**
    data collection and, 184
    literature reviews and, 126
    meta-analysis and, 356
    paradigms and, 7–8, 7*t*
    research reports and, 65
    statements of purpose and, 104
    statistical decision-making and, 228
Observation, 184, 189–191, 292–295
    bias and, 191, 255*t*, 295
    categories and checklists, 190
    equipment for, 189
    ethical issues and, 85, 191
    evaluation of method, 191
    participant, 269, 292, **387**
    persistent, 326, **387**
    qualitative research and, 54, 292–295
    quantitative research and, 51, 184, 189–191
    sampling and, 191
    structured, 180, 190–191
    unstructured, 292–295
Observational notes, 294, 294*b*, **386**
Observational research, 47, 159–162, **386**. *See also* Nonexperimental research
Observed frequency, 235
Observed score, 201, **386**
Observer
    bias, 191, 255*t*, 295
    interobserver reliability, 204, 209, **383**
    training and assessment of, 191
Obtained score, 201, **386**
Odds, 225, 240, **386**
Odds ratio (OR), 225, 240, **386**
    effect size index, 237, 360
One-group pretest-posttest design, 158, 168
Online literature search, 120

Open coding, 311, 314, 314*t*, **386**
Open-ended question, 184–185, **386**
Operational definition, 44, **386**. *See also* Data collection; Measurement
Operationalization, 44, **386**
  interpretation and, 251
Ordinal measurement, 200, 238*t*, **386**
Outcome variable, 43, **386**. *See also* Dependent variable
  experiment and, 154
  hypotheses and, 109
  keywords and, 119
  PICO questions and, 29–30, 31*t*, 105
  relationships and, 46
  research questions and, 105
Outcomes research, 346–347, **386**

**P**

*p* value, 64, 231, 241–242, 256, **387**. *See also* Level of significance
Paired *t*-test, 233
Pair matching, 165–166
Paradigm, 6–11, **387**
  methods and, 8–10
  research problem and, 100–101, 111
Paradigm case, 310–311, **387**
Parameter, 215, 226, **387**
  estimation of, 227–228
Parametric statistical test, 231, 236, **387**. *See also* Statistic(s)
PARIHS model, 27
Parse's Theory of Human Becoming, 133
Participant. *See* Study participant
Participant observation, 269, 292–293, **387**
Participatory action research (PAR), 277, **387**
Paterson et al. metasynthesis approach, 366
Path analysis, **387**
Patient preferences, EBP and, 33
Pattern of association, qualitative research, 47
  qualitative analysis and, 305, 307
Pearson's *r*, 222, 236, 238*t*, **387**. *See also* Correlation
  effect size index, 237, 360
Peer debriefing, 325*t*, 330, **387**
Peer reviewer, 62, 67, **387**
Pender's Health Promotion Model (HPM), 134–135, 134*f*, 137, 144–145
Pentadic dramatism, 274, **387**
Per protocol analysis, **387**
Percentages, 215, 216*t*
Perfect relationship, 222, **387**
Persistent observation, 324*t*, 325–326, **387**
Person triangulation, 327, **387**
Personal (face to face) interviews, 186, 347, **387**. *See also* Interview; Self-report(s)
Personal notes, 294, 295*b*, **387**
Phenomenology, 48–49, 270–271, **387**
  artistic expressions and, 287, 310
  data analysis and, 308–311
  data collection and, 289*t*
  descriptive, 270–271
  Duquesne school, 308
  hermeneutics and, 271, 310–311
  interpretive, 271, 310

  literature reviews and, 117
  problem statements and, 104
  research questions and, 106
  sampling and, 287
  statement of purpose and, 104–105
  Utrecht school, 308–309
Phenomenon, 7, 41, 41*t*, 42
Photo elicitation, 291, **387**
Photographs, as data, 269, 273
Photovoice, 291
Physiologic measure, 51, 184, 192
PICO components, 29–30, 31*t*
  experimental design and, 153, 154
  hypotheses and, 107
  independent variables and, 43
  interventions and, 29, 153
  keywords and, 119
  literature search and, 30, 119
  outcome variables and, 29, 43
  populations and, 29, 177
  research questions and, 105
PICO question, 29–30, 31*t*, **387**
Pilot study, 35–36, 346, **387**
Pilot test, 35, 345
Placebo, 155, **387**
Placebo effect, **387**
Plagiarism, 92
Planning phase of study
  qualitative research, 53–54, 53*f*
  quantitative research, 50*f*, 51–52
Point estimation, 227, **387**
Population, 50*f*, 51, 177, **387**. *See also* Sampling
  estimation of values for, 227–228. *See also* Inferential statistics
  parameters and, 215
  PICO component and, 29, 31*t*, 177
Positive relationship, 222, **387–388**
Positive results, 257, **388**
Positively skewed distribution, 216, 218*f*, **388**
Positivism, 6
Positivist paradigm, 6–8, 7*t*, **388**
*Post hoc* test, 234, **388**
Poster session, 62, **388**
Postpositivist paradigm, 8
Posttest, 154, **388**
Posttest-only design, 154, **388**
Power, 167, **388**
  meta-analysis and, 356
  sample size and, 181–182
  statistical conclusion validity and, 167
  Type II errors and, 229
Power analysis, 181, 229, 230, **388**
Practical (pragmatic) clinical trial, 345, **388**
Practice guidelines, 25–26
Pragmatism, 340
Preappraised evidence, 24–26
Precision, 32, **388**
  confidence intervals and, 227, 233. *See also* Confidence intervals
  interpretation of results and, 256
Prediction, as research purpose, 13, **388**

Predictive validity, 206, **388**
Predictor variable, 239
Pregnant women, as a vulnerable group, 91
Pretest, 154, **388**
Pretest-posttest design, 154, **388**
Prevalence, 160, 347, **388**
Primary source, 117, **388**
Primary study, 24, 355, 357, **388**
Priorities for nursing research, 5, 110
Priority, mixed methods research and, 342, **388**
Privacy, study participants and, 85–86
Probability, 8, 72, 225–231
Probability level. *See* Level of significance
Probability sampling, 180–181, **388**. *See also*
    Sampling
Probing, 328, **388**
Problem statement, 100, 100*t*, 102–104, 103*b*, **388**.
    *See also* Hypothesis; Research problem
Process analysis, 345, **388**
Process consent, 87, **388**
Prochaska's Transtheoretical Model, 138
Producer of nursing research, 3
Product-moment correlation coefficient (*r*), 222, **388**.
    *See also* Correlation; Pearson's *r*
Professional conference, 36, 62
Prognosis questions, 14–15, 14*t*, 23*f*, 31*t*, 152*t*, 160
Program of research, 101
Prolonged engagement, 324*t*, 325–326, **388–389**
Proposal, 52, **389**
Prospective design, 151, 160, **389**
    longitudinal research vs., 164
Protocol
    intervention, 51, 155, 346, **383**
    literature review, 124, 124*f*
Psychometric assessment, 205, **389**
Psychometrics, **389**
Publication bias, 358, **389**
PubMed, 122, 123*f*
Purpose, statement of, 100, 100*t*, 104–105
Purposive sampling, 179–180, 285, **389**

**Q**

Q-sort, 189, **389**
Qualitative analysis, 54–55, **389**. *See also* Qualitative
    research
    analytic overview, 305–306
    analytic procedures, 304–315
    coding and, 302*b*, 303, 303*b*, 304*f*, 306, 329
    computers and, 304
    content analysis, 275, 306–307, **377**
    critiquing, 315–316, 316*b*
    data management and organization, 301–304
    ethnographic analysis, 307–308
    grounded theory analysis, 311–315
    literature reviews and, 125
    phenomenological analysis, 308–311
    trustworthiness and, 324*t*–325*t*, 328–331
Qualitative content analysis, 306–307
Qualitative data, 45, 45*b*, **389**. *See also* Unstructured
    data collection
    analysis of. *See* Qualitative analysis

    coding of, 302*b*, 303, 303*b*, 304*f*, 306, 329
    enhancement of quality, 325–328
    methods of data collection, 288–296, 289*t*
    mixed methods research and, 342–343
    organization of, 301–304
    secondary analysis, 348
Qualitative research, 8–10, **389**. *See also*
    Qualitative data
    activities in, 53–55
    analysis and, 300–317. *See also* Qualitative analysis
    case studies, 273–274
    causality in, 267–268
    credibility of results, 332
    critical research and, 276*t*
    critiquing, 333–334
    data collection and, 288–296, 289*t*. *See also*
        Unstructured data collection
    descriptive studies, 275
    disciplinary traditions and, 48–49, 268*t*
    ethical issues and, 54, 87, 89
    ethnography, 49, 268–270. *See also* Ethnography
    grounded theory, 48, 272–273. *See also* Grounded
        theory
    historical research, 273
    hypotheses and, 107
    ideological perspectives and, 275–277
    interpretation of findings, 332–333
    literature reviews and, 54, 117
    metasynthesis, 25, 362–367. *See also* Metasynthesis
    mixed methods and, 339–344
    narrative analysis, 274
    paradigms and, 8–10, 100–101
    phenomenology, 48–49, 270–271. *See also*
        Phenomenology
    problem statement and, 104
    quality and integrity in, 321–332
    research design and, 54, 265–281. *See also* Research
        design, qualitative studies
    research questions and, 106–107
    statement of purpose and, 104–105
    systematic reviews and, 25, 362–367
    theory and, 139–141, 366. *See also* Theory
    triangulation in, 72, 324*t*, 325*t*, 326–327, 329. *See also*
        Triangulation
    trustworthiness and, 72, 321–332. *See also*
        Trustworthiness
Quality Health Outcomes Model, 347
Quality improvement and risk data, 6
Quality, in qualitative research, 321–332. *See also*
    Trustworthiness
Quantitative analysis, 52, **389**. *See also* Hypothesis
    testing; Statistic(s); Statistical test
    credibility of results, 251–255
    critiquing, 243–244, 243*b*
    descriptive statistics, 215–225. *See also* Descriptive
        statistics
    inferential statistics, 225–237, 238*t*. *See also* Inferential
        statistics
    interpretation of results, 249–264
    measurement levels and, 200–201
    multivariate statistics, 237–240, 241*t*

Quantitative data, 45, **389**. *See also* Measurement; Quantitative analysis; Structured data collection
analysis of, 214–247. *See also* Quantitative analysis; Statistic(s)
assessment of data quality, 201–209
measurement and, 199–202. *See also* Measurement
methods of data collections, 183–194
secondary analysis, 348
Quantitative research, 8–10, **389**. *See also* Quantitative analysis; Quantitative data
data collection and, 183–194. *See also* Structured data collection
experimental vs. nonexperimental, 47–48. *See also* Experiment; Nonexperimental research
hypotheses and, 107–110
measurement and, 199–209
mixed methods research and, 339–344
research designs and, 51–52, 149–170
research problems and, 100–102
research questions and, 105–107
sampling in, 177–183
scientific method and, 8–9
statement of purpose and, 104
steps in, 49–53
theory and, 141–142. *See also* Theory
Quasi-experiments, 157–159, **389**
advantages and disadvantages, 158–159
evidence hierarchy and, 23, 152*t*
internal validity, 167–169
Quasi-statistics, 306, 325*t*, **389**
Question(s). *See also* Item(s); Scale; *specific question types*
background, 29
clinical, 29–30
closed-ended vs. open-ended, 184, 185
EBP and, 14, 14*t*, 23*f*, 31*t*
foreground, 29
grand tour, 290, **381**
PICO, 29–30, 31*t*, 105, **387**. *See also* PICO components
research, 105–107
types of, structured, 184–185, 185*t*
Questionnaire, 185–186, **389**. *See also* Self-report(s)
anonymity and, 89, 186
implied consent and, 87
Internet, 186, 348
interviews vs., 185–186
mailed, 186
scales and, 186. *See also* Scale
surveys and, 348
Quota sampling, 178–179, 179*t*, **389**

**R**
*R*, 239, **389**
*r*, 222, 236, 237, 238*t*, 360, **389**. *See also* Correlation
*R*², 239, **389**
Random assignment, 154, **389**. *See also* Randomization
Random bias, 73
Random effects model, 361, **389**
Random number table, 154, **390**
Random sampling, 180, **390**. *See also* Probability sampling
Random selection, 180
random assignment vs., 180

Randomization, 74, 154, **390**. *See also* Experiment
constraints on, 158
experimental designs and, 154–156
internal validity and, 167, 168
quasi-experimental design and, 157
random selection vs., 180
research control and, 165
Randomized controlled trial (RCT), 22–23, 153–157, 345, **390**. *See also* Clinical trial; Experiment; Intervention
evidence hierarchies and, 22, 23, 23*f*, 152*t*
Randomness, 74, **390**
Range, 219, **390**
Rank-order question, 185*t*
Rating question, 185*t*
Rating scale, 190–191, **390**. *See also* Scale
Ratio measurement, 201, 238*t*, 241*t*, **390**
Raw data, 64, 327, **390**
RCT. *See* Randomized controlled trial (RCT)
Reactivity, 189, 255*t*, **390**
Readability, 51, **390**
Reasoning. *See* Logical reasoning
Recall bias, 255*t*
Receiver operating characteristic curve (ROC curve), **390**
Records, as data sources, 183–184, 269, 273
Refereed journal, **390**. *See also* Peer reviewer
References
in research report, 65
screening for literature review, 123
Reflective (reflexive) notes, 294, 326, 327, **390**
Reflexive journal, 270, 324*t*, 326
Reflexivity, 75, 324*t*, 325*t*, 326, 331, 332, **390**
Regression analysis, 238–239, **390**
Relationality, 270
Relationship, 46–47, **390**. *See also* Causal (cause-and-effect) relationship
correlation and, 222–223. *See also* Correlation
hypotheses and, 50, 107–110
qualitative analysis and, 47, 305, 307
statistical analysis of, 222, 236
theories and, 133
Relative risk (RR), 225, **390**
Reliability, 202–205, **390**
definition of, 72, 202
intercoder, 204, 324*t*, **383**
internal consistency, 203–204, **383**
interrater, 204, 329, 360, **383**
stability and, 202
statistical, 72
test-retest, 202–203, **393**
validity and, 205
Reliability coefficient, 202, **390**
interpretation of, 204
Repeated measures ANOVA, 234–235, 238*t*, **390**
Replication, 4, 169, 255, **390**
Report. *See* Research report
Representativeness, 75
Representative sample, 75, 177–178, 180, 181, 284, **390**
Research, 2, 6, **390**
aims of, 100, 104, 113
basic vs. applied, 11

challenges in, 71–75
clinical, 2, 21, **376**
correlational, 159–160, 162, **378**
critical theory and, 275
critiquing of, 67–71. *See also* Critique, research
descriptive, 160–161, **379**
evidence-based practice and, 2–3, 21–24. *See also* Evidence-based practice
experimental, 47–48, 153–157. *See also* Experiment
health services, 346–347
intervention,14, 344–346, **383**. *See also* Clinical trial; Experiment
methodologic, 349, **385**
mixed methods (MM), 339–353, **385**
nonexperimental, 47–48, 159–162, **386**. *See also* Nonexperimental research
outcomes, 346–347
purposes of, 11–15
qualitative, 8–10, **389**. *See also* Qualitative research
quantitative, 8–10, **389**. *See also* Quantitative research
quasi-experimental, 157–159. *See also* Quasi-experiments
secondary analysis, 348
survey, 347–348, **393**
terminology of, 40–47
theory and, 139–142
Research, nursing. *See* Nursing research
Research control. *See* Control, research
Research critique. *See* Critique, research
Research design, 51, **390**. *See also* Research design, mixed methods studies; Research design, qualitative studies; Research design, quantitative studies
Research design, mixed methods studies, 342–344. *See also* Mixed methods research
notation for, 342
priority and, 342, 343
sampling and data collection, 343–344
sequencing and, 342
Research design, qualitative studies, 54, 266–275. *See also* Qualitative research
characteristics of, 266
critiquing, 277–278, 278b
disciplinary traditions and, 268–273
ethnographic, 268–270
features of, 266–267
grounded theory, 272–273
ideological perspectives and, 275–277, 276t
mixed methods and, 342–344
phenomenologic, 270–271
planning and, 51–52, 266
Research design, quantitative studies, 51, 149–174
causality and, 151–152
characteristics of good design, 166–170
construct validity and, 169–170, 254
controls for external confounding factors, 162–164
controls for intrinsic confounding factors, 164–166
critiquing, 170, 170b
EBP questions and, 152
ethics and, 156
evidence hierarchy and, 23f, 152t
experimental designs, 153–157
external validity and, 169, 254

internal validity and, 168–169, 254
key features, 150–151, 150t
longitudinal vs. cross-sectional, 162–163
mixed methods and, 342–344
nonexperimental research, 159–162
quasi-experimental design, 158
statistical conclusion validity and, 167, 254
Research Ethics Board, 91
Research findings, 63. *See also* Interpretation of results; Results
Research hypothesis, 109, 228, **390**. *See also* Hypothesis; Hypothesis testing
Research methods, 8–10, **390**. *See also* Methods, research
Research misconduct, 92, **390**
Research, nursing. *See* Nursing research
Research problem, 49, 53–54, 99–107, **391**
communication of, 102–107
critique of, 110–111, 111b
development and refinement of, 101–102
paradigms and, 100–101, 111
qualitative studies and, 53–54, 101
quantitative studies and, 49, 100–101
significance of, 110, 111b
sources of, 101
terms relating to, 100
Research program, 101
Research question, 100, 105–107, **391**. *See also* Research problem
Research report, 52, 62–66, **391**. *See also* Dissemination
abstracts in, 62
content of, 62–65
critiquing, 66–71, 69t, 70t. *See also* Critique, research
discussion section in, 65
IMRAD format, 62
introduction in, 62–63
journal article, 62–65. *See also* Journal article
locating, 118–123
method section in, 63
qualitative studies and, 55
quantitative studies and, 52
reading, 66
references in, 65
results section in, 63–65
as source of research questions, 101
style of, 65–66
tips on reading, 66
titles of, 62
types of, 61–62
Research review. *See* Literature review
Research setting, 41. *See also* Setting, research
Research utilization, 4, 21, 52–53, **391**. *See also* Evidence-based practice
Researcher, 41, 41t
Researcher credibility, 325t, 331–332, **391**
Respect for human dignity, 84–85
Respondent, 89, 184–186, 189, **391**. *See also* Study participant
Response alternative, 184
Response bias, 183
Response rate, 183, **391**
nonresponse bias and, 183
questionnaires vs. interviews, 186

Response set bias, 188, 202, 255*t*, **391**
Results, 52, 55, **391**
 credibility of, 251–255
 dissemination of, 4, 52–53. *See also* Dissemination of
  research results; Research report
 evidence-based practice and, 22–24. *See also*
  Evidence-based practice
 generalizability of, 8, 75, 260. *See also* Generalizability
 hypothesized, 257–258
 interpretation of, 52, 249–264, 322–323. *See also*
  Interpretation of results
 mixed, 259
 nonsignificant, 258
 qualitative, 64–65, 322–333
 statistical, 63–64, 240–242
 transferability and, 35, 75, 323, 333
 unhypothesized, 259
 utilization of, 21
Results section, research report, 63–65
Retrospective design, 151, 160, **391**
Review. *See also* Critique, research
 blind, 62, **375**
 ethical issues and, 91
 literature, 49, 116–130, **384**. *See also* Literature review
 peer, 62, 67, 330
 systematic, 4, 25, 355–368. *See also* Systematic review
Rights, human subjects, 51, 54, 83–92. *See also* Ethics,
  research
Rigor
 qualitative research and, 321–322. *See also*
  Trustworthiness
 quantitative research and, 249–250. *See also* Reliability;
  Validity
Risk
 description of, 223–225
 indexes of, 224*t*. *See also* Odds ratio
 minimal, 87
Risk ratio (RR), 225, **390**
Risk-benefit ratio, 86–87, **391**
Rival hypothesis, 159, 168, **391**
ROC curve, **391**
Rogers' Diffusion of Innovations Theory, 27
Roy's Adaptation Model, 137

**S**

Sample, 51, 177, 284, **391**. *See also* Sample size; Sampling
 representativeness of, 75, 177–178, 180, 181, 284
Sample size, 181–182, 286
 power analysis and, 181, 229, **388**
 qualitative studies, 286
 quantitative studies, 181–182
 standard errors and, 226
 statistical conclusion validity, 182
 statistical power, 167
 Type II errors and, 229, 256, 258–259
Sampling, 177–183, **391**. *See also* Sample size
 basic concepts, 177–178
 bias and, 178, 183
 consecutive, 179, **377**
 construct validity and, 254
 convenience, 178, **377**
 critiquing, 182–183, 183*b*, 288, 289*b*

 ethnography and, 287
 external validity and, 169
 grounded theory studies and, 287–288
 inference and, 251, 251*f*, 252*t*
 items, in measuring instruments, 202
 in meta-analysis, 357–358
 in metasynthesis, 364
 mixed methods research, 343–344
 nonprobability, 178–180, 181, **386**
 observational, 191
 phenomenological studies and, 287
 probability, 180–181, **388**
 purposive, 179–180, 285, **389**
 qualitative research and, 283–288
 quantitative research and, 177–183
 quota, 178–179, **389**
 random, 180, **390**
 sample size and, 181–182, 286. *See also* Sample size
 snowball, 284–285, **392**
 strata and, 178
 systematic, 181, **393**
 theoretical, 286, 287, **393**
Sampling bias, 178, 183, **391**
Sampling distribution, 225–227, 226*f*, 230*f*, **391**
Sampling error, 181, 226, 255*t*, **391**
Sampling frame, 180, **391**
Sampling interval, 181
Sampling plan, 51, 177–183, **391**. *See also* Sampling
 critiquing, 182–183, 183*b*
Sandelowski and Barroso metasynthesis approach,
  366–367
Saturation, data, 55, 286, 324*t*, **391**
Scale, 186–188, **391**
 internal consistency and, 203–204
 Likert, 186–188, 187*t*, **384**
 rating, observational, 190–191
 response set bias and, 188
 summated rating, 187, **393**
 visual analog, 188, **394**
Schematic model, 134
Scientific merit, 72, **391**. *See also* Reliability; Validity
Scientific method, 8–9, **391**. *See also* Quantitative
  research
Scientific research. *See* Research
Scientist. *See* Researcher
Score(s), 186–188
 obtained (observed), 201, **386**
 scales and, 186–188, 187*t*
 true, 201, **394**
Screening instrument, 208, **391**
Search, electronic literature, 119–123
Search engine, Internet, 118
Secondary analysis, 348, **391**
Secondary source, 117, **391–392**
Selection, random, 180
Selection threat (self-selection), 161, 168, 255*t*, **392**
Selective approach, phenomenological analysis, 309–310
Selective coding, grounded theory, 311–312, **392**
Self-administered questionnaire, 348. *See also*
  Questionnaire
Self-determination, 84, **392**
Self-efficacy theory, 138, 141

Self-report(s), 51, 184–189, 290–292, 347, **392**. *See also* Interview; Questionnaire; Scale
  critiquing, 193*b*, 296*b*
  evaluation of method, 189, 292
  interviews, 184, 288
  Q sort, 189
  qualitative methods and, 290–291
  quantitative methods and, 51, 184–189
  questionnaires vs. interviews, 186
  response bias and, 188
  scales, 186–188. *See also* Scale
  structured, 184–189
  types of question, 184–185
  unstructured and semistructured, 290–291
  vignettes, 189
Self-selection (selection bias), 161, **392**
Semistructured interviews, 290, **392**
Sensitivity, 208–209, 208*t*, **392**
Sensitivity analysis, 361, 362, **392**
Sequential design, mixed methods, 342, **392**
Setting, research, 41, 151, 267, **392**
  qualitative research and, 267
  quantitative research and, 151
Shared theory, 139
Significance level, 64, 229–231, **392**
Significance of research problems, 110, 111*b*
Significance, statistical, 64, 230–231. *See also* Statistical significance
Simple hypothesis, 109
Simple random sampling, 180, **392**
Single positioning, 293
Site, 41, **392**
Skewed distribution, 216, 218*f*, **392**
Snowball sampling, 284–285, **392**
Social Cognitive Theory (Bandura), 138, 141
Social desirability response bias, 188, 255*t*, **392**
Social issues, source of research problem, 101
Social-psychological scales, 186–188. *See also* Scale
Space triangulation, 327, **392**
Spatiality, 270
Spearman's rank-order correlation (Spearman's rho), **392**
Specificity, screening instruments and, 208–209, 208*t*, **392**
Spradley's ethnographic method, 307–308
Stability of measures, 202–203
Stakeholder, 346
Standard deviation (SD), 219–220, **392**
Standard error, **392**
Standard error of the mean (SEM), 226–227
Standardized mean difference (SMD), 360, **392**
Statement of purpose, 100, 104–105, **392**
Statistic(s), 215–243, **392**
  bivariate, 221–225, 232–237, **375**
  critique of, 243–244
  descriptive, 215–225, **379**. *See also* Descriptive statistics
  inferential, 225–237, **382**. *See also* Inferential statistics
  multivariate, 237–240, **385**. *See also* Multivariate statistics
  parametric vs. nonparametric, 231, 236
  tips on understanding, 240–243
Statistical analysis, 52, 63–64, **392**. *See also* Quantitative analysis; Statistic(s); Statistical test
Statistical conclusion validity, 167, 182, 254, **392**. *See also* Power

Statistical control, 166, 239, 244, **392**
Statistical heterogeneity, meta-analysis, 358, 361, 361*f*, **392**
Statistical hypothesis. *See* Null hypothesis
Statistical inference, 109, 228, **393**. *See also* Inferential statistics
Statistical power, 167, 229, **393**. *See also* Power
Statistical reliability, 72
Statistical significance, 64, 230–231, **393**
  clinical significance vs., 256
  interpretation and, 257–259
  level of, 64, 229–231, **392**
  power analysis and, 229
  statistical conclusion validity, 167
  tests of, 230–231. *See also* Statistical test
Statistical tables, 242–243
Statistical test, 228, 230–231, **393**. *See also* Inferential statistics; Multivariate statistics; *specific tests*
  guide to bivariate tests, 237, 238*t*
  guide to multivariate tests, 240, 241*t*
  Type I and Type II errors, 228–229
Stepwise replication, 325*t*, 329
Stetler model of research utilization, 27
Stipend, 84, **393**
Strata, 178, **393**
Stratified random sampling, 180, **393**
Strauss and Corbin's grounded theory method, 272–273, 313–314, 314*t*
Structured (quantitative) data collection, 184–194, **393**. *See also* Measurement
  biophysiologic measures, 184, 192. *See also* Biophysiologic measures
  observations and, 189–192. *See also* Observation
  self-reports, 184–189. *See also* Self-report(s)
Study, 41. *See also* Research
Study participant, 41, **393**
  communication with, 164
  controlling intrinsic factors and, 164–166
  rights of, 83–85, 92–93
Style. *See* Writing style
Subgroup analysis, 362
Subject(s), 41, **393**. *See also* Study participant
Subject heading, literature search
  description of, 119
  MeSH, 122, 364
Subjectivity. *See* Objectivity
Subject search, literature review, 119
Subscale, 205
Substantive theory, 139, 272
Summated rating scale, 187–188, **393**
Survey research, 347–348, **393**. *See also* Self-report(s)
  sampling and, 181
Symbolic interactionism, 140, 272
Symmetric distribution, 216, 217*f*, **393**
Systematic bias, 73
Systematic review, 4, 355–372, **393**
  critiquing, 367–369, 368*b*
  evidence-based practice and, 25, 355–356
  meta-analyses, 356–362. *See also* Meta-analysis
  metasyntheses, 362–367. *See also* Metasynthesis
Systematic sampling, 181, **393**

**T**

Table
  crosstabs (contingency), 221–222, 221*t*, 223, 224*t*,
    **377, 378**
  of random numbers, 154
  statistical, tips on reading, 242–243
Tacit knowledge, 269, **393**
Target population, 177, 251, 252*t*, **393**
Taxonomic analysis, 307
Taxonomy, 307, **393**
Telephone interview, 186, 348
Temporal ambiguity, internal validity and, 167
Temporality, 270
Terminally ill patients as a vulnerable group, 90
Test statistic, 230, 231, **393**. *See also* Statistic(s);
    Statistical test
Test-retest reliability, 202–203, 203*t*, **393**
Textword search, 119
Theme, 55, **393**
  cultural, 307–308
  in literature reviews, 125
  method slurring and, 315
  phenomenology and, 308–311
  in qualitative analysis, 55, 64, 305, 306
Theoretical code, grounded theory, 312
Theoretical distribution, 230, 231
Theoretical framework, 50, 135, 142–144. *See also*
    Conceptual model; Theory
Theoretical notes, 294, 294*b*, 295
Theoretical sampling, 286, 287, **393**
Theory, 42, 133, **393**. *See also* Conceptual model;
  *specific theory*
  borrowed, 139
  construct validity and, 207
  critiquing, 143–144, 143*b*
  development of, 139–142
  explanatory research and, 42
  grounded, 48, 140, **381**. *See also* Grounded theory
  hypotheses and, 107, 141
  intervention, 346, **383**
  metatheory, 366
  mixed methods research and, 341–342
  nursing and, 136–138
  phenomenology and, 139
  qualitative research and, 139–141
  quantitative research and, 141–142
  research and, 139–142
  shared, 139
  as source of research problems, 101
  substantive, 139
  testing, 141
Theory of Human Becoming (Parse), 133
Theory of Planned Behavior (Ajzen), 138–139
Theory of Reasoned Action, 138–139
Theory of Stress and Coping (Lazarus and Folkman), 139
Theory triangulation, 325*t*, 329, **394**
Therapy questions, 14, 14*t*, 23*f*, 31*t*, 152*t*. *See also* Clinical
    trial; Experiment
Thick description, 288, 294, 331, 325*t*, 334, **393**
Threat to internal validity, 167–168
Time sampling, 191, **393**

Time series design, 158, 168, **393**
Time triangulation, 327, **393**
Title, research report, 62
Tool. *See* Instrument
Topic guide, 290, **393**
Topic, research, 100, 100*t*. *See also* Research problem
Tradition, as knowledge source, 5
Tradition, disciplinary, 48
Transcriptions, of interviews, 291, 324*t*, 327
Transferability, **393**
  definition of, 75
  EBP and, 35
  literature themes, 125
  qualitative findings and, 288
  trustworthiness of qualitative research and, 323, 324*t*,
    325*t*, 333
Translating Research Into Practice (TRIP) database, 26
Transtheoretical Model (Prochaska), 138
Treatment, 153, **394**. *See also* Experiment; Intervention;
    Therapy questions
Treatment group, 154, **394**
Trial and error, 6
Triangulation, 72, 326, **394**
  corroborating evidence and, 255
  data, 324*t*, 326–327, **379**
  of data collection methods, 193, 326–327
  definition, 72
  investigator, 325*t*, 329, **383**
  method, 325*t*, 326–327, **385**
  mixed methods designs, 340
  person, 327, **387**
  space, 327, **392**
  time, 327, **393**
  theory, 325*t*, 329
Triangulation design, 342, **394**
True score, 201, **394**
Trustworthiness, in qualitative research, 55, 72,
    321–334, **394**
  critiquing, 333–334, 334*b*
  definition of, 72, 322
  interpretation of findings, 332–333
  Lincoln and Guba's standards, 322–323
  strategies for enhancing, 324–332, 324*t*–325*t*
*t*-test, 232–233, 232*t*, 238*t*, **394**
Two-way ANOVA, 234
Type I error, 228–229, 229*f*, 255*t*, 257, **394**
Type II error, 228–230, 229*f*, 255*t*, 256, 258, **394**
Typical case sampling, 285

**U**

Uncertainty in Illness Theory (Mishel), 137–138
Unhypothesized significant results, interpretation, 259
Unimodal distribution, 216, **394**
Unit of analysis, 25, **394**
Univariate statistics, 215–221, **394**
Unstructured (qualitative) data collection, 54, 288–296
  critiquing, 295–296, 296*b*
  evaluation of, 292, 295
  observation and, 292–294, 294*b*, 295*b*
  self-reports and, 290–292
Unstructured interview, 290, **394**

Unstructured observation, 292–294, 295*b*, **394**. *See also* Participant observation
Utilization. *See* Research utilization
Utrecht school of phenomenology, 308–310

## V

Validity, 72, **394**
  concurrent, 206, **376**
  construct, 169–170, 206–207, 254, 346, **377**
  content, 205–206, **377**
  credibility and, 253–254
  criterion-related, 206, **378**
  external, 169, 254, **380**. *See also* Generalizability
  face, 205, **380**
  inference and, 253
  internal, 167–169, 254, 255*t*, **383**
  measurement and, 205–207
  mixed methods research and, 340
  predictive, 206, **388**
  qualitative research and, 321–322
  reliability and, 205
  statistical conclusion, 167, 182, 254, **392**. *See also* Power
Validity coefficient, 206, 222, **394**
Van Kaam's phenomenological method, 308, 309*t*
Van Manen's phenomenological method, 308–310, 309*t*
Variability, 218–221, **394**. *See also* Heterogeneity; Homogeneity; Variable
  control over. *See* Control, research
Variable(s), 42–44, **394**
  conceptual definition of, 44, 50, 135, **376**

  confounding, 73, 151, 152, **377**. *See also* Confounding variable
  core, 48, 272, 314, **378**
  dependent, 43–44, **379**. *See also* Dependent variable
  extraneous, 73, 151, **380**. *See also* Confounding variable
  independent, 43–44, **382**. *See also* Independent variable
  mediating, 74, **384**
  operational definition of, 44, **386**
Variance, 219, **394**
  analysis of, 233–235, **374**
  multivariate analysis of, 239
VAS. *See* Visual analog scale (VAS)
Vignette, 189, **394**
Visual analog scale (VAS), 188, 188*f*, **394**
Vivid recording, qualitative integrity and, 325*t*, 327–328
Volunteer sample, 284
Vulnerable groups, 90–91, **394**

## W

Web-based survey, **394**
Wait-listed control group, 155
Wildcard character, 120
Writing style
  of literature review, 126, 127*t*
  of journal articles, 65–66
  qualitative reports and, 65, 325*t*, 331
  quantitative reports and, 65–66

## Y

Yea-sayer, 188

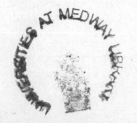